Orthopaedic Surgery
Examination and
Board Review

Orthopaedic Surgery Examination and Board Review

Editor

Manish K. Sethi, MD

Associate Professor of Orthopaedics & Rehabilitation
Department of Orthopaedic Trauma
Vanderbilt University Medical Center
Nashville, Tennessee

Associate Editors

Ashley C. Dodd, BS

Research Analyst
Department of Orthopaedic Trauma
Vanderbilt University Medical Center
Nashville, Tennessee

Basem Attum, MD, MS

Vanderbilt Orthopaedic Institute Center for Health Policy
Vanderbilt University Medical Center
Nashville, Tennessee

McGraw Hill Education

New York   Chicago   San Francisco   Athens   London   Madrid   Mexico City
Milan   New Delhi   Singapore   Sydney   Toronto

Orthopaedic Surgery Examination and Board Review

1 2 3 4 5 6 7 8 9 0   DSS/DSS   20 19 18 17 16

ISBN 978-0-07-183280-9
MHID 0-07-183280-7

This book was set in Minion Pro by Aptara, Inc.
The editors were Brian Belval and Regina Y. Brown.
The production supervisor was Catherine H. Saggese.
Production management was provided by Aptara.
RR Donnelley was printer and binder.

This book is printed on acid-free paper.

Library of Congress Cataloging-in-Publication Data

Names: Sethi, Manish K., author.
Title: Orthopaedic surgery : examination and board review / Manish Sethi.
Description: First edition. | New York : McGraw-Hill Education, [2016] |
    Includes index.
Identifiers: LCCN 2015039470 | ISBN 9780071832809 (pbk. : alk. paper) | ISBN
    0071832807 (pbk. : alk. paper)
Subjects: | MESH: Orthopaedic Procedures—Case Reports. | Orthopaedic
    Procedures—Examination Questions.
Classification: LCC RD755 | NLM WE 18.2 | DDC 617.9—dc23 LC record available at http://lccn.loc.gov/2015039470

McGraw-Hill books are available at special quantity discounts to use as premiums and sales promotions, or for use in corporate training programs. To contact a representative please visit the Contact Us pages at www.mhprofessional.com.

*This book is dedicated to my parents Dr. Brahm D. Sethi (1941–2003)
and Dr. Chander M. Sethi.*

Without the sacrifices they made for my future I would not be here today.
—MKS

Contents

8. ORTHOPAEDIC ONCOLOGY
John A. Abraham, Christina Gutowski, William Morrison, and Wei Jiang

Page 449

9. SPORTS MEDICINE
Joseph DeAngelis

Page 506

10. PEDIATRICS
Coleen S. Sabatini

Page 528

Contributors

Ayesha Abdeen, MD
Instructor in Orthopaedic Surgery at Beth Israel
    Deaconess Medical Center
Beth Israel Deaconess Medical Center
Boston, Massachusetts

John A. Abraham, MD
Associate Professor of Orthopaedic Surgery and
    Radiation Oncology
Thomas Jefferson University
Director, Center for Musculoskeletal Oncology
Kimmel Cancer Center, Thomas Jefferson University
Chief, Division of Orthopaedic Oncology
Rothman Institute
Philadelphia, Pennsylvania

Basem Attum, MD, MS
Vanderbilt Orthopaedic Institute Center for Health
    Policy
Vanderbilt University Medical Center
Nashville, Tennessee

Bryce A. Basques, BS
Department of Orthopaedics and Rehabilitation
Yale University School of Medicine
New Haven, Connecticut

Andrea S. Bauer, MD
Assistant Clinical Professor of Orthopaedics
Shriners Hospitals for Children—Northern
    California
University of California
Davis School of Medicine

Daniel D. Bohl, MPH
Department of Orthopaedics and Rehabilitation
Yale University School of Medicine
New Haven, Connecticut

Christopher M. Bono, MD
Chief, Orthopaedic Spine Service, Brigham and
    Women's Hospital
Associate Professor of Orthopaedic Surgery
Harvard Medical School
Boston, Massachusetts

Adrienne Bonvini, PA-C
Department of Orthopaedics
University of Vermont Medical Center
Burlington, Vermont

Michael R. Briseno, MD
Orthopedic Spine Surgeon
North Texas Orthopaedics
Grapevine, Texas

Cordelia W. Carter, MD
Assistant Professor of Orthopaedics and
    Rehabilitation
Yale School of Medicine
Yale-New Haven Hospital
New Haven, Connecticut

Thomas D. Cha, MD, MBA
Department of Orthopaedics
Instructor in Orthopaedic Surgery
Harvard Medical School
Boston, Massachusetts

Saad B. Chaudhary, MD, MBA
Assistant Professor at Rutgers—New Jersey Medical
    School
Newark, New Jersey
Christ Hospital
Hackensack University Medical Center
Hackensack, New Jersey

Ivan Cheng, MD
Associate Professor
Department of Orthopaedic Surgery
Stanford University
Redwood city, California

Christopher P. Chiodo, MD
Department of Orthopaedic Surgery
Brigham and Women's Hospital
Harvard Medical School
Boston, Massachusetts

Joseph Cohen, MD
Department of Orthopaedic Surgery
University of Chicago Medicine
Chicago, Illinois

Joseph P. DeAngelis, MD
Assistant Professor of Orthopaedics
Harvard Medical School
Director of Sports Medicine Research
Department of Orthopaedics
Beth Israel Deaconess Medical Center
Boston, Massachusetts

Richard J. De Asla, MD
Orthopaedic Surgeon, Foot and Ankle
Excel Orthopaedic Specialists
Woburn, Massachusetts

Ashley C. Dodd, BS
Research Analyst
Department of Orthopaedic Trauma
Vanderbilt University Medical Center
Nashville, Tennessee

Tom Douglas, MD
Naval Medical Center Portsmouth
Uniformed Services University of the
   Health Sciences
Portsmouth, Virginia

Thomas Dowd, MD
Department of Orthopaedics
San Antonio Military Medical Center
Sam Houston, Texas

Kyle R. Eberlin, MD
Division of Plastic and Reconstructive Surgery
Hand Surgery Service
Massachusetts General Hospital
Harvard Medical School
Boston, Massachusetts

Jason Eck, DO, MS
Orthopaedic Spine Surgeon
Center for Sports Medicine and Orthopaedics
Chattanooga, Tennessee

Islam Elboghdady, BS
Research Assistant
Department of Orthopaedic Surgery
Rush University Medical Center
Chicago, Illinois

John Paul Elton, MD
Vail Summit Orthopaedics
Vail Summit Orthopaedic Foundation
Vail, Colorado

Marco L. Ferrone, MD
Brigham and Women's Hospital
Boston, Massachusetts

James N. Foster, MD
Department of Orthopaedic Surgery
San Antonio Military Medical Center
Fort Sam Houston, Texas

Nicholas S. Golinvaux, BA
Department of Orthopaedics and Rehabilitation
Yale University School of Medicine
New Haven, Connecticut

Jonathan N. Grauer, MD
Associate Professor of Orthopaedics and
   Rehabilitation and of Pediatrics;
Co-Director, Orthopaedic Spine Service;
Co-Director, Yale New Haven Hospital Spine Center

Daniel Guss, MD, MBA
Department of Orthopaedic Surgery
Massachusetts General Hospital
Harvard Medical School
Boston, Massachusetts

Christina J. Gutowski, MD, MPH
Orthopaedic Chief Resident
Thomas Jefferson University Hospital
Philadelphia, Pennsylvania

Mitchel B. Harris, MD
Professor, Department of Orthopaedic Surgery
Harvard Medical School
Brigham and Women's Hospital
Boston, Massachusetts

Hamid Hassanzadeh, MD
Spine Surgery Fellow
Department of Orthopaedic Surgery
Rush University Medical Center
Chicago, Illinois

Scott D. Hodges, DO
Center for Sports Medicine and Orthopaedics
Chattanooga, Tennessee

Christina M. Hylden, MD
San Antonio Military Medical Center
Department of Orthopaedics
Fort Sam Houston, Texas

Mark E. Jacobson, MD
Shoreline Orthopaedic & Sports Medicine Clinic
Zeeland, Michigan
Holland Hospital Medical Staff Spectrum Health
    Zeeland Community Hospital
Holland, Michigan

Wei Jiang, MD, PhD
Assistant Professor of Pathology
Thomas Jefferson University
Director, Translational Research/Pathology Core Facility
Kimmel Cancer Center, Thomas Jefferson University
Philadelphia, Pennsylvania

Jeffrey R. Jockel, MD
Colorado Permanente Medical Group
Denver, Colorado

Anton Jorgensen, MD
Spine Surgery Fellow
Department of Orthopaedic Surgery
Rush University Medical Center
Chicago, Illinois

David Kim, MD
Director of Medical Education
New England Baptist Hospital for Spinal Surgery
Associate Clinical Professor of Orthopaedic Surgery
Tufts University Medical School
Boston, Massachusetts

Melissa Klausmeyer, MD
Department of Plastic Surgery
Kaiser Permanente Hospital, Southern California
Assistant Clinical Professor
University of Southern California
Los Angeles, California

Joshua Lamb, MD
Department of Orthopaedic Surgery
Beth Israel Deaconess Medical Center
Harvard Medical School
Boston, Massachusetts

Drew Lansdown, MD
Department of Orthopaedic Surgery
University of California
San Francisco, California

Bryan K. Lawson, MD
Department of Orthopaedic Surgery
San Antonio Military Medical Center
Fort Sam Houston, Texas

Darren Lebl, MF, FAAOS
Assistant Attending Orthopaedic Surgeon
Assistant Scientist, Research Division
Hospital for Special Surgery
Assistant Professor of Orthopaedic Surgery
Weill Medical College of Cornell University
New York, New York

Alejandro Marquez-Lara, MD
Research Coordinator
Department of Orthopaedic Surgery
Rush University Medical Center
Chicago, Illinois

Jasmin McGinty, MD
SLUCare Physician Group
Saint Louis University Hospital
SSM Cardinal Glennon Children's Medical Center
St. Louis, Missouri

William B. Morrison, MD
President, Society of Skeletal Radiology
Professor of Radiology
Director, Division of Musculoskeletal Radiology
Thomas Jefferson University Hospital
Philadelphia, Pennsylvania

Chaitanya S. Mudgal, MD, MS (Orth.), MCh (Orth.)
Assistant Professor in Orthopaedic Surgery,
    Harvard Medical School
Program Director, Hand Surgery Fellowship
Massachusetts General Hospital
Boston, Massachusetts

Sreeharsha V. Nandyala, BA
Research Coordinator
Department of Orthopaedic Surgery
Rush University Medical Center
Chicago, Illinois

Ali Al-Omari, MD
Division of Orthopaedic Surgery
Children's Hospital of Philadelphia
Philadelphia, Pennsylvania

Nirav K. Pandya, MD
Children's Hospital and Research Center in
    Oakland (CHRCO)
UCSF Benioff Children's Hospital
Director of the Orthopaedic Surgery Service

Peter Passias, MD
New York Spine Institute
NYU Medical Center-Hospital for Joint Diseases
New York, New York

Alpesh Patel, MD
Director, Orthopaedic Spine Surgery
Associate Professor
Department of Orthopaedic Surgery
Co-Director, Northwestern Spine Center
Chicago, Illinois

Adam Pearson, MD
Assistant Professor of Orthopaedics
Geisel School of Medicine, Dartmouth
Dartmouth-Hitchcock Medical Center
    Orthopaedic Surgery
Lebanon, New Hampshire

Coleen S. Sabatini, MD, MPH
Children's Hospital and Research Center in
    Oakland (CHRCO)
UCSF Benioff Children's Hospital
Director of the Orthopaedic Surgery Service

Andrew Schoenfeld, MD, MSc
Director of Spine Surgical Research
Department of Orthopaedic Surgery
Brigham and Women's Hospital
Harvard Medical School
Boston, Massachusetts

Manish K. Sethi, MD
Associate Professor of Orthopaedics &
    Rehabilitation
Department of Orthopaedic Trauma
Vanderbilt University Medical Center
Nashville, Tennessee

Melinda Sharkey, MD
Assistant Professor of Orthopaedics and
    Rehabilitation
Assistant Clinical Professor of Nursing and of
    Pediatrics
Yale School of Medicine
Yale-New Haven Hospital
New Haven, Connecticut

Andrew J. Sheean, MD
Department of Orthopaedic Surgery
San Antonio Military Medical Center
Fort Sam Houston, Texas

Lewis Shi, MD
Assistant Professor, Shoulder and Elbow Surgery
Department of Orthopaedic Surgery and
    Rehabilitation Medicine
University of Chicago medicine and Biological
    Sciences
Chicago, Illinois

Kern Singh, MD
Associate Professor
Department of Orthopaedic Surgery
Rush University Medical Center
Chicago, Illinois

Jeremy T. Smith, MD
Orthopaedic Surgeon, Foot and Ankle
Department of Orthopaedic Surgery
Brigham and Women's Hospital
Boston, Massachusetts

Daniel J. Stinner, MD
The Department of Regenerative Medicine United
    States Army Institute of Surgical Research
Department of Orthopaedics and Rehabilitation

Eric Sundberg, MD
Spine Surgery Fellow
Department of Orthopaedic Surgery
Rush University Medical Center
Chicago, Illinois

Jennifer Tangtiphaiboontana, MD
Department of Orthopaedic Surgery
University of California
San Francisco, California

David J. Tennent, MD
Department of Orthopaedic Surgery
San Antonio Military Medical Center
Fort Sam Houston, Texas

Alexander A. Theologis, MD
Department of Orthopaedic Surgery
University of California
San Francisco, California

Sunil Thirkannad, MD
Attending Hand Surgeon, Kleinert-Kutz
    Hand Care Center and Christine M Kleinert
    Institute for Hand and Microsurgery Clinical
Associate Professor of Hand Surgery
    (General Surgery)
Clinical Associate Professor of Orthopaedic Surgery
University of Louisville
Louisville, Kentucky

Michael J. Vives, MD
Associate Professor
Department of Orthopaedics
Chief, Spine Division
Rutgers, the State University of New Jersey
New Jersey Medical School
Newark, New Jersey

Amanda T. Whitaker, MD
Department of Orthopaedic Surgery
University of California
San Francisco, California

Lee Yu-Po, MD
Associate Clinical Professor
UCSD Department of Orthopaedic Surgery
San Diego, California

Preface

Welcome to the First Edition of *Orthopaedic Surgery: Examination and Board Review.*

We recall the stress of the OITE, ABOS Part 1 and recertification examinations. While the tests have evolved over time, one fact remains the same—preparation is the key. This book is very different than all other board review textbooks for multiple reasons:

1. **The format is case based**

   This book simulates the American Board of Orthopaedic Surgery (ABOS) Part 1 format with one clinical vignette followed by a series of questions and answers.

2. **Clinical interpretation is emphasized**

   With the transition to computerized testing for both the OITE, ABOS 1 and recertification examinations, test takers are increasingly being asked to interpret clinical scenarios with complex imaging, clinical photographs, and intraoperative findings. Older Orthopaedic board preparation materials have focused on basic knowledge as the "paper test" could not as effectively assess more complex clinical interpretation and decision making. This book focuses on reinforcing basic concepts in the context of making clinical decisions with clinical pictures, intraoperative photos, and complex imaging. Our work is very unique in this regard.

3. **The cases push the test taker for time**

   Along with the computer format and longer clinical vignettes with imaging and photos, the test taker is now pushed for time. Our cases are structured in a similar fashion to encourage the test taker to focus on the important details and focus less upon the extraneous details that are often provided on the Orthopaedic boards. Surgeons can time themselves and prepare with some time pressure to simulate the actual test.

4. **Authors understand OITE, ABOS, and recertification test writers**

   Many of our contributors in the book have participated in the process of writing questions for the ABOS Part 1 and the OITE and understand the rigor of test writing and the knowledge that examiners expect.

5. **Basic science concepts are included across all sections**

   In most orthopaedic review texts, basic science is included as a separate section without being incorporated into a clinical context. In this book, basic science is integrated across 10 chapters for each subspecialty.

In closing we would like to thank all of our contributors who have worked on this project over 2 years. It is our sincere hope that our work positions you to succeed on the OITE, ABOS 1, and recertification examinations as well as your career as an orthopaedic surgeon making clinical decisions about patients.

1

Spine

Mitchel B. Harris and Christopher M. Bono

CASE 1

Dr. Thomas D. Cha; Dr. Ali Al-Omari

A 63-year-old male sustained a hyperextension injury to his neck while diving into a pool. Upon presentation, he reports decreased sensation in his hands and decreased strength in his arms and wrists, but no lower extremity complaints. On motor examination, he has 5/5 strength in his deltoids and elbow flexors and 4/5 strength in the elbow extensors, wrist extensors, and finger flexors. Lower extremity motor examination is normal. Sensation is decreased to light touch in both hands. Otherwise his sensation is preserved. Images of his cervical spine are shown in Figures 1–1 to 1–3.

Injury to which of the following spinal cord tracts is most likely to be responsible for this patient's motor deficit?

A. Fasciculus gracilis
B. Lateral corticospinal tract
C. Anterior corticospinal tract
D. Lateral spinothalamic tract

Discussion

The correct answer is (B). The clinical scenario describes a patient with central cord syndrome (CCS). CCS continues to be the most common incomplete spinal cord

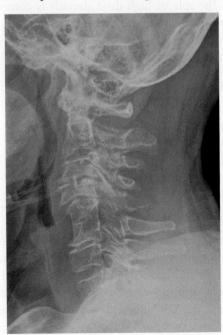

Figure 1–1

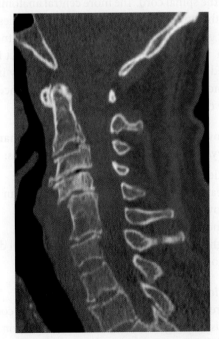

Figure 1–2

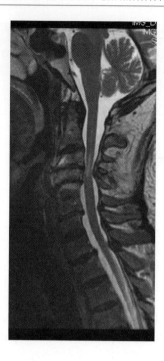

Figure 1–3

injury accounting for 15.7% to 25% of all spinal cord injuries. The characteristic presentation is an extension moment injury in a previously spondylotic and stenotic spine. Figures 1–1 to 1–3 demonstrate a spondylotic spine with central narrowing and CSF effacement that is worst at the C3–4 level. Bleeding, edema, and/or Wallerian degeneration lead to damage of the lateral corticospinal tract which is the main descending motor tract in the spinal cord. The more central anatomic position of the homunculus to the upper extremities places them at greater risk than those to the lower extremities. As such, injury to the lateral corticospinal tract is characterized by upper more than lower extremity involvement and motor deficits being more pronounced than sensory deficits.

The above patient is inquiring about his chances of recovery. He should be informed that there is:

A. Little chance of motor recovery
B. Greater chance of sensory recovery than motor recovery
C. Good chance of motor recovery
D. High likelihood of secondary neurological deterioration

Discussion

The correct answer is (C). Patients with central cord syndrome usually regain bowel and bladder function as well as the ability to ambulate. The progression of neurologic

and motor recovery usually begins in the lower extremities than the upper extremities. Prognostic factors predictive of long-term improvement include: age, severity of initial injury, early neurologic improvement, absence of spinal cord signal, and formal education level of the patient. In general, central cord injuries have good prognoses for motor recovery. Neurological deterioration is possible but unlikely with central cord injuries. Most of the recovery with central cord injuries is motor, not sensory.

During the first 24 hours of admission, the patient's neurological examination worsens, demonstrating only 1/5 strength in the elbow flexors, extensors, wrist, and hands. The lower extremities demonstrate 3/5 strength in all groups. Treatment at this time should be:

A. Observation
B. High-dose steroids
C. Surgical decompression
D. Repeat imaging

Discussion

The correct answer is (C). The patient presented with a mild central cord syndrome. In such instances, observation and nonoperative treatment is a reasonable treatment option, provided the patient remains neurologically stable or improves. Long-term clinical outcomes of surgical and nonoperative treatment are comparable. However, in the setting of a progressively worsening neurological deficit, early/urgent surgical decompression is more prudent than continued observation. The role of high-dose steroids is controversial for acute spinal cord injuries. While repeat imaging can be performed, it is likely to be unchanged and will not significantly affect the treatment plan.

Objectives: Did you learn…?

- The clinical presentation and responsible pathological injury for central cord syndrome?
- Prognosis of central cord syndrome?
- Indications for surgery for this disorder?

CASE 2

Dr. Thomas D. Cha; Dr. Michael R. Briseno

A 56-year-old man presents to you with a chief complaint of severe right buttock, posterior thigh, and lower leg pain for 12 weeks. It radiates to the lateral aspect of his foot, and it is worse with sitting or standing for prolonged periods and with walking. Now over the past 2 weeks, he reports difficulty with toe push-off on the right side. Treatment so far has been nonsteroidal

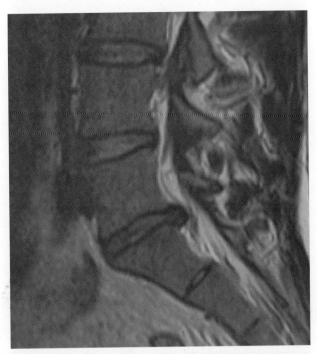

Figure 1–4

anti-inflammatory drugs (NSAID), physical therapy, and an epidural injection without significant relief. Physical examination findings include 4/5 right ankle plantar flexion, a positive straight leg raise on the right, and an absent right Achilles tendon reflex. Images of his lumbar spine are shown in Figures 1–4 and 1–5.

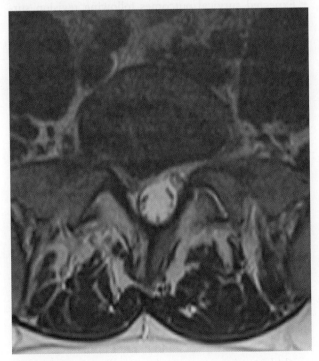

Figure 1–5

The next most appropriate step in management of this patient is:

A. Continued physical therapy
B. Another epidural injection
C. Lumbar discectomy
D. Decompression and fusion

Discussion

The correct answer is (C). The patient presents with classic right S1 radiculopathy and new onset plantar flexion weakness. The images demonstrate a right-sided paracentral disc herniation at L5/S1 compressing the traversing S1 nerve root. Despite nonoperative management, he continues to have severe pain and new weakness. Continued physical therapy or an epidural injection is unlikely to improve the patient's pain at this time. In the setting of neurological decline, surgery is more strongly indicated. Lumbar discectomy is the most appropriate procedure for this patient. Fusion would only be indicated if there were radiographic signs of instability, which are not present.

The patient re-presents to you in 9 months. He reports that surgery was successful in decreasing his leg pain and weakness until 2 months ago. He now reports recurrent low back pain and right leg pain, similar to his first episode. Physical examination demonstrates slightly decreased sensation on the lateral foot but no motor deficits. He demonstrates a positive straight leg raise test. The patient reports no fevers or chills and has a well-healed incision. Images from a gadolinium-enhanced magnetic resonance imaging (MRI) of his lumbar spine are shown in Figures 1–6 and 1–7.

What is the most likely cause of the patient's recurrent symptoms?

A. Perineural scar around the S1 nerve root
B. Ventral epidural abscess
C. Recurrent disc herniation
D. Arachnoiditis

Discussion

The correct answer is (C). The patient's history and imaging are most consistent with a recurrent disc herniation. He had a period of time after surgery during which symptoms were substantially improved and a clear episode marking recurrent pain. The MRI with gadolinium helps to differentiate recurrent disc herniation versus perineural fibrosis. The key radiographic findings on MRI for perineural fibrosis include: intermediate signal intensity, enhancement after contrast, irregular borders,

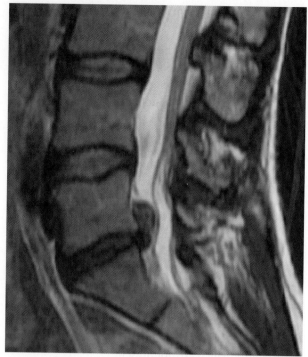

Figure 1–6

and a retracted dura. This contrasts with the MRI findings of recurrent herniation of low signal intensity on T1 and T2, no enhancement after contrast, smooth margins and displaced dura. The radiographic findings demonstrate a clear disc herniation, making perineural fibrosis less likely to be the primary pathology. Supported by the fact that the patient denies any constitutional symptoms such as fevers and/or chills, the MRI is not consistent with

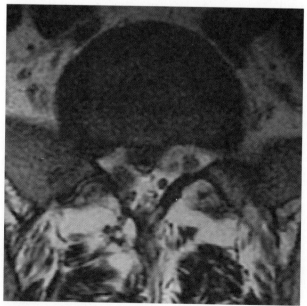

Figure 1–7

an epidural abscess. While arachnoiditis can be related to neural pain following surgery, the MRI does not demonstrate the classic signs of nerve root clumping.

The patient has failed a 3-month course of nonoperative treatment for his problem. You have offered him surgical treatment. Compared to his initial surgery, he should be informed that the second surgery will likely be associated with:

A. Worse clinical result
B. Greater chance for neurological injury
C. Lower risk of dural tear
D. Equivalent outcomes

Discussion

The correct answer is (D). Several studies have demonstrated that patients undergoing a revision discectomy have similar clinical outcomes as those undergoing an index discectomy. If anything, there is a higher risk of dural tear with a revision procedure. A higher chance for neurological injury with surgery has not been reported.

Objectives: Did you learn...?

• To utilize appropriate algorithm for treatment of primary disc herniation?
• The differential diagnosis of postoperative radicular pain following discectomy?
• MRI characteristics of recurrent disc herniation versus perineural fibrosis?
• Expected surgical outcomes following revision surgery for recurrent disc herniation?

CASE 3

Dr. Thomas D. Cha; Dr. Mark E. Jacobson

A 27-year-old previously healthy woman is transferred directly to your trauma center with severe low back pain after jumping from an overpass in an apparent suicide attempt. The trauma team completes the primary survey, and the patient is hemodynamically stabilized with fluid resuscitation. On secondary survey she is found to have significant pain with examination/manipulation of her pelvis. Lower extremity examination demonstrates multiple superficial abrasions and grade 4/5 strength with great toe extension and ankle dorsiflexion on the left. Inspection of the perineum shows no blood at the urethral meatus or rectum; however, rectal tone and perianal sensation are decreased. The remainder of the examination is unremarkable. An anteroposterior view of the pelvis demonstrates unilateral superior and inferior rami fractures and a right L5 transverse process fracture.

The next most appropriate imaging study that should be obtained is:

A. Inlet and outlet pelvic radiographs
B. Lateral sacral radiograph
C. Pelvic CT
D. Angiogram

Discussion

The correct answer is (C). It is important to recognize that plain radiographs may only detect 30% of sacral injuries. This patient's plain x-ray findings are highly suggestive of more substantial injuries than isolated rami fractures and transverse process fractures. In fact, the transverse process fracture should be assumed to have occurred by avulsion via the lumbosacral ligaments, which suggests large displacement of the hemipelvis. While plain radiographs may demonstrate sagittal displacement of sacral fractures, they are often of poor quality and do not enable delineation of the entire fracture pattern. A pelvic computed tomography (CT) scan is indicated to better evaluate the bony injury as well as canal encroachment, particularly in the setting of a neurological deficit. An angiogram might be indicated if the patient was hemodynamically unstable and an intrapelvic bleed was suspected.

CT scan images of the above patient are shown in Figures 1–8 and 1–9. Definitive management of this injury should be:

A. 3 months of bed rest followed by progressive mobilization
B. Open reduction and posterior plating of the sacrum

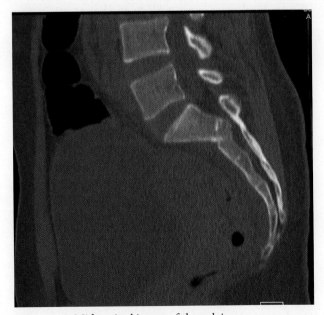

Figure 1–8 Mid-sagittal image of the pelvis.

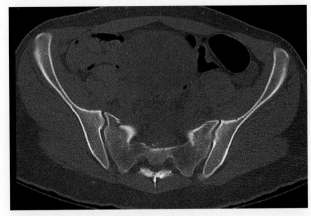

Figure 1–9 Axial image of the pelvis.

C. Laminectomy and bilateral iliosacral screw fixation
D. Laminectomy and lumbopelvic stabilization

Discussion

The correct answer is (D). Critical steps in decision-making include determination of neurologic status, presence of associated pelvic ring injuries, and stability of the lumbopelvic junction. The neurologic examination demonstrates a deficit that is at least in part localized to the sacral nerve roots. In the presence of sacral canal compromise, decompression via laminectomy is indicated. The CT scan demonstrates a U-type injury with a high transverse sacral fracture and bilateral vertical extension through the sacral foramen. In the descriptive classification of sacral fractures in Denis zone 3, H-type and U-type sacral fractures represent spinopelvic dissociation and must be distinguished from fractures localized to the posterior pelvic ring, which are vertically unstable. The spinopelvic junction serves as a critical transitional zone as the axial load of the upper body is distributed from the upper sacrum to the ilium and finally the acetabulum. Surgery is indicated to prevent progressive deformity and chronic pain. Reconstruction should include stabilization from the lumbar spine to the pelvis using a pedicle screw/iliac screw construct. Nonoperative treatment with progressive mobilization is not appropriate for this type of fracture. Plating of the sacrum is not sufficient to restore stability of this injury; nor are sacroiliac screws.

At the 6-week follow-up visit, the above patient reports she has difficulty controlling her bladder. Regarding prognosis, she should be informed this condition is likely to:

A. Remain unchanged
B. Worsen
C. Improve
D. Completely recover

Discussion

The correct answer is (C). Injuries through Denis Zone 3 have a high incidence of neurologic injury. With or without decompression, up to 80% of patients have neurologic improvement. Incomplete injuries, as exhibited by the patient in this case, have a better prognosis for recovery than complete injuries. Though the prognosis is generally good, complete recovery is unlikely.

Objectives: Did you learn...?

• Choose appropriate imaging studies for suspected sacral fractures?
• Recognize the hallmarks of vertically unstable sacral fractures?
• Determine optimal definitive treatment for spinopelvic dissociation?

CASE 4

Dr. Ivan Cheng

You are called to the emergency department to evaluate a 32-year-old man with a history of intravenous drug use who presents with a 2-week history of increasing neck pain and a 2-day history of fevers and progressive weakness in his arms and legs. On examination, he has 3/5 strength globally in his upper and lower extremities and is unable to ambulate without assistance.

Of the following, which is the most appropriate diagnostic test to confirm the suspected diagnosis?

A. Plain radiographs
B. CT scan
C. MRI
D. Bone scan

Discussion

The correct answer is (C). While x-rays and a CT scan may be helpful in evaluating overall alignment of the cervical spine as well as possible bony changes, an MRI would be the best imaging modality to visualize any neurologic involvement leading to the patient's deficit. With the patient's history, an infectious etiology is highly likely. While a bone scan can demonstrate increased activity in an area of infection, it does not help localize the exact location and extension of neurological involvement. In the event that an MRI is contraindicated, a CT scan, ideally with intrathecal contrast, would be a reasonable alternative.

Advanced imaging is shown in Figure 1–10. What is the most likely diagnosis?

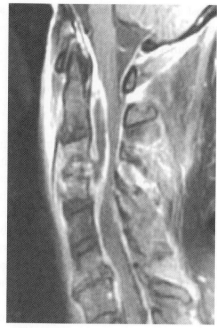

Figure 1–10

A. Ossification of the posterior longitudinal ligament
B. Epidural abscess
C. Tumor
D. Disc herniation

Discussion

The correct answer is (B). The T1 sagittal MRI demonstrates an epidural process that extends behind the C2, C3, and C4 vertebral bodies. There is destruction of the C3–4 disc space, which likely represents discitis/osteomyelitis. The epidural mass is most likely an abscess originating from the C3–4 disc space. OPLL, or ossification of the posterior longitudinal ligament, would typically be seen as an intermediate signal along the posterior aspect of the disc space/vertebral bodies and would not be associated with disc space destruction. Metastatic tumors and primary bone tumors more commonly involve the vertebral bodies themselves and do not typically cause increased signal within the disc space itself. Extruded disc herniations can extend behind the vertebral bodies but are not as large as depicted in these images and do not lead to signal changes within the disc space with bony involvement.

What is the next step in the management of this patient?

A. CT-guided aspiration
B. Empiric antibiotics
C. Anterior corpectomy
D. Laminectomy

Discussion

The correct answer is (C). An anterior corpectomy will achieve a number of surgical goals. First, it will remove the infected bone and disc space material, which is the source of infection. Second, it will allow direct drainage and debridement of the epidural abscess. Finally, it will enable reconstruction of the spine to restore stability. CT-guided aspiration and empiric antibiotics are not appropriate in a patient with a neurologic deficit. A posterior laminectomy alone is not useful in removing a ventral abscess and may lead to postoperative kyphosis from destabilization given the amount of disc and bony involvement in the anterior column. Empiric antibiotics would be a last resort for a patient who is medically unfit for surgery.

Which of the following is the most likely organism to be identified from this patient?

A. *Staphylococcus aureus*
B. *Staphylococcus epidermidis*
C. *Salmonella*
D. *Haemophilus influenzae*

Discussion

The correct answer is (A). The most common organism is methicillin-sensitive *S. aureus* followed by methicillin-resistant *S. aureus*. *Salmonella* is more common in patients with sickle cell disease. *H. influenzae* is more common in the pediatric population.

Objectives: Did you learn...?

- The ideal imaging study to determine the source of acute neurologic compromise in the setting of atraumatic neck pain?
- Treatment of an epidural abscess with neurological involvement?
- The most common organisms causing spinal epidural abscesses?

CASE 5

Dr. Ivan Chang

A 62-year-old otherwise healthy woman presents to your clinic with complaints of both chronic low back pain and difficulty ambulating distances secondary to pain radiating into her buttocks and posterior thighs. She reports her pain is relieved with forward flexion. On examination, the patient has a forward flexed posture and 4/5 strength in her bilateral EHLs and left tibialis anterior muscle. She has failed nonoperative treatment including extensive physical therapy and

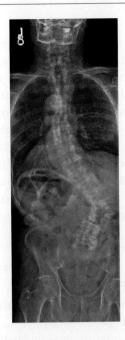

Figure 1–11

epidural injections. Plain radiographs are shown in Figures 1–11 and 1–12. In addition, an MRI demonstrates significant central stenosis at L4–5 (not shown).

Which of the following is the ideal surgical option for this patient?

A. L4–5 laminectomy
B. L4–5 laminectomy and fusion
C. L4–5 laminectomy, L3–5 fusion
D. L4–5 laminectomy, T10 to S1 fusion

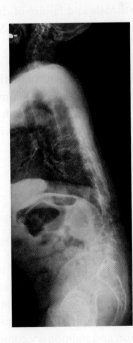

Figure 1–12

Discussion

The best answer is (D). Both decompression (laminectomy) alone and a selective decompression and L4–5 (or L3–5) fusion have a high risk of worsening both the coronal and sagittal plane alignment. The long plate films demonstrate a typical de novo degenerative scoliosis with a coronal curve apex at L2–3, rotatory subluxation at L3–4, a fractional curve at L4–S1, and loss of lumbar lordosis. The most reliable method of treating this patient's neurogenic claudication, sagittal imbalance, and listhesis is decompression and fusion with instrumentation from the thoracic spine to sacrum.

What construct would be most appropriate for the surgical treatment of this patient?

A. Segmental posterior instrumentation and fusion from T10–S1
B. Segmental posterior instrumentation and fusion from T10–S1 plus iliac fixation
C. Segmental posterior instrumentation and fusion from T10–S1 and L5–S1 interbody fusion
D. Segmental posterior instrumentation and fusion from T10–S1 and L5–S1 interbody fusion plus iliac fixation

Discussion

The correct answer is (D). With long constructs extending to the sacrum, the highest risk for failure lies at the lumbosacral junction. The best method to prevent pseudarthrosis and failure of distal fixation is to include an interbody fusion at L5–S1 and include iliac fixation.

In discussing the potential complications of a long posterior spinal fusion with instrumentation and decompression for deformities in the older adult population, the patient should be advised that most likely complication is:

A. Surgical site infection
B. Dural tear
C. Neurologic deficit
D. Cardiac event

Discussion

The correct answer is (B). While all of the choices are known complications from the surgical treatment of spinal deformities in the older population, the most commonly reported complication is dural tear followed by wound infection and pulmonary complications.

Objectives: Did you learn...?

- Ideal treatment of high-grade degenerative scoliosis with stenosis and sagittal imbalance?
- Optimal instrumentation construct for the surgical treatment of this condition?
- The most likely complications following surgery of this kind?

CASE 6

Dr. Ivan Chang

You are evaluating a 15-year-old otherwise healthy boy in your clinic who has a primary complaint of low back pain. On examination, he has significant hamstring tightness but is otherwise neurologically normal. A lateral radiograph and sagittal T2 MRI are shown in Figures 1–13 and 1–14.

What is the most common nerve root deficit following surgical reduction of this condition?

A. L3
B. L4
C. L5
D. S1

Discussion

The correct answer is (C). The course of the L5 nerve root is subjected to compression within the neuroforamen in high-grade slips, and tension of the root over the ventral surface of the sacrum places it at the highest risk for dysfunction following surgical reduction maneuvers.

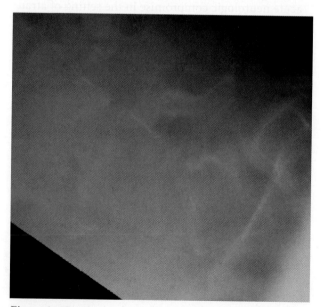

Figure 1–13

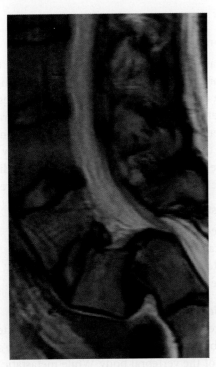

Figure 1–14

During the surgical reduction, neuromonitoring motor signals significantly diminish in the bilateral tibialis anterior muscles. What is the next most appropriate step?

A. Continue reduction
B. Halt reduction, fuse in that position
C. Return preoperative position and fuse in that position
D. Reverse reduction, reassess decompression, attempt reduction again if signals return

Discussion

The correct answer is (D). Neurophysiologic monitoring during surgical reduction of high-grade spondylolisthesis is critical in the prevention of postoperative neurologic deficits. If neuromonitoring changes are encountered, general recommendations include reversal of the last surgical steps including lessening the reduction. This is followed by reassessment of the decompression, which may prompt proceeding with an osteotomy of the sacral dome to facilitate more efficient slip reduction without nerve root tension. In the setting described, reduction should not be continued or maintained. While returning to the preoperative position and fusing is an option, one should first ensure that the signals have returned and that the decompression is adequate.

Of the following, which is the most important surgical treatment of this deformity?

A. Reducing translation
B. Improving slip angle
C. Changing pelvic incidence
D. Restoring lumbar lordosis

Discussion

The correct answer is (B). Reduction of high-grade spondylolisthesis remains controversial. Pelvic incidence remains constant in the skeletally mature patient and thus cannot be changed. Patients with high-grade spondylolisthesis are typically hyperlordotic, thus restoring lumbar lordosis is not an important goal. The radiographic factor most highly associated with improved long-term outcomes appears to be improvement of the slip angle.

Objectives: Did you learn...?

- Which nerve root is at most risk during reductions of high-grade spondylolisthesis?
- The steps that should be taken if neuromonitoring signals are lost during surgical reduction maneuvers?
- The radiographic parameters that is most correlated with outcomes in the surgical treatment of high-grade spondylolisthesis?

CASE 7

Dr. Jason Eck; Dr. Scott D. Hodges

A 64-year-old woman underwent an uncomplicated anterior C4 and 5 corpectomy followed by a C3–7 laminectomy and C2–T2 posterior instrumented fusion for cervical spondylotic myelopathy (CSM). On postoperative day 2, the patient was found to have new onset, significant weakness in right deltoid (1/5) and biceps (2/5) strength. Her examination otherwise was unchanged from her preoperative examination, with normal lower extremity strength and sensation. The incision was benign appearing and her laboratory studies were normal.

The most likely diagnosis is:

A. Central cord syndrome
B. Epidural abscess
C. Screw misplacement
D. C5 nerve root palsy

Discussion

The correct answer is (D). C5 nerve root palsy is a well-known potential complication of cervical spine decompression with reported rates ranging from 0% to 30%, but most studies suggest an incidence of approximately

7%. The case presentation is typical with significant uni-lateral weakness in the muscles innervated by the C5 nerve, which includes the deltoid and biceps, that has a delayed onset days after surgery. Central cord syndrome is unlikely as it would present with diffuse upper more than lower extremity weakness. A postoperative epidural abscess is possible but less likely to develop so early after surgery, particularly in the setting of normal laboratory values. Postoperative imaging studies did not reveal the presence of aberrant screw position, but a CT scan could be obtained to rule this out more definitively.

What is the most appropriate treatment for this patient?

A.   Observation
B.   Epidural steroid injection
C.   Nerve transfer
D.   Cervical foraminotomy

Discussion

The correct answer is (A). The large majority of patients have complete recovery with a mean time of 4 to 5 months. Recovery is spontaneous and no specific treatment has been shown to shorten the time of recovery. If there was any question on the placement of instrumentation based on the postoperative radiographs, a CT scan could be obtained. In rare cases that fail to recover function, nerve transfer procedures can be used to restore function to the arm, but these are never performed as an initial treatment. An epidural steroid injection would be ineffective. A cervical foraminotomy is usually not recommended considering the favorable natural history.

Which of the following has been demonstrated to be a risk factor for this condition?

A.   Age
B.   Surgical duration
C.   Use of instrumentation
D.   Severity of stenosis
E.   Width of laminectomy

Discussion

The correct answer is (A). Advanced patient age has been reported to increase the risk of C5 nerve palsy, with data suggesting patients older than 65 years being at a particularly higher risk. The other factors listed have not been reported to be risk factors for C5 nerve root palsy.

Objectives: Did you learn to …

• Identify patient symptoms that suggest the presence of postoperative C5 nerve palsy?
• Treat a patient with postoperative C5 nerve palsy?
• Identify risk factors for postoperative C5 nerve palsy?

CASE 8

Dr. Jason Eck; Dr. Scott D. Hodges

A 78-year-old woman is complaining of a new onset of mid-thoracic back pain after a fall from standing 2 days ago. She denies any radiating pain or paresthesias into the extremities. Physical examination demonstrates that she is neurologically intact and has localized tenderness over the thoracic spine. She remains ambulatory and has adequate pain relief with over-the-counter medications. Thoracic spine radiographs are shown in Figure 1–15.

The most likely diagnosis is:

A.   Osteoporotic compression fracture
B.   Metastatic pathologic fracture
C.   Vertebral osteomyelitis
D.   Scheuermann's kyphosis

Discussion

The correct answer is (A). The patient has an osteoporotic vertebral compression fracture involving the anterior portion of the vertebral body. While metastatic disease is common at this age, it is more likely that this represents a benign compression fracture. The disc spaces are preserved, indicating that this is likely not discitis with osteomyelitis. Scheuermann's kyphosis characteristically presents with wedging of the vertebral bodies and typically presents in young, adolescent males.

Treatment at this time should be:

A.   Observation
B.   Bracing and bedrest

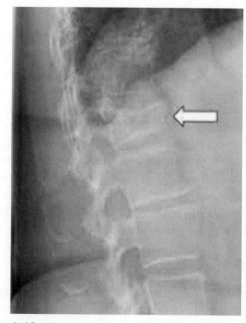

Figure 1–15

C. Vertebroplasty

D. Kyphoplasty

Discussion

The correct answer is (A). If the pain is adequately controlled with nonprescription medication and activity modification, the fracture can heal without other treatment. Bracing with a thoracolumbarsacral orthosis (TLSO) can provide improved pain control if needed but is not required from a structural standpoint. Furthermore, forced bedrest would be detrimental to a patient who is currently ambulatory. Cement augmentation, either by vertebroplasty or kyphoplasty, is an option as it can provide more immediate pain relief. However, in a patient with only 2 days of pain who remains ambulatory, noninvasive treatment should be the first option.

The above patient is undergoing a vertebroplasty of the fractured level. During the procedure, you note that cement has extravasated posterior to the vertebral body. The next most appropriate step in management is:

A. Immediate laminectomy

B. Physical examination

C. Urgent MRI

D. Anterior corpectomy

Discussion

The correct answer is (B). There is a defined rate of cement extravasation with vertebroplasty (20–30%).

The vast majority of cases of cement extravasation into the spinal canal are fortunately asymptomatic. Thus, it is highly likely that the noted cement will not result in a clinically significant deficit. No further cement should be injected and the patient should undergo a careful neurological examination. If there are any noted deficits, the patient should undergo advanced imaging and an appropriate decompressive procedure if warranted.

Objectives: Did you learn...?

• Diagnose a vertebral compression fracture?

• Understand the natural history of osteoporotic compression fractures?

• Understand the risks and benefits of cement augmentation for osteoporotic compression fractures?

CASE 9

Dr. Marco L. Ferrone

A 46-year-old male presents with a 1-year history of worsening low back and left leg pain. Despite having been treated for sciatica with physical therapy and manipulation, his symptoms are worse. He denies lower extremity weakness and bowel and bladder dysfunction. He does report increasing night pain and weight loss. On physical examination he has no deficits, but has a palpable, firm, fixed, nontender mass at the lumbosacral junction on the left. He presents with the following imaging studies, CT and MRI (Figs. 1–16 and 1–17).

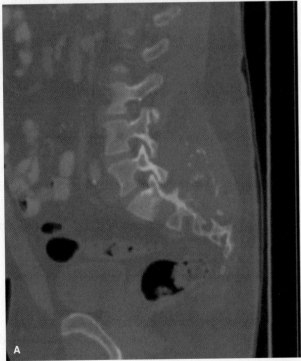
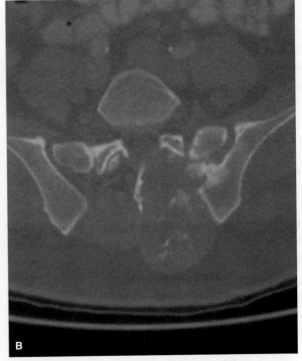

Figure 1–16 Sagittal CT image through lumbar spine (**A**), Axial CT image through the lumbosacral junction (**B**).

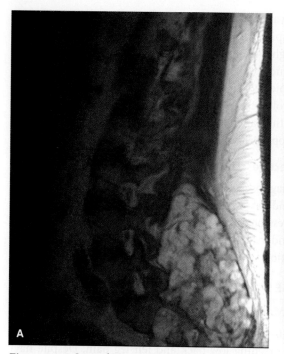
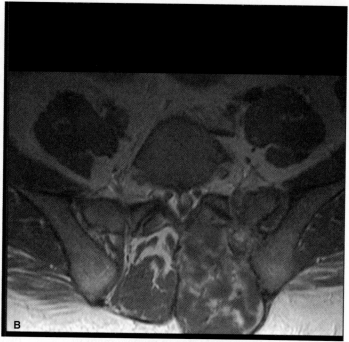

Figure 1–17 Sagittal T2 weighted MRI of lumbar spine (**A**), axial T1-weighted image post-contrast of lumbar spine (**B**).

Based on the above vignette the next most appropriate step in evaluation of this patient would be:

A. Surgical resection
B. Observation
C. Staging studies
D. Chemotherapy and radiation
E. Radiation only

Discussion

The best answer is (C). This is most likely a malignant process given his age, weight loss, presence of night pain, as well as the imaging characteristics. Workup for a bone lesion should include local and remote imaging, as well as laboratory work, including complete blood count, chemistry, and alkaline phosphatase. In certain circumstances, serum protein immunoelectrophoresis, prostate specific antigen, and carcinoembryonic antigen may be appropriate.

The local staging has been completed with CT and MRI of the entire lesion; what is needed to complete the remote staging?

A. Whole body bone scan with Technetium 99 (^{99}Tc)
B. CT chest/abdomen/pelvis
C. Whole body MRI
D. None of the above
E. A and B only

Discussion

The best answer is (E). Remote staging accomplishes the task of establishing the presence or absence of metastases. Lung is the most common site of metastasis. In addition, the CT scan of the abdomen and pelvis will evaluate for the presence of retroperitoneal metastases in the case of small round cell tumors, as well as to evaluate lymph nodes in the case of lymphoma. In addition, the studies would exclude another solid organ as the primary site of disease. Whole body bone scan with Technetium 99 (^{99}Tc) is often ordered to rule out skip metastasis. When considering lesions like multiple myeloma or renal cell cancer metastases, a skeletal survey can be considered as these lesions can be silent on bone scan.

Local and remote staging reveal an isolated lesion. The next most appropriate step in managing this patient is:

A. Core needle biopsy by patients primary care provider
B. Incisional biopsy at closest community hospital
C. Biopsy directed by operating surgeon
D. Excisional biopsy by surgeon
E. None of the above

Discussion

The best answer is (C). The biopsy is a critical step and should be done with the coordination of the treating surgeon who will resect the tumor. The biopsy tract needs to be resectable at the time of definitive surgery. Errant biopsies can lead to contamination of the field and spread of the tumor resulting in increased morbidity and mortality. When biopsies done at referring institutions are compared to those done at treatment centers, Mankin showed that errors in diagnosis, 27.4% versus 12.3%, were significantly higher as were the adverse effects on outcome, 17.4% versus 3.5%. Excisional biopsy is reserved for small superficial tumors.

A core needle biopsy is performed by interventional radiology, after the biopsy trajectory was discussed with the surgeon. The following are histologic images of the biopsy (Figs. 1–18A–C). The most likely diagnosis is:

A. Liposarcoma
B. Aneurysmal bone cyst
C. Osteosarcoma
D. Chondrosarcoma
E. Chordoma

Discussion

The best answer is (D). The slides show grade I chondrosarcoma. There is cellular tumor cartilage infiltrating the normal osteoid. Seen are plump nuclei with more than one cell per lacunae.

The best treatment would be:

A. Radiation then resection
B. Chemotherapy then resection
C. Chemotherapy and radiation then resection
D. Resection
E. Chemotherapy and radiation

Discussion

The best answer is (D). Chondrosarcoma is treated with surgery, en bloc wide margin resection, without chemotherapy and radiation. Chondrosarcoma is thought to be resistant to both chemotherapy and radiation. Osteosarcoma is treated with neoadjuvant chemotherapy, surgery, and adjuvant chemotherapy. Ewing's sarcoma can be treated similarly with neoadjuvant chemotherapy,

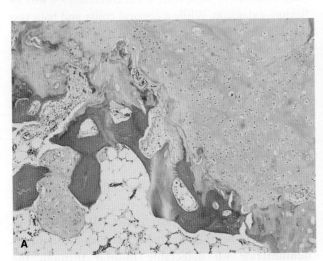

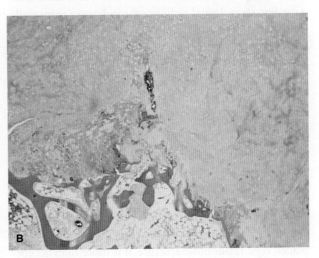

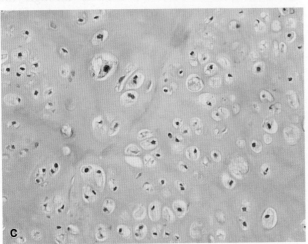

Figure 1–18 Cartilaginous neoplasm invading through bone into marrow space (**A**), Highlights bone destruction and abnormal cellularity and atypia within the cartilage tumor (**B**), Tumor cells exhibit clear atypia (large, middle cell) and occasional binucleate forms (**C**). Images taken by David M. Meredith MD, Brigham & Women's Hospital, Department of Pathology.

surgery, and adjuvant chemotherapy or alternatively with chemotherapy and radiation only.

Objectives: Did you learn...?

- Identify patient symptoms that suggest the presence of a malignant lesion?
- Stage primary bone tumors?
- Biopsy protocol?
- Identify and treat chondrosarcoma?

CASE 10

Nicholas S. Golinvaux; Bryce A. Basques; Daniel D. Bohl; Dr. Jonathan N. Grauer

You are called to the emergency department to evaluate an 87-year-old woman who became confused in the middle of the night and fell while getting out of bed. She resides in an assisted living facility. Her current medical history includes Alzheimer's dementia, diabetes, hypertension, and hyperlipidemia. Her son reports that 7 years ago she had a heart attack that was treated with a cardiac stent. Initial radiographs indicate a minimally displaced type II odontoid fracture.

The optimal treatment for this patient's fracture is:

A. Halo-vest immobilization
B. Cervical collar
C. Odontoid screw
D. Posterior C1–2 fusion
E. Posterior occiput-C3 fusion

Discussion

The correct answer is (B). This patient has multiple comorbidities that make her a suboptimal surgical candidate. Furthermore, in the case of a minimally displaced type II odontoid fracture, it is more than acceptable to definitively treat an elderly, demented patient with a rigid cervical collar for 6 to 12 weeks. Though treatment with a cervical collar can have lower rates of bone healing than surgery, fibrous union is generally sufficient in a low-demand individual. Use of a halo vest is associated with high rates of complications, especially aspiration, in the elderly population and has not demonstrated superior outcomes to cervical collars. As stated above, this patient is a poor surgical candidate, owing to her significant past medical history, making choices C through E less than ideal. Moreover, an odontoid screw requires adequate bone density for proper fixation, and this patient is likely to have osteoporotic bone given her age, gender, and history of diabetes. A

posterior C1–2 fusion may be a reasonable option for this injury type, particularly if any significant displacement or instability was identified. However, this would be rather aggressive in a low-demand, demented, and medically compromised patient. Posterior occiput to C3 fusion is more extensive than would generally be indicated to surgically treat this injury.

Which of the following treatments would result in a decrease of cervical rotation by approximately 55% and of cervical flexion–extension by 15%?

A. Cervical collar
B. Anterior odontoid screw
C. Posterior C1–2 fusion
D. Posterior occiput to C3 fusion
E. Halo vest

Discussion

The correct answer is (C). A posterior C1–2 fusion has been shown to lead to an approximate decrease in cervical rotation of 55% with a concordant 15% loss of flexion–extension. While a cervical collar and halo vest would likely lead to some stiffening of the neck, they would be unlikely to yield a marked decrease in motion. Similarly, it would be unlikely for an anterior odontoid screw to cause a marked decrease in cervical range of motion as it is not a fusion procedure and does not cross a motion segment. In contrast, posterior occiput to C3 fusion is associated with a much more significant decrease in cervical rotation and flexion/extension.

The patient has been in a cervical collar following this injury for 3 months. She has no complaint of pain and remains neurologically intact. Though there is lack of bone healing, flexion–extension radiographs demonstrate no detectable motion through the fracture site. The next step in management should be:

A. Continued collar immobilization
B. Anterior odontoid screw
C. Posterior C1–2 fusion
D. Discontinue collar
E. Switch to halo vest

Discussion

The correct answer is (D). In an elderly patient with a minimally displaced odontoid fracture for whom the decision was made to treat nonoperatively with a rigid cervical collar, the chances of nonunion are high (as high as 30–70% failure of radiographic union). However, these patients generally develop a fibrous union that provides sufficient functional stability for a patient in this demographic. The patient in the current case demonstrates no motion on flexion/extension films and is asymptomatic, so she may discontinue her use of a collar. Close clinical and radiographic follow-up is sufficient to monitor for new-onset instability or symptoms. Continued collar immobilization, an anterior odontoid screw, posterior C1–2 fusion, and switch to a halo vest are all unnecessary interventions in an asymptomatic patient with a stable nonunion without motion on follow-up flexion/extension films.

Objectives: Did you learn...?

- Manage a type II odontoid fracture in an elderly patient with several medical comorbidities?
- Understand the resulting loss of cervical motion following C1–2 fusion?
- Manage asymptomatic nonunion of a type II odontoid fracture?

CASE 11

Nicholas S. Golinvaux; Bryce A. Basques; Daniel D. Bohl; Dr. Jonathan N. Grauer

A 45-year-old man is brought to the trauma bay after falling from his roof while cleaning his gutters. He complains of severe lower back pain but is neurologically intact. Initial CT images demonstrate an L1 burst fracture with a fracture through the lamina, 50% canal compromise from bony retropulsion, and 25 degrees of segmental kyphosis. An MRI demonstrates discontinuity of the ligamentum flavum and interspinous ligaments at the injured level.

What is the rate of noncontiguous spine fractures in a scenario such as this?

A. 0%
B. 15%
C. 40%
D. 60%

Discussion

The correct answer is (B). Several studies have reported the incidence of noncontinuous spinal fractures to range from 3.7% to 22%. Some specific injury patterns also have increased risks of nonspinal fractures. For example, burst fractures that result from a fall from height have increased risk of calcaneus fractures. Flexion–distraction injuries that occur after motor vehicle accidents with lap belts have increased risk of intra-abdominal injuries. Thoracolumbar fractures have also been noted to be associated with pelvic fractures.

Which of the following features is the strongest indicator of instability of this injury?

A. 25 degrees of kyphosis
B. 50% canal compromise
C. Posterior ligamentous disruption
D. Posterior arch fracture

Discussion

The correct answer is (C). Historically, a number of radiographic parameters have been used to suggest that a thoracolumbar burst fracture is unstable. Even today, textbooks continue to publish the so-called 50–50–25 rule, which indicates that a fracture with at least 50% of canal compromise, 50% of vertebral body height loss, and 25 degrees of kyphosis is unstable. Over the past decade, a number of studies have clearly shown that all of these radiographic features can be present in a stable injury that can be successfully treated nonoperatively. With the advent of MRI, direct visualization of the posterior ligamentous complex can reveal whether or not there is disruption of these stabilizing structures, which includes the facet joint capsule, interspinous ligaments, and supraspinous ligaments. Disruption of the ligamentum flavum, though not significant structurally by itself, suggests that a large flexion moment was delivered to the spine at the moment of injury. Thus, the correct answer is posterior ligamentous disruption, as was indicated by the MRI findings described in the case. A lamina fracture at the thoracolumbar junction in the presence of a neurological injury can be an indication of entrapped nerve roots and a traumatic dural tear. However, by itself it does not constitute posterior column disruption.

Which of the following would be the best option for definitive treatment of this injury?

A. Custom-molded thoracolumbar orthosis
B. Anterior corpectomy
C. Laminectomy and noninstrumented fusion
D. Instrumented posterior fusion

Discussion

The correct answer is (D). The patient has an unstable thoracolumbar burst fracture. Nonoperative treatment in an orthosis would not be desirable. Operative stabilization would be the mainstay of treatment. While an anterior corpectomy would be an ideal method of decompressing the patient, it is not necessary in a patient who is neurologically intact. Furthermore, an anterior corpectomy alone without any type of stabilization or fusion would leave the patient less stable after surgery than before. A laminectomy also further destabilizes the patient. Though a noninstrumented fusion may eventually lead to stability once bony union is achieved, this could take months and would require prolonged immobilization. The best option would be an instrumented posterior fusion, which would both stabilize the patient immediately and allow immediate mobilization.

Objectives: Did you learn...?

- Identify the rates of noncontiguous spine fractures?
- Understand the factors that suggest instability in a lumbar burst fracture?
- Manage a lumbar burst fracture?

CASE 12

Nicholas S. Golinvaux; Bryce A. Basques; Daniel D. Bohl; Dr. Jonathan N. Grauer

A 67-year-old woman presents to your office complaining of progressive back pain over the past year. She also reports unintentional weight loss and occasional night sweats. Upon examination, she is neurologically intact but has some localized tenderness in the mid-thoracic spine. MRI with contrast demonstrates a large, uniformly enhancing epidural lesion with a significant amount of cord compression at T7 and some involvement of the posterolateral aspect of the vertebral body extending into the pedicle. Her intervertebral discs appear uninvolved. Initial blood tests are normal, including a white blood count of 7,200 WBCs/μL and an erythrocyte sedimentation rate (ESR) of 5 mm/h (normal range 0–20).

What is the next most appropriate step in management?

A. Biopsy of the lesion
B. IV antibiotics
C. Repeat CBC
D. Irrigation and debridement

Discussion

The correct answer is (A). The patient's history is concerning for some type of neoplastic process. The MRI indicates an epidural lesion with bone involvement but no involvement of the discs. Typical pyogenic infections usually start in the disc spaces. Thus, it would be unlikely that this patient has discitis with an associated epidural abscess, though this is certainly in the differential diagnosis. The exact MRI characteristics described in this patient are also of interest. Epidural lymphoma

appears isointense or hypointense on T1 and a hyperintense or hypointense appearance on T2. There tends to be uniform and diffuse gadolinium enhancement. When epidural lymphoma is suspected, tissue is needed to confirm and refine the diagnosis. Hence, a biopsy should be obtained. In this case, biopsy would probably be of the pedicle/posterolateral vertebral body. The MRI appearance of an epidural abscess is heterogeneously enhancing epidural collection that is isointense or hypointense on T1 images but hyperintense on T2 images. If the lesion is large, there may be rim enhancement if an epidural abscess is present. Regarding irrigation and debridement, it would be preferable to obtain a diagnosis prior to initiating care, especially given that the patient is neurologically intact and likely has a tumor.

A biopsy of the lesion is performed. The pathology report states that the tissue is consistent with stage II (early) Hodgkin's lymphoma. Which of the following factors would indicate the need for surgical treatment at this time?

A. Positive disease identified in lymph nodes adjacent to the lesion
B. Epidural collection spanning more than one vertebral level
C. Imminent pathologic collapse
D. Significant cord compression

Discussion

The correct answer is (C). An unstable pathologic vertebral body fracture or what is determined to be a pending pathologic collapse poses the threat of neurological decline and should be addressed surgically, provided the patient is medically fit for an operation. The other choices in this question are not clear indications for surgery. Spinal cord compression in the absence of neurological deficit is not an immediate indication for surgery. Because lymphomas (and in particular Hodgkin's lymphoma) are usually highly sensitive to chemotherapy and radiation, these treatments should be attempted first. Surgical decompression may become necessary, but it should be reserved for those very few patients who do not exhibit a good response to chemotherapy and radiation or who have a progressive neurological deficit.

The patient remains neurologically intact following biopsy. What is the next step in treatment?

A. Immunotherapy
B. Chemotherapy and radiation

C. Anterior decompression and fusion

D. Posterior decompression and fusion

Discussion

The correct answer is (B). Standard chemotherapy regimens for Hodgkin's disease are highly effective at reducing the tumor burden and producing a complete clinical response. Chemotherapy is often followed with time-dose radiation therapy. With respect to immunotherapy, multiple antibody-based agents are being investigated, but none have established efficacy that is as high as that with chemotherapy and radiation. With respect to surgical options, these may become necessary should pathologic fracture of the vertebral body occur, if there is onset of neurologic symptoms or if the tumor is not responding to initial therapy. However, in most other scenarios, chemotherapy and radiation therapy should be able to sufficiently reduce the tumor burden, rendering surgical intervention unnecessary. Furthermore, the case scenario does not provide enough information from which one can determine the ideal surgical approach should it be indicated.

Objectives: Did you learn...?

- Evaluate a thoracic epidural lesion?
- Recognize surgical and nonsurgical indications for a thoracic lymphoma?
- Definitively manage a thoracic lymphoma?

CASE 13

Dr. Jason Eck; Dr. Scott D. Hodges

A 23-year-old man was involved in a high-speed motor vehicle accident. On presentation to the trauma bay, his chief complaint was neck pain. Physical examination demonstrated that he was neurologically intact. Images of the cervical spine are shown in Figure 1–19A–B. Full workup demonstrated no other injuries.

The patient's injury is best characterized as which of the following?

A. Jefferson fracture

B. Hangman's fracture

C. Burst fracture

D. Facet dislocation

Discussion

The correct answer is (B). The imaging clearly demonstrates a Hangman's fracture, also known as a C2 traumatic spondylolisthesis. The hallmark of this injury is a fracture through the pars interarticularis of C2, which effectively dissociates the anterior elements from the posterior arch and facet joints. A Jefferson fracture refers to C1 ring fractures that can have varying degrees of lateral displacement. There is no evidence of vertebral body comminution with posterior vertebral body

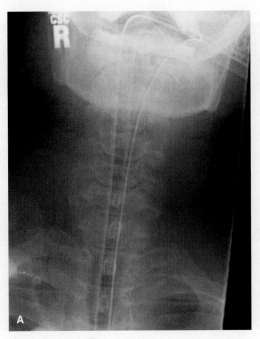
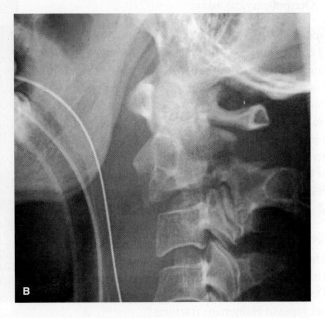

Figure 1–19 **A–B**

involvement, which would be characteristic of a burst fracture. While some Hangman's fractures can be associated with facet dislocation, there is no evidence of this on the imaging.

What is the classification for this fracture?

A. Type I
B. Type II
C. Type IIA
D. Type III

Discussion

The correct answer is (B). Type I fractures have minimal horizontal displacement, no angulation, and the C2–3 disc remains intact. Type II fractures are both displaced and angulated, presumably hinging around the anterior longitudinal ligament. Importantly, these fractures reduce with longitudinal traction. Type IIA fractures have minimal horizontal displacement but are significantly angulated. It is presumed that the anterior fragment rotates in place, most likely disrupting the anterior longitudinal ligament. These injuries are worsened by traction and reduced with axial compression. Type III fractures have bilateral C2–3 facet dislocations.

What is the most appropriate definitive treatment for this patient?

A. Hard collar
B. Traction and halo immobilization
C. Anterior and posterior C2–3 fusion
D. Occipitocervical fusion

Discussion

The correct answer is (B). While type I fractures can be treated immediately in a hard collar, type II fractures are best treated initially with traction to achieve fracture reduction. After a short period of traction, the patient should be placed in a halo vest to allow mobilization. As indicated above, type IIA fractures should not be placed in traction; patients should be placed in a halo vest with some axial compression applied. Type III fractures require surgical reduction of the facet dislocation and internal stabilization.

Objectives: Did you learn…?

• Identify a Hangman's fracture based on imaging?
• Understand the classification of Hangman's fractures?
• Determine the most appropriate treatment of different types of Hangman's fractures?

CASE 14

Dr. David Kim

A 70-year-old retired, funeral director presents with symptoms of right upper extremity numbness and weakness. He reports that he developed acute neck and right upper arm pain while undergoing a dental procedure. Treatment so far has been nonsteroidal anti-inflammatory medication and physical therapy with cervical traction. While his pain improved with this course of treatment, he has ongoing paresthesias radiating into his right hand and weakness affecting his right upper extremity. Figures 1–20 and 1–21 show a midsagittal and axial image through C6–7, respectively.

Based on the information provided, which of the following is the most likely diagnosis?

A. Radiculopathy
B. Intradural tumor
C. Myelopathy
D. Central cord syndrome

Discussion

The correct answer is (A). Considering the patient's complaints and the imaging, he most likely has radiculopathy, probably secondary to a disc-osteophyte complex associated with foraminal stenosis at the C6–7 level. There is no suggestion in the history of walking imbalance or dexterity issues in the upper extremities. Thus, a diagnosis of myelopathy is less likely. Further-

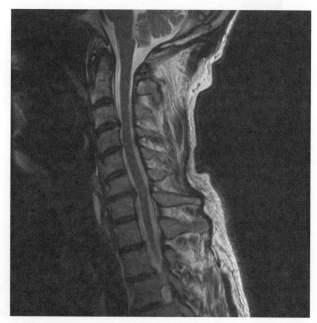

Figure 1–20

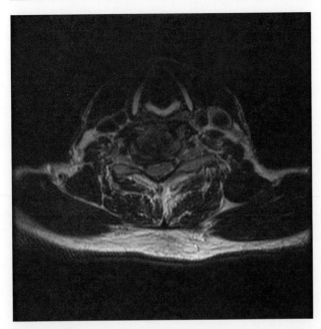

Figure 1–21

more, the degree of spinal compression is mild and not likely (though not impossible) to cause spinal cord dysfunction. An intradural tumor would have a different MRI appearance, likely demonstrating an area of high signal within the parenchymal tissue of the spinal cord itself. A central cord syndrome is an acute spinal cord injury with upper extremities being affected more than lower extremities.

Which of the following physical examination findings would you most likely find in this patient?

A. Weakness of right elbow flexion and wrist extension with sensory loss of the thumb
B. Weakness of right elbow flexion and wrist flexion with sensory loss of the thumb
C. Weakness of right elbow extension and wrist flexion with sensory loss of the middle finger
D. Weakness of right elbow extension and wrist extension with sensory loss of the middle finger

Discussion

The correct answer is (C). The patient has nerve root compression at the C6–7 level, which would affect the exiting C7 nerve. Weakness of right elbow extension and wrist flexion with sensory loss of the middle finger are the most likely findings.

Despite 12 weeks of supervised, nonoperative treatment, the patient reports ongoing moderate pain, paresthesia, and weakness that limits his physical activity and affects his quality of life. Physical examination reveals no change in his right upper extremity weakness or sensory deficit. As he is considering surgery, the patient inquires about the relative benefit of anterior versus posterior surgery. Relative to posterior surgery, he should be advised that anterior surgery results in:

A. Inferior clinical outcomes
B. Unacceptable clinical outcomes
C. Superior clinical outcomes
D. Equivalent clinical outcomes

Discussion

The correct answer is (D). Both anterior and posterior surgical approaches have been associated with consistently good clinical outcomes in this patient population having single level radiculopathy from foraminal stenosis secondary to a disc-osteophyte complex.

Objectives: Did you learn...?

- Recognize the clinical presentation of cervical radiculopathy associated with a disc-osteophyte complex?
- Understand the physical examination findings most commonly associated with C7 nerve root compression?
- Appreciate the relative outcomes of different surgical approaches to this problem?

CASE 15

Dr. David Kim

A 62-year-old woman underwent a routine single-level L4–5 laminectomy and posterior instrumented fusion for spinal stenosis with degenerative spondylolisthesis. She reports substantial symptomatic improvement for 10 years but now presents with recurrent low back pain and increasing leg pain when walking distances. Figure 1–22 shows a lateral plain radiograph taken 1 year after surgery. Figure 1–23 shows the same view at 10-year follow-up.

The patient's recurrent symptoms are most likely associated with which of the following?

A. L4–5 nonunion
B. L3 spondylolysis
C. Adjacent segment disease
D. Flatback syndrome

Discussion

The correct answer is (C). The two radiographs depict interval development of an L3–4 spondylolisthesis immediately proximal to an L4–5 spinal fusion. In the setting of a patient with recurrent back pain and claudication

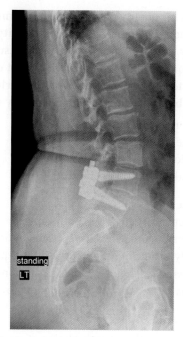

Figure 1–22

symptoms several years after initially successful lumbar laminectomy and fusion surgery, the radiographic findings strongly suggest development of adjacent segment degeneration and imply symptomatic spinal stenosis at the L3–4 level (though not appreciable on plain films). L4–5 nonunion can present in delayed fashion several years

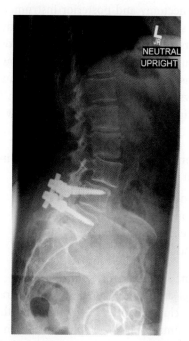

Figure 1–23

after surgery but is more often associated with mechanical back pain as opposed to recurrent claudication. In addition, a plain lateral radiograph would not be sufficient to make this determination. L3 spondylolysis can result from weakness of the pars interarticularis following laminectomy. However, the L3 pars is clearly seen and appears to be intact. This would also not be associated with claudicant-type symptoms. Finally, flatback syndrome can result in back pain and bilateral thigh cramping secondary to postoperative sagittal imbalance but does not cause claudication. This patient's lordosis appears to be preserved.

The risk of adjacent segment degeneration 10 years following surgery is approximately:

A. 5%
B. 15%
C. 25%
D. 45%

Discussion

The correct answer is (C). Overall, the incidence of adjacent segment disease appears to be approximately 25% to 30% within 10 years of the index surgery. The relative risk based on specific spinal level appears to vary directly with relative segmental motion and is therefore greatest at the L4–5 level. Of all surgery-related risk factors studied to date, one of the most consistently demonstrated risk factors for increased adjacent segment stress and degeneration appears to be sagittal plane imbalance, specifically kyphotic malalignment.

Which of the following surgical techniques has eliminated the risk of adjacent segment disease?

A. Artificial disc replacement
B. Dynamic stabilization with flexible rods
C. Anterior lumbar interbody fusion
D. None of the above

Discussion

The correct answer is (D). To date, no surgical fusion technique or alternative so-called "motion-sparing" technology has successfully reduced or eliminate the overall rate of adjacent segment degeneration and disease. Both artificial disc replacements and dynamic stabilization devices were initially developed with the specific goal of reducing the rate of adjacent segment degeneration, but clinical studies have so far shown no advantage over fusion surgery and have shown potentially increased rates of device-related complications. Interbody fusion demonstrates increased stiffness in biomechanical models, but clinical studies have not proven superiority of one fusion technique over another. Of note, adjacent segment degeneration refers to the appearance of radiologic degeneration involving the level(s) adjacent to a fused spinal segment. Adjacent segment disease is the term used when such degeneration is associated with actual symptoms such as pain, weakness, or sensory changes. The major cause of these entities, whether natural history or iatrogenic, remains a matter of intense ongoing debate, and the question remains largely unanswered.

Objectives: Did you learn...?

- To identify clinical occurrence of adjacent segment degeneration and disease?
- The incidence of adjacent segment degeneration?
- The inadequacy of modern surgical techniques to reduce or eliminate adjacent segment degeneration?

CASE 16

Dr. David Kim

A 51-year-old fireman whose primary complaint was chronic low back pain and right-sided leg pain underwent an L4–5 lumbar laminectomy and posterior instrumented spinal fusion for a diagnosis of L4–5 lumbar stenosis and degenerative spondylolisthesis. During surgery, bilateral pedicle screw instrumentation is placed at the L4 and L5 levels. There were no apparent complications and intraoperative radiographs including anteroposterior and lateral views were unremarkable. Immediately following surgery, the patient reported substantial relief of his right lower extremity pain, numbness, and weakness but now has difficulty sitting and walking due to new onset of severe left lower extremity pain, numbness, and weakness. Physical examination reveals a positive straight leg raise test on the left side, dense numbness in the left great toe, and new focal weakness in left ankle and great toe dorsiflexion.

What is the next most appropriate step in managing this patient?

A. Continued observation
B. Repeat radiographs
C. MRI with contrast
D. CT

Discussion

The correct answer is (D). The patient has new severe postoperative sciatica and a new neurological deficit, so simple observation is not appropriate. Intraopera-

tive radiographs revealed no apparent abnormalities, so repeated plain radiographs are unlikely to provide additional useful information. An MRI study would be indicated if the concern was for a potential postoperative epidural hematoma, but with complete relief of pain and symptoms in one lower extremity, a hematoma becomes less likely. The most likely etiology is direct nerve root impingement from a malpositioned pedicle screw. A CT scan with sagittal and coronal reconstructions is most likely to identify this problem.

Imaging of this patient shows an inferomedial left L5 pedicle breach and likely impingement of the adjacent nerve root by the pedicle screw. What is the next most appropriate step in managing this patient?

A. Continued observation
B. Narcotic pain medication
C. Epidural injection
D. Surgery

Discussion

The correct answer is (D). Additional surgery is required to directly examine the position of the left L5 pedicle screw with respect to the adjacent nerve root. If potential impingement is observed, the screw must be removed and repositioned. Alternatively, if stable screw fixation cannot be achieved, and there is no gross spinal instability, the implants can be removed altogether and a noninstrumented in situ fusion can be performed. An epidural injection might improve pain but would not be advised so soon after surgery. Furthermore, it would not address the neurological deficit. Continued observation and narcotic medications alone would also not address the underlying issue.

During surgery, a malpositioned left L5 pedicle screw appears to be directly impinging upon the adjacent nerve root. Despite multiple attempts to reposition the screw, stable fixation cannot be achieved, and the surgeon elects to remove all implants and perform a noninstrumented in situ fusion instead. Following surgery, the patient should be advised that, relative to an instrumented fusion, a noninstrumented fusion has:

A. Equivalent long-term nonunion rates
B. Poorer short- and long-term clinical outcomes
C. Poorer short-term outcomes
D. Equivalent short- and long-term clinical outcomes

Discussion

The correct answer is (D). Noninstrumented so-called "in situ" fusions are associated with a significantly lower fusion rate compared with instrumented spinal fusions. Despite this fact, both in situ and instrumented fusions achieve comparable short- and long-term clinical outcomes, although some investigators believe that the long-term increased nonunion rate of in situ fusions results in overall marginally worse outcomes in terms of pain and disability scores. Of note, the literature suggests that pedicle screws with 2 mm or less of a cortical breech are unlikely to be associated with significant clinical problems, whereas medial or caudal breeches of 5 mm or more are considered more likely to be associated with neurological symptoms. Nevertheless, in the setting of a new neurological deficit in the immediate postoperative period, early radiologic assessment and treatment of potentially malpositioned pedicle screws are recommended.

Objectives: Did you learn...?

* Identify the signs and symptoms of a malpositioned lumbar pedicle screw?
* Select appropriate treatment for malpositioned pedicle screws associated with neurological symptoms?
* The potential outcomes associated with instrumented versus noninstrumented lumbar spinal fusions?

CASE 17

Dr. Darren Lebl

You are evaluating a 28-year-old male patient in the trauma bay who was a restrained driver in a car that was "T-boned" by another vehicle traveling approximately 35 miles per hour. His injuries include a pulmonary contusion, severe ecchymosis on his chest wall, and three rib fractures. He smells of alcohol; yet he is cooperative with your instructions. There is no midline spine tenderness and he is neurologically intact. His blood alcohol level is 0.21%. The patient is being admitted for observation of his pulmonary contusions before transfer to police custody for driving under the influence.

The trauma team is requesting a spine consult to "clear the patient's cervical spine." The next most appropriate step is:

A. Flexion–extension views
B. CT scan cervical spine
C. MRI cervical spine
D. Remove the collar and clear the spine

Discussion

The correct answer is (B). In a patient in whom you cannot rely on the clinical examination (because of intoxi-

cation or other reason for altered mental status), clinical examination by itself is not sufficient to clear the cervical spine. If the patient is not expected to be examinable within 48 hours, the most sensitive method to detect a bony cervical spine injury is the CT scan. A patient who is intoxicated should be examinable within 24 hours (provided there are no other reasons for altered mental status). Flexion–extension views have fallen out of favor for a number of reasons. First, it relies on the patient being awake, examinable, and cooperative. Second, it often misses the lower cervical spine, particularly the cervicothoracic junction, which is better seen on other imaging methods. Removing the collar and clearing the spine in this patient who is intoxicated and has other distracting injuries is not recommended. The remaining controversy is whether a negative CT scan is sufficient alone to "clear" the cervical spine. Regardless, the first-line test remains the CT scan.

Two days later, you are making rounds on the patient. He has been sober and ambulatory in the observation unit for the past 24 hours and remains in a hard cervical collar. The advanced imaging ordered does not show any evidence of fracture, dislocation, or malalignment. He does not complain of pain or tenderness upon palpation of the spinous processes and is neurologically intact. The next step in management for the cervical spine should be:

A. Maintain the collar for 6 weeks
B. Remove the collar
C. MRI cervical spine
D. Flexion–extension views under anesthesia

Discussion

The correct answer is (B). The patient is now awake and examinable. If the primary advance imaging (CT) is negative, the patient's collar may be removed if there is no pain or tenderness in the neck and the patient is neurologically intact. Keeping the collar in place for 6 weeks is not indicated. An MRI would be suggested if the patient was still not examinable at this time. Flexion–extension views would have limited utility and, in particular, should not be performed under anesthesia.

The passenger in the car was a 28-year-old female who was wearing a seat belt. She was ambulatory immediately after the accident, though she has a small abrasion on her right forearm. She denies neck pain. Her toxicology screen is negative, she's alert, oriented, cooperative, and

neurologically intact. When the paramedics arrived at the scene, they placed her on a backboard and in a field cervical collar. The backboard has since been removed, and she is sitting upright in the emergency department in the cervical collar. Plain radiographs of the right upper extremity are negative. There is no midline spine tenderness. The patient is able to rotate her head 45 degrees to each side and actively flex/extend her neck without pain. The next most appropriate step in the management of her cervical spine is:

A. Obtain five plain radiographic views of the cervical spine
B. CT scan of the cervical spine
C. MRI cervical spine
D. Remove the field collar

Discussion

The correct answer is (D). The patient fulfills all of the requirements to be clinically cleared. She is neurologically intact, awake, alert, examinable, and has no distracting injuries. She has no pain or tenderness of the cervical spine. Imaging of this patient is not necessary in order to clear her spine.

Objectives: Did you learn...?

• A systematic approach to evaluation of the patient with suspected cervical spine injury?
• The radiographic imaging required in patients suspected of having a cervical spine injury?
• The timing and role of CT and MRI in cervical trauma patients?

CASE 18

Dr. Darren Lebl

A 63-year-old man presents to your office with complaints of diminished hand dexterity. He reports difficulty using his cellular phone, buttoning buttons on his shirt, and writing over the past 6 to 9 months. His wife reports that he is increasingly more unsteady on his feet and has fallen several times. He has had low back pain for 20 years and axial neck pain for the last 5 years. Plain radiographs of the cervical spine show degenerative disks at several different levels in the subaxial spine. Physical examination demonstrates that he has 5/5 strength in his bilateral upper and lower extremities. Pertinent positives include a Hoffman's sign in the right upper extremity, hyperreflexia in the biceps and triceps reflex bilaterally, and five to six beats of clonus bilaterally. He has intact sensation to light touch throughout and normal rectal tone.

Which of the following diagnostic tests should be obtained at this time?

A. MRI
B. CT
C. EMG
D. Lumbar puncture

Discussion

The correct answer is (A). The patient has a history that is consistent with cervical spondylotic myelopathy (CSM). Plain films confirm the presence of spondylosis. His history and examination indicates spinal cord dysfunction. The next study that should be ordered is an MRI of the cervical spine. A CT would be a reasonable alternative if the patient had a contraindication for MRI. That being said, a CT myelogram would be preferred. An EMG is not likely to be positive or useful in the diagnosis of myelopathy. A lumbar puncture is also not likely to be useful in making the diagnosis as there are usually no associated hallmark changes of the cerebrospinal fluid (CSF) in a patient with myelopathy.

Advanced images of the patient's cervical spine (Fig. 1–24) are reviewed. Of the following, which surgical treatment is most appropriate?

A. Laminectomy C3–6
B. Anterior cervical discectomy and fusion C4–5, C5–6
C. C5 corpectomy, C4–7 fusion
D. Laminectomy and fusion C2–6

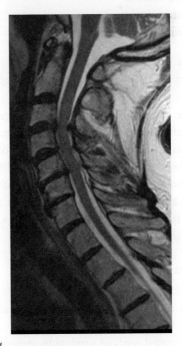

Figure 1–24

Discussion

The correct answer is (D). The sagittal T2-weighted MRI demonstrates a relatively lordotic spine with multilevel degeneration and cord compression at C3–4, C4–5, and C5–6. There is both anterior and posterior effacement of the CSF. Anterior or posterior procedures might be appropriate. Of note, a posterior procedure, such as laminectomy and fusion or laminoplasty is a reasonable option because of the preserved lordosis. In fact, it has been suggested that either procedure can be performed in a cervical spine with no more than 13 degrees of kyphosis. Effective posterior decompression relies on directly removing the posterior compressive structures (i.e., infolded ligamentum flavum, facet joints) and indirect decompression from the anterior structures (i.e., discs, vertebral body osteophytes) via the spinal cord drifting posteriorly. In this specific case, of the choices, laminectomy and fusion of C2–6 would decompress the stenotic segments. A laminectomy of C3–6 might achieve adequate decompression, but it is not recommended to perform a laminectomy alone as it may result in post-laminectomy kyphosis. An anterior cervical discetomy and fusion (ACDF) might be appropriate, but choice B does not include the most stenotic level, C3–4. Likewise, a corpectomy can be appropriate, but choice C does not include the most stenotic level.

The primary goal of this surgical procedure is to:

A. Prevent complete quadriplegia
B. Improve balance
C. Prevent progression
D. Improve neck pain

Discussion

The correct answer is (C). The primary goal of surgery for CSM is to prevent progression of the disorder. In general, the natural history of CSM is for stepwise progression, left untreated. That being said, many studies have demonstrated improvements of some of the symptoms and signs of CSM, such as balance difficulty and dexterity issues. Neck pain improvement may occur but is variable and unreliable. Quadriplegia is usually not part of the natural history of CSM, though possible with secondary injuries.

Objectives: Did you learn...?

• The clinical presentation of CSM?
• Decision-making and options for surgical treatment of CSM?
• The anticipated goals of surgical treatment of CSM?

CASE 19

Dr. Darren Lebl

A 22-year-old male construction worker falls from a roof. He has midline spine tenderness at his thoracolumbar junction and describes severe pain in his back. His examination demonstrates no lower extremity deformities, full range of motion of arms and legs, 5/5 motor strength in the upper and lower extremities, intact sensation to light touch in arms and legs, normal rectal tone, no saddle anesthesia, and a present bulbocavernosus reflex.

The next step in evaluation should be:

A. CT scan of the thoracic and lumbar spine
B. Long cassette (36″) standing plain radiographs
C. MRI of the cervical, thoracic, and lumbar spine
D. CT myelogram of the cervical, thoracic, and lumbar spine

Discussion

The correct answer is (A). As the case scenario strongly suggests an injury to the spine at the thoracolumbar junction, a CT scan of both the thoracic and lumbar regions is indicated. An MRI should not be the first imaging study obtained. Standing films should not be obtained in a trauma patient with a potentially unstable spine injury. A CT myelogram would only be obtained if an MRI was indicated but the patient had a contraindication to an MRI.

Images of the above patient are shown in Figures 1–25 and 1–26. This injury is best characterized as which of the following?

A. Compression fracture
B. Burst fracture
C. Chance fracture
D. Fracture-dislocation

Discussion

The correct answer is (B). The images demonstrate an L1 vertebral body fracture with a small degree of kyphosis. There is comminution of the vertebral body with a posterior vertebral body fragment that is slightly retropulsed into the spinal canal. This separate posterior vertebral body fragment (which is noncontiguous with the pedicles) is the hallmark of a burst fracture. Compression fractures do not have any posterior vertebral body involvement. A Chance fracture, also known as a seat belt fracture or flexion–distraction injury, will exhibit distraction of the posterior elements through bone, bone-ligament, or purely ligament structures, with an

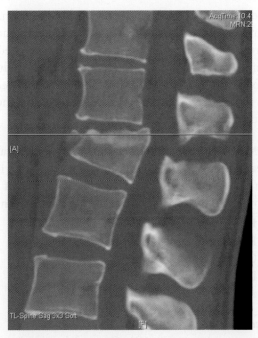

Figure 1–25

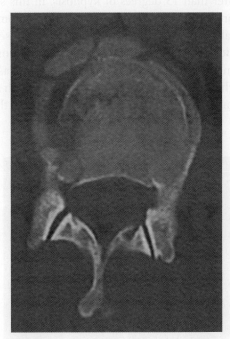

Figure 1–26

axis of rotation somewhere within the anterior vertebral body or anterior to the vertebral body. A fracture dislocation exhibits translational deformities between the injured levels. While there appears to be a translational deformity on the sagittal CT, the vertebral bodies of the uninjured levels above and below are actually well aligned.

An MRI was obtained of this patient. Your review as well as the radiologist's review clearly demonstrate that there is no posterior ligamentous disruption. The next step in management should be:

A. L1 corpectomy and instrumented fusion
B. T12 to L2 posterior instrumented fusion
C. T11 to L3 posterior instrumented fusion
D. Nonoperative management with option for an orthosis

Discussion

The correct answer is (D). Considering that the posterior ligamentous complex is not disrupted, which is generally held to be the key to fracture stability, this injury would be best characterized as a stable thoracolumbar burst fracture. Randomized controlled trials have demonstrated that operative and nonoperative treatment of this injury results in equivalent clinical results. Surgical treatment, as described in choices A, B, or C, would be options if the patient had an unstable fracture, that is, posterior ligamentous complex disruption or a neurological injury that would benefit from decompression. With equivalent clinical outcomes and the avoidance of operative complications, nonoperative treatment would be best. The patient may benefit from a thoracolumbosacral orthosis (TLSO); mostly by comfort. It is usually prudent to get a set of upright radiographs (in the brace) to confirm stability of the fracture prior to discharge.

Objectives: Did you learn…?

• To evaluate patients with suspected thoracolumbar spinal trauma?
• How to use imaging studies to confirm diagnosis of suspected thoracolumbar spinal trauma?
• How to use decision-making skills for operative versus nonoperative treatment of thoracolumbar burst fractures?

CASE 20

Dr. Peter Passias

A 57-year-old woman is being seen in your office for the first time. She has a chief complaint of a progressive decline in her ability to walk over the past few years due to weakness in her legs and a sense of unsteadiness. She has recently begun using a cane and also noticed that she has been dropping objects more frequently. She states she does not have the same strength she used to have in her hands. Occasionally, her fingers feel diffusely numb. She does have a history of occasional neck pain that is moderate. No difficulty with speech or swallowing is appreciated. She was given a prescription for physical therapy by her primary care physician but is not happy with her progress.

Based on the information presented, which of the following is the most likely diagnosis?

A. Amyotrophic lateral sclerosis
B. Cervical spondylotic myelopathy
C. Cervical radiculopathy
D. Lumbar spinal stenosis

Discussion

The correct answer is (B). CSM is the most common spinal cord disorder in older adults. Typical symptoms are neck stiffness, arm pain, numbness, and weakness in the upper and lower extremities. MRI of the cervical spine is highly recommended in patients with suspected CSM. CSM can be confused with amyotrophic lateral sclerosis (ALS); the key distinguishing factor between the two is the absence of sensory abnormalities in the extremities and the presence of fasciculations in ALS patients. Cervical radiculopathy does not result in gait instability or dexterity issues. Lumbar spinal stenosis would not affect the upper extremities.

Physical examination of the patient is significant for limited neck flexion and extension. The patient reports increased pain when looking up. Motor examination demonstrates 3/5 strength in the upper extremities bilaterally and 4/5 strength in the lower extremities, though sensation was intact. The patient demonstrates an ataxic, broad-based shuffling gait and is unable to walk on her toes or heels. When flicking the nail of her index finger, flexion is noted in her thumb and index finger. This finding is best described as:

A. Normal
B. Hoffman's sign
C. Inverted radial reflex
D. Pectoralis reflex

Discussion

The correct answer is (B). The Hoffman's sign is present in about 80% of patients with cervical myelopathy accordingly. The Hoffman's sign is commonly used in clinical practice to assess cervical spine disease. A positive Hoffman's sign reflects the presence of an upper,

motor neuron lesion from spinal cord compression. An inverted radial reflex can also be a sign of upper, motor neuron compression and dysfunction. It is elicited by tapping the brachioradialis tendon, which produces reflexive flexion in the thumb and index finger. A pectoralis reflex is elicited by tapping the tendon in the shoulder/chest region.

An MRI is obtained (Fig. 1–27). Plain radiographs reveal a relatively fixed alignment on dynamic views with no evidence of gross instability. Which of the following is the most appropriate treatment plan for this patient?

A. Physical therapy
B. Cervical laminoplasty C3–7
C. Laminectomy and fusion C3–7
D. Anterior corpectomies of C5–6

Discussion

The correct answer is (D). Cervical laminoplasty or laminectomy is not recommended in the presence of greater than 13 degrees of kyphosis. In this setting, anterior decompression is preferred. Corpectomy is a reasonable option. When performing three consecutive corpectomies (in this case only two; C5 and 6), posterior instrumentation and fusion are recommended as there is a high risk of anterior strut dislodgement with stand-alone anterior constructs. Continued physical therapy

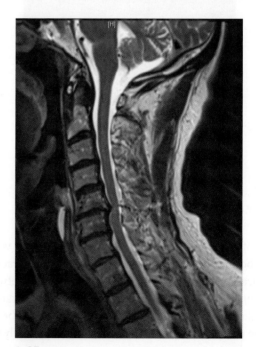

Figure 1–27

(i.e., nonoperative treatment) is not recommended as CSM has a poor natural history.

Objectives: Did you learn...?

- The differential diagnosis of a patient presenting with symptoms and signs of CSM?
- The physical examination signs of a patient with CSM?
- Management of CSM in the setting of fixed kyphosis greater than 13 degrees?

CASE 21

Dr. Peter Passias

A 15-year-old high school football linebacker is seen in your office for the first time. He has been complaining of pain in his lower back for the past 6 months. Initially it was mild and only present at the end of games. Recently it has begun occurring more frequently. He denies weakness or numbness in his legs but has experienced pain in the left posterior buttock when his pain is most intense. He has not had any treatment to date.

The symptoms experienced by this patient are most likely related to which of the following conditions?

A. Lumbar herniated disc
B. Spinal stenosis
C. Spondylolysis
D. Degenerative spondylolisthesis

Discussion

The correct answer is (C). Many athletes experience acute, low back pain with or without a specific injury to the lumbar spine during their careers. It is particularly prevalent in athletes whose sport involves repetitive hyperextension, twisting, axial loading and direct contact, such as football or gymnastics. Adolescent football players often experience lower back pain that can be related to spondylolysis (i.e., pars fracture/nonunion/stress reaction) with or without spondylolisthesis. Symptoms of spondylolysis at this age are usually exclusively low back pain; there are typically no lower extremity symptoms. Of the other choices listed, a herniated disc is possible in a younger person but would more likely present with lower extremity radicular pain. Spinal stenosis is rare at this age and again would present with more lower extremity symptoms. Degenerative spondylolisthesis would be exceedingly rare in a 15-year-old boy.

Plain radiographs are obtained, which demonstrate bilateral bony defects of the L5 pars interarticularis

without spondylolisthesis. There is preservation of the L5–S1 disk space height. Treatment at this time should be:

A. Bracing in extension along with extension exercises
B. Pars interarticularis repair utilizing a screw-rod construct
C. Posterior spinal fusion L5–S1
D. Rigid bracing in flexion

Discussion

The correct answer is (D). There is general agreement that an initial course of nonoperative treatment of at least 3 to 6 months consisting of a rigid lumbar brace (e.g., Boston flexion type brace) is prudent. Bracing in extension is usually not recommended, as are extension exercises as they aggravate the pain. If nonoperative treatment fails and the patient continues to experience chronic low back pain, direct surgical repair of the pars interarticularis or L5–S1 fusion might be indicated.

The patient above refused treatment after the consultation. He presented back to you 5 years later. Currently he is experiencing severe constant pain in his lower back radiating to his left posterior buttock and lateral thigh. He presents with an MRI that now demonstrates a grade 2 spondylolisthesis at L5–S1. Which of the following treatment should be recommended at this time?

A. Posterior L5–S1 fusion
B. Laminectomy of L5
C. Anterior and posterior L3–S1 fusion with reduction
D. Pars repair

Discussion

The correct answer is (A). With a documented progression of a slip with symptoms that have persisted for 5 years, surgical treatment is indicated. Of the choices, a posterior L5–S1 fusion is the most reasonable choice. With prone positioning, the slip might reduce and the fusion can be performed with instrumentation in this position. Choice B is incorrect because laminectomy alone can lead to worsening of the slippage. Anterior and posterior L3–S1 fusion is an aggressive procedure; it might be recommended for patients with higher grade slips. Direct repair of the pars fracture is reserved for patients with no slip and no disc degeneration.

Objectives: Did you learn...?

- The typical presentation, signs, and symptoms of a patient with spondylolysis?

- Appropriate initial management of spondylolysis without spondylolisthesis?
- The surgical options for a patient with longstanding spondylolysis and spondylolisthesis?

CASE 22

Dr. Peter Passias

A 53-year-old man with a 30-year history of smoking was admitted to the emergency department with complaints of weakness in his legs for the past week and pain in the mid-lumbar region. He does not report perianal sensory loss, bowel, or bladder incontinence. Prior to this episode he was a highly functioning administrator with no physical limitations. MRI image is shown in Figure 1–28.

The next most appropriate step in management is:

A. Surgical decompression and fusion
B. PET scan
C. Vertebroplasty
D. CT-guided biopsy

Discussion

The correct answer is (D). In patients with suspected metastatic disease, it is important to perform a thorough radiographic workup to understand the primary cancer site and to visualize the extent of the metastasis unless the patient has a rapidly progressing condition.

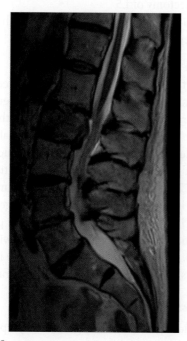

Figure 1–28

This patient began having neurological symptoms 1 week ago, and there is a concern about cauda equina syndrome. Although positron emission tomography (PET) CT allows for rapid screening and staging that would help guide the aggressiveness of surgical management of metastatic disease to the spine, it would first be advised that the patient undergo a CT-guided biopsy of the most accessible lesion (which may not be in the spine) to determine the type of cancer and tissue of origin. If the patient has a rapidly progressive neurological deficit, then surgical decompression and fusion might be appropriate, at which time tissue can be sent for pathological examination. A vertebroplasty is not indicated in the setting of a neurological deficit and spinal cord compression.

Initial workup confirms that the lesion in the spine is a metastatic renal cell carcinoma. No other metastatic lesions are identified and you are planning to offer surgery. Which of the following preoperative maneuvers would be most appropriate?

A. External beam radiation
B. Stereotactic radiation
C. Chemotherapy
D. Embolization

Discussion

The correct answer is (D). As you have already made the decision to proceed with surgery, external beam or stereotactic radiation would be best postponed until after surgery if indicated. Preoperative radiation is a risk factor for wound complication such as dehiscence and infection. In fact, renal cell carcinoma is in general radioresistant and would not be indicated. Chemotherapy should also be delayed until after surgery, if indicated. Embolization would be a reasonable consideration prior to surgery in order to find and possibly embolize a feeder vessel to the tumor. This could potentially decrease blood loss during surgery.

The most appropriate surgical treatment is:

A. Laminectomy
B. Laminectomy and fusion
C. Corpectomy
D. Kyphoplasty

Discussion

The correct answer is (C). The image demonstrates a lesion of the L2 vertebral body with involvement of the spinal canal. Of the choices, a corpectomy, either performed through an anterior or posterolateral approach, would be the most effective method of removing the tumor-involved bone and achieving decompression. A laminectomy by itself would not be recommended as it will destabilize the spine. A laminectomy and fusion would be an option, although this would not allow maximal decompression of the spinal canal via removal of the involved bone. Kyphoplasty would be contraindicated in the setting of retropulsed bone/tumor and a neurological deficit.

Objectives: Did you learn...?

- Appropriate management of cancer patients with metastasis to the bone?
- Preoperative measures prior to surgery for a metastatic lesion?
- Appropriate surgical treatment?

CASE 23

Dr. Alpesh Patel

A 40-year-old, right-hand dominant man presents to the emergency room with neck pain following a fall down a flight of stairs at work 2 hours ago. He reports that he does not remember the entire incident. Currently, he is complaining of severe neck pain, right arm weakness, and right-hand numbness; he is awake, alert, oriented, and cooperative. Physical examination demonstrates 2/5 strength of the right elbow extension while all other motor groups in the upper and lower extremities have full strength. Rectal tone is intact. Sensation is decreased in the right, long finger and dorsal forearm; it is intact in all other areas.

Which of the following imaging studies should be obtained first?

A. MRI of the entire spine
B. Flexion and extension views
C. CT scan of the cervical spine
D. CT scan of the entire spine

Discussion

The correct answer is (D). The patient's history of a traumatic event, neck pain, and upper extremity weakness is concerning for a cervical spine injury. The mechanism of injury was a fall down the stairs associated with loss of consciousness. Assuming that the patient has a cervical spine injury, there is 10% to 15% chance that he has a noncontiguous concomitant fracture elsewhere in the spine. Thus, obtaining imaging of only the cervical

spine would not be prudent. Multidetector CT scans have largely become the initial imaging modality in most trauma centers. A head-to-toe scan can be acquired in a short period of time and can be used to evaluate the cervical, thoracic, and lumbar spine as a screening tool. A CT scan of the cervical spine would be inadequate as one can miss concomitant injuries. An MRI might be useful in the setting of a neurological injury, but it would not be the initial imaging test. Furthermore, an MRI of other regions of the spine would not be indicated unless an injury was detected on CT. Flexion–extension views are generally not advisable due to their lack of sensitivity in the acute setting. The cervicothoracic junction is also quite difficult to visualize in the flexion–extension views.

CT scan images of his cervical spine are shown in Figures 1–29 to 1–31. The next step in management should be:

A. High-dose methylprednisolone
B. Upright cervical spine MRI
C. Awake, closed reduction
D. Surgical stabilization

Discussion

The correct answer is (C). The patient has a unilateral right C7 facet dislocation with a small associated fracture. The use of high-dose methylprednisolone for acute spinal cord injury, while frequently discussed, remains controversial with

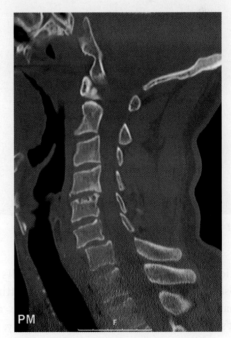

Figure 1–29

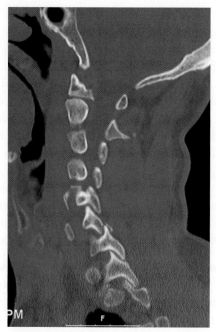

Figure 1–30

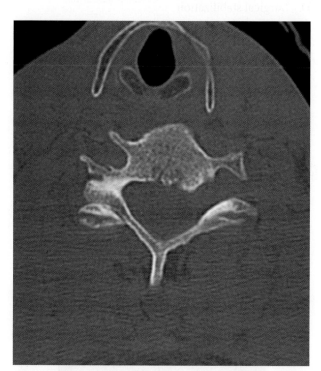

Figure 1–31

limitations in the evidence supporting its use. At most, it is a treatment option in the setting of a spinal cord injury. That being said, the above patient's examination reveals a C7 root injury, not a spinal cord injury. A reduction of the dislocation

would be a reasonable next step in this patient as he is awake, alert, and able to cooperate with an examination. An awake closed reduction has been demonstrated to be both safe and effective in treating cervical dislocations. While a successful closed reduction would not obviate the need for surgical stabilization, it can provide expeditious neurological decompression (via realignment) and enable surgery to be performed in a less urgent manner on a reduced spine. One reported risk of closed reduction is the risk of disc herniation and subsequent neurological deterioration. This has led some surgeons to obtain a prereduction MRI to determine if a disc herniation is present with the dislocation. For some, the presence of a disc herniation prompts an anterior discectomy prior to reduction. However, an upright MRI would not be advisable. The patient may eventually undergo surgical stabilization but not until the spine is reduced. Stabilization in a nonreduced position would not be ideal.

Following placement of cranial tongs, you have added 15 lb of weight. After a few minutes, the patient's examination remains unchanged and he continues to complain of neck pain and spasms. The next step in management should be:

A. Add another 10 lb of weight
B. Obtain a lateral cervical radiograph
C. Perform a manual reduction maneuver
D. Administer a muscle relaxer

Discussion

The correct answer is (B). The decision has been made to perform a closed reduction in this patient using cranial tongs. Once the tongs are in place and the initial weight applied, a lateral cervical radiograph must be obtained to ensure that there are no occult ligamentous injuries, such as an occipitoatlantal dissociation, which may be worsened by traction. Adding an additional 10 lb of weight is reasonable after an initial x-ray has been taken. A manual reduction maneuver has been described and can be effective. However, it should be reserved for select cases in which traction alone has not been effective and should not be performed with only 15 lb of weight. Despite the patient's complaint of muscle spasms, muscle relaxers, which also act as central nervous system depressants, should not be given as they can alter sensorium and affect the patient's ability to participate in an examination.

With 90 lb of weight, a lateral cervical radiograph confirms a successful reduction. The patient notes less pain in his neck and arm, and his examination is unchanged. The weight is reduced to 20 lb, the patient is placed into a cervical collar, and the reduction is maintained. An MRI is obtained and shows reasonable alignment and no disc herniations. Which of the following is the best treatment for this patient?

A. Halo-vest immobilization
B. Rigid cervical collar
C. C6–7 anterior discectomy and instrumented fusion
D. C6–7 laminectomy

Discussion

The correct answer is (C). Continued nonsurgical treatment, either through a halo-vest orthosis or rigid cervical collar, would provide insufficient support for the patient's unstable injury. This would risk redislocation, chronic pain, and/or neurological decline. Surgical stabilization is preferred. Either anterior or posterior surgery can be appropriate. An acceptable posterior procedure would be a posterior C6–7 instrumented fusion. A C6–7 laminectomy alone would lead to further destabilization of the spine. Furthermore, a laminectomy is not needed as the reduction has effected decompression via realignment. An acceptable anterior procedure would be an anterior discectomy and fusion with instrumentation for stabilization. This procedure is facilitated by the fact that the patient's injury has already been reduced.

Objectives: Did you learn…?

- The radiographic imaging indicated in the setting of suspected cervical spine trauma?
- The indications for and application of closed cervical reduction for a facet dislocation?
- The options for definitive treatment of cervical facet dislocations?

CASE 24

Dr. Alpesh Patel

A 23-year-old man presents to your emergency room with severe back pain after a 30-foot fall out of a tree while intoxicated 3 hours earlier. He reports no neck pain, no upper extremity weakness or numbness, though he states that he feels weak in his legs and numbness in his groin. Currently, he is awake, alert, oriented, and cooperative and does not appear to be intoxicated. Vital signs included a blood pressure of 100/60 and heart rate of 95 beats per minute. Physical examination demonstrates midline tenderness of the lumbar spine with no palpable gap or step-off. Upper extremities show full strength and sensation. Lower extremities examination shows 2/5 bilateral strength in hip flexion and knee extension, 3/5 bilateral strength of ankle dorsiflexion, big toe extension, and ankle plantar flexion. Rectal tone is normal. Sensation to light touch and pin prick is diffusely decreased in both lower extremities and in the perineum. Bulbocavernosus reflex is present. A CT scan of his cervical and thoracic spine is negative. CT images of his lumbar spine are shown in Figures 1–32 and 1–33.

The injury of L2 is best described as which of the following?

A. Compression fracture
B. Burst fracture
C. Flexion–distraction injury
D. Fracture-dislocation

Discussion

The correct answer is (B). The CT images reveal a comminuted fracture of the L2 vertebral body with involvement of its posterior aspect. The distinguishing feature between a burst fracture and a compression fracture is involvement of the posterior aspect of the vertebral body. Furthermore, burst fractures demonstrate that the posterior body fragments are no longer in continuity with

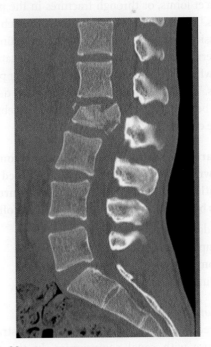

Figure 1–32

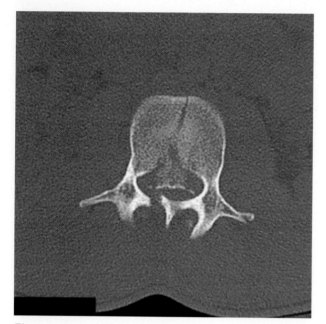

Figure 1–33

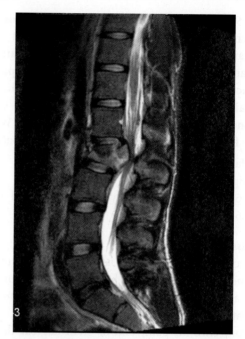

Figure 1–34

the posterior elements (i.e., pedicles). Thus, they are free fragments that often are retropulsed into the spinal canal. Lamina fractures are often concomitant at the level of a burst fracture. By themselves, they do not infer injury to the posterior ligamentous complex. They can, however, be associated with dural tears and nerve root entrapment. Flexion–distraction injuries, also known as Chance or seat belt injuries, demonstrate widening of the posterior elements, either between the spinous processes, gapping at the facet joints, or through fractures in the posterior elements. There can be varying degrees of vertebral body compression, though typically not with comminution of the posterior vertebral margin. Fracture-dislocations can present with various fractures of the anterior or posterior elements. The hallmark feature is a translation deformity that can be noted by misalignment of the vertebral bodies in the coronal and/or sagittal planes.

A lumbar spine MRI is obtained, images from which are shown in Figures 1–34 and 1–35. Based on the information presented, the type of neurological injury is best characterized as which of the following?

A. Cauda equina injury
B. Complete spinal cord injury
C. Incomplete spinal cord injury
D. Conus medullaris injury

Discussion

The correct answer is (A). The MRI demonstrates the L2 fracture with canal compromise. In this patient,

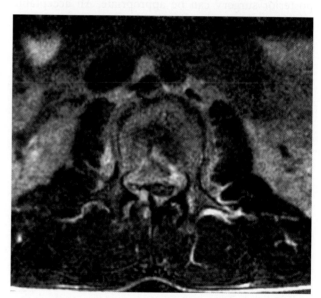

Figure 1–35

the conus medullaris of the spinal cord terminates at the T12–L1 level. The fracture is at the L2 level. Thus, the neurological injury is at the level of the cauda equina, distal to the conus medullaris and spinal cord. The patient's neurological examination is consistent with this type of injury with the presence of lower extremity weakness, intact rectal tone, and perineal numbness, though this can vary.

The trauma team has determined that the patient has no other injuries besides the L2 fracture. The

next best step in management for this patient should be:

A. High-dose methylprednisolone
B. Lumbosacral orthosis
C. Immobilization on a rotating bed
D. Surgical treatment

Discussion

The correct answer is (D). This patient has an L2 burst fracture with a profound neurological deficit in the presence of canal compromise. These injury features warrant surgical management for decompression of the neural elements, realignment of the spine, and stabilization. As the patient is not medically compromised and has no other injuries, there would be little reason to think that he would not be a surgical candidate. An orthosis should be reserved for patients with stable burst fractures without neurological deficit. Prolonged immobilization in a rotating bed (e.g., Rotorest bed) would be reserved only for those patients who are medically unfit for surgery. The use of high-dose methylprednisolone, previously considered standard of care, is currently only a treatment option for spinal cord level injuries. Regardless, the patient has a cauda equina level injury, which was excluded in the original NASCIS study protocols.

Objectives: Did you learn...?

• To characterize the radiographic imaging findings of thoracolumbar spine trauma?
• To accurately describe the type and level of neurological injury with a lumbar burst fracture?
• The treatment for thoracolumbar burst fractures with neurological injury?

CASE 25

Dr. Adam Pearson

A 60-year-old man presents with neck and right arm pain radiating to his posteromedial arm, medial forearm, and ulnar aspect of the hand. He notes numbness in the ulnar aspect of the forearm and hand, though he notes no dexterity issues or gait imbalance. He gets some relief from right shoulder abduction. The symptoms developed insidiously about 2 months ago and are not associated with any constitutional symptoms. Physical examination reveals weakness of his hand intrinsic muscles, numbness of the ulnar aspect of the forearm and hand, normal upper and lower extremity reflexes, a positive Spurling's sign on the right, and a negative Hoffman's sign.

What is the most likely diagnosis?

A. Ulnar neuropathy
B. C5–6 foraminal stenosis
C. C7–T1 disk herniation
D. Cervical myelopathy

Discussion

The correct answer is (C). The patient presents with upper extremity symptoms that can be recreated with a Spurling's maneuver (lateral flexion/side bending and axial rotation towards the side of the pathology) and classic signs and symptoms of C8 radiculopathy (ulnar forearm and hand numbness, hand intrinsic weakness, normal reflexes). The C8 dermatome includes the ulnar forearm and hand, and the C8 nerve innervates the intrinsic hand musculature. The C8 nerve exits from the C7–T1 foramen and can be compressed by a C7–T1 disk herniation. Ulnar neuropathy can cause similar symptoms but would not be associated with a positive Spurling's sign or neck pain. C5–6 foraminal stenosis would affect the C6 nerve root and its associated innervated structures (elbow flexion, radial aspect of the forearm and hand). Cervical myelopathy is possible and can have a variable presentation which can include numbness and weakness. However, this patient does not have any complaints of dexterity or gait dysfunction nor does he have any long tract signs (i.e., no Hoffman's sign).

Which of the following is the most appropriate diagnostic test to obtain at this time?

A. Plain radiographs with flexion–extension views
B. Magnetic resonance imaging (MRI) scan
C. Computed tomography (CT) myelogram
D. Nerve Conduction Studies/Electromyography (EMG)

Discussion

The correct answer is (B). The neural structures in the cervical spine are best imaged by MRI. MRI is the diagnostic modality of choice to detect cervical disc herniations. In patients with contraindications to an MRI, a CT myelogram is a reasonable alternative, but owing to its invasiveness, should not be considered a first choice for all patients. Plain radiographs with or without flexion-extension views are useful for preoperative planning but are not helpful for diagnosis of a herniated disk. If there is a question about the diagnosis, nerve conduction studies and EMG can be helpful to rule out peripheral nerve entrapment, peripheral neuropathy, or to narrow down a symptomatic level in the setting of multilevel compression on imaging. It is not necessary to have electrodiagnostic to make the diagnosis of cervical radiculopathy.

Imaging of the above demonstrated a large paracentral disk herniation compressing the right side of the spinal cord and the exiting nerve root. You had enrolled the patient in a physical therapy program Despite this and treatment with anti-inflammatory medications, he continues to have substantial symptoms and is interested in surgical treatment. Which of the following is the most appropriate surgical technique?

A. Posterior C7–T1 foraminotomy
B. Posterior C7–T1 laminectomy and fusion
C. C7–T1 anterior cervical discectomy and fusion (ACDF) with anterior plate
D. C7–T1 anterior cervical discectomy and fusion (ACDF) with anterior plate and manubriotomy in order to access the cervicothoracic junction

Discussion

The correct answer is (C). Given that the disc is large and compressing the spinal cord, an anterior approach is favored. This would most commonly involve an anterior cervical discectomy and fusion. Plate stabilization would be preferred in order to increase fusion rates as well as to afford greater construct stability at the cervicothoracic junction. A posterior foraminotomy can be effective for soft disc material that is in the foramen but does not allow for safe removal of disc located more centrally and anterior to the spinal cord. A posterior laminectomy and fusion at C7–T1 would not necessarily address the disc herniation and anterior compression; this procedure is best reserved for cases of central stenosis or severe foraminal stenosis. Manubriotomy is almost never needed to access C7–T1, though it can be necessary to reach levels caudal to T1 from an anterior approach. Anterior approaches to the cervicothoracic junction and upper thoracic spine can put structures such as the recurrent laryngeal nerve, thoracic duct, and great vessels at risk. The recurrent laryngeal nerve originates in the carotid sheath as a branch of the vagus nerve and then returns to the larynx in the groove between the trachea and esophagus after looping inferior to the right subclavian artery or the aorta on the left. It theoretically has a more predictable course on the left side, prompting some surgeons to favor left-sided approaches, though no study has ever demonstrated an increased

risk of recurrent laryngeal nerve problems with right-sided approaches. The thoracic duct carries lymph and ascends through the thorax to empty into the left subclavian vein and is thus theoretically at risk with left-sided approaches, especially below T1.

Objectives: Did you learn…?
- Recognize the signs and symptoms of C8 radiculopathy?
- Understand the options for imaging workup of cervical disc herniations?
- Determine the optimal surgical approach for a C7–T1 disc herniation?

CASE 26

Dr. Adam Pearson

A 75-year-old woman presents with 1 month of low back pain radiating to her bilateral buttocks and posterolateral thighs with some diffuse pain and numbness below her knees. This pain comes on with standing and walking and resolves with sitting down and low back flexion. She notes it is easier to walk uphill than downhill and finds leaning on a shopping cart helpful. She has no significant medical comorbidities. Neurological examination is normal with no numbness or weakness, though she has mildly decreased yet symmetric, lower extremity, deep tendon reflexes. She has palpable distal pulses in the lower extremities and has had no treatment for this condition.

What is the most likely diagnosis for this patient?

A. Peripheral neuropathy
B. Lumbar spinal stenosis
C. Vascular claudication
D. Trochanteric bursitis

Discussion

The correct answer is (B). Neurogenic claudication from lumbar spinal stenosis classically presents with back pain radiating to the buttocks and lower extremities in a nonradicular pattern and is brought on with standing and extension. Sitting and flexion tend to relieve the pain as the spinal canal has a greater volume in this position. The physical examination is frequently normal. Peripheral neuropathy should be in the differential diagnosis; however, it is more commonly associated with constant symptoms that are not necessarily aggravated by activity. Vascular claudication can be exacerbated by activity but usually presents with decreased lower extremity pulses. In addition, walking uphill would not necessarily be less troublesome than walking downhill, nor would leaning on a shopping cart be helpful. Trochanteric bursitis can become more symptomatic with activity, but again would not be relieved with leaning on a shopping cart or lumbar flexion.

Which of the following diagnostic tests would best help confirm the patient's diagnosis?

A. Plain radiographs
B. MRI
C. CT
D. EMG

Discussion

The correct answer is (B). MRI scan best demonstrates neural compression from spinal stenosis. CT is an option but is best when acquired with intrathecal contrast (i.e., CT myelogram). However, this test requires an invasive step and should be considered as a second choice in patients with contraindications to MRI. Plain radiographs can help better to define bony anatomy and identify potential instability during the surgical planning phase but are not critical for diagnosis. EMG can be helpful to rule out peripheral neuropathy but are not typically helpful in the diagnosis of spinal stenosis. In fact, they are often negative in such cases.

Imaging shows moderate to severe central and lateral recess stenosis at L4–5. There is no spondylolisthesis or scoliosis evident on upright radiographs. What is the most appropriate treatment at this point in time?

A. Physical therapy
B. Epidural steroid injections
C. Laminectomy
D. Laminectomy and fusion

Discussion

The correct answer is (A). With just 1 month of symptoms and no prior treatment, nonoperative, noninvasive treatment is indicated. While there is no strong evidence supporting physical therapy's ability to change the natural history of symptomatic spinal stenosis and neurogenic claudication, it is still maintained as a reasonable first step for treatment. Injections may be considered if physical therapy is not helping. Surgery can be considered if symptoms persist despite an appropriate course of nonoperative treatment. In the absence of spondylolisthesis or scoliosis, laminectomy without fusion is the most appropriate surgical intervention.

Objectives: Did you learn...?

• Recognize the signs and symptoms of neurogenic claudication from spinal stenosis?
• Order the appropriate imaging?
• Determine the most appropriate treatment?

CASE 27

Dr. Adam Pearson

A 65-year-old man with cervical spondylotic myelopathy (CSM) underwent a C3–7 laminetomy and fusion. On postoperative day 1, he reported that his preoperative symptoms were substantially improved. On postoperative day 2, he developed shortness of breath and was subsequently diagnosed with a pulmonary embolism. For this, intravenous heparin was started. Ten hours following the start of heparin, he reported increased neck pain as well as increased numbness in his arms and legs. Examination demonstrated marked upper and lower extremity weakness. An MRI is obtained and shown in Figure 1–36.

The most likely diagnosis for this patient is:

A. Infection
B. Epidural hematoma
C. Spinal fluid leak
D. Spinal cord infarct

Discussion

The correct answer is (B). The patient is at risk for epidural hematoma due to anticoagulation in the acute postoperative period. He presents with classic findings of pain and progressive neurological deficit. The MRI

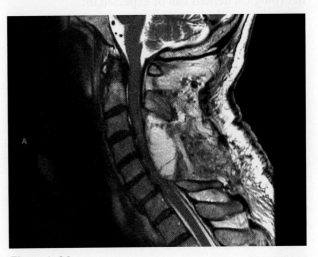

Figure 1–36

shows a T2 hyperintense fluid collection in the laminectomy site causing cord compression. While spinal fluid, seroma, and blood all have similar appearance on MRI, the former two are under low pressure and would not likely cause this degree of cord compression. An infection would be highly unlikely on postoperative day 2. A spinal cord infarct is possible but would not be associated with the start of anticoagulation.

Treatment at this point should be:

A. Percutaneous drainage
B. Anticoagulation reversal and observation
C. Blood patch
D. Urgent surgical evacuation

Discussion

The correct answer is (D). Among the strongest predictors of neurological recovery following a symptomatic epidural hematoma is time to surgery after development of neurological deficit. Data suggests greater chance of recovery in patients undergoing surgical decompression within 12 hours compared to after 12 hours. When a patient presents with a neurological deficit and an epidural hematoma, this is a surgical emergency. Percutaneous drainage would not be appropriate as it would likely be inadequate in removing the hematoma. A blood patch involves injecting more blood into the spinal canal and might be an effective treatment for a CSF leak. While the anticoagulation may be reversed, observation without surgery and evacuation of the hematoma would not be appropriate.

The above patient returns to the operating room 4 hours from symptom onset. Long-term, his neurological deficits can be expected to:

A. Recover
B. Not worsen
C. Worsen
D. First recover, then worsen

Discussion

The correct answer is (A). Data has indicated complete or partial functional recovery in the vast majority of patients who were emergently returned to the operating room for evacuation of an epidural hematoma. The strongest predictors of complete neurological recovery are the severity of initial deficit and time to surgical decompression. Patients would rarely worsen following surgery. If surgery is delayed, they would be less likely to improve.

Objectives: Did you learn...?

- Recognize the signs and symptoms of epidural hematoma?
- Select the appropriate treatment and timing of treatment?
- Understand the predictors and prognosis of neurological recovery following an epidural hematoma?

CASE 28

Dr. Andrew Schoenfeld

The trauma team at your hospital asks you to consult on the case of a 78-year-old male who was brought to the hospital following a fall at his house. During the fall, the patient's son reports that his father's head struck the refrigerator, and that he then became unresponsive. CT scan of the patient's head demonstrated a subdural hematoma. The patient is obtunded and cannot be meaningfully examined. He is in a cervical collar placed by the paramedics at the time of transport. Plain films were obtained in the ER, but no other radiographic studies were performed. The plain film lateral demonstrates a diffusely osteopenic cervical spine, loss of the normal lordotic posture, and disc space ossification via marginal osteophytes along the vertebral bodies. The film was interpreted as negative for fracture by the attending radiologist.

The next best step in management for this patient is:

A. Remove the cervical collar
B. Leave the cervical collar until the patient is conscious
C. Obtain a cervical spine CT
D. Apply cranial tongs and cervical traction

Discussion

The correct answer is (C). The patient has ankylosing spondylitis. In this population, fractures may be difficult to detect using only plain films. The patient is also obtunded and should be presumed to have a cervical injury until proven otherwise. The rigid, immobile spine that occurs as a result of ankylosing spondylitis is prone to unstable, three-column fracture even with low energy mechanisms, such as a fall from standing. A CT scan is the imaging modality of choice to detect cervical spine fractures in patients with hyperostotic disease as well as any individual suspected of cervical spine trauma.

Further imaging demonstrates an extension-type fracture involving the ankylosed disc space at C5–6.

The trauma team wishes to admit the patient to the intensive care unit to monitor his subdural hematoma. While in the ICU, which of the recommendations is most appropriate?

A. The patient should be placed in a halo-thoracic vest and maintained with the head of bed at a 45-degree angle.
B. The patient should be placed on log-roll precautions with his cervical spine immobilized close to the preinjury position.
C. The patient should be placed on log-roll precautions with his cervical spine immobilized in a flexed position with 70 lb of traction via cranial tongs.
D. The patient should be placed on log-roll precautions with 50 lb of longitudinal traction.

Discussion

The correct answer is (B). Patients with a fractured ankylosed spine should be immobilized in the best approximation of their preinjury cervical posture. This can be achieved with low-weight cervical traction with or without a well-fitting cervical collar supported by pillows or blankets. Log-roll precautions should also be employed. Substantial traction weight should be avoided in patients with ankylosing spondylitis fractures as it can cause undue distraction through the injury site. Longitudinal traction would effectively create an extension moment on the previously kyphotic spine and would not be advised.

Definitive treatment of this previously active and independent man should be:

A. Immobilization in a halo-thoracic vest for a period of 3 months
B. Anterior plate fixation across the fracture site at C5–6
C. Posterior instrumented fusion at C5–6
D. Long posterior instrumented fusion

Discussion

The correct answer is (D). The rigid, ankylosed spine behaves biomechanically like a long-bone rather than a series of vertebral segments as in the normal cervical spine. This necessitates an approach similar to the treatment of extremity fractures. Short constructs may be exquisitely prone to failure. Of the choices, a long posterior instrumented fusion offers the most stability and chance for healing. Halo-thoracic immobilization is associated with poor outcomes and high mortality rates in the elderly population.

Following surgery, the patient's family inquires about the long-term impact of this fracture on his physical function and survival. They should be advised that his mortality risk is:

A. No different than for a non-ankylosed patient
B. Lower than a non-ankylosed patient
C. Equivalent to a similarly aged patient with an osteoporotic fracture
D. Higher than a non-ankylosed patient

Discussion

The correct answer is (D). A number of investigations have found that post-treatment mortality rates are high for patients with ankylosing spondylitis and a spinal fracture. A recent analysis, comparing patients with ankylosing spondylitis and cervical spine fracture to age- and sex-matched controls, confirmed that this risk persisted for up to 2 years after the fracture event. In that study, the mortality rate for individuals with cervical fracture in the setting of ankylosing spondylitis was 37.5% and 62.5% at 3 months and 2 years post-fracture, respectively, as compared to 7% and 20.9% in control group.

Objectives: Did you learn...?

- Indications for the initial radiographic imaging and diagnostic evaluation for patients with ankylosing spondylitis and a suspected fracture?
- The appropriate approach to positioning and monitoring for patients with ankylosing spondylitis and a known fracture?
- The appropriate approach to surgical intervention for patients with ankylosing spondylitis and a known fracture?
- The influence of ankylosing spondylitis on long-term survival in patients treated for spinal fractures?

CASE 29

Dr. Andrew Schoenfeld

A 29-year-old athletic male presents to you office with a 4-week history of back pain and right lower extremity radiating pain that extends to the lateral aspect of his foot. His symptoms were precipitated by a cross-training workout. He was referred to your office after MRI obtained by his primary care manager revealed a 1.0 cm L5–S1 paracentral disc herniation impinging the right S1 nerve root in the lateral recess. He denies saddle anesthesia and reports no episodes of bowel or bladder incontinence. He has only received naprosyn from his family physician for pain control and no other treatment has been prescribed. The patient has little reproducible back pain via palpation. Sensory and motor functions are intact via manual testing, but the patient has difficulty performing a single-stance leg raise on the right. Deep tendon reflexes are 1+/4+ at S1 on the right as compared to 2+/4+ elsewhere. The patient demonstrates a positive straight leg raise and a positive Lasegue sign on the right.

The next best step in management for this patient is:

A. Schedule the patient for a L5–S1 discectomy.
B. Have the patient return to his primary care manager and return to your clinic only if symptoms progress.
C. Refer the patient to physical therapy.
D. Schedule the patient for a transforaminal lumbar interbody fusion at L5–S1.

Discussion

The correct answer is (C). The patient has an acute disc herniation with associated radiculopathy. There are no indications for urgent surgical decompression. Most instances of acute radiculopathy from disc herniation in young patients will resolve within 6 weeks of onset. Only following 6 weeks of persistent symptomatology should consideration be given for epidural injections or more invasive treatment options.

The patient returns to your clinic after 4 weeks of intense physical therapy. His symptoms have remained constant and no progression has occurred. His examination remains unchanged from that obtained at initial presentation. He is an avid runner and weight lifter and would like to return to physical activity as soon as possible. He is concerned that delaying surgical intervention will result in permanent "nerve damage."

Based on the available literature, your opinion is that:

A. Duration of radicular symptoms has no impact on long-term functional outcomes.
B. Symptom duration may impair postsurgical recovery but has no long-term impact on function.
C. Symptom duration may adversely impact recovery but only if symptoms have been present for periods upwards of 2 years.
D. Symptom duration may adversely impact recovery but only if symptoms have been present for periods upwards of 6 months.

Discussion

The correct answer is (D). A number of studies support the contention that symptom duration can adversely impact postsurgical recovery, principally in the areas of chronic

pain and physical function. Most large works support the fact that outcomes are not compromised as long as surgery is performed within 6 to 12 months of symptom onset. Surgery performed for patients whose symptoms have been present for periods of 12 months or greater have been found to have inferior results as compared to those who received surgical intervention at an earlier time-point.

You decide to offer the patient a right-sided L5–S1 discectomy, using an operative microscope. The patient wishes to know how successful the surgery is likely to be in terms of relieving his predominant symptom, which is radicular leg pain.

You tell him that:

A. The surgery is likely to be successful given the fact that he is young, male, healthy, and has a herniation greater than 6.0 mm in size.
B. The surgery is likely to be successful given the fact that he is active, male, and has no motor deficits by manual testing.
C. The surgery is likely to be unsuccessful given the fact that he is physically active and male.
D. The surgery is likely to be unsuccessful given the fact that he has a herniation less than 1.5 cm in size.

Discussion

The correct answer is (A). Previous work has identified female gender, multiple medical comorbidities, and unemployment as predictors of inferior outcome following lumbar discectomy. The size of the disc herniation has also been found to play an important role in influencing outcome. Disc herniations of a size 6.0 mm or greater were found to have superior outcomes as compared to those with fragments sized 5.9 mm or less.

The patient also asks about his back pain, which is not his major concern but still troublesome. He desires to know whether the surgery you propose is likely to "cure" his back pain symptoms.

Based on the available literature, you tell him that:

A. The surgery is solely intended for his leg related symptoms. The surgery will not impact his back pain at all.
B. While primarily intended to relieve his leg related symptoms, the surgery may also improve his back pain to a certain extent although it is unlikely to be complete.
C. While primarily intended to relieve his leg related symptoms, the surgery may also completely relieve his back pain.

D. The surgery is intended to treat his back pain. Whether his leg-related symptoms improve depends on the size of the disc fragment and whether there has been vascular insult to the S1 nerve root.

Discussion

The correct answer is (B). Lumbar discectomy is primarily designed to relieve radicular pain symptoms. Nonetheless, a number of studies, including the Maine Lumbar Spine Study's 10-year follow-up results, have found that many patients experience substantial relief of their preoperative, low back pain symptoms following surgery. However, the relief of back pain following such an intervention is rarely complete, and residual back pain is often experienced.

As you are scheduling the case, your colleague suggests that you try to perform the procedure "Minimally Invasively," using a tubular retractor system.

When compared to microsurgical procedures, tubular discectomy has been found to:

A. Have superior results in terms of functional outcomes
B. Have inferior results in terms of chronic back pain but superior outcomes for leg-related symptoms
C. Have no difference in outcomes
D. Higher blood loss and longer operative times but superior results for relief of radicular symptoms

Discussion

The correct answer is (C). Most comparative studies have found no difference in outcomes between tubular discectomy and microsurgical lumbar discectomy. A randomized prospective trial comparing the two types of interventions found that patients had similar functional and clinical outcomes. Patients treated with tubular discectomy in this study were found to have greater leg and back pain as well as lower rates of satisfaction and higher rates of repeat surgery, although none of these findings were statistically significant.

Objectives: Did you learn...?

- Indications for the initial management of patients who present with acute radicular findings in the setting of a lumbar disc herniation?
- The influence of symptom duration on functional outcome following surgical intervention?
- Factors predictive of successful surgical outcome after lumbar discectomy?

- The impact of lumbar discectomy on leg and back pain–related symptoms in the setting of a disc herniation?
- The difference between the use of minimally invasive techniques and microsurgical decompression in terms of functional outcomes following surgery?

CASE 30

Dr. Andrew Schoenfeld

You are asked to evaluate a 48-year-old obese woman who presented to the emergency department 48 hours ago with severe low back pain, fevers, and chills of several days duration. CT and MRI demonstrated discitis involving the L4–5 disc space and adjacent osteomyelitis of the L4 and L5 vertebral bodies. No epidural abscess was appreciated on imaging. Standing radiographs demonstrate relatively normal alignment in the affected area. She denies saddle anesthesia and has had no episodes of bowel or bladder incontinence. Her body mass index is 43 and she is diabetic, but she has no other medical conditions; she was found to be HIV-negative at the time of admission. Physical examination demonstrates reproducible back pain with palpation diffusely throughout the lumbar region, but her sensory and motor functions are normal. No upper motor neuron findings are present. Blood cultures obtained before starting vancomycin are growing methicillin-sensitive *S. aureus*.

The next best step in management is:

A. Request a CT-guided biopsy
B. Surgical debridement and instrumented fusion
C. Infectious disease consultation for antibiotic management
D. Lumbar corset

Discussion

The correct answer is (C). The patient has a spondylodiscitis with no evidence of neurologic deficit, epidural abscess, or gross deformity. Blood cultures may identify the responsible organism for infection in as many as 85% of cases of discitis/osteomyelitis. In the current case, the cultures indicate a methicillin-sensitive organism, thus vancomycin would not be necessary. Infectious disease consultation is important in order to optimize the choice of antibiotic. If there is any suggestion that the cultures are unreliable or were not growing an organism, then a CT-directed biopsy should be obtained. While immobilization in the form of a rigid orthosis might be effective in decreasing pain, a lumbar corset would not. Surgical debridement and instrumented fusion are not indicated at this time unless the patient develops a deformity, fails a course of antibiotic treatment, develops a neurological deficit, or has intractable pain that is unresponsive to other measures.

The patient is eventually discharged from the hospital on parenteral antibiotics. She returns to your office for follow-up 6 weeks after discharge. Her back pain has diminished but has not completely resolved. She remains neurologically intact without any subjective complaints or objective deficits noted on examination. Plain film imaging, obtained in your office, shows no evidence of vertebral body collapse or instability. Laboratory tests, ordered by infectious disease doctor, show that her white blood cell count, ESR, and C-reactive protein are now within normal limits. Treatment at this time should be:

A. Surgical intervention
B. Stop antibiotics
C. Follow-up as needed
D. Continue antibiotics for another 6 weeks

Discussion

The correct answer is (D). Her laboratory values are indicative of a favorable response to the current antibiotic regimen. Vertebral osteomyelitis typically requires a total of 12 weeks of antibiotic treatment. At the 6-week mark, infectious disease doctors often recommend conversion to oral antibiotics (if available). However, antibiotics should not be stopped altogether. The patient will probably avoid surgery with this type of positive response but should continue to be followed until there is radiographic evidence of autofusion of the disc space.

Six weeks later, the patient returns to the emergency department with a marked increase in her back pain. She remains neurologically intact. An MRI shows increasing bone destruction of the L4 and L5 vertebral bodies. Plain films demonstrate 20 degrees of segmental kyphosis in this area, though there is no evidence of epidural abscess. The next most appropriate step in treatment should be:

A. 12 more weeks of antibiotics
B. Debridement and circumferential fusion
C. CT-guided biopsy and blood cultures
D. L4 and L5 laminectomy

Discussion

The correct answer is (B). The patient has evidence of spinal instability which is an indication for surgical intervention. In light of the evidence of increasing bone destruction and kyphosis, the most appropriate

approach is to thoroughly debride the infected vertebral bone and then reconstruct the spine using an interbody strut followed by posterior instrumentation and fusion. Another 12 weeks of antibiotics is not likely to eradicate the infection or treat the underlying instability. A CT-guided biopsy and blood cultures would be indicated if surgery was not planned. A laminectomy would be contraindicated as it will result in greater instability.

Objectives: Did you learn...?

- Indications for the initial management and diagnostic evaluation of patients with vertebral osteomyelitis in the absence of epidural abscess?
- The appropriate duration of intravenous antibiotic therapy and indications for surgical intervention?
- The approach to surgical management in the setting of failed response to an appropriate course of antibiotic therapy?

CASE 31

Islam Elboghdady; Dr. Anton Jorgensen; Dr. Kern Signh

A 44-year-old construction worker presents to the office with reports of neck pain and sharp arm pain that radiates to the left middle finger. Symptoms began 2 weeks prior. Physical examination demonstrates 5/5 motor strength in both upper extremities except for 4/5 strength in the left triceps. There also is noted a positive Spurling's sign to the left, reproducing the patients arm pain that radiates into his long finger. The patient obtains an MRI, shown in Figure 1–36 and Figure 1–37.

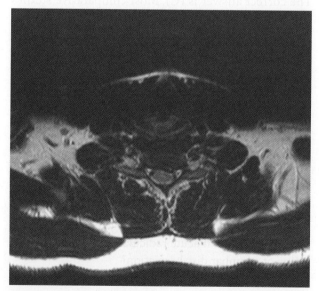

Figure 1–37 Axial MRI demonstrating a left paracentral herniated nucleus pulposus at C6–7. (Courtesy of Dr. Kern Singh)

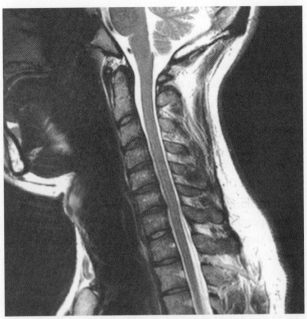

Figure 1–38 Sagittal MRI demonstrating a posterior intervertebral disc fragment at the C6–7 level. (Courtesy of Dr. Kern Singh)

What is the most likely etiology to explain this patient's symptoms?

A. Burst fracture of the C6 vertebrae causing spinal stenosis and nerve root impingement

B. C6–7 herniated nucleus pulposus with neuroforaminal compromise

C. Ossification of the posterior longitudinal ligament

D. Cervical spinal stenosis causing myelopathy and spinal cord compression

Discussion

The correct answer is (B). This patient most likely has a foraminal herniated intervertebral disc at the C6–7 level causing compression of the exiting C7 nerve root. Disc degeneration is associated with the loss of proteoglycans, water, and cellularity. The outer and inner layers of the annulus fibrosus become incompetent. This structural alteration lessens the threshold of pressure required for the nucleus pulposus to herniate through the annulus fibrosus. Labor intense activities or high impact sports may result in transiently high increases in disc pressure, increasing the likelihood for a potential disc herniation. Cervical radiculopathy is a clinical diagnosis made based on history and physical examination. The MRI images are included in Figure 1–37 and Figure 1–38.

What is the best next step in management for this patient?

A. Anterior cervical discectomy and fusion

B. Posterior cervical foraminotomy and discectomy

C. Transforaminal epidural steroid injections

D. Pharmacologic management (NSAIDs)

Discussion

The correct answer is (D). The majority of disc herniations will resolve spontaneously. The herniated nucleus pulpous (HNP) will be resorbed, as demonstrated on long-term radiographic assessment of patients who underwent nonoperative treatment. The first step involves pharmacologic treatment with non-steroidal anti-inflammatory drugs (NSAIDs). Similarly, corticosteroids may also be utilized to minimize the symptoms being experienced by the patient. It should be noted that corticosteroids have not been demonstrated to provide long-term pain relief. There are no randomized controlled trials to support the routine utilization of muscle relaxants for the initial management of HNP. Opiates may be utilized for initial pain control but the dosing should be short-term, as long-term narcotic utilization is not indicated.

Physical therapy should also be encouraged in addition to pharmacologic management. Although PT has not been demonstrated to improve outcomes associated with cervical HNP, it may provide symptomatic relief.

If pharmacologic management and physical therapy are ineffective, epidural steroid injections (ESI) may be attempted. Some evidence suggests that corticosteroid ESIs carry greater efficacy than anesthetic or saline injections and may limit surgical intervention. Similarly, selective nerve root blocks (SNRB) can be utilized for diagnostic purposes or therapeutic relief. Improvement following SNRB localizes the source of pain to the irritated nerve root. Unlike ESIs, SNRBs function by local steroid deposition near the nerve root as it exits the foramen without infiltration into the spinal canal.

Following 3 months of nonoperative management, the patient reports worsening left arm weakness. Physical examination demonstrates numbness over the left third digit and 3/5 muscle strength with elbow extension in the left arm. The patient has exhausted NSAIDs, physical therapy, and epidural steroid injections.

What is the next best step in management?

A. Selective nerve root block

B. Anterior cervical discectomy and fusion

C. Continued nonoperative management

D. Laminectomy

Discussion

The correct answer is (B). The majority of disc herniations resolve spontaneously with time, and therefore, nonoperative management should be encouraged even after 3 months. However, this patient demonstrates worsening motor strength. As such, this patient will likely benefit from an anterior cervical discectomy and fusion (ACDF) to limit the progression of symptoms. ACDF will serve to maintain the segmental cervical lordosis and restore disk height to decompress the C7 nerve root. The limitations of ACDF include diminished motion at the fused spinal segment and potential risk of adjacent segment degeneration and instability. One alternative to ACDF includes cervical disc arthroplasty (CDA), which is proven to be noninferior to ACDF for the management of degenerative disk disease. An additional option is a posterior cervical foraminotomy and discectomy. A foraminotomy is not indicated for central disc herniations but can be an effective, motion-sparing procedure for patients with foraminal compromise secondary to osteophytes and/or disc herniation.

Which of the following complications are specific to anterior cervical spine surgery?

1. Dysphagia
2. Dysphonia
3. Cervical soft tissue swelling
4. Recurrent laryngeal nerve injury
5. Horner's syndrome
6. Infection
7. Excessive blood loss
8. Incidental durotomy

    A. 1, 2, 3, 4, 5
    B. 1, 3, 5, 7, 8
    C. 3, 5, 6, 8, 8
    D. 5, 6, 7, 8
    E. 2, 4, 5, 7, 8

Discussion

The correct answer is (A). Dysphagia is a unique complication that is specific to anterior cervical spine surgery. Retraction of the recurrent laryngeal nerve and the esophagus can contribute to impaired swallowing. Dysphagia typically improves and resolves within days following the anterior cervical procedure. Dysphonia is the result of injury or compression of the recurrent laryngeal nerve, which is essential for vocal cord function. Prevertebral soft tissue swelling typically peaks on the second and third days postoperatively and dissipates by 6 weeks. Horner's syndrome is a very rare complication of ACDF that results from injury to the cervical sympathetic trunk (CST). The CST lies superficial to the longus coli, excessive retraction may result in injury presenting as a triad of ptosis, miosis, and anhydrosis. Infection and blood loss are complications inherent to any surgical procedure. Vertebral artery injury and incidental durotomies are more likely with a posterior cervical spine procedure than an anterior cervical approach.

Objectives: Did you learn...?

- Initial management of a cervical HNP; importance of nonoperative management?
- Next steps after failure of nonoperative management?
- The complications specific to an ACDF?

CASE 32

Dr. Alejandro Marquez-Lara; Dr. Eric Sundberg; Dr. Kern Singh

A 62-year-old, overweight (BMI = 28.9 kg/m^2) female with no significant medical or surgical history presents complaining of progressive lower back pain for the past 3 months. Her symptoms worsen with prolonged walking/standing and improve with sitting. The neurovascular examination is unremarkable and no motor deficit is appreciated. Imaging studies are obtained (Figs. 1–39 to 1–42).

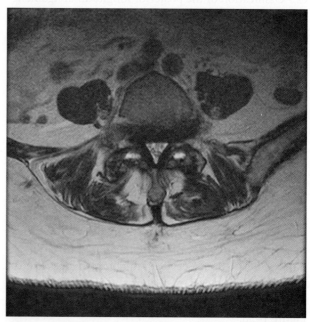

Figure 1–39 Axial T2-weighted MRI demonstrating central spinal stenosis at the L4–5 disc level. (Courtesy of Dr. Kern Singh)

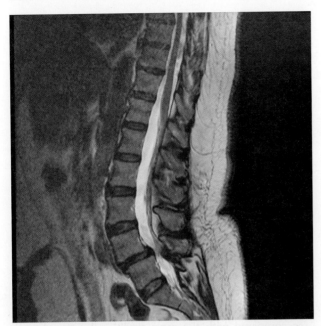

Figure 1–40 Sagittal T2-weighted MRI demonstrating L4–5 spondylolisthesis with canal narrowing. (Courtesy of Dr. Kern Singh)

What is the next step in management?

A. Counsel the patient to lose weight and return in 3 months
B. Nonsteroidal anti-inflammatory medication, physical therapy, and weight loss
C. Epidural steroid injection
D. Lumbar total disc replacement

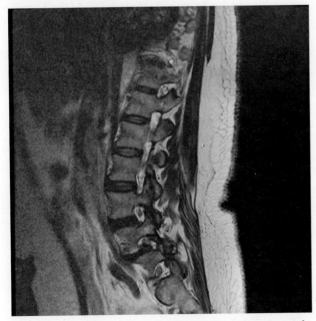

Figure 1–41 Sagittal T1-weighted MRI demonstrating right foraminal narrowing. (Courtesy of Dr. Kern Singh)

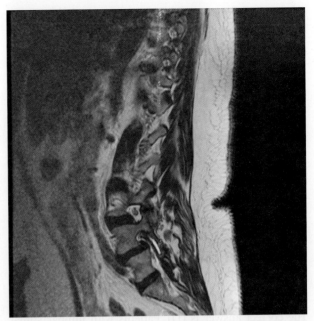

Figure 1–42 Sagittal T1-weighted MRI demonstrating left foraminal narrowing.

Discussion

The correct answer is (B). This patient demonstrates symptoms of back pain associated with an L4–5 spondylolisthesis and spinal stenosis. Most patients (76%) with degenerative spondylolisthesis and spinal stenosis without radicular symptoms respond well to nonoperative management. Directionally specific physical therapy, namely flexion-based Williams' exercises, may have some benefit in patients with positional specific symptomatology.

After 6 months, the patient has minimal relief of symptoms. She continues to complain of back pain aggravated by standing and walking and improving with flexion and sitting. In addition, she mentions intermittent lower extremity pain, numbness, and tingling that radiates to the dorsum of her foot. Her walking and standing tolerance have also diminished.

What is the next step in management?

A. Microscopic lumbar discectomy
B. Continue nonoperative management for another 6 months
C. Epidural steroid injection (ESI)
D. None of the above

Discussion

The correct answer is (D). The patient continues to have back pain and now complains of neurogenic claudication. In this case, recent evidence from the Spine Patient

Outcomes Research Trial (SPORT) suggests that non-operative management in a symptomatic patient with spondylolisthesis and spinal stenosis will benefit greater from surgical intervention than nonoperative management (ESIs).

On physical examination, sensation to light touch over the dorsal foot and lateral aspect of the leg is diminished and you notice weakness with great toe extension on the right side compared to the left.

What surgical option is best for this patient at this time?

A. Limited decompression (e.g., laminoforaminotomy)
B. Laminectomy
C. Decompression and fusion without instrumentation
D. Decompression and fusion with instrumentation

Discussion

The correct answer is (D). Patients with lumbar spinal stenosis from spondylolisthesis who have failed conservative management for 3 to 6 months are associated with better outcomes with surgical decompression and fusion than continued nonoperative management. The surgical technique should aim to decompress the neural structures and stabilize the affected segment. Instrumented fixation is associated with higher fusion rates than noninstrumented techniques. Flexion–extension radiographs may be obtained to help determine the severity of instability. In those patients with nonmobile spondylolisthesis and collapsed disc spaces, it is reasonable to offer the patient a laminectomy with preservation of the midline structures. In these cases, the risk of progression of the spondylolisthesis may be low, and a surgical fusion may be obviated.

What are the potential benefits of an interbody fusion?

A. Better restoration of disc and foraminal height
B. Higher fusion rates than posterolateral fusions
C. Better short- and long-term clinical outcomes
D. Both A and B
E. A, B, and C

Discussion

The correct answer is (D). Interbody fusion procedures including anterior, transforaminal, and posterior interbody fusions improve disc and foraminal height. In addition, some studies have reported higher fusion rates with interbody implants due to the higher surface area for bone graft incorporation. Currently, there is no evidence that demonstrates better outcomes with interbody techniques compared to traditional posterolateral fusions in patients with degenerative spondylolisthesis.

There is an increased risk of injury to neural elements from the retraction required for disc excision and placement of the interbody device. The additional costs, potentially greater operative times, and blood loss should also be taken into consideration.

Objectives: Did you learn...?

- Nonoperative treatment with directionally specific physical therapy is an acceptable, initial treatment option in the setting of spondylolisthesis with spinal stenosis?
- Decompression and instrumented fusion is the most accepted surgical technique to treat spondylolisthesis with spinal stenosis after exhausting nonoperative management?
- The addition of an interbody fusion device can help restore the disc height and promote a stable fusion. However, further research is warranted to characterize the short- and long-term outcomes with this technique as compared with the more traditional posterolateral fusion?

CASE 33

Sreeharsha V. Nandyala; Dr. Hamid Hassanzadeh; Dr. Kern Singh

A 55-year-old patient with a history of smoking and congestive heart failure sustained a traumatic spondylolisthesis at L4–5 following a motor vehicle accident. Due to the degree of instability, an anterior and posterior spinal fusion was performed from L3–5. The procedural time was prolonged due to extensive instability. At the 3-week follow-up, the patient reports severe back pain, fever, and drainage from the surgical wound-site. The ESR was 100 mm/h with a white blood cell count of 15,000/mm^3. Plain film radiographs demonstrated a stable construct and no evidence of segmental deformity.

Which of the following are published risk factors for the patient's current state?

1. History of smoking
2. Congestive heart failure
3. Male gender
4. Multilevel fusion
5. Longer duration of surgery

A. 1 and 2
B. 1, 2, 3
C. 1, 4, 5
D. 1, 3, 4, 5
E. 1, 2, 3, 5
F. 1, 2, 3, 4, 5

Discussion

The correct answer is (C). The elevated ESR and WBC at 3 weeks with concomitant fever and wound drainage are suspicious signs for postoperative wound infection. The ESR typically peaks at 1 week following surgical intervention. Postoperative infections can be attributed to multiple patient- and surgical-related risk factors. In this scenario, the surgical risk factors include a multilevel fusion secondary to greater tissue dissection, operative time, and instrumentation. In addition, this patient carries a history of smoking, which is a published risk factor for postoperative complications including infection, pseudarthrosis, and poor wound healing. Conversely, male gender and a history of congestive heart failure are not published risk factors for postoperative spinal infection.

Which of the following imaging modalities should be obtained?

A. Contrasted CT
B. Noncontrasted MRI
C. Contrasted MRI
D. Bone scintigraphy
E. Ultrasound

Discussion

The correct answer is (C). MRI with gadolinium enhancement is the best radiographic modality to detect surgical site infections (SSIs). If spinal instrumentation is present, MRI should be utilized with metal artifact reduction sequences. Vertebral and soft tissue changes on imaging must be differentiated between two different states: normal postoperative changes and vertebral osteomyelitis. Both states are associated with type 1 end plate changes that are characterized by adjacent marrow edema and hypointense signal on T1 imaging. Vertebral osteomyelitis may also be associated with high signal intensity in the disc space. In addition, gadolinium contrast serves to demonstrate areas of enhancement in the disc space. Vertebral osteomyelitis is associated with circumferential disc enhancement whereas linear areas of enhancement are more resemblant of normal postoperative changes.

CT can be utilized to assess for implant failure and bony remodeling/destruction. Bone scintigraphy will not differentiate between the normal postoperative state versus infection, as both states are associated with increased metabolism and uptake. Gadolinium contrast is essential to visualize the pattern of disc enhancement.

Imaging studies indicated a subfascial infection at L4–5 with bony destruction and fluid collection. Which of the following should be the next course of action?

A. IV antibiotics
B. Bedside incision and drainage
C. Surgical debridement and irrigation with retention of instrumentation
D. Surgical debridement and irrigation with removal of instrumentation
E. CT-guided aspiration and drainage

Discussion

The correct answer is (C). The type of postoperative spinal infection dictates the next appropriate course of action. Superficial SSIs often respond to a course of IV antibiotics and/or surgical drainage. Conversely, medical therapy alone is likely unsuccessful with subfascial infections due to poor tissue vascularity and penetration of antibiotics. Deep SSIs typically warrant extensive debridement of infected and necrotic tissue with removal of extraneous bone or graft pieces. The surgeon should aim to retain instrumentation in an effort to maintain the stability of the spinal column. If implants are loose, they can be removed and replaced; however, the patient must be monitored closely for potential pseudarthrosis or spinal instability. In this patient's case, the infection developed at 3 weeks and is considered an early postoperative infection. In cases of a late deep SSI (6 months to 1 year), the surgeon may elect to remove instrumentation to adequately clear the infection, as bony arthrodesis is likely forthcoming if not already achieved. The surgeon must be cognizant that in cases of deep infection, serial surgical debridements are likely necessary to effectively clear the infection. In addition, there is some evidence promoting the utilization of antibiotic impregnated beads or grafts following surgical debridement in order to address the issue of poor IV antibiotic penetrance to the infection site.

What is the best course for antibiotic therapy in this patient?

A. No antibiotic therapy is warranted following surgical debridement
B. Course of oral antibiotic therapy
C. Course of intravenous antibiotic therapy
D. Course of IV antibiotic therapy followed by course of oral antibiotics
E. Lifetime oral antibiotics

Discussion

The correct answer is (D). Initially patients with postoperative spinal infections should be placed on broad spectrum antibiotics following surgical debridement until a culture and sensitivity profile of the organism(s) is obtained. The most common pathogen is *S. aureus*. Typically, a 6-week course of intravenous antibiotic therapy is recommended followed by a course of oral antibiotics. Infectious disease specialists should be consulted to determine the type, dosage, and duration of antibiosis appropriate for each patient. For patients with methicillin-resistant *S. aureus* infections, new guidelines recommend 6 weeks of intravenous antibiotic therapy followed by oral antibiotics until fusion is achieved. Some physicians advocate removal of the hardware once the arthrodesis has been obtained in order to eradicate any potential for infectious recurrence.

Objectives: Did you learn…?

- The risk factors for postoperative spinal infection include smoking, multilevel fusion procedures, and prolonged duration of surgery among other factors?
- Contrasted MRI is paramount for the diagnosis of a postoperative spinal infection?
- The management of a postoperative spinal infection is dependent upon the extent of infection?
- Antibiotics carry an integral role for the management of postoperative spine infections. Infectious disease specialists should be consulted to aid in selection and length of therapy?

CASE 34

Dr. Michael J. Vives; Dr. Saad B. Chaudhary

A 20-year-old man presents to the trauma bay after striking his head while diving into a shallow pool. He was not able to get out of the pool himself and was extricated by others. Upon presentation, he is alert and oriented. Physical examination of his upper extremities demonstrates 5/5 strength in shoulder abduction and elbow flexion, 4/5 in the wrist extension, and 1/5 strength of elbow extension, wrist flexion, and finger abduction/flexion. Lower extremity strength is 1/5 in all groups. Sensation is intact along the lateral shoulder, arm, and forearm, but decreased along the middle finger and medial forearm and arm. Lower extremity sensation is globally decreased. Figure 1–43A–C are axial and sagittal CT images of his cervical spine. Figure 1–43D is a sagittal MRI of his cervical spine.

The patient's cervical spine injury is best described as which of the following?

A. Hangman's fracture
B. Lateral mass fracture
C. Flexion teardrop fracture
D. Facet dislocation

Discussion

The correct answer is (C). The imaging studies demonstrate a flexion teardrop injury. The important injury characteristics include a triangular fracture fragment along the anteroinferior aspect of the vertebral body that is thought to be produced by shear forces via a flexion–compression moment. The paramedian CT images demonstrate gapping in the facet joints which indicates that the facet capsule has been disrupted. Flexion teardrop injuries should be distinguished from anterior avulsion fractures, often called extension teardrop fractures, which also can involve the anteroinferior corner of the vertebral body. However, the fracture is produced by failure in tension and is more commonly seen in elderly patients who sustain an extension injury mechanism. A Hangman's fracture refers to an injury specifically of the pars interarticularis of C2. A Chance fracture, also known as a flexion–distraction or seat belt injury, occurs in the thoracolumbar region and exhibits evidence of both posterior and anterior structure failing under tension. Though the facet joints do appear to be gapped on the CT images, they are not dislocated, thus the injury should not be described as a facet dislocation.

This injury most likely occurs via which of the following mechanisms?

A. Hyperextension
B. Flexion–compression
C. Flexion–distraction
D. Forced rotational

Discussion

The correct answer is (B). This injury pattern is most commonly produced by a compressive force imparted on a flexed spine. Compression–flexion injuries, as described by Allen and Ferguson, can present in varying stages ranging from simple blunting of the anterior vertebral body (best described as a compression fracture) to unstable injures with teardrop fragments and a characteristic sagittal split, pronounced kyphosis, and facet gapping as exhibited in the above injury. Hyperextension injuries may show widening anterior with associated fracture of the posterior elements but would not be likely to present with kyphotic deformity. Flexion–distraction injuries in the cervical spine, the prototype of which is bilateral facet

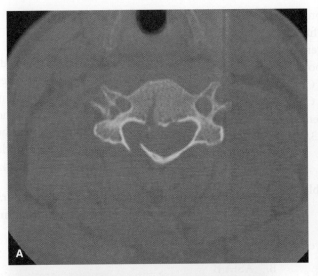

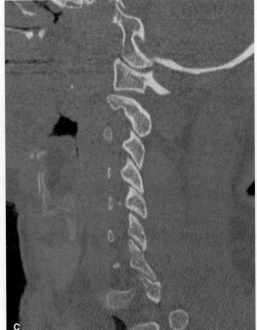

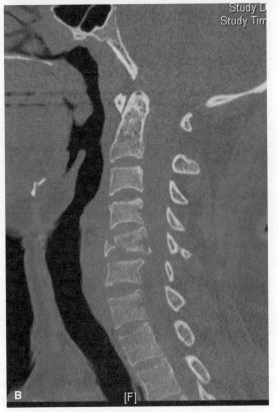

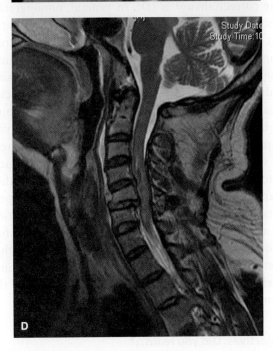

Figure 1–43 **A–D**

dislocations, show substantial widening posteriorly with subluxation, dislocation, or fracture dislocation of one or both facet joints. Rotational injuries most commonly present with unilateral pedicle or articular process fractures with varying degrees of translational deformity.

Based on the patient's examination findings, his motor level would best be described as:

A. C5

B. C6

C. C7

D. T1

Discussion

The correct answer is (B). Utilizing international standards, the motor level is defined as the lowest (most caudal) level with key muscle strength of at least grade 3/5, provided that muscle function cranial to this segment is full (5/5). This patient's elbow flexion is 5/5 and wrist extension is 4/5, both of which represent C6 function. Elbow extension and wrist flexion are 1/5, which represent C7 function. Finger flexion and abduction represent C8 and T1 function, both of which are 1/5 in this patient. Thus, this patient's most caudal segment with at least 3/5 strength is C6.

Provided that the patient is medically stable, definitive treatment should be:

A. Immobilization in a hard cervical collar
B. 6 weeks of cervical traction followed by halo-vest application
C. Laminectomy of C3 through C7
D. C5 corpectomy and instrumented fusion

Discussion

The correct answer is (D). In general, nonoperative treatment of a patient with a neurological deficit is not ideal. With the surgical goals being decompression of the spinal canal, realignment, and stabilization, anterior corpectomy and instrumented fusion addresses all three. Closed treatment with a hard cervical collar would not adequately stabilize the spine or be able to maintain alignment. While halo-vest immobilization has been described for the treatment of this injury type with comparable neurological outcomes as anterior corpectomy and fusion, radiographic outcomes are inferior, that is, kyphosis persists. Notwithstanding, 6 weeks of cervical traction would not be advisable in a patient who is fit to safely undergo surgery. A laminectomy would cause further destabilization of the spine in this case and would likely not results in substantial decompression of the spinal cord.

Objectives: Did you learn...?

- The imaging findings suggestive of a cervical flexion teardrop fracture, including the nuances that distinguish it from other more stable injuries?
- The typical injury mechanism associated with teardrop injuries and spectrum of injury patterns produced by this mechanism?
- How to determine the motor level of a spinal cord injury based on evaluation of key muscle function?
- Appropriate treatment considerations for this injury pattern?

CASE 35

Dr. Michael J. Vives; Dr. Saad B. Chaudhary

A 43-year-old man was struck by a car while walking along the road. Neurologic examination demonstrates 5/5 strength in all muscle groups in his upper extremities but 0/5 strength throughout the lower extremities. Though sensation throughout the lower extremities is absent, he has diminished yet present perianal sensation to light touch and pinprick. His imaging studies are shown in Figure 1–44A–C.

The patient's neurologic injury can be best described by which of the following American Spinal Injury Association (ASIA) impairment scale grades?

A. ASIA A
B. ASIA B
C. ASIA C
D. ASIA D

Discussion

The correct answer is (B). The ASIA impairment scale helps to characterize the severity of a spinal cord injury. It relies on determining the degree of motor and sensory function below the level of injury. ASIA A refers to a patient with no motor or sensory function below the injury level. ASIA B denotes that some sensory function is preserved below the level of injury. ASIA C denotes that there is some motor function below the injury level, but that it is less than 3/5. ASIA D indicates that motor function below the injury level is at least 3/5. ASIA E is normal motor and sensory function below the level of injury. In the above case, there is some, albeit diminished, sensation in the perianal region. This indicates an ASIA B grade. While this is certainly not useful function at this time, it is an important prognosticator of neurological recovery as the patient demonstrates some function of the spinal cord below the level injury.

In the trauma bay, the patient's blood pressure suddenly drops to 80/50 mm Hg while his pulse increases to 120 bpm. A 1-L fluid bolus of lactated Ringers is infused which normalizes his blood pressure and pulse. This clinical phenomenon is best characterized as which of the following?

A. Hypovolemic shock
B. Spinal shock
C. Neurogenic shock
D. Autonomic dysreflexia

Discussion

The correct answer is (A). The patient's hypotension was combined with tachycardia that responded well

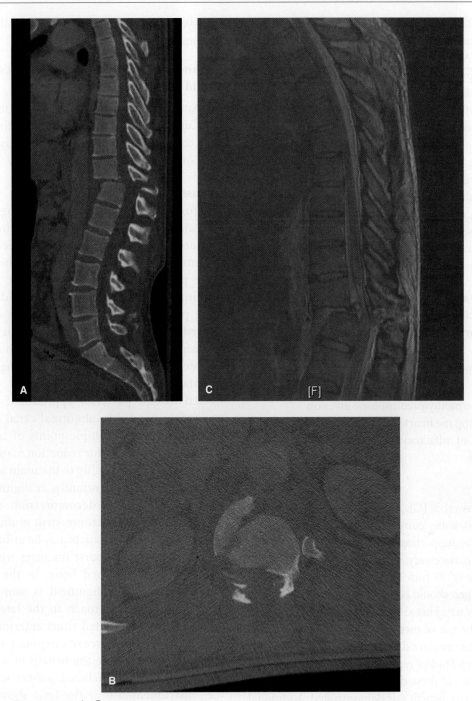

Figure 1–44 **A–C**

to judicious fluid administration. This suggests that he was experiencing hypovolemic shock. Neurogenic shock, often following a spinal cord injury, typically manifests with hypotension combined with bradycardia. Neurogenic shock is more frequently associated with cervical level spinal cord injury, and fluid resus-

citation should be administered carefully as to avoid volume overload. After achieving euvolemia, vasopressors should be used to support blood pressure in lieu of delivering more fluid. Neurogenic shock occurs as a result of the lack of sympathetic tone in the peripheral vasculature. Spinal shock refers to a transient syndrome of flaccid areflexic paralysis and anesthesia after spinal cord injury which hinders accurate determination of ASIA grade and prognosis. It does not affect blood pressure or heart rate. The resolution of spinal shock is heralded by the return of the bulbocavernosus reflex. Importantly, conus level injury can result in persistent loss of the bulbocavernosus reflex in the absence of spinal shock. Autonomic dysreflexia is a syndrome involving massive imbalance of sympathetic discharge in response to pain below the level of neurologic injury. It often manifests as severe headache, flushing, and extreme elevation of blood pressure with compensatory bradycardia and can be life-threatening. The most common triggering source is severe bladder distension.

During early management and resuscitation of this patient, which of the following is currently recommended in order to maximize neurological recovery?

A. Systemic hypothermia using an intravenous cooling system
B. High-dose methylprednisolone infusion
C. Maintaining mean arterial pressure of 85 mm Hg
D. Injection of olfactory ensheathing cells into the injury site

Discussion

The correct answer is (C). Although there are no level I studies on this issue, current consensus among spinal surgeons is that supporting spinal cord perfusion using vasopressors, if necessary, to maintain a mean arterial blood pressure of 85 mm Hg is ideal. In addition, supplemental oxygen should be used as necessary to ensure that adequately oxygenated blood is perfusing the injured spinal cord. The use of methylprednisolone had become widespread after the second and third National Acute Spinal Cord Injury Studies reported a positive effect. Subsequent analyses of these data, however, have suggested that no conclusive benefit was demonstrated. Additional concerns over risks of infection, bleeding, and pulmonary complications as well as an effect on fusion have resulted in high-dose steroids being considered a treatment option rather than a recommendation at this time. In fact, many major trauma centers in the United States and Canada no longer routinely use high-dose steroids for spinal cord injured patients. Systemic hypothermia is currently an experimental therapy under study in the acute setting. Injection of olfactory ensheathing cells is also an experimental intervention that might be used in a delayed setting but not immediately following a spinal cord injury.

Definitive management of this patient's spinal injury should be:

A. Anterior corpectomy, strut graft, and instrumentation
B. Custom-molded thoracolumbar orthosis
C. Laminectomy and short-segment fusion
D. Long-segment instrumented fusion

Discussion

The correct answer is (D). The imaging studies demonstrate a thoracic fracture-dislocation. Using the Thoracolumbar Injury Classification Scale this would be considered a translational injury which is assigned three points for injury morphology. The patient's incomplete spinal cord injury would be assigned three points in the neurologic status category. The injured posterior ligamentous complex would also be assigned three points. Injuries with overall scores greater than four are generally managed surgically. Translational or rotational injuries are typically treated from a posterior approach if the vertebral translation has led to abnormal canal alignment, as seen in this case. Multiple points of transpedicular fixation can be useful for reduction maneuvers and to provide sufficient stability to maintain alignment and promote fusion. Importantly, realignment in such cases usually effects decompression of the spinal canal. Anterior corpectomy, strut graft, and anterior instrumentation constructs may be utilized in the setting of comminuted burst fractures with neurologic injury from retropulsed bone. In the translational injury presented, realignment is more challenging from an anterior approach in the lateral decubitus position, and an isolated short anterior construct is not ideal with the degree of circumferential ligamentous disruption. While the benefit of a laminectomy in such a case can be debated, a short-segment fusion (i.e., instrumented only the level above and below) does not offer sufficient strength to reduce and stabilize the injury. Nonoperative treatment in a custom-molded brace would not be advised.

Objectives: Did you learn...?

• Essential distinguishing features of complete versus incomplete spinal cord injuries?
• Definitions and characteristics of hemodynamic shock, neurogenic shock, and spinal shock, which are commonly confused entities?

- Current recommendations for early supportive management of spinal cord-injured patients?
- A strategy for evaluating the essential features of thoracolumbar injuries to determine relative stability and the benefit of surgery?

CASE 36

Dr. Lee Yu-Po

A 57-year-old woman with a 20-year history of rheumatoid arthritis presents with progressively severe neck pain, clunking, and suboccipital headaches. Pain slightly improves with use of a soft collar. No loss of fine motor dexterity, balance, or bowel/bladder function is noted. Her flexion–extension lateral radiographs are shown in Figure 1–45A and B.

The patient's imaging studies demonstrate which of the following conditions?

A. Atlantoaxial instability
B. Subaxial subluxation
C. Basilar invagination
D. Diffuse idiopathic skeletal hyperostosis

Discussion

The correct answer is (A). Atlantoaxial instability is the most common pattern of affliction in the rheumatoid spine. Rheumatoid synovitis at the C1–2 joints and around the stabilizing transverse, apical, and alar

ligaments leads to atlantoaxial instability. In the figures provided, there is a substantial gap in the atlantodens interval noted with the neck in flexion as compared to extension, in which the subluxation reduces. Subaxial subluxation results from rheumatoid induced laxity and inflammatory involvement of the subaxial facet and uncovertebral joints. This commonly manifests as a step ladder–type sagittal deformity, often at C3–4 and C4–5. Considering that the films provided do not demonstrate this area of the spine, one cannot make this diagnosis. Basilar invagination occurs from rheumatoid-induced bony and cartilaginous destruction of the occipitoatlantal and atlantoaxial joints, occipital condyles, and C1 lateral masses. Vertical translation of the odontoid can result in brainstem compression or excessive kyphosis of the cervicomedullary junction. Significant neurologic compromise or sudden death can occur. Based on the lateral views of the spine, the tip of the odontoid process does not appear to protrude into the foramen magnum. Diffuse idiopathic skeletal hyperosto (DISH) is an ossifying diathesis of the spine that is unrelated to rheumatoid arthritis. It manifests as large flowing osteophytes bridging three or more relatively well-preserved disc spaces of the cervical spine. This patient's radiographs do not demonstrate evidence of DISH.

Which of the following measurements most strongly indicates that surgical management is warranted

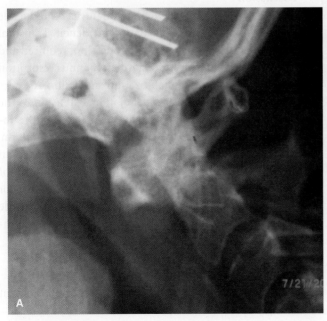

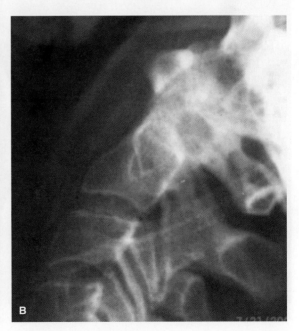

Figure 1–45 **A–B**

in a patient with C1-2 instability from rheumatoid arthritis? (AADI, anterior atlantodens interval; PADI, posterior atlantodens interval)

A. AADI of 4 mm
B. AADI of 6 mm
C. PADI of 18 mm
D. PADI of 12 mm

Discussion

The correct answer is (D). The anterior atlantodens interval (AADI) is measured on a lateral view from the anterior odontoid to the posterior surface of the anterior ring of C1. Normal AADI in adults is less than 3 mm. The posterior atlantodental interval (PADI) is measured from the posterior odontoid to the anterior surface of the posterior ring of C1. The normal PADI is greater than 14 mm. The PADI has been found to be a better predictor for the development of paralysis than the AADI. Patients with PADI less than 14 mm have increased risk of neurologic deficit and should therefore be recommended for surgery, even if asymptomatic. Patients undergoing surgery who have a PADI less than 10 mm are less likely to experience postoperative recovery of neurologic deficit.

Figure 1–45C shows a sagittal MRI of the cervical spine of the patient. The white line that is drawn

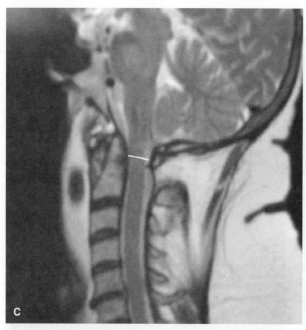

Figure 1–45 **C**

measures 12 mm. This line demonstrates which of the following parameters?

A. Posterior atlanto dens interval
B. Space available for the cord
C. MacGregor's line
D. Powers ratio

Discussion

The correct answer is (B). The line is demonstrating the actual space available for the cord (SAC) which can only be accurately measured by MRI since some patients may have significant pannus extending posterior to the odontoid (aka dens) that will not be visible by radiographs. A true SAC less than 13 mm is generally considered an indication for surgery. The posterior atlantodental interval (PADI) is measured on a lateral plain x-ray. MacGregor's line is drawn from the hard palate to the base of the occiput. Basilar invagination (BI) is defined as migration of the superior odontoid more than 4.5 mm above this line. Power's ratio is used to evaluate for possible traumatic occipitocervical dissociation.

Which of the following is the best surgical option for the described patient?

A. Transoral dens resection and C1–2 fusion
B. Occipitocervical fusion
C. C1–2 fusion with screw stabilization
D. C1–2 Gallie fusion

Discussion

The correct answer is (C). The patient has a reducible C1–2 subluxation without neurologic deficit. Transoral removal of the odontoid and pannus is not required and has significant morbidity. Regardless, pannus resorption is frequently seen after stabilization and fusion. As there is no evidence of basilar invagination, extension to the occiput is not required. Posterior C1–2 fusion with sublaminar wires, such as the Gallie technique, is an option, but usually requires postoperative halo immobilization and has fallen out of favor recently. More rigid forms of internal fixation, such as transarticular C1–2 screws or C1 lateral mass screws with C2 pedicle screws, provide more rigid fixation and higher fusion rates when combined with bone grafting.

Objectives: Did you learn...?

• The different patterns of cervical spine involvement in patients with rheumatoid arthritis?

- The difference between the AADI and PADI and associated treatment recommendations?
- The concept of the SAC, the impact of periodontoid pannus, and the role of MRI?
- The surgical treatment considerations for patients with AAI?

CASE 37

Dr. Lee Yu-Po

You are called to the trauma bay to evaluate a 47-year-old male who was a restrained driver in a high speed motor vehicle accident. Vital signs: BP 120/80, HR 100, SaO₂ 95%. On your initial evaluation, his Glasgow coma scale score is 15 and he is cooperative with the examination. He has ecchymosis in his chest. He complains of chest, back, and abdominal pain. He has normal sensation with 5/5 motor strength but the iliopsoas is 3/5 on the left side. AP and lateral radiographs are shown Figure 1–46A–B.

What is your next course of action?

A. Place patient in a TLSO brace.
B. Mobilize the patient with physical therapy.

C. Start trauma dose steroids.
D. Send patient for spiral CT of the thoracolumbar spine.

Discussion

The correct answer is (D). The patient was involved in a high-speed accident with significant force. A compression fracture is noted at L1. Better visualization is needed to determine the stability of this injury. CT is becoming the study of choice in these cases because the high sensitivity and specificity of CT in detecting thoracolumbar injuries.

CT of the thoracolumbar spine shows a burst fracture at L1 with 20% height loss and 30% canal compromise (Fig. 1–47). There is also widening of the interspinous space between T12 and L1. He has not lost any additional motor strength.

What is your next course of action?

A. Order MRI lumbar spine.
B. Place patient in a TLSO brace.
C. Start trauma dose steroids.
D. Strengthen his left leg with physical therapy.

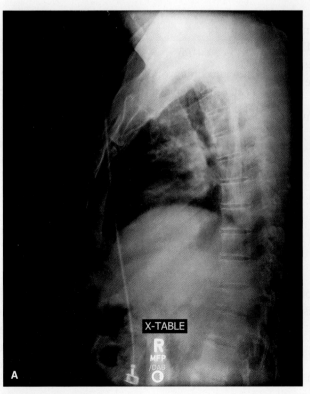
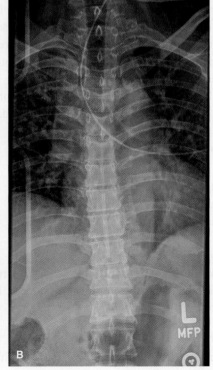

Figure 1–46 **A–B**

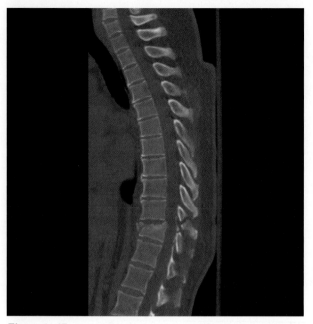

Figure 1–47

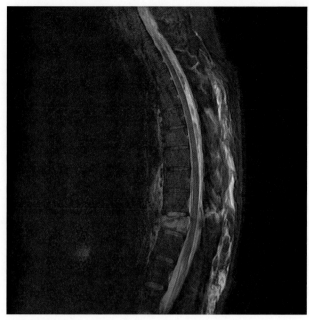

Figure 1–48

Discussion

The correct answer is (A). In this case, better visualization is necessary because the patient has a neurologic injury. Even though his neurologic injury has not progressed, better visualization with MRI is recommended to determine how much compression exists and also to evaluate for any other potential lesions such as a disc herniation.

An MRI is obtained and there is a 50% canal compromise seen (Fig. 1–48). No other injuries are noted.

What is your next course of action?

A. Place patient is a TLSO brace.
B. Start trauma dose steroids.
C. Strengthen his left leg with physical therapy.
D. Discuss surgery with the patient.

Discussion

The correct answer is (D). In the setting of neurologic compromise with canal compression, surgery is the most appropriate answer.

Objectives: Did you learn…?

• The correct order of ordering CT versus MRI in flexion/distraction injuries?

• When it is appropriate to consider closed versus open treatment in flexion/distraction injuries?

CASE 38

Dr. Lee Yu-Po

In your clinic, you see your first patient of the day. He is an otherwise healthy 34-year-old male. He complains of pain that begins in his mid-back and clearly radiates across his back into his abdomen. Examination shows normal sensation and 5/5 motor strength. His knee and ankle jerk reflex is 2+.

What is your next course of action?

A. Place patient in a lumbar corset.
B. Initiate physical therapy for lumbar strengthening.
C. Obtain MRI of the lumbar spine.
D. Obtain MRI of the thoracic spine.

Discussion

The correct answer is (D). In this case, there is suspicion of a compressive lesion on the spinal cord or nerve root in the thoracic spine. Advanced imaging is suggested here versus a corset or physical therapy because a diagnosis is warranted prior to initiating any treatments. MRI of the thoracic spine is more appropriate than MRI of the lumbar spine because the radiation of the pain to the abdomen is more suggestive of a thoracic lesion versus a lumbar lesion.

MRI reveals an acute thoracic disc herniation, your next course of action is:

A. Place patient in a lumbar corset.
B. Send the patient for thoracic epidural or nerve root injection.
C. Admit the patient for emergent discectomy.
D. Recommend a discectomy via a transthoracic approach.

Discussion

The correct answer is (B). At this time, his symptoms are relatively stable. Most acute thoracic disc herniations may be treated nonoperatively. Relative surgical indications include myelopathy, lower extremity weakness or paralysis, bowel or bladder symptoms, or chronic radiculopathy that is refractory to conservative measures. Treatment may include a course of nonsteroidal anti-inflammatories, rest, modification of activities, and physical therapy. In this case, the patient is having radicular pain and injections are an option.

He has had his epidural injections and his pain was improved for a few weeks. But he twisted his back over the weekend and now has complains of progressive numbness and subjective weakness in his legs. He also complains of worsening pain that radiates across his back and to his abdomen. Examination shows patchy areas of decreased sensation and 4/5 motor strength in both lower extremities. The knee and ankle jerk reflex is 3+ whereas biceps is 2+. Babinski is mildly positive and he demonstrates three beats of clonus.

What is your next course of action?

A. Initiate physical therapy for lower extremity strengthening.
B. Place patient in a lumbar corset.
C. Discuss surgical decompression.
D. Send for another epidural injection.

Discussion

The correct answer is (C). In most instances, thoracic disc herniations may be treated nonoperatively. Surgical indications in this case include progressive myelopathy and lower extremity weakness.

Objectives: Did you learn...?

• Appropriate imaging in detecting disc herniations?
• When nonoperative versus operative treatment is most appropriate in thoracic disc herniations?

BIBLIOGRAPHY

An HS, Seldomridge JA. Spinal infections: diagnostic tests and imaging studies. *Clin Orthop Relat Res.* 2006;444: 27–33.

Anderson DG, Vaccaro AR. *Decision Making in Spinal Care.* Thieme; 2012. p. 364.

Angtuaco EJ, McConnell JR, Chadduck WM, et al. MR imaging of spinal epidural sepsis. *Am J Neuroradiol.* 1987;8(5):879–883.

Atlas SJ, Keller RB, Wu YA, et al. Long-term outcomes of surgical and nonsurgical management of lumbar spinal stenosis: 8 to 10 year results from the main lumbar spine study. *Spine (Phila Pa 1976).* 2005;30(8):936–943.

Ayhan S, Nelson C, Gok B, et al. Transthoracic surgical treatment for centrally located thoracic disc herniations presenting with myelopathy: a 5-year institutional experience. *J Spinal Disord Tech.* 2010;23(2):79–88.

Berry GE, Adams S, Harris MB, et al. Are plain radiographs of the spine necessary during evaluation after blunt trauma? Accuracy of screening torso computed tomography in thoracic/lumbar spine fracture diagnosis. *J Trauma.* 2005;59(6):1410–1413.

Beyer CA, Cabanela ME, Berquist TH. Unilateral facet dislocations and fracture-dislocations of the cervical spine. *J Bone Joint Surg Br.* 1991;73(6):977–981.

Boriani S, Bandiera S, Donthineni R, et al. Morbidity of en bloc resections in the spine. *Eur Spine J.* 2010;19(2):231–241.

Boyer MI. *AAOS Comprehensive Orthopaedic Review 2.* Rosemont, IL: American Academy of Orthopaedic Surgeons. Copyright; 2014; p. 868.

Bradford, DS, Mcbride GG. Surgical management of thoracolumbar spine fractures with incomplete neurologic deficits. *Clin Orthop Relat Res.* 1987;218:201–216.

Bubendorf L, Schöpfer A, Wagner U, et al. Metastatic patterns of prostate cancer: an autopsy study of 1,589 patients. *Hum Pathol.* 2000;31(5):578–583.

Burke JT, John H, Harris Jr. Acute injuries of the axis vertebra. *Skelet Radiol.* 1989;18(5):335–346.

Cannada LK. *Orthopaedic Knowledge Update 11.* Rosemont, IL: American Academy of Orthopaedic Surgeons; Copyright, 2014: p. 831.

Cannada LK. *Orthopaedic Knowledge Update 11.* Rosemont, IL: American Academy of Orthopaedic Surgeons; Copyright, 2014: p. 719.

Cannada LK. *Orthopaedic Knowledge Update 11.* Rosemont, IL: American Academy of Orthopaedic Surgeons; Copyright, 2014: p. 455.

Cannada LK. *Orthopaedic Knowledge Update 11.* Rosemont, IL: American Academy of Orthopaedic Surgeons; Copyright, 2014: p. 740.

Cannada LK. *Orthopaedic Knowledge Update 11*. Rosemont, IL: American Academy of Orthopaedic Surgeons; Copyright, 2014.

Cannada LK. *Orthopaedic Knowledge Update 11*. Rosemont, IL: American Academy of Orthopaedic Surgeons; Copyright, 2014: pp. 677–678.

Cannada LK. *Orthopaedic Knowledge Update 11*. Rosemont, IL: American Academy of Orthopaedic Surgeons; Copyright, 2014: p. 679.

Cannada LK. *Orthopaedic Knowledge Update 11*. Rosemont, IL: American Academy of Orthopaedic Surgeons; Copyright, 2014: p. 697.

Capaul M, Zollinger H, Satz N, Dietz V, Lehmann D, Schurch B. Analyses of 94 consecutive spinal cord injury patients using ASIA definition and modified Frankel score classification. *Spinal Cord*. 1994;32(9):583–587.

Carragee EJ. Pyogenic vertebral osteomyelitis. *J Bone Joint Surg*. 1997;79(6):874–880.

Castro WHM, Halm H, Jerosch J, Malms J, Steinbeck J, Blasius S. Accuracy of pedicle screw placement in lumbar vertebrae. *Spine (Phila Pa 1976)*. 1996;21(11):1320–1324.

Chen YC, Sosnoski DM, Mastro AM. Breast cancer metastasis to the bone: mechanisms of bone loss. *Breast Cancer Res*. 2010;12(6):215.

Connolly PJ, Esses SI, Kostuik JP. Anterior cervical fusion: outcome analysis of patients fused with and without anterior cervical plates. *J Spinal Disord*. 1996;9(3):202–206.

Coscia M, Thomas L, Daniel C. Acute cauda equina syndrome: diagnostic advantage of MRI. *Spine (Phila Pa 1976)*. 1994;19(4):475–478.

Deguchi M, Rapoff AJ, Zdeblick TA. Posterolateral fusion for isthmic spondylolisthesis in adults: analysis of fusion rate and clinical results. *J Spin Disord*. 1998;11(6):459–464.

Denis F, Steven D, Thomas C. Sacral fractures: an important problem retrospective analysis of 236 cases. *Clin Orthop Relat Res*. 1988;227:67–81.

Denis F. The three column spine and its significance in the classification of acute thoracolumbar spinal injuries. *Spine (Phila Pa 1976)*. 1983;8(8):817–831.

DiPaola C P, Molinari RW. Posterior lumbar interbody fusion. *J Am Acad Orthop Surg*. 2008;16(3):130–139.

Emery SE. Cervical spondylotic myelopathy: diagnosis and treatment. *J Am Acad Orthop Surg*. 2001;9(6):376–388.

Fisher CG, Dvorak MF, Leith J, Wing PC. Comparison of outcomes for unstable lower cervical flexion teardrop fractures managed with halo thoracic vest versus anterior corpectomy and plating. *Spine (Phila Pa 1976)*. 2002;27(2):160–166.

Flesch SA, William HL Jr, Nabil JA. *Neuromonitoring During Spine Surgery. Monitoring Technologies in Acute Care Environments*. New York: Springer; 2014:267–274.

Fountas KN, Kapsalaki EZ, Nikolakakos LG, et al. Anterior cervical discectomy and fusion associated complications. *Spine (Phila Pa 1976)*. 2007;32(21):2310–2317.

France JC, Yaszemski MJ, Lauerman WC, et al. A randomized prospective study of posterolateral lumbar fusion: outcomes with and without pedicle screw instrumentation. *Spine (Phila Pa 1976)*. 1999;24(6):553–560.

Fujimori T, Inoue S, Le H, et al. Long fusion from sacrum to thoracic spine for adult spinal deformity with sagittal imbalance: upper versus lower thoracic spine as site of upper instrumented vertebra. *Neurosurg Focus*. 2014;36(5):E9.

Garfin SR, Harry NH, Srdjan M. Instructional Course Lectures, The American Academy of Orthopaedic Surgeons-Spinal Stenosis. *J Bone Joint Surg*. 1999;81(4):572–586.

Gibbons KJ, Soloniuk DS, Razack N. Neurological injury and patterns of sacral fractures. *J Neurosurg*. 1990;72(6):889–893.

Gouliouris T, Aliyu SH, Brown NM. Spondylodiscitis: update on diagnosis and management. *J Antimicrob Chemother*. 2010;65(suppl 3):iii11–iii24.

Greenleaf R, Harris MB. *Lumbar Burst Fractures. Orthopedic Traumatology*. New York: Springer; 2013:55–68.

Guzman JZ, Baird EO, Fields AC, et al. C5 nerve root palsy following decompression of the cervical spine a systematic evaluation of the literature. *Bone Joint J*. 2014;96-B(7):950–955.

Haid RW Jr, Subach BR, McLaughlin MR, Rodts GE Jr, Wahlig JB Jr. C1–C2 transarticular screw fixation for atlantoaxial instability: a 6-year experience. *Neurosurgery*. 2001;49(1):65–70.

Halliday AL, Henderson BR, Hart BL, Benzel EC. The management of unilateral lateral mass/facet fractures of the subaxial cervical spine: the use of magnetic resonance imaging to predict instability. *Spine (Phila Pa 1976)*. 1997;22(22):2614–2621.

Hee HT, Majd ME, Holt RT, Pienkowski D. Better treatment of vertebral osteomyelitis using posterior stabilization and titanium mesh cages. *J Spinal Disord Tech*. 2002;15(2):149–156.

Holland JF. *Cancer Medicine*. 5th ed. Hamilton, Ontario; New York: B.C. Decker; 2000.

Inoue S, Watanabe T, Goto S, Takahashi K, Takata K, Sho E. Degenerative spondylolisthesis pathophysiology and results of anterior interbody fusion. *Clin Orthop Relat Res*. 1988;227:90–98.

Kaneda K, Abumi K, Fujiya M. Burst fractures with neurologic deficits of the thoracolumbar-lumbar spine results of anterior decompression and stabilization with anterior instrumentation. *Spine (Phila Pa 1976)*. 1984;9(8):788–795.

Kang M, Gupta S, Khandelwal N, Shankar S, Gulati M, Suri S. CT-guided fine-needle aspiration biopsy of spinal lesions. *Acta Radiol*. 1999;40(5):474–478.

Kim DH, Vaccaro AR. Osteoporotic compression fractures of the spine; current options and considerations for treatment. *Spine J*. 2006;6(5):479–487.

Kim WJ, Choy WS, Lee CK, Chang BS, Kang JW. Leakage of cement in percutaneous transpedicular vertebroplasty for painful osteoporotic compression fractures. *J Bone Joint Surg Br*. 2003;85(1):83–89.

Kumar VG, Rea GL, Mervis LJ, McGregor JM. Cervical spondylotic myelopathy: functional and radiographic long-term outcome after laminectomy and posterior fusion. *Neurosurgery.* 1999;44(4):771–777.

Laufer I, Rubin DG, Lis E, et al. The NOMS framework: approach to the treatment of spinal metastatic tumors. *Oncologist.* 2013;18(6):744–751.

Malanga GA. The diagnosis and treatment of cervical radiculopathy. *Med Sci Sports Exerc.* 1997;29(7 Suppl):S236–S245.

Mankin HJ, Mankin CJ, Simon MA. The hazards of the biopsy, revisited. Members of the Musculoskeletal Tumor Society. *J Bone Joint Surg Am.* 1996;78(5):656–663.

Massie JB, Heller JG, Abitbol JJ, McPherson D, Garfin SR. Postoperative posterior spinal wound infections. *Clin Orthopaed Relat Res.* 1992;284:99–108.

Matsumura A, Namikawa T, Hashimoto R, et al. Clinical management for spontaneous spinal epidural hematoma: diagnosis and treatment. *Spine J.* 2008;8(3):534–537.

Miller MD, ed. *Review of Orthopaedics.* 6th ed. Philadelphia, PA: WB Saunders; 2012:597.

Miller MD, ed. *Review of Orthopaedics.* 6th ed. Philadelphia, PA: WB Saunders; 2012:599–603.

Miller MD, ed. *Review of Orthopaedics.* 6th ed. Philadelphia, PA: WB Saunders; 2012:593–594.

Millikan JS, Cain TL, Hansbrough J. Rapid volume replacement for hypovolemic shock: a comparison of techniques and equipment. *J Trauma.* 1984;24(5):428–431.

Nelson DW, Martin MJ, Martin ND, Beekley A. Evaluation of the risk of noncontiguous fractures of the spine in blunt trauma. *J Trauma Acute Care Surg.* 2013;75(1):135–139.

Nguyen QN, Shiu AS, Rhines LD, et al. Management of spinal metastases from renal cell carcinoma using stereotactic body radiotherapy. *Int J Radiat Oncol Biol Phys.* 2010;76(4):1185–1192.

Olerud C, Jónsson H Jr, Löfberg AM, Lörelius LE, Sjöström L. Embolization of spinal metastases reduces peroperative blood loss: 21 patients operated on for renal cell carcinoma. *Acta Orthop Scanda.* 1993;64(1):9–12.

Onel D, Sari H, Dönmez C. Lumbar spinal stenosis: clinical/radiologic therapeutic evaluation in 145 patients-conservative treatment or surgical intervention?. *Spine (Phila Pa 1976).* 1993;18(2):291–298.

Patel AA, Dailey A, Brodke DS, et al; Spine Trauma Study Group. Thoracolumbar spine trauma classification: the Thoracolumbar Injury Classification and Severity Score system and case examples. *J Neurosurg Spine.* 2009;10(3):201–206.

Porter RW. Spinal stenosis and neurogenic claudication. *Spine (Phila Pa 1976).* 1996;21(17):2046–2052.

Reid DC, Hu R, Davis LA, Saboe LA. The nonoperative treatment of burst fractures of the thoracolumbar junction. *J Trauma.* 1988;28(8):1188–1194.

Saal JA, Saal JS. Nonoperative treatment of herniated lumbar intervertebral disc with radiculopathy: an outcome study. *Spine (Phila Pa 1976).* 1989;14(4):431–437.

Sakaura H, Hosono N, Mukai Y, Ishii T, Yonenobu K, Yoshikawa H. Outcome of total en bloc spondylectomy for solitary metastasis of the thoracolumbar spine. *J Spinal Disord Tech.* 2004;17(4):297–300.

Sakaura H, Hosono N, Mukai Y, Ishii T, Yoshikawa H. C5 palsy after decompression surgery for cervical myelopathy: review of the literature. *Spine (Phila Pa 1976).* 2003;28(21):2447–2451.

Sakaura H, Hosono N, Mukai Y, Ishii T, Yoshikawa H. C5 palsy after decompression surgery for cervical myelopathy: review of the literature. *Spine (Phila Pa 1976).* 2003;28(21):2447–2451.

Schaeren S, Broger I, Jeanneret B. Minimum four-year follow-up of spinal stenosis with degenerative spondylolisthesis treated with decompression and dynamic stabilization. *Spine (Phila Pa 1976).* 2008;33(18):E636–E642.

Scherping SC Jr. Cervical disc disease in the athlete. *Clin Sports Med.* 2002;21(1):37–47.

Schoenfeld AJ, Bono CM. Cervical spine fractures and dislocations. In: Court-Brown CM, Heckman JD, McQueen MM, Ricci WM, Tornetta P III (Eds.). *Rockwood and Green's Fractures in Adults,* 8th ed. Philadelphia, PA: Wolters Kluwer, 2015:1677–1756.

Schoenfeld AJ, Harris MB, McGuire KJ, Warholic N, Wood KB, Bono CM. Mortality in elderly patients with hyperostotic disease of the cervical spine following fracture: An age- and sex-matched study. *Spine J.* 2011;11:257–264.

Simpson AK, Harris MB. *Cervical Spine Clearance. Orthopedic Traumatology.* Springer, New York, 2013:23–39.

Steiner ME, Micheli LJ. Treatment of symptomatic spondylolysis and spondylolisthesis with the modified Boston brace. *Spine.* 1985;10(10):937–943.

Taggard DA, Traynelis VC. Management of cervical spinal fractures in ankylosing spondylitis with posterior fixation. *Spine.* 2000;25(16):2035–2039.

Takami M, Nohda K, Sakanaka J, Nakamura M, Yoshida M. Usefulness of full spine computed tomography in cases of high-energy trauma: a prospective study. *Eur J Orthop Surg Traumatol.* 2014;24(Suppl 1):S167–S171.

Thompson C. Hyperextension injury of the cervical spine with central cord syndrome. Diss University of Cape Town, 2013.

Tokuhashi Y, Matsuzaki H, Oda H, Oshima M, Junnosuke R. A revised scoring system for preoperative evaluation of metastatic spine tumor prognosis. *Spine.* 2005;30(19):2186–2191.

Truumees E, Herkowitz HN. Cervical spondylotic myelopathy and radiculopathy. *Instr Course Lect.* 1999;49:339–360.

Vahldiek MJ, Panjabi MM. Stability potential of spinal instrumentations in tumor vertebral body replacement surgery. *Spine.* 1998;23(5):543–550.

Veeravagu A, Patil CG, Lad SP, Boakye M. Risk factors for postoperative spinal wound infections after spinal decompression and fusion surgeries. *Spine.* 2009;34(17):1869–1872.

Wainner RS, Fritz JM, Irrgang JJ, Boninger ML, Delitto A, Allison S. Reliability and diagnostic accuracy of the clinical examination and patient self-report measures for cervical radiculopathy. *Spine.* 2003;28(1):52–62.

Weinstein JN, Lurie JD, Tosteson TD, et al. Surgical versus non-operative treatment for lumbar disc herniation: four-year results for the Spine Patient Outcomes Research Trial (SPORT). *Spine*. 2008;33(25):2789–2800.

Weinstein JN, Lurie JD, Tosteson TD, et al. Surgical vs non-operative treatment for lumbar disk herniation: the Spine Patient Outcomes Research Trial (SPORT) observational cohort. *JAMA*. 2006;296(20):2451–2459.

Wolf A, Levi L, Mirvis S, et al. Operative management of bilateral facet dislocation. *J Neurosurg*. 1991;75(6):883–890.

2

Shoulder and Elbow

Lewis Shi

CASE 1

Dr. Joseph Statz

A 76-year-old, right-hand-dominant man presents to clinic complaining of right shoulder pain. The pain started several months ago, has gotten progressively worse, and is located diffusely over his deltoid region. He has night pain and pain with overhead activity. On examination, there is no visible muscle atrophy, and he has full passive and near full active range of motion. He experiences pain and some weakness with resisted shoulder forward flexion and abduction.

What is the most likely diagnosis?

A. Acromioclavicular joint arthritis
B. Full-thickness rotator cuff tear
C. Adhesive capsulitis
D. Glenohumeral labral tear
E. Partial-thickness rotator cuff tear

Discussion

The correct answer is (E). Chronic, degenerative rotator cuff tears are very common in older patients. They usually present with insidious onset of diffuse pain over the deltoid that can radiate partially down the upper arm or into the trapezius. This pain is exacerbated with overhead activities, and night pain is common, which is a predictor of poor outcome with nonoperative treatment. These tears are thought to be the result of a combination of chronic impingement and rotator cuff degeneration from normal aging. The physical examination findings in this case are typical of rotator cuff tears and will be discussed more extensively below.

The scenario given is not one of the acromioclavicular (AC) joint arthritis (Answer A), which would manifest as pain localized directly at the AC joint, especially with palpation and cross-body adduction testing during examination. Classically, when asking a patient with shoulder pain to localize the pain, if he has AC joint arthritis, he will point with one finger directly over the AC joint. If he has a rotator cuff tear, he will take his hand and lay it over the deltoid due to the diffuse nature of the pain.

Differentiating between partial- and full-thickness tears (Answer B) on examination is difficult, but in general, if a patient is able to flex his or her shoulder through a full or nearly full active range of motion, the tear is not full thickness. A full-thickness tear would generally be associated with significantly decreased active range of motion because the rotator cuff is not able to actively move and stabilize the glenohumeral joint. With a partial-thickness tear, there is still continuous rotator cuff muscle that is able to move and stabilize the shoulder. There is usually not significant weakness with resisted active shoulder flexion but there is pain with it. Other signs of chronic full-thickness tears include weakness, visible atrophy of cuff musculature, and other findings depending on the location of the tear. These signs are almost never seen with partial-thickness tears. With the patient in this case, the physical examination findings are not severe enough to make one suspect a full-thickness tear, so it is more likely that he has a partial-thickness tear.

Adhesive capsulitis (Answer C) causes diffuse shoulder pain with restriction of active and passive range of motion. This patient has near full range of motion of his shoulder.

A labral tear (Answer D) does not classically present with the signs or symptoms seen in this case. Labral tears usually occur acutely with a compression or distraction injury, are associated with mechanical symptoms like clicking and catching, and are diagnosed clinically with different physical examination maneuvers than those for rotator cuff tears.

In the general population, what is the most commonly torn rotator cuff muscle?

A. Supraspinatus
B. Infraspinatus
C. Teres minor
D. Subscapularis
E. Teres major

Discussion

The correct answer is (A). It has been shown that it is the most commonly torn tendon, likely as the result of anatomic, vascular, and biomechanical factors. None of the other rotator cuff tendons, the infraspinatus, teres minor, or subscapularis (Answers B–D) tear as often as the supraspinatus. The teres major (Answer E) is not part of the rotator cuff.

What physical examination maneuver best tests for a supraspinatus tear?

A. Belly press test
B. Hornblower test
C. Jobe test
D. Lift-off test
E. External rotation lag

Discussion

The correct answer is (C). Each RC tendon has specific tests for pathology. The supraspinatus strength test (aka Jobe test) is performed by abducting the shoulder to 90 degrees, bringing the arm in the scapular plane (30 degrees forward), and maximally internally rotating the arm (thumb pointing to the floor) (Fig. 2–1). The test is positive if weakness is found or if pain is experienced. Another test for the supraspinatus is the drop arm test. In the drop arm test, the arm is passively elevated by the examiner to the Jobe position, the patient is asked to attempt to keep it there, and the arm is released by the examiner. The test is positive if the patient is not able to keep the arm elevated and the arm drops.

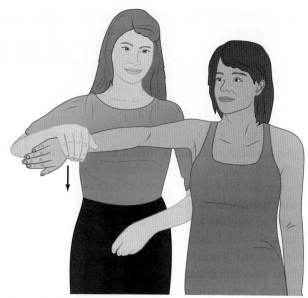

Figure 2–1 Jobe test.

The belly press test (Answer A) and lift off test (Answer D) are used to evaluate for subscapularis pathology (Figs. 2–3 and 2–4). The hornblower test (Answer B) assesses the teres minor (Fig. 2–2). The external rotation lag test (Answer E) evaluates the infraspinatus.

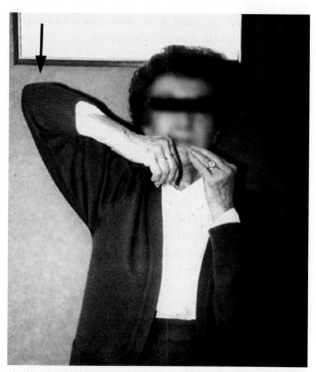

Figure 2–2 Positive hornblower's sign. (From Kuzel BR, Grindel S, Papandrea R, Ziegler D. Fatty infiltration and rotator cuff atrophy. *J Am Acad Orthop Surg.* 2013;21(10):613–623.)

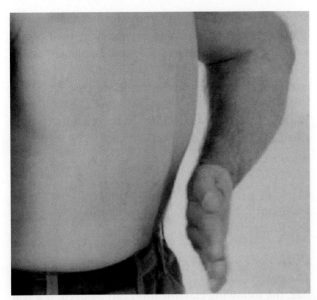
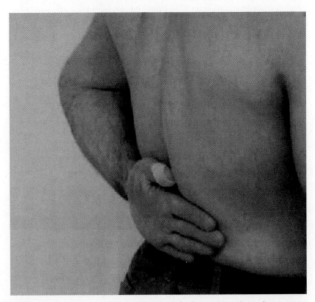

Figure 2–3 Positive lift-off test with the patient's left arm in the right picture. Negative lift-off test with the patient's right arm in the left picture. (From Lyons RP, Green A. Subscapularis tendon tears. *J Am Acad Orthop Surg.* 2005;13(5):353–363.)

What radiologic test should be used to confirm the diagnosis in this patient?

A. Shoulder CT
B. Shoulder MRI
C. Shoulder roentgenogram
D. Shoulder arthrogram
E. Shoulder MR arthrogram

Discussion

The correct answer is (B). An MRI showing a rotator cuff tear is considered diagnostic of a rotator cuff tear because of its high sensitivity, specificity, and accuracy. It has superb soft tissue imaging abilities (see Fig. 2–5). However, it should be noted that while MRI usually can differentiate between partial- and full-thickness rotator

cuff tears, this varies with the power and accuracy of the MRI facility. This is also true with the ability of MRI to differentiate between partial-thickness rotator cuff tears and subacromial bursitis. An arthroscopy is needed for definitive differentiation of these pathologies.

Shoulder CT scans (Answer A) are not typically used to diagnose rotator cuff tears. X-rays, aka roentgenograms (Answer C), can show signs of rotator cuff pathology but are not diagnostic. Some signs of chronic rotator cuff tears that are sometimes seen on AP view x-rays include calcific tendonitis, calcification of the coracohumeral ligament, proximal migration of the humerus, and cystic changes of the greater tuberosity. An outlet view x-ray can show a type III (hooked) acromion, which is correlated with a higher rate of rota-

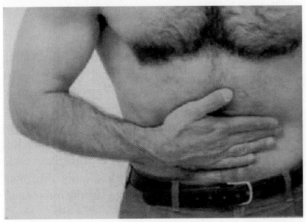
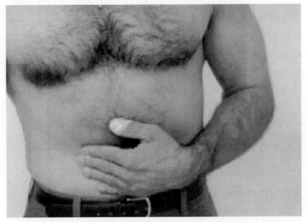

Figure 2–4 Positive belly-press test with the patient's left arm in the right picture. Negative belly-press test with the patient's right arm in the left picture. (From Lyons RP, Green A. Subscapularis tendon tears. *J Am Acad Orthop Surg.* 2005;13(5):353–363.)

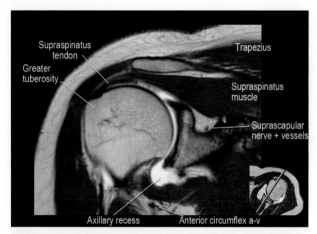

Figure 2–5 Coronal oblique view MRI slice of a left shoulder. (Reproduced with permission from Smithius R and van de Woude HJ. Shoulder MR Anatomy: Normal Anatomy, Variants, and Checklist. *Radiology Assistant.* April 2, 2012.)

tor cuff tears, or an OS acromiale, which would require special consideration for surgical treatment. Shoulder arthrograms (Answer D) are used primarily only when MRI is contraindicated and are considered positive for a rotator cuff tear if dye leaks from the glenohumeral joint into the subacromial space. MR arthrogram (Answer E) has been shown to have equivalent diagnostic ability compared with standard MRI and can be used to diagnose rotator cuff tears. However, it adds an additional step and cost to a standard MRI, and it does not offer any additional diagnostic benefit for rotator cuff pathology. Therefore, standard MRI is preferred to MR arthrogram.

Shoulder ultrasound is another modality that can be used to diagnose rotator cuff tears. It is generally less expensive than MRI but the sensitivity and specificity are more operator-dependent.

Objectives: Did you learn...?

• Clinically diagnose a rotator cuff tear?
• Identify the most commonly torn rotator cuff muscle?
• Perform the physical examination maneuvers to isolate and test each rotator cuff muscle?
• Radiologically diagnose a rotator cuff tear?

CASE 2

Dr. Joseph Statz

A 65-year-old, left-hand-dominant woman returns to clinic complaining of persistent left shoulder pain. She has a chronic, degenerative rotator cuff tear of her left shoulder and has persistent symptoms after 2 months of physical therapy, corticosteroid injections, and NSAID use. An MRI of the left shoulder is obtained, which shows a medium-sized, full-thickness tear of the supraspinatus and part of the infraspinatus with no retraction, no atrophy, and no fatty infiltration.

Which of the following widths of tears would be classified as a medium-sized rotator cuff tear?

A. 0.5 cm
B. 2 cm
C. 4 cm
D. 7 cm
E. 10 cm

Discussion

The correct answer is (B). When classifying tears by size, the following classification can be used. If a tear is less than 1 cm, it is considered a small tear (Answer A). If a tear is between 1 and 3 cm, it is considered a medium tear (Answer B). If a tear is between 3 and 5 cm, it is considered a large tear (Answer C). If a tear is greater than 5 cm, it is considered a massive tear (Answers D and E). In Europe, tears that involve two or more rotator cuff tendons are also considered massive tears.

During diagnostic arthroscopy, a thick band of tissue is seen just before the insertion of the supraspinatus and infraspinatus that is running perpendicular to the direction of the muscle fibers. What is this structure called?

A. Rotator crescent
B. Rotator interval
C. Rotator cable
D. Rotator cuff
E. Rotator bridge

Discussion

The correct answer is (C). This structure is a thickening of the coracohumeral ligament that starts anteriorly just posterior to the short head of the biceps tendon on the coracoid process, extends posteriorly through the edge of the avascular zone of the supraspinatus and infraspinatus, and ends at the inferior edge of the infraspinatus. One proposed function of the cable is to act like a cable in a suspension bridge, helping to evenly distribute forces on the humeral head produced by the rotator cuff (see Fig. 2–6).

The rotator crescent (Answer A) is the thin tissue that exists lateral to the rotator cable medial to the

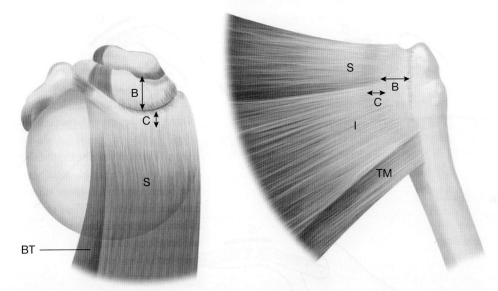

Figure 2–6 Illustration showing the rotator cable and rotator crescent. B, rotator crescent; C, rotator cable; BT, biceps tendon; I, infraspinatus; S, supraspinatus; TM, teres minor. (Redrawn from Burkhart SS, Lo IKY. Arthroscopic rotator cuff repair. *J Am Acad Orthop Surg.* 2006;14(6):333–346.)

attachment of the supraspinatus and infraspinatus. It is composed on the tendons of these two rotator cuff muscles (see Fig. 2–6).

The rotator interval (Answer B) is the area on the anterior shoulder bordered by the subscapularis inferiorly and the supraspinatus superiorly.

The rotator cuff (Answer D) is composed of all four rotator cuff muscles, the supraspinatus, infraspinatus, teres minor, and subscapularis.

What is the most likely shape of this patient's rotator cuff tear?

A. U shaped
B. L shaped
C. V shaped
D. Crescent shaped
E. Massive and immobile

Discussion

The correct answer is (D). Rotator cuff tears come in different shapes. Crescent-shaped tears are tears where the edge of the torn rotator cuff tendons form a crescent shape with an apex that points medially along the tension line of the rotator cuff muscles but is not retracted. Since this patient's tear is not retracted, the tear is likely to be crescent shaped.

U-shaped tears (Answer A) look similar to crescent-shaped tears but the apex of the U extends further medially, usually to the edge of the glenoid in the sagittal plane.

An L-shaped tear (Answer B) resembles a tear that can be thought of as partially a crescent-shaped tear and partially a U-shaped tear. One leg of the L is the more mobile, less retracted, crescent-shaped tear which transitions into the other leg of the L, which is a less mobile, more retracted part of the tear which resembles a U-shaped tear.

Finally, a massive and immobile tear (Answer E) can be either U-shaped or longitudinal. These tears are greater than 5 cm in size and cannot be mobilized to the greater tuberosity.

A V-shaped tear (Answer C) is not a type of rotator cuff tear.

What muscles make up the anterior and posterior force-couples, respectively?

A. Anterior: subscapularis. Posterior: supraspinatus
B. Anterior: pectoralis major. Posterior: infraspinatus
C. Anterior: latissimus dorsi. Posterior: infraspinatus
D. Anterior: subscapularis. Posterior: infraspinatus and teres minor
E. Anterior: pectoralis major. Posterior: infraspinatus and teres minor

Discussion

The correct answer is (D). One of the functions of the rotator cuff is to dynamically stabilize the humeral head in the glenoid, providing a fulcrum so that the shoulder can articulate properly. In order to do this, forces around the center of rotation must be equal in

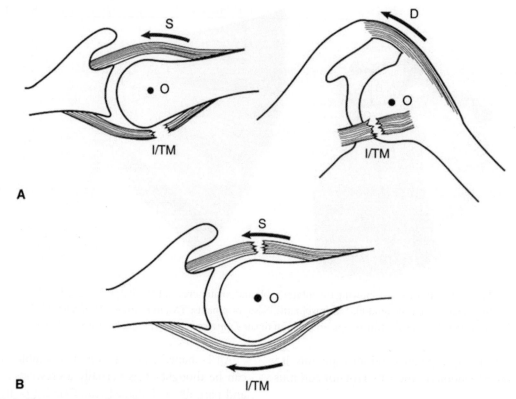

Figure 2–7 **A.** The transverse plane force couple (left) and the coronal plane force couple (right) are disrupted by a massive rotator cuff tear involving the posterior rotator cuff, infraspinatus, and teres minor. **B.** An alternative pattern of disruption of the transverse plane force couple. The transverse plane force couple is disrupted by a massive tear involving the anterior rotator cuff (ie, subscapularis). D = deltoid, I = infraspinatus, O = center of rotation, S = subscapularis, TM = teres minor. (From Burkhart SS, Lo IKY. Arthroscopic rotator cuff repair. *J Am Acad Orthop Surg.* 2006;14(6):333–346.)

the transverse and coronal planes. In the transverse plane, the humeral head is relatively unconstrained by the glenoid anteriorly and posteriorly. Any anterior and posterior forces placed on the humeral head must be balanced so that it does not sublux or dislocate in an anterior or posterior direction. This is accomplished by the subscapularis pulling the humeral head anteriorly with the same force that the infraspinatus and teres minor pull it posteriorly. All of these muscles also act to pull the humeral head medially into the concavity of the glenoid, stabilizing it in a medial-lateral dimension. When a patient has a rotator cuff tear, these force couples become uneven and can lead to instability (see Fig. 2–7).

What muscles make up the superior and inferior force-couples, respectively?

A. Superior: deltoid. Inferior: supraspinatus and infraspinatus
B. Superior: trapezius. Inferior: subscapularis, infraspinatus, and teres minor
C. Superior: deltoid. Inferior: subscapularis, infraspinatus, and teres minor
D. Superior: deltoid. Inferior: supraspinatus, infraspinatus, and teres minor
E. Superior: deltoid. Inferior: supraspinatus

Discussion

The correct answer is (C). As stated above, the rotator cuff is needed to stabilize the humeral head in the glenoid and provide a fulcrum to allow the humeral head to rotate properly. In the coronal plane, the humeral head is relatively unconstrained by the glenoid superiorly and inferiorly, so forces on the humeral head in these directions must be balanced. This is accomplished by the combined inferior forces of the subscapularis, infraspinatus, and teres minor equaling the superior force of the deltoid. When a patient has a rotator cuff tear, these force couples can be uneven, causing instability (see Fig. 2–7 above).

Objectives: Did you learn…?

• Classify full-thickness rotator cuff tears based on size, shape, and retraction?
• Identify the rotator cable and crescent?
• Identify the muscles that compose the force couples in the transverse and coronal planes?

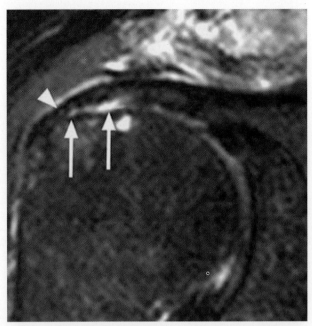

Figure 2–8 Reproduced with permission from Stadnick ME. *Partial Rotator Cuff Tears.* MRI Web Clinic. 2007 (Apr).

CASE 3

Dr. Joseph Statz

A 35-year-old male has had left shoulder pain for 4 months, ever since a low-speed motor vehicle accident (MVA). Physical examination demonstrates preserved range of motion but pain and some weakness with Jobe's testing. His imaging is shown in Figure 2–8.

What is the most likely diagnosis?

A. Partial articular surface tendon avulsion (PASTA)
B. Full-thickness rotator cuff tear
C. Superior labrum anterior to posterior tear (SLAP)
D. Anterior labral periosteal sleeve avulsion (ALPSA)

Discussion

The correct answer is (A). These are best diagnosed on an MRI as seen in the imaging provided; addition of intra-articular contrast can further improve this study. Answer B, full-thickness rotator cuff tear, is incorrect as the bursal side of the tendon can be seen to be in continuity. Answer C, a SLAP lesion, will be visualized as a labral tear on a coronal MRI and will be found at the biceps root. Answer D, an ALPSA lesion, will be most clearly seen on an axial MRI. It is a variant of a Bankart lesion where the labrum is displaced medially and inferiorly rolling down the glenoid neck underneath the periosteum.

Rotator cuff tears are a common reason for shoulder pain and a common reason to obtain shoulder imag-

ing. As a result, numerous different imaging modalities exist offering different pros and cons. Plain films are still the initial imaging modality of choice. These are most useful in ruling out other possible diagnosis but can help with the diagnosis of a rotator cuff tear as well. Changes to the tendon itself may appear as calcific tendinosis, which would most commonly be seen at the bone–tendon interface. A decrease in the acromio-humeral distance (less than 2 mm) may also be indicative of a cuff tear. In late cases of rotator cuff tears, superior subluxation of the humerus may be evident. Certain variations in acromial anatomy, including spurs or a hook-shaped (type 3) acromions, may be associated with rotator cuff tears as well. With progression of rotator cuff tears, degenerative changes including spurs, cysts, and sclerosis may be evident at the greater tuberosity. In late, massive tears one may see degenerative changes consistent with rotator cuff arthropathy.

Ultrasound has been gaining popularity recently as it is extremely cost effective when compared to MRI and allows a dynamic assessment of the tendons. It has been shown to have greater than 90% specificity and sensitivity when performed by an experienced operator.

MRI remains the most popular imaging modality for diagnosing rotator cuff tears. Normal rotator cuff tendon appears dark on both T1 and T2 sequences. Tears may be noted as being full-thickness, articular-sided, bursal-sided, or intrasubstance. They are visualized as a disruption in the regular contour of the tendon and increased signal intensity on T2 sequences. Occasionally, an MR arthrogram may provide additional information regarding a cuff tear, although this is not routinely ordered.

What MRI sequence and plane is best for viewing supraspinatus rotator cuff tears?

A. T1 coronal
B. T1 sagittal
C. T2 sagittal
D. T2 coronal
E. T2 axial

Discussion

The correct answer is (D). T2 sequence causes most soft tissues, including muscle and tendon, to appear dark and inflammation, such as at the site of a tear, to appear bright. This means that if there is a rotator cuff tear, there will be a bright spot along the course of the dark rotator cuff tendon. This is easiest to pick out in the coronal plane because the tendon runs in this plane, allowing one to view the entire supraspinatus tendon and tear in one cut.

A T1 sequence coronal view (Answer A) would allow you to view the entire tendon and tear in one cut, but will not provide as much contrast between the tear and tendon as a T2 sequence. A T1 sequence sagittal view (Answer B) would not provide the best sequence or plane for viewing a rotator cuff tear. T1 sequence is useful to visualize Hill–Sachs lesions more than rotator cuff tears. Neither a T2 sequence sagittal view nor a T2 sequence axial view (Answers C and E) would allow one to view a rotator cuff tear in the optimal plane.

What percentage of asymptomatic patients older than 60 year of age will have a rotator cuff tear?

A. 0 to 10
B. 10 to 30
C. 30 to 60
D. 60 to 80
E. 80 to 100

Discussion

The correct answer is (C). Numerous studies have shown that the rate of asymptomatic rotator cuff tears is between 30% and 60% in patients older than 60 years of age. The frequency of tears tends to increase with advanced age.

A 45-year-old carpenter presents with shoulder pain that has been ongoing for the last 3 months. He denies any significant injury. He describes night pain and significant discomfort at work. His imaging is shown in Figure 2–9. What is the most likely diagnosis?

A. Subscapularis tear
B. Supraspinatus tear
C. Labral tear
D. Anterior labral periosteal sleeve avulsion (ALPSA)
E. Shoulder instability

Discussion

The correct answer is (A). Medial subluxation of the biceps tendon as seen in this MRI is commonly associated with a tear of the subscapularis tendon which attaches to the lesser tuberosity. This patient's pain may in part be attributable to the subscapular tear and this should be evaluated for during physical examination. Supraspinatus tears (Answer B) cannot be easily visualized on axial views and are not associated with medial biceps subluxations. A labral tear and ALPSA lesion (Answers C and D) are not seen on the images provided. The question stem and MRI are not suggestive of shoulder instability (Answer E).

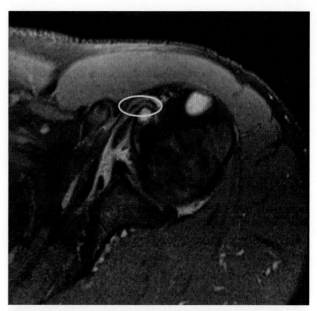

Figure 2–9 From Shi LL, Mullen MG, Freehill MT, et al. Accuracy of Long Head of the Biceps Subluxation as a Predictor for Subscapularis Tears. *Arthroscopy* 2015;32(4):615–619.

Objectives: Did you learn...?

- Diagnose and treat acute rotator cuff tears?
- Acquire advanced imaging at the appropriate time for rotator cuff tears?
- Use the correct MRI sequence and plane for imaging rotator cuff tears?
- Diagnose a subscapularis tear based on medial biceps tendon subluxation?

CASE 4

Dr. Joseph Statz

A 59-year-old, right-hand-dominant man presents to clinic complaining of right shoulder pain due to a worker's compensation injury. He has night pain and pain with overhead movement. He takes no medications, is otherwise healthy, and works as a mechanical engineer. His examination shows normal passive and active range of motion, a positive Neer impingement sign, positive Hawkins test, and a positive Jobe test with pain and weakness. His right arm is neurovascularly intact. Plain radiographs are normal.

What is the first step in treatment in this patient?

A. Arthroscopic rotator cuff repair
B. Physical therapy to strengthen the rotator cuff and stabilize the scapula
C. Subacromial corticosteroid injection
D. Expectant management
E. Arthroscopic rotator cuff debridement

Discussion

The correct answer is (B). Several factors are involved when deciding whether a patient should receive operative treatment versus a trial of nonoperative treatment for their rotator cuff injury. Some of these include: age and functional demands of the patient, duration of tear, mechanism of injury (if any), size and type of tear, retraction of tendons, atrophy of muscles, etc. In the majority of cases, however, conservative therapy is the initial modality of choice.

This patient has been clinically diagnosed with a chronic, degenerative rotator cuff tear. Chronic degenerative tears almost always should receive a trial of nonoperative, conservative treatment; the less active and older the patient is, the more one should consider a conservative approach. In this situation, conservative treatment should be instituted prior to obtaining an MRI as advanced imaging is extremely unlikely to change your decision.

The first step in conservative treatment is a regimen of physical therapy to strengthen the rotator cuff muscles and the periscapular muscles in order to restore normal biomechanical shoulder movement. Additional nonoperative modalities include: NSAIDs, activity modification, ice, heat, iontophoresis, massage, transcutaneous electrical nerve stimulation (TENS), pulsed electromagnetic field (PEMF), and phonophoresis (ultrasound). A recent AAOS Guideline found that no recommendation can be made for or against the use of these modalities.

Medications include NSAIDs and subacromial corticosteroid injections (Answer C). NSAIDs and corticosteroid injections serve to reduce inflammation and associated pain. They not only alleviate pain but also allow for more efficacious physical therapy. Corticosteroid injections are particularly used if there is thought to be rotator cuff tendon impingement. While commonly used, the AAOS guidelines once again state that no recommendation can be made for or against the use of corticosteroid injections.

Arthroscopic rotator cuff repair or debridement (Answers A and E) can be performed after failure of physical therapy to alleviate pain and restore function with subsequent MRI diagnosis of a rotator cuff tear. The choice of which operation to perform depends on the characteristics of the tear such as depth, retraction, and atrophy, which will be discussed in more detail below. However, one instance in which surgery should be considered before conservative treatment is in the case of acute, traumatic avulsion rotator cuff tears. Acute, traumatic avulsion tears should be surgically repaired if they are less than 3 weeks old because at that time they will not have retracted or atrophied. They can thus be relatively easily repaired to the greater tuberosity with good outcomes. If a person has an acute avulsion tear but waits longer than 4 to 6 weeks to present to an orthopaedic surgeon, this should then be treated like a chronic, degenerative tear because the tear will have had time to atrophy and retract.

Offering the patient no treatment (Answer D) would be inappropriate because the treatments discussed above would be helpful in alleviating pain and restoring function.

After consistently receiving physical therapy, taking NSAIDs, and having subacromial corticosteroid injections for 3 months, the patient's symptoms continue to worsen. An MRI confirms a full-thickness rotator cuff tear, and the decision is made to perform an arthroscopic rotator cuff repair. Compared to a nonworker's compensation patient, what are workers' compensation patients more likely to experience postoperatively?

A. Lower rate of returning to work and lower patient satisfaction

B. Higher rate of returning to work and lower patient satisfaction

C. Lower rate of returning to work and higher patient satisfaction

D. Higher rate of returning to work and higher patient satisfaction

E. Lower rate of returning to work and similar patient satisfaction

Discussion

The correct answer is (A). One study by Misamore et al. found that 94% of nonworker's compensation patients returned to work postoperatively compared to 42% of worker's compensation patients. They also found that 92% of nonworkers' compensation patients rated their shoulder as good or excellent postoperatively compared to 54% of worker's compensation patients.

Objectives: Did you learn...?

• Conservatively treat a chronic, rotator cuff tear?
• Identify postoperative differences in workers' compensation patients?

CASE 5

Dr. Joseph Statz

A 70-year-old, right-hand-dominant woman returns to clinic complaining of persistent, right shoulder pain. She has been clinically diagnosed with a chronic, degenerative rotator cuff tear of her right shoulder. Despite 2 months of consistent physical therapy, injections, and NSAID use, she has worsening pain and weakness. She takes no medications, is otherwise healthy, and is a retired accountant. Her examination shows no obvious atrophy of the supraspinatus or infraspinatus. She has 140 degrees of active shoulder flexion and abduction compared to 160 and 180 with the contralateral side, normal passive range of motion, a positive Neer impingement sign, a positive Hawkins test, as well as pain and weakness with Jobe test. The rest of the examination is normal. Plain radiographs are normal. MRI of the right shoulder shows a tear of the supraspinatus with minimal retraction, no atrophy, and no fatty infiltration. The patient is scheduled for arthroscopy.

If during diagnostic arthroscopy, the tear is determined to be a partial-thickness tear that is 5 mm deep, how would you now treat this patient?

A. Arthroscopic rotator cuff debridement
B. No further operative intervention at this time and an additional trial of physical therapy, NSAIDs, and corticosteroid injection
C. Arthroscopic rotator cuff repair
D. Mini-open rotator cuff repair
E. No further treatment

Discussion

The correct answer is (C). Although treatment algorithms are debated, a generally accepted rule is that with chronic, rotator cuff tears, if the tear does not respond to a trial of conservative treatment, operative treatment is warranted. For partial-thickness tears, the type of operation that should be performed is often controversial. One useful decision-making tool for patients with partial-thickness tears is the Ellman classification.

The Ellman classification differentiates between bursal-sided tears (Ellman classification B) and articular-sided tears (Ellman classification A), and also between those that are less than 3 mm in depth (Ellman classification I), between 3 and 6 mm in depth (Ellman classification II), and greater than 6 mm in depth (Ellman classification III). If a tear is bursal-sided and less than 3 mm in depth (BI), this can be treated with arthroscopic debridement of the tear (Answer A). If it is bursal-sided and greater than 3 mm in depth (BII as in this patient or BIII), this should be treated with arthroscopic rotator cuff repair (Answer C). In addition, subacromial decompression should be considered with all bursal-sided tears, and acromioplasty should be performed if the patient

Table 2–1 SUMMARY OF ELLMAN CLASSIFICATION TEARS AND THEIR TREATMENTS

Ellman Classification	Articular or Bursal Sided?	Depth (mm)	Treatment
AI	Articular	<3	Debridement
AII	Articular	3–6	Debridement
AIII	Articular	>6	Repair
BI	Bursal	<3	Debridement
BII	Bursal	3–6	Repair
BIII	Bursal	>6	Repair

Data from From Wolff AB, Sethi P, Sutton KM, Covey AS, Magit DP, Medvecky M. Partial-thickness rotator cuff tears. *J Am Acad Orthop Surg.* 2006;14(13):715–725.

has a type II or type III acromion or has anterior acromion bone spurs. If the tear is articular-sided and less than 6 mm (Ellman classification AI or AII), this can be debrided. If the tear is articular-sided and greater than 6 mm in depth (Ellman classification AIII), this should be repaired. Subacromial decompression and acromioplasty may not be necessary in the case of articular-sided tears. Refer to Table 2–1 and Figure 2–10 for a summary of the Ellman classifications and the indicated surgical treatment after failure of conservative treatment.

An additional trial of physical therapy, NSAIDs, and corticosteroid injections (Answer B) would be inappropriate in this case. If the patient failed to improve with this therapy the first time, it is unlikely that a second course of conservative management would be valuable. In these circumstances, operative treatment is warranted and the type of operation should be decided as described above.

A mini-open rotator cuff repair (Answer D) can be performed with similar long-term outcomes as arthroscopic repair, but arthroscopic repair has the potential for faster, short-term recovery postoperatively and is preferred.

Offering the patient no further treatment (Answer E) would be inappropriate in this case because an operation would be helpful in alleviating her pain and restoring function.

It should be noted that with chronic, rotator cuff tears, advanced imaging should not be acquired until after conservative management has failed. The only indication for early advanced imaging would be to differentiate the diagnosis from either infection or tumor. If conservative management cannot manage the patient's symptoms, then an MRI should be obtained to characterize the tear in order to help with operative planning. With *acute* tears – where there is a clear

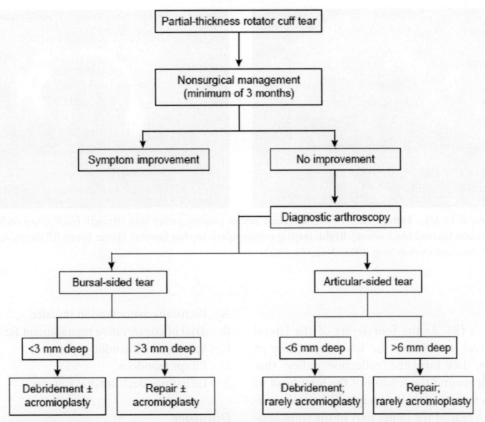

Figure 2-10 Potential treatment algorithm for partial-thickness rotator cuff tears. (Reproduced with permission from Shi LL, Mullen MG, Freehill MT, et al. Accuracy of Long Head of the Biceps Subluxation as a Predictor for Subscapularis Tears. Arthroscopy 2015;32(4):615-619.)

traumatic mechanism preceding symptoms – obtaining an MRI immediately is justifiable because surgery within 3 weeks of injury has much better outcome than surgery done after the first 3 weeks.

In the above patient, if during diagnostic arthroscopy, the tear is determined to be a full-thickness tear, how would you now treat this patient?

A. Arthroscopic rotator cuff debridement
B. Additional trial of physical therapy, NSAIDs, and corticosteroid injections
C. Arthroscopic rotator cuff repair
D. Mini-open rotator cuff repair
E. No further treatment

Discussion
The correct answer is (C). All full-thickness rotator cuff tears that fail conservative treatment and can be repaired arthroscopically should be repaired arthroscopically. They should not be debrided (Answer A).

An additional trial of physical therapy, NSAIDs, and corticosteroid injections (Answer B) would be inappro-

priate in this case. If the patient failed to improve with this therapy the first time, it is unlikely that it would work the second time. In these circumstances, operative treatment is warranted and the type of operation should be decided as described above.

A mini-open rotator cuff repair (Answer D) can be performed with similar long-term outcomes as arthroscopic repair, but arthroscopic repair has the potential for faster, short-term recovery postoperatively and is preferred.

Offering the patient no further treatment (Answer E) would be inappropriate in this case because an operation would be helpful in alleviating her pain and restoring function.

Which of the following findings is indicative of a subscapularis tendon tear?

A. High riding humeral head on plain radiographs
B. An empty intertubercular groove on MRI
C. Posterior shoulder dislocation
D. A type III acromion
E. Medial scapular winging

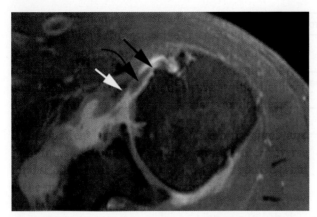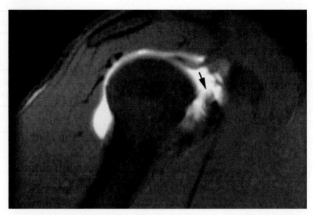

Figure 2–11 Axial T1 MRI. **Left:** an empty intertubercular sulcus, positive pulley sign (straight *black arrow* on left), and dislocated biceps tendon (curved *black arrow*). **Right:** fraying subscapularis tendon (*arrow*). (From Lyons RP, Green A. Subscapularis tendon tears. *J Am Acad Orthop Surg.* 2005;13(5):353–363.)

Discussion

The answer is (B). As the four layers of the lateral rotator interval insert onto the lesser tuberosity of the humerus, they form the "reflection pulley" that forms a sling around the tendon of the long head of the biceps before it enters the bicipital (intertubercular) groove. A tear of the upper part of the subscapularis can disrupt this reflection pulley and destabilize the biceps tendon, allowing it to sublux or even dislocate out of its groove, usually in a medial direction. If this happens, the intertubercular groove will be empty on MRI. Often, a "pulley sign" will also be seen on MRI when this occurs. This is when contrast material extravasates extra-articularly just over the superior border of the subscapularis tendon on axial images (see Fig. 2–11).

A high riding humeral head on plain films (Answer A) is associated with a massive rotator cuff tear and is the first sign of progression to cuff tear arthropathy that is seen on plain film.

Anterior, not posterior, shoulder dislocations (Answer C) are associated with subscapular tendon tears.

A type III acromion (Answer D) has been shown to be associated with rotator cuff tears of the supraspinatus, not the subscapularis.

Medial scapular winging (Answer E) results from dysfunction of the serratus anterior muscle, most commonly due to iatrogenic injury to the long thoracic nerve, which innervates the serratus anterior.

What is the best initial treatment for a healthy, 40-year-old patient with an acute subscapularis tendon tear?

A. Pectoralis major tendon transfer
B. Trial of conservative management for 6 weeks
C. Subscapularis tendon repair
D. Biceps tenodesis
E. Latissimus dorsi tendon transfer

Discussion

The correct answer is (C). Because of the acute nature of the tear, immediate surgical repair of the torn subscapularis tendon is indicated. Early surgical repair within 6 months of injury of acute tears is associated with better functional outcomes that repair after 6 months of injury. Waiting could lead to muscle atrophy, fatty infiltration, and retraction; all of which make surgery more challenging and worse outcomes. For these reasons, a trial of conservative management (Answer B) would be inappropriate.

A pectoralis major tendon transfer (Answer A) is one option to fix a torn subscapularis, but it is reserved for tears that are irreparable. Repair of the native subscapularis has better outcomes than using a tendon transfer. A biceps tenodesis (Answer D) may be performed along with a subscapularis tendon repair, but it will not treat the main problem, which is a torn subscapularis tendon. A latissimus dorsi tendon transfer (Answer E) is used for irreparable tears of the posterosuperior rotator cuff (supraspinatus and infraspinatus) in certain patients. However, no tendon transfer would be used in an acute, repairable tear of the rotator cuff.

During arthroscopy of a patient with a chronic subscapularis rotator cuff tear, the superior glenohumeral ligament (SGHL) is noted to be avulsed off of

the glenoid. What intra-articular landmark can be used to identify the superolateral border of the tear?

A. Comma sign
B. ALPSA lesion
C. Terry–Thomas sign
D. Sulcus sign
E. Piano key sign

Discussion

The correct answer is (A). When a chronic, retracted subscapularis tendon tear is present, the superolateral border of the tear can be identified by a comma-shaped ligamentous structure that exists at this border. This is composed of an avulsed superior glenohumeral ligament blending with the coracohumeral ligament and is called the comma sign (see Fig. 2–12).

ALPSA lesion (Answer B) is an anterior labral periosteal sleeve avulsion. It occurs when there is an injury to the anterior labrum that causes it to be pulled off of the glenoid. In this pathology, when the labrum comes off it takes with it part of the periosteum covering the anterior glenoid.

A Terry–Thomas sign (Answer C) is when, on AP wrist x-ray, there is an enlarged space between the scaphoid and lunate and is a sign of a scapholunate dislocation.

A sulcus sign (Answer D) can be found with shoulder instability. On physical examination, if downward traction is put on a shoulder with the arm at the side, a depression can be found between the acromion and the humeral head, indicating ligamentous laxity of the shoulder.

A piano key sign (Answer E) can signify distal radioulnar joint (DRUJ) instability. If the distal ulna protrudes dorsally at the DRUJ, can be translated volarly on examination, springs back dorsally after released from volar translation, and is more impressive than the contralateral wrist, this is a positive piano key sign.

Objectives: Did you learn...?

- Classify and surgically treat partial-thickness rotator cuff tears?
- Surgically treat full-thickness rotator cuff tears?
- Recognize the significance of an empty bicipital groove?
- Treat an acute subscapularis tear?
- Recognize a comma sign?

CASE 6

Dr. Joseph Statz

A 70-year-old, right-hand-dominant woman presents to clinic with right shoulder pain and weakness. She has had progressive weakness and severe pain with overhead motions for the last several years to the point where she is no longer able to reach overhead. She endures severe night pain as well. Conservative treatment with physical therapy, NSAIDs, and corticosteroids used to help but do not anymore. She is otherwise healthy and takes no medications. On examination, she has visible atrophy of the supraspinatus and infraspinatus muscles. She has very limited active flexion and abduction of 30 degrees, external rotation of 10 degrees, and internal rotation to T12. She has full passive range of motion (ROM) with positive Neer, Hawkins, and Jobe test; a positive drop arm test; and a positive external rotation lag sign. The rest of the examination is normal. Plain films are normal. An MRI reveals a massive rotator cuff tear involving the supraspinatus and infraspinatus. The supraspinatus and infraspinatus both show signs of minimal atrophy, minimal fatty infiltration, and retraction to the glenoid.

During arthroscopy, it is confirmed that the patient has a massive and immobile tear with a small part of

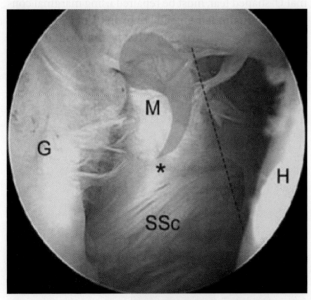

Figure 2–12 Comma sign, indicating the superior border of a chronic, retracted subscapularis tendon tear. G, glenoid; H, humerus; SSc, subscapularis; M, medial sling of biceps (comma); *, junction of medial sling of biceps and subscapularis tendon. (Redrawn from Burkhart SS, Lo IKY. Arthroscopic rotator cuff repair. *J Am Acad Orthop Surg.* 2006;14(6):333–346.)

the anterior supraspinatus still attached to the greater tuberosity. What technique will likely need to be used in order to repair the rotator cuff to the greater tuberosity?

A. Anterior interval slide
B. Posterior interval slide
C. Krackow stitch
D. Double-bundle reconstruction
E. Marginal convergence

Discussion

The correct answer is (A). Massive and immobile tears can be either U-shaped or longitudinal. These can sometimes be repaired using an anterior or posterior interval slide technique. In an anterior interval slide technique, there is some anterior portion of the supraspinatus still attached to the greater tuberosity laterally and rotator interval anteriorly. The greater tuberosity attachment can be incised and the rotator interval attachment can be detached by incising the coracohumeral ligament. In a posterior interval slide technique, there is some posterior portion of the supraspinatus still attached to the infraspinatus. This can be detached by incising the interval between the supraspinatus and infraspinatus (Answer B). These interval slide techniques decrease the tension and improve lateral mobilization, allowing the supraspinatus to be more easily repaired to the greater tuberosity. The posterior leaf of the tear is then brought together with the anterior leaf through marginal convergence, leaving you with a small crescent-shaped tear that can be repaired to the greater tuberosity (see Fig. 2–16).

Crescent-shaped tears are not retracted much medially, can be mobilized laterally relatively easily, and thus can be relatively easily repaired to humeral bone (see Fig. 2–13).

U-shaped tears can be repaired using marginal convergence (Answer E). U-shaped tears have an apex that extends further medially, usually to the edge of the glenoid in the sagittal plane, and this part cannot be mobilized all the way to the greater tuberosity. Because of this lack of mobility, these tears have to be repaired using marginal convergence, which is essentially zipping up the U from the apex toward the greater tuberosity using side to side sutures to bring together the anterior and posterior leaves of the U-shaped tear. In performing this marginal convergence, you essentially are converting a U-shaped tear into a crescent-shaped tear that can be relatively easily mobilized to the greater tuberosity, allowing it to be repaired (see Fig. 2–14).

Finally, an L-shaped tear resembles a tear that can be thought of as partially a crescent-shaped tear and partially a U-shaped tear. One leg of the L is the more mobile, less retracted, crescent-shaped tear which transitions into the other leg of the L, a less mobile, more retracted part of the tear which mechanically and visually resembles a U-shaped tear. The retracted U-shaped part, like a normal U-shaped tear, must be repaired using marginal convergence. Then the remaining crescent-shaped part, like a normal crescent-shaped tear, can be mobilized laterally and repaired to bone (see Fig. 2–15).

A Krackow stitch (Answer C) is a locking stitch that can be used in various tendinous repairs, including

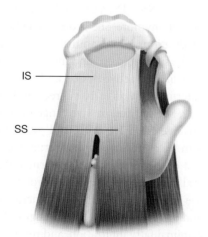
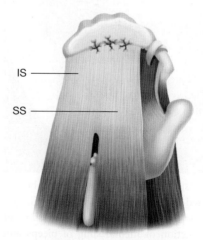

Figure 2–13 Crescent-shaped rotator cuff tear and repair. SS, supraspinatus; IS, infraspinatus. (Redrawn from Burkhart SS, Lo IKY. Arthroscopic rotator cuff repair. *J Am Acad Orthop Surg.* 2006;14(6):333–346.)

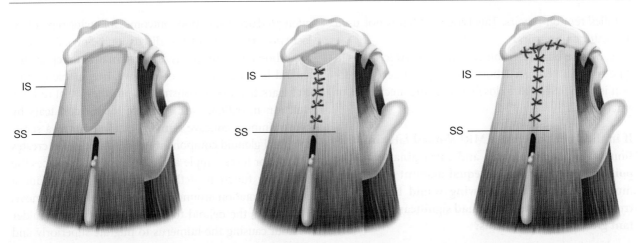

Figure 2-14 U-shaped rotator cuff tear and repair using marginal convergence. SS, supraspinatus; IS, infraspinatus. (Redrawn from Burkhart SS, Lo IKY. Arthroscopic rotator cuff repair. *J Am Acad Orthop Surg.* 2006;14(6):333–346.)

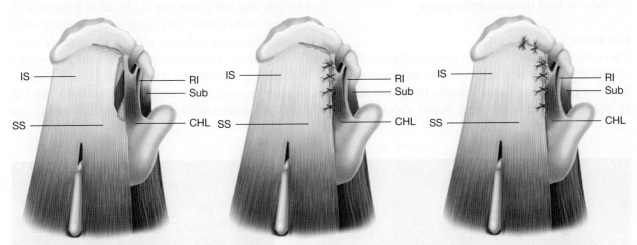

Figure 2-15 L-shaped rotator cuff tear and repair using marginal convergence. SS, supraspinatus; IS, infraspinatus; RI, rotator interval; CHL, coracohumeral ligament; Sub, subscapularis. (Redrawn from Burkhart SS, Lo IKY. Arthroscopic rotator cuff repair. *J Am Acad Orthop Surg.* 2006;14(6):333–346.)

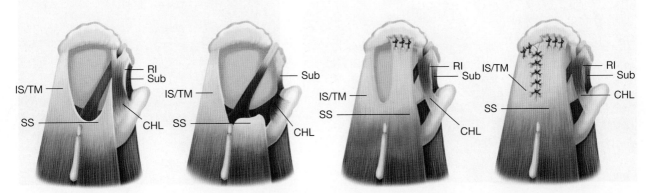

Figure 2-16 Massive, immobile rotator cuff tear and repair using anterior interval slide followed by marginal convergence. SS, supraspinatus; IS/TM, infraspinatus/teres minor; RI, rotator interval; CHL, coracohumeral ligament; Sub, subscapularis. (Redrawn from Burkhart SS, Lo IKY. Arthroscopic rotator cuff repair. *J Am Acad Orthop Surg.* 2006;14(6):333–346.)

Achilles' tendon repairs. This type of stitch is not used in rotator cuff repairs.

A double-bundle reconstruction (Answer D) is a type of ACL reconstruction. This type of reconstruction is thought to more closely mimic the mechanics of a native ACL.

If in the same patient the MRI showed fatty infiltration of the supraspinatus and infraspinatus to the point where there was an equal amount of fat and muscle, which of the following would be the best treatment if the patient also had significant concomitant glenohumeral arthritis?

A. Hemiarthroplasty
B. Total shoulder arthroplasty
C. Latissimus dorsi tendon transfer
D. Arthroscopic rotator cuff repair
E. Reverse total shoulder arthroplasty

Discussion

The correct answer is (E). Given that her rotator cuff has atrophied and has fatty infiltration to the point where there are equal parts fat and muscle, this is considered an irreparable rotator cuff tear. Repair should not be attempted because of poor outcomes following repair (see last two paragraphs of this discussion below). A reverse total shoulder arthroplasty is an alternative to repair that should be used in cases of massive, irreparable rotator cuff tears. It is a semi-constrained prosthesis that restores function in patients with massive rotator cuff tears by constraining a concave humeral cap inferior to a semi-spherical glenoid component (glenosphere). This creates an inferior force-couple and a fulcrum that replaces the stabilizing function of the infraspinatus maintaining a center of rotation around which the shoulder can move. This allows the deltoid to abduct and flex the shoulder without causing the humerus to migrate superiorly and about the acromion. In an elderly patient with a massive, irreparable rotator cuff tear (as in this patient), a reverse total shoulder arthroplasty is the procedure of choice.

It should be noted that reverse total shoulder arthroplasty is also the procedure of choice in patients with cuff-tear arthropathy (aka rotator cuff arthropathy). Characteristics of cuff-tear arthropathy include superior migration of the humerus due to a massive rotator cuff tear, glenohumeral joint destruction, subchondral osteoporosis, and humeral head collapse (see Fig. 2–17). A reverse total shoulder arthroplasty in this case

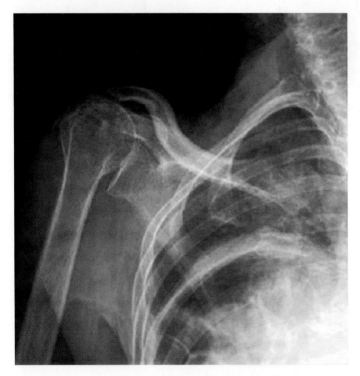
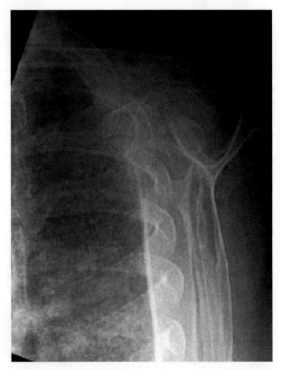

Figure 2–17 X-rays of a patient showing evidence of cuff tear arthropathy. The humerus is migrated superiorly, the glenohumeral joint is destroyed, there is subchondral osteoporosis, and the humeral head is collapsed. (From Ecklund KJ, Lee TQ, Tibone J, Gupta R. Rotator cuff tear arthropathy. *J Am Acad Orthop Surg.* 2007;15(6):340–349.)

serves the purpose of eliminating pain caused by glenohumeral joint arthritis while restoring functional motion and is the procedure of choice in patients with cuff-tear arthropathy.

A hemiarthroplasty (Answer A) was previously the procedure of choice for cuff-tear arthropathy until the reverse total shoulder prosthesis was developed. A hemiarthroplasty reliably relieves pain, but it does not restore function as well as the reverse total shoulder. Also, if the patient had a previous coracoacromial ligament release or anterior deltoid detachment, they are at risk for anterosuperior escape of the humeral head after hemiarthroplasty.

A total shoulder arthroplasty (Answer B) is contraindicated in the case of cuff-tear arthropathy because of glenoid component loosening. If a glenoid component is used in this patient, the superior translation of the humeral head component on the glenoid component could cause it to loosen and rock, producing a "rocking-horse" glenoid component.

A latissimus dorsi tendon transfer (Answer C) would be a good option if this patient still had a normal glenohumeral joint and were young (less than 50 years old). But this patient has cuff-tear arthropathy, so his glenohumeral joint is destroyed. Performing a latissimus dorsi tendon transfer might restore some range of motion, but the patient would still have pain from arthritis in his shoulder.

An arthroscopic rotator cuff repair (Answer D) would be a poor choice in this patient given the characteristics of her tear. With massive rotator cuff tears, Goutallier et al. showed that the degree of fatty degeneration of the infraspinatus correlated directly with the time between onset of shoulder pain and the rotator cuff repair (meaning people who waited longer to present and undergo surgery had more fatty degeneration of their infraspinatus tears), with the loss of active external rotation of the shoulder both pre- and postoperatively (meaning that more fatty degeneration predicts less function before and after repair), and with a higher rate of repair failure (meaning that more fatty degeneration predicts greater risk of operative failure). They also did not find any reversal of infraspinatus fatty degeneration after rotator cuff repair.

In addition, Goutallier et al. formulated a classification system for rotator cuff tears that is helpful in determining whether a massive rotator cuff tear is reparable or not based on fatty degeneration. Progressive atrophy and fatty degeneration occurs as the length of time the rotator cuff has been torn increases. The fat to muscle

Table 2–2   GOUTALLIER CLASSIFICATION

Goutallier Classification	Description
Stage 0	Normal
Stage 1	Minimal fatty streaks
Stage 2	Significant amount of fatty streaks but more muscle than fat
Stage 3	Equal amounts of fat and muscle
Stage 4	More fat than muscle

Data from Kuzel BR, Grindel S, Papandrea R, Ziegler D. Fatty infiltration and rotator cuff atrophy. *J Am Acad Orthop Surg.* 2013;21(10):613–623.

ratio is used in the Goutallier classification. The cause of this atrophy and degeneration is not fully understood but is likely due to a combination of loss of mechanical tension of the muscle and muscle denervation.

This classification was originally based on CT imaging but is now applied to MRI imaging and uses sagittal oblique views at the most lateral slice in which the scapular spine is continuous with the scapular body. There are five categories that range from stage 0 to stage 4. A classification of stage 0 is normal, stage 1 is some fatty streaks, stage 2 is more muscle than fat, stage 3 is equal amounts of fat and muscle, and stage 4 is more fat than muscle. This patient's rotator cuff tear involves the supraspinatus and infraspinatus, and both have atrophied to the point of having equal amounts of fat and muscle, giving her tear a Goutallier classification of stage 3 (see Table 2–2 and Fig. 2–18). As a general rule, if there is stage 3 or 4 fatty atrophy, rotator cuff repair will not be successful and a reverse total shoulder or tendon transfer would be a better operation.

If a patient had the same tear but was a healthy, active 50 year old with no glenohumeral arthritis, which of the following choices would be the best treatment?

A. Latissimus dorsi tendon transfer
B. Arthroscopic rotator cuff repair
C. Subscapularis tendon transfer
D. Trapezius tendon transfer
E. Reverse total shoulder arthroplasty

Discussion

The correct answer is (A). In young, active patients with a massive, irreparable rotator cuff tear without

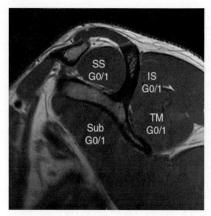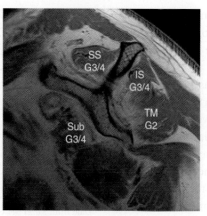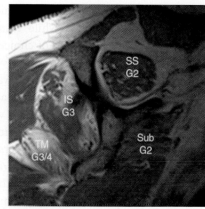

Figure 2–18 Three different patients showing different stages of fatty degeneration with Goutallier stages. Higher stages are predictive of worse outcomes after rotator cuff repair. SS, supraspinatus; IS, infraspinatus; TM, teres minor; Sub, subscapularis. (From Kuzel BR, Grindel S, Papandrea R, Ziegler D. Fatty infiltration and rotator cuff atrophy. *J Am Acad Orthop Surg.* 2013;21(10):613–623.)

glenohumeral arthritis, a tendon transfer is the most reasonable option to attempt to restore function of the shoulder. In a tear involving the supraspinatus and infraspinatus, the posterior and inferior force-couples in the transaxial and coronal planes, respectively, are out of balance because of the involvement of the infraspinatus in both of those. Because of this, the humerus cannot be dynamically stabilized in the glenoid during active movement of the shoulder. The most popular way to restore this in a young, healthy patient is through a latissimus dorsi tendon transfer in which the insertion of the tendon is transferred from the humeral shaft to the greater tuberosity (see Fig. 2–19). This creates a new posterior and inferior force-couple and creates an external rotation force.

It should be noted that due to the differences in the length and force vector magnitude and direction between the infraspinatus and latissimus dorsi, the force couple is not perfectly restored, and thus the shoulder after a tendon transfer never works as well as with a successful repair of the native cuff. The latissimus force vector is much more vertical and greater in magnitude than the infraspinatus. This transfer thus has variable results in restoring function. Factors associated with poor outcome include subscapularis dysfunction, deltoid dysfunction, osteoarthritis of the glenohumeral or acromioclavicular joint, and loss of teres minor function, none of which are present in this patient.

An arthroscopic rotator cuff repair (Answer B) would be a poor choice in this patient given the characteristics of her tear. The degree of fatty degeneration of the

rotator cuff in this case puts the patient at risk for poor outcomes after rotator cuff repair.

A subscapularis tendon transfer (Answer C) has been used by some orthopedists to attempt to restore

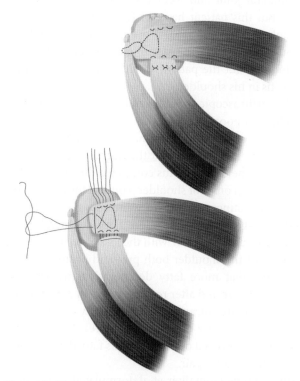

Figure 2–19 Latissimus dorsi tendon transfer on a right shoulder viewed from superiorly with anterior being the left side of the image. **Top:** final appearance. **Bottom:** final sutures being thrown through the latissimus dorsi. (From Omid R, Lee B. Tendon transfers for irreparable rotator cuff tears. *J Am Acad Orthop Surg.* 2013;21(8):492–501.)

an inferior force couple and abduction force by transferring the superior portion of the subscapularis more superiorly to the greater tuberosity. It would likely not be a successful procedure in this patient, though, because there would still be a lack of posterior and inferior force-couple due to the torn infraspinatus. The transfer would help to make up for the loss of function of the supraspinatus abduction force but would not help with the loss of the infraspinatus.

A trapezius tendon transfer (Answer D) is used by some orthopaedic surgeons with good success in restoring external rotation for brachial plexopathy and has some renewed interest in general, but it has not been reported in the literature as a surgical technique for rotator cuff tears and is not as popular as the latissimus dorsi transfer. The inferior trapezius force vector is similar in magnitude and direction to the infraspinatus, so using this transfer makes good biomechanical sense, but other issues exist such as the need to use an Achilles tendon allograft to bridge the distance between the trapezius tendon and the greater tuberosity.

A reverse total shoulder arthroplasty (Answer E) restores range of motion in a shoulder with an irreparable rotator cuff, but it has significant limitations of lifting activities and a higher risk of needing revisions in younger patients like this 50 year old. The goal of surgery in this young, active patient would be to increase function of his shoulder without the limitations of a reverse total shoulder arthroplasty.

If this patient had been diagnosed with a chronic, irreparable tear of the subscapularis and had failed a trial of physical therapy, corticosteroid injections, and NSAIDs, what would be the most reasonable next step in treatment?

A. Subscapularis tendon repair
B. Biceps tenotomy
C. Pectoralis major tendon transfer
D. Reverse total shoulder arthroplasty
E. Supraspinatus tendon transfer

Discussion

The correct answer is (C). When the native rotator cuff is irreparable, using a tendon transfer is the next step. Since the force vector of the pectoralis major muscle is similar to that of the subscapularis, this tendon can be used as an effective tendon transfer, restoring internal rotation and humeral head centering and compression. The surgery is performed by detaching the pectoralis major from its humeral insertion and moving the insertion to the lesser tuberosity. The tendon of the pectoralis major can run anterior to the conjoined tendon or can be transposed posterior to the conjoined tendon but anterior to the musculocutaneous nerve. This latter method more closely replicates the force vector direction of the subscapularis, but has not been shown to lead to better outcomes (see Fig. 2–20). A latissimus dorsi tendon transfer is also sometimes used for irreparable subscapularis tendon tears.

Subscapularis tendon repair is by definition impossible since this is an irreparable subscapularis tendon tear (Answer A). A tenotomy of the long head of the biceps (Answer B) would likely be performed as a part of the tendon transfer surgery, but would not by itself help in

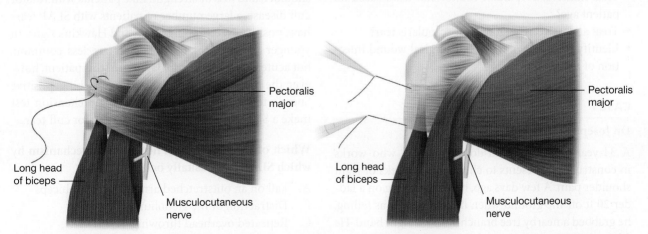

Figure 2–20 Pectoralis major tendon transfer. **Left:** partial tendon transfer. **Right:** complete tendon transfer. Both use a subcoracoid approach. (From Omid R, Lee B. Tendon transfers for irreparable rotator cuff tears. *J Am Acad Orthop Surg.* 2013;21(8):492–501.)

restoring function. A reverse total shoulder arthroplasty (Answer D) is used for massive, irreparable rotator cuff tears of the anterosuperior rotator cuff but not for subscapularis tears, as in this question. A supraspinatus tendon transfer (Answer E) is not a surgery that has been described for irreparable subscapularis tendon tears.

If the patient presents with concerning signs and symptoms of wound infection 1 month after reverse total shoulder surgery but cultures are negative, what is the most likely causative organism?

A. *Staphylococcus aureus*
B. *Streptococcus pyogenes*
C. *Propionibacterium acnes*
D. *Pseudomonas aeruginosa*
E. *Trichophyton rubrum*

Discussion

The correct answer is (C). This bacterium is the most common cause of delayed or indolent infections of surgical wounds. Cultures are often negative because it takes a long time, about 14 to 21 days for it to grow out on cultures. *Staphylococcus aureus* (Answer A), *Streptococcus pyogenes* (Answer B), and *Pseudomonas aeruginosa* (Answer D) are some bacterial causes of acute wound infections but would likely present within a week or two of surgery and would likely grow out on cultures. *Trichophyton rubrum* (Answer E) is a fungus that is the leading cause of ringworm and is not commonly a cause of surgical wound infection.

Objectives: Did you learn...?

* Surgically repair full-thickness rotator cuff tears based on tear shape?
* Treat massive, irreparable rotator cuff tears based on patient age?
* Treat a massive, irreparable subscapularis tear?
* Identify the cause of a delayed surgical wound infection of the shoulder?

CASE 7

Dr. Joseph Statz

A 34-year-old, right-hand-dominant man who works in construction presents to clinic with 3 weeks of right shoulder pain. A few days ago, he was working on a ladder 20 ft off the ground when he fell. As he was falling, he grabbed a nearby tree branch with his right hand. He felt immediate pain in his right shoulder and is now having pain, clicking, and catching with overhead activity.

He is otherwise healthy and takes no medications. On examination, his right, upper extremity is neurovascularly intact; his active and passive shoulder range of motion is limited by clicking and catching; and he has a positive compression–rotation test, Neer impingement sign, Hawkin's sign, and Speed's test. He also has pain with anterior apprehension test. The rest of the examination is normal. X-rays are normal.

What is the most likely diagnosis?

A. Acromioclavicular joint arthritis
B. Full-thickness rotator cuff tear
C. Subacromial bursitis
D. Superior labral tear from anterior to posterior (SLAP tear)
E. Partial-thickness rotator cuff tear

Discussion

The correct answer is (D). In an acute shoulder injury caused by a traction mechanism with pain associated with overhead motion and mechanical symptoms such as popping, catching, clicking, or grinding, the most likely injury is a SLAP tear. A SLAP tear is identified in about 6% of all shoulder arthroscopies. Of these, about 12% to 30% are isolated SLAP tears and 70% to 88% are associated with other shoulder pathologies.

Acromioclavicular (AC) joint arthritis (Answer A) does not usually occur in an acute injury. It typically has an insidious onset and is more common in patients who are weight lifters or overhead throwing athletes. Mechanical symptoms are not typical.

Rotator cuff tears, subacromial bursitis (Answers B, C, and E), and SLAP tears can present almost identically, with pain in overhead motion, pain when lying on the shoulder, and loss of strength. Like patients with rotator cuff disease, a large number of patients with SLAP tears have positive Neer impingement and Hawkin's signs. In younger patients, rotator cuff tears are less common, but acute avulsion tears do happen. In this patient, however, the presence of the clicking and catching, positive Speed's test, and pain with anterior apprehension test make a SLAP tear more likely than a rotator cuff tear.

Which of the following is not a usual mechanism by which SLAP tears usually occur?

A. Fall on an outstretched arm with tensed biceps
B. Distraction of the glenohumeral joint
C. Repeated overhead throwing
D. Military press weight lifting
E. Shoulder dislocation

Discussion

The correct answer is (D). This is a common mechanism of AC joint pathology including distal clavicular osteolysis.

The most common mechanisms by which a SLAP tear occurs are compression (Answer A) and traction (Answer B). Compression generally occurs when a person falls on an outstretched arm that is slightly flexed and abducted with a tensed biceps. Traction can occur in an anterior, superior, or inferior direction. In the case of this patient, he was falling and caught a tree branch, causing traction in a superior direction. Traction can also occur with overhead throwing (Answer C) or with shoulder dislocation (Answer E). Up to 33% of slap tears, however, have insidious onset.

Many studies have been conducted to investigate SLAP tears in the context of overhead throwing. It appears that SLAP tears are most likely to occur during the late cocking and deceleration phases of throwing due to the increased stress and strain at the superior glenoid/biceps tendon interface and decreased strength of the biceps tendon in these positions. In addition, posterior capsule contracture with consequential increased external rotation and decreased internal rotation of shoulders of overhead throwing athletes can lead to a peel-back phenomenon of the biceps anchor and internal impingement of the rotator cuff between the humerus and the posterosuperior labrum in the late cocking phase, leading to SLAP tears. This is especially true in patients who have over 25 to 30 degrees less internal rotation as compared to the contralateral shoulder.

Which one of the following physical examination maneuvers is not used to diagnose a SLAP tear?

A. Crank test
B. Load and shift test
C. O'Brien's test
D. Anterior slide test
E. Anterior apprehension test

Discussion

The correct answer is (B). This test is used to diagnose shoulder instability.

At this time, there is no highly sensitive or specific physical examination finding for SLAP tears. Authors who first describe the findings report good accuracy, but these findings are not replicated by independent examiners. However, there have been many maneuvers described to test for a SLAP tear including the Crank (Answer A), O'Brien (Answer C), anterior slide (Answer D), and anterior apprehension (Answer E) tests.

The O'Brien is one of the most common and is conducted as follows: the shoulder is flexed 90 degrees, internally rotated, and slightly adducted. Resisted shoulder flexion is performed in this position and then repeated with the shoulder externally rotated but still in 90 degrees of flexion and slightly adducted. If pain is experienced with internal rotation that is deep, anterior, and decreased with external rotation, the test is considered positive (see Fig. 2–21A–B).

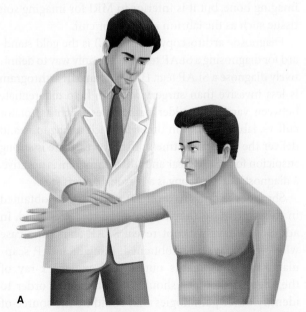 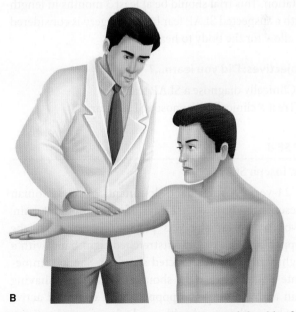

Figure 2–21 **(A–B)** O'Brien's active compression test. **Left:** resisted shoulder flexion in pronation. **Right:** resisted shoulder flexion in supination. (From Tennent TD, Beach WR, Meyers JF. A review of the special tests associated with shoulder examination. Part II: laxity, instability, and superior labral anterior and posterior (SLAP) lesions. *Am J Sports Med.* 2003;31(2):301–307.)

What is the next step in management?

A. Physical therapy and NSAIDs
B. Diagnostic arthroscopy
C. Arthroscopic debridement
D. Arthroscopic repair
E. Arthroscopic biceps tenodesis

Discussion

The correct answer is (A). Although there have been few studies that have reported on the efficacy of conservative treatment of SLAP tears, it is a good first step in treatment because of the low risk when compared with surgical treatment (Answers C, D, and E) and high potential benefit. Also, as stated above, it is difficult to diagnose a SLAP tear on physical examination, and other shoulder injuries can often exist concomitantly with SLAP tears. Attempting a trial of physical therapy could result in complete resolution of symptoms whether the symptoms are due to a SLAP tear, a different pathology, or multiple pathologies.

A trial of physical therapy should also be attempted before any additional diagnostic testing is performed, such as MRI, MR arthrogram, or diagnostic arthroscopy (Answer B) unless an injury is suspected that requires acute diagnosis and treatment, which is not the case with this patient.

Physical therapy should focus on strengthening the rotator cuff muscles and scapular stabilizers while restoring normal range of motion, especially internal rotation. This trial should be at least 3 months in length with a suspected SLAP tear before surgery is considered to allow for the body to heal itself.

Objectives: Did you learn...?

• Clinically diagnose a SLAP tear?
• Treat a clinically-diagnosed SLAP tear?

CASE 8

Dr. Joseph Statz

A 24-year-old, left-hand-dominant, businesswoman presents to clinic with 2 days of right shoulder pain. Two days prior she was playing soccer when she tripped and fell on an outstretched right hand with a slightly flexed and abducted shoulder. She felt immediate pain in her right shoulder and is now having pain and grinding and popping with overhead activity. She is otherwise healthy and takes no medications. On examination, she has grinding and popping with shoulder motion and a positive O'Brien's test, Hawkin's sign, Speed's test, and pain with anterior apprehension

testing. The rest of the examination is normal. X-rays are normal.

If conservative management with 6 weeks of physical therapy (PT) and NSAIDs fails, what is the next step in management?

A. CT arthrography
B. Diagnostic MRI
C. Diagnostic arthroscopy
D. Shoulder x-rays
E. Diagnostic MR arthrogram

Discussion

The correct answer is (E). MRI (Answer B) is the best type of imaging modality for imaging soft tissues, such as the labrum. In a labrum tear, there will be high signal intensity in the area of the tear usually around the biceps anchor, and sometimes a glenoid labral cyst can be found which has been found to be highly sensitive and specific for a labrum tear. MRI has been shown to have an 84% to 98% sensitivity, 63% to 91% specificity, and 74% to 96% accuracy. An MR arthrogram (Answer E) involves adding intra-articular contrast to an MRI, which increases visual contrast between the intra-articular soft tissue structures and synovial fluid, improving the sensitivity and specificity of MRI for diagnosing SLAP tears. Because of this increased benefit and with a high suspicion for a labral tear, an MR arthrogram should be obtained.

CT arthrography (Answer A) is better than MRI for imaging bone, but it is inferior to MRI for imaging soft tissue such as the labrum and rotator cuff.

Diagnostic arthroscopy (Answer C) is the gold standard for diagnosing a SLAP tear. It is the only way to definitively diagnose a SLAP tear. However, an MR arthrogram is less invasive than surgery and can help differentiate between various shoulder pathologies (such as rotator cuff vs. labrum tears) in order to reach a diagnosis and deliver the correct treatment. If, however, there is strong suspicion for a SLAP tear and MR arthrogram is negative, a diagnostic arthroscopy is a reasonable next step.

Shoulder x-rays (Answer D) were already obtained in this patient, so they do not need to be repeated. In addition, x-rays will not reveal SLAP tears. In a case where no x-rays were obtained, though, an AP, scapular AP, supraspinatus outlet, and axillary x-ray of the affected shoulder should be obtained in order to identify other pathologies that could be the source of shoulder pain.

An MR arthrogram shows the superior labrum is detached from the superior glenoid, and the biceps

tendon anchor is disrupted. How would this tear be classified according to the Snyder classification?

A. Type I
B. Type II
C. Type III
D. Type IV
E. Type V

Discussion

The correct answer is (B). The Snyder classification of SLAP tears is the first widely used classification systems for SLAP tears and consists of types I to IV (see Fig. 2–22A–B and Table 2–3). In type I tears (Answer A), there is fraying of the glenoid edge of the superior labrum, but the biceps tendon and superior labrum are both firmly attached to the biceps anchor and glenoid edge. In type II tears (Answer B), the biceps tendon and the superior labrum are detached from the superior glenoid edge and biceps anchor. In type III tears (Answer C), there is a bucket-handle tear of the superior labrum, but the remainder of the superior labrum and biceps tendon remain firmly attached to the glenoid rim and biceps anchor. In type IV tears (Answer D), there is a bucket-handle tear of the superior labrum that extends into the biceps tendon with extension of parts of the labral flap or biceps tendon into the joint space, and the remainder of the labrum and biceps tendon remain firmly attached to the glenoid rim and biceps anchor. Type V tears (Answer E) do not exist. Complex lesions do exist and typically consist of a combination of type II and IV tears.

If a type II tear is confirmed during diagnostic arthroscopy in the above patient, what treatment should be administered?

A. Labrum debridement
B. Biceps tenodesis
C. Labrum repair
D. Labrum reconstruction
E. Biceps tenotomy

Discussion

The correct answer is (C). Correct treatment of SLAP tears follows correct tear classification. If a patient has an unstable type II tear and are <25 to 30 years old, they should have a labrum repair, and that is the case in this patient. If a patient has an unstable type II tear and are >30 to 35 years old, they should have a biceps tenodesis. If they have a degenerative type II tear that is associated with other lesions, a labrum debridement (Answer A) can be performed and repair is usually unnecessary, especially if the patient is old and less active. This

patient has an acute, unstable Type II labrum tear and is young, so she should have a labrum repair.

If a patient has a type I or III tear, they should have a labrum debridement (Answer A). With a type III tear, this involves resecting the unstable labrum fragment and repairing the middle glenohumeral ligament (MGHL) to the labrum if it became detached with the unstable fragment.

If a patient is young or old and has a type IV tear, and if the tear involves less than 30% of the biceps tendon (meaning that greater than 70% of the biceps tendon is still intact), the unstable parts of the labrum and biceps tendon should be debrided. If a patient is old and has a type IV tear that involves more than 30% of the biceps tendon, a labrum debridement and biceps tenodesis/tenotomy should be performed (Answers B and E). If a patient is young and has a type IV tear that involves more than 30% of the biceps tendon, a repair of the labrum and biceps tenodesis/tenotomy should be performed. Labral reconstructions (Answer D) are rarely performed (see Table 2–3).

If, during diagnostic arthroscopy, the only significant finding is a cord-like, middle glenohumeral ligament that attaches to the base of the biceps anchor, and there is no labral tissue attached to the anterosuperior glenoid rim, what should be done?

A. Labrum repair by attaching the middle glenohumeral ligament to the glenoid rim
B. Nothing
C. Labrum reconstruction
D. Biceps tenodesis
E. Biceps tenotomy

Discussion

The correct answer is (B). This arthroscopic finding described is a Buford complex (Fig. 2–23B), and it is a normal anatomic variant that occurs in about 1.5% of shoulders. It consists of a cord-like middle glenohumeral ligament (MGHL) that attaches to the biceps anchor with a lack of labral tissue at the anterosuperior glenoid rim. If a Buford complex is misdiagnosed as a SLAP tear and the MGHL were anchored to the glenoid rim (Answer A), the patient could have significantly restricted range of motion, especially in external rotation.

There is no need to reconstruct the labrum (Answer C) or to tenodese or tenotomize the biceps tendon (Answers D and E) in this case because there is no pathology of these structures.

Other normal variants found in the shoulder that should be known include a sublabral foramen (Fig. 2–23A)

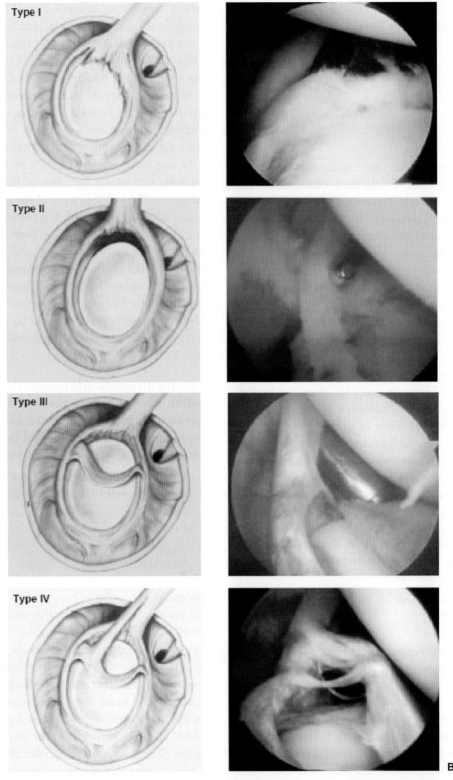

Figure 2-22 **(A–B)** Snyder classification of rotator cuff tears in cartoon and arthroscopic views. (From Mileski RA, Snyder SJ. Superior labral lesions in the shoulder: pathoanatomy and surgical management. *J Am Acad Orthop Surg.* 1998;6(2):121–131.)

Table 2–3   SNYDER CLASSIFICATION DESCRIPTION AND TREATMENT

Snyder Classification	Description of Labrum	Description of Biceps Tendon	Treatment
Type I	Fraying of glenoid edge	Intact	Labrum debridement
Type II	Detached from glenoid	Detached from anchor	Labrum repair if unstable and <25–30 y/o Biceps tenodesis if unstable and >30–35 y/o Labrum debridement if degenerative at any age
Type III	Bucket-handle tear	Intact	Labrum debridement with MGHL repair if detached
Type IV	Bucket-handle tear	Tear extends into biceps	If young or old and <30% biceps torn, labrum and biceps debridement If young and >30% biceps torn, labrum repair and biceps tenodesis/tenotomy If old and >30% biceps torn, labrum debridement and biceps tenodesis/tenotomy

From Mileski RA, Snyder SJ. Superior labral lesions in the shoulder: pathoanatomy and surgical management. *J Am Acad Orthop Surg.* (1998);6(2):121–131.

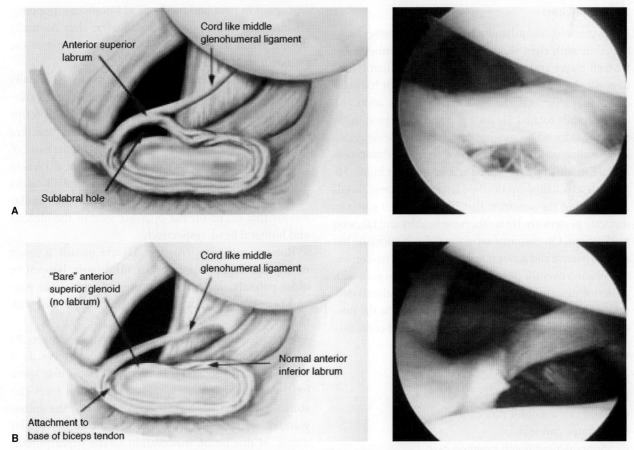

Figure 2–23 Two normal variants of labral anatomy. **A, Top:** sublabral foramen at 2 o'clock position. **B, Bottom:** Buford complex. (From Mileski RA, Snyder SJ. Superior labral lesions in the shoulder: pathoanatomy and surgical management. *J Am Acad Orthop Surg.* 1998;6(2):121–131.)

at about 2 o'clock position on a right shoulder that occurs in about 3.3% of shoulders and a sublabral foramen with a cord-like MGHL that occurs in about 8.6% of shoulders. Another normal variant is a meniscoid superior labrum in which the inner lip of the labrum partially covers the glenoid articular cartilage. True SLAP tears can be differentiated from these normal variants because they show hemorrhage or granulation tissue at the base of the biceps tendon or under the labrum, and there is a space between the glenoid articular cartilage and the superior labrum/biceps tendon that can be mobilized 3 to 4 mm with traction of the biceps tendon.

Objectives: Did you learn...?

- Diagnose a SLAP tear through imaging?
- Classify SLAP tears?
- Recognize normal labrum variants that can resemble SLAP tears?

CASE 9

Dr. Joseph Statz

A 25-year-old, right-hand-dominant man presents to the clinic with right shoulder pain. He is a professional football player and plays as an offensive lineman. Three days ago, he was blocking with his hands with his right elbow fully extended and his shoulder flexed, adducted, and internally rotated. He felt a pop and sharp pain in his right shoulder when making contact with the defender. He was diagnosed with a posterior shoulder dislocation in the ER, which was relocated and he was sent home. He presents as a follow-up in clinic having persistent shoulder pain and the sensation that his shoulder is going to dislocate posteriorly. He is otherwise healthy and takes no medications. On examination of the right shoulder, he has normal passive and active range of motion, but tenderness to palpation over the posterior joint line. He has pain with posterior stress test, and the rest of the examination is normal. X-rays show a small bone fragment next to the posterior glenoid rim with a normal humeral head contour.

What is the most likely diagnosis?

A. Posterior labrum tear
B. SLAP tear
C. Anterior shoulder dislocation
D. Rotator cuff tear
E. Supraglenoid notch ganglion cyst

Discussion

The correct answer is (A). Posterior shoulder dislocations classically occur when the patient's shoulder is the recipient of trauma while it is flexed, adducted, and internally rotated (as in this case). When the shoulder dislocates posteriorly or when the shoulder relocates, the humeral head can tear the posterior labrum and sometimes avulse off part of the posterior glenoid with the labrum (reverse Bankart lesion), which is present in this case as shown by the small bone fragment on the x-ray. The glenoid can also collapse part of the anterior humeral head articular surface, resulting in a reverse Hill–Sachs lesion, which is not present in this case as shown by the normal humeral head contour on the x-ray. This can lead to posterior instability due to the lack of a functional posterior labrum, which normally helps to deepen the joint and act as a mechanical block, preventing the humeral head from displacing posteriorly. Patients also experience shoulder pain over the posterior joint line, where the tear is located.

SLAP tears (Answer B) occur usually due to compression or traction injuries, not posterior dislocations, and result in pain and mechanical symptoms (popping, clicking, and catching) of the shoulder. They normally do not result in posterior instability or pain over the posterior joint line.

Anterior shoulder dislocations (Answer C) usually occur with the shoulder flexed, abducted, and externally rotated. They can result in or be caused by anterior instability, and one may find a Bankart (chip fracture of the anterior glenoid) or Hill–Sachs (compression of posterior articular surface of the humeral head) lesion on radiographs. Reverse Bankart and reverse Hill–Sachs lesions are called "reverse" because they are similar lesions that occur on the opposite side of the glenoid and humeral head, respectively.

Rotator cuff tears (Answer D) are usually a result of chronic degeneration, occur insidiously, happen in older patients, and classically present with night pain and pain with overhead motion. This does not fit with the picture presented in the current case.

Supraglenoid notch ganglion cysts (Answer E) cause compression of the suprascapular nerve as it passes around the lateral border of the scapular spine by the spinoglenoid notch. Posterior labral tears can sometimes result in formation of a cyst in the spinoglenoid notch, which can compress the suprascapular nerve. At this point, innervation to the supraspinatus has already occurred, so compression at the spinoglenoid notch would result in infraspinatus dysfunction with normal supraspinatus function. This patient has normal motion with no evidence of neuropathy or infraspinatus pathology. He likely has a posterior labral tear with a reverse Bankart and not a compressive spinoglenoid notch cyst.

Which of the following physical examination maneuvers is not used to diagnose a posterior labrum tear?

A.   Posterior stress test
B.   Jerk test
C.   Posterior load and shift test
D.   Kim test
E.   Apprehension test

Discussion

The correct answer is (E). The apprehension test is used to diagnose anterior instability. It is performed by having the patient lie supine and the examiner passively abduct and externally rotate the patient's shoulder. If the patient feels as if the shoulder is going to dislocate anteriorly, the test is positive.

Physical examination maneuvers to test for a posterior labral tear overlap with those for posterior instability because the former can be one of the causes of the latter. The posterior stress test is performed by: lying the patient supine, flexing the shoulder and elbow to 90 degrees, internally rotating the shoulder then putting a posteriorly directed force on the flexed elbow down the shaft of the humerus with one hand, and palpating any posterior subluxation or dislocation of the humerus out of the glenoid with the other hand against the posterior shoulder (see Fig. 2–24). The test is positive if any subluxation or dislocation is palpated.

The jerk test (Answer B) is performed with the patient in a sitting position. The examiner flexes the shoulder to 90 degrees, fully internally rotates the shoulder,

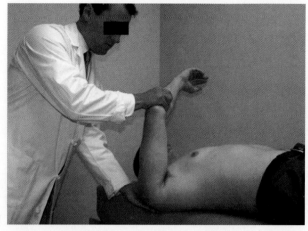

Figure 2–24 Posterior stress test. (From Millett PJ, Clavert P, Hatch GFR, Warner JJP. Recurrent posterior shoulder instability. *J Am Acad Orthop Surg.* 2006;14(8):464–476.)

and flexes the elbow to 90 degrees. The examiner then pushes on the flexed elbow in a posterior direction down the shaft of the humerus (see Fig. 2–25). A positive test is when the shoulder subluxes or dislocates posteriorly. If the shoulder dislocates, the shoulder is then extended, and the humeral head will relocate with a jerking motion, hence the name of the test.

The posterior load and shift test (Answer C) is performed with the patient seated and the arm at the side. The examiner holds with one hand the patient's humerus by gripping anteriorly and posteriorly just below the greater tuberosity. The examiner pushes the humeral head into the glenoid while attempting to displace the humerus posteriorly (see Fig. 2–26). The test is positive if there is a greater than 50% displacement of the humeral head out of the glenoid.

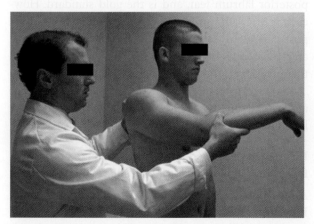

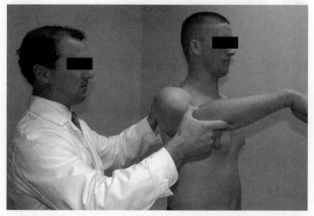

Figure 2–25 Jerk test. (From Millett PJ, Clavert P, Hatch GFR, Warner JJP. Recurrent posterior shoulder instability. *J Am Acad Orthop Surg.* 2006;14(8):464–476.)

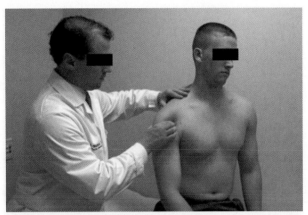 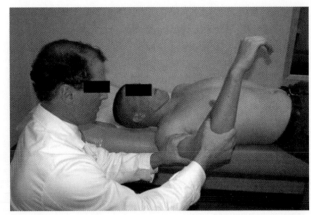

Figure 2–26 Load and shift test. (From Millett PJ, Clavert P, Hatch GFR, Warner JJP. Recurrent posterior shoulder instability. *J Am Acad Orthop Surg.* 2006;14(8):464–476.)

What is the diagnostic study of choice for a posterior labrum tear?

A. CT scan
B. Arthroscopy
C. MRI
D. MR arthrogram
E. X-ray

Discussion

The correct answer is (D). MRI (Answer C) is exceptional at imaging soft tissue structures, including the

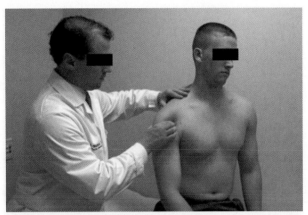

Figure 2–27 Axial T1 MR arthrogram of right shoulder showing posterior Bankart lesion. (From Rouleau DM, Hebert-Davies J, Robinson CM. Acute traumatic posterior shoulder dislocation. *J Am Acad Orthop Surg.* 2014;22(3):145–152.)

labrum (see Fig. 2–27). Adding contrast dye into the glenohumeral joint with an MR arthrogram increases the sensitivity, specificity, and accuracy for diagnosis of a labral tear even further, making this the test of choice. In a patient with a posterior dislocation without an associated fracture of the humerus, obtaining an MRI/MR arthrogram is essential. Injury to the posterior labrum occurs in 58% of these cases. If a patient has an irreducible, posterior shoulder dislocation, it is usually due to soft tissue interposition, and MRI/MR arthrogram can identify what structure is blocking the relocation.

A CT scan (Answer A) is very useful for preoperative planning in case of fractures associated with dislocations or if there is a reverse Hill–Sachs lesion. This would not be as good as MRI for imaging soft tissues.

Arthroscopy (Answer B) would be more invasive than MR arthrogram, carrying with it surgical risks. MR arthrogram is an excellent modality for diagnosing posterior labrum tear, and is the gold standard. However, if MR arthrogram fails to make a diagnosis and a posterior labral tear is still highly suspected, performing an arthroscopy should be considered for diagnostic and therapeutic purposes.

X-rays (Answer E) were already obtained in this case and would not be helpful in diagnosing a posterior labral tear.

If surgery is required, what is the preferred treatment for an isolated, posterior labrum tear?

A. Arthroscopic labrum repair
B. Open repair
C. Physical therapy, NSAIDs, and glenohumeral joint corticosteroid injections

D. Arthroscopic capsular shift

E. Open reconstruction

Discussion

The correct answer is (A). Of patients with posterior shoulder instability, those with reverse Bankart lesions are ideal candidates for arthroscopic repair. Arthroscopic repair is relatively contraindicated in those who have had prior arthroscopic repairs that failed, avulsion of the glenohumeral ligaments off of the humerus, and those with symptomatic multidirectional instability in patients with connective tissue disease such as Ehlers–Danlos. This is not contraindicated, however, if a patient with a connective tissue disease is symptomatic only posteriorly. In patients with posterior instability who have malformed glenoid bone, either eroded or retroverted, arthroscopic repair is absolutely contraindicated because a bone-altering surgery is required.

One can perform the arthroscopy with three or four portals, putting one or two posteriorly and two anteriorly, making sure the posterior portal is lateral enough to access the posterior glenoid rim. An anterosuperior portal is used for the camera and a mid-anterior portal is used for instruments and suture passing. Both anterior portals are placed in the rotator interval. To repair the reverse Bankart, suture anchors are passed through the mid-anterior portal and used to reattach the labrum.

Open repair (Answer B) can be used to repair many causes of posterior shoulder instability including posterior capsular shifts or bony repairs but is not the preferred method to repair a posterior labral injury. Conservative treatment (Answer C) should not be tried if surgical treatment is required, as the question stem stated. However, a trial conservative treatment should be tried in patients with posterior instability because of its low morbidity and high efficacy. Studies have shown that nonsurgical treatment is effective for 65% to 80% of cases of posterior instability.

Arthroscopic shifts (Answer D) can be used to tighten the posterior capsule if that is the etiology of posterior instability. However, in this case, the patient has instability due to a posterior labrum tear, so tightening the posterior capsule would not be as effective as repairing the labrum tear.

Reconstructive surgeries (Answer E) are not normally required to treat cases of posterior instability associated with posterior labrum tears because the labrum can normally be repaired. They can be used if there is a focal defect in the glenoid bone, though.

Objectives: Did you learn…?

- Diagnose a posterior labrum tear based on history and physical examination?
- Surgically treat a posterior labrum tear?

CASE 10

Dr. Joseph Statz

A 30-year-old, right-hand-dominant man presents to clinic complaining of anterior right shoulder pain. There is pain mostly with overhead movement that radiates to the biceps muscle belly. He takes no medications, is otherwise healthy, and works as a car mechanic. He is an avid volleyball player. His examination includes a positive Hawkins test, positive Yerguson's test, tenderness to palpation over the intertubercular sulcus, and a negative Speed's test. The rest of the examination is normal. Plain radiographs are normal.

What is the most likely diagnosis?

A. Long head of the biceps tendonitis

B. Subscapularis tendon tear

C. SLAP tear

D. Subacromial bursitis

E. Anterior labroligamentous periosteal sleave avulsion (ALPSA)

Discussion

The correct answer is (A). Isolated biceps tendonitis tends to occur in young patients who participate in overhead sports. In older patients, it almost always occurs in associations with other pathologies, such as rotator cuff disease, labral pathology, or AC joint problems. Regardless of age, though, biceps tendonitis tends to present with anterior to anteromedial shoulder pain that can radiate to the biceps and is worse with repetitive use.

Subscapularis tendon tears (Answer B) can lead to biceps tendon subluxation out of the intertubercular sulcus, which can lead to irritation and inflammation of the biceps tendon. However, this patient does not have any other symptoms or signs of a subscapularis tear.

A SLAP tear (Answer C) can also be found with biceps tendonitis as the long head of the biceps tendon originates proximally at the superior labrum. However, this patient is not having mechanical symptoms that would be associated with a SLAP tear, and his presentation is more consistent with biceps tendonitis.

Subacromial bursitis (Answer D) is another pathology often found with biceps tendonitis, but the patient's presentation resembles biceps tendonitis more so than subacromial bursitis.

Anterior labral periosteal sleeve avulsion (ALPSA) (Answer D) occurs most commonly with an anterior shoulder dislocation when the humeral head causes a Bankart lesion that also pulls the glenoid periosteum off the glenoid bone. This can result in anterior shoulder pain. This patient does not have any evidence of shoulder dislocation, and the presentation is consistent with biceps tendonitis.

Which of the following is not a physical examination finding in biceps tendon pathology?

A. Positive Speed's test
B. Positive Yerguson's test
C. Tenderness to palpation over the intertubercular sulcus
D. Positive apprehension test
E. Popeye deformity

Discussion

The correct answer is (D). The apprehension test is used to help diagnose anterior shoulder instability. It is performed with the patient supine. The examiner abducts the shoulder to 90 degrees, flexes the elbow to 90 degrees, and then externally rotates the shoulder. If the patient experiences a sensation that the shoulder is going to dislocate anteriorly, the test is positive.

Speed's test (Answer A) is performed by having the patient flex the shoulder to 90 degrees with an extended elbow and supinated forearm. He is then asked to flex the shoulder against resistance. A positive test is when the patient feels pain in the bicipital groove. This test is specific but not sensitive for biceps tendonitis, SLAP lesions, and biceps rupture.

Yerguson's test (Answer B) is performed with the elbow flexed to 90 degrees at the patient's side. The examiner grasps the patient's hand as if giving a hand shake and asks the patient to supinate against resistance. The examiner then palpates the patient's proximal biceps. If the patient feels pain in the bicipital groove, the test is positive. This test, like Speed's test, is specific but not sensitive for biceps tendonitis, SLAP lesions, and biceps rupture.

Tenderness to palpation over the intertubercular groove (Answer C) is indicative of biceps tendonitis.

A Popeye deformity (Answer E) occurs when the patient is asked to flex the elbow, and the biceps is seen to bunch up much more than the contralateral biceps. This is indicative of biceps tendon rupture, which can happen rarely in severe cases of biceps tendonitis.

If the above patient is clinically diagnosed with biceps tendonitis, what is the preferred initial management?

A. Biceps tenotomy
B. Biceps tenodesis
C. Reconstruction of the transverse humeral ligament
D. Physical therapy, rest, NSAIDs, cryotherapy, and corticosteroid injections
E. Biceps repair

Discussion

The correct answer is (D). Like many shoulder injuries, first line treatment is conservative since it is better to treat noninvasively if there is a good chance the treatment is successful. Any type of surgery (Answers A, B, C, and E) carries with it significant risk and should be carried out only after failure of several weeks of conservative treatment. Injections can be given in the glenohumeral joint, since the biceps runs through it, or in the biceps tendon sheath in the intertubercular groove. When given in the groove, though, the injection should ideally be placed in the sheath around the tendon and not in the tendon itself.

Which of the following is not an indication for surgical intervention with long head of the biceps tendon pathology?

A. "Hourglass" biceps tendon on arthroscopy
B. 20% thickness tear
C. Subscapularis tear with biceps tendon subluxation
D. Isolated medial biceps tendon subluxation
E. Inflamed "lipstick" biceps tendon on arthroscopy

Discussion

The correct answer is (B). Tears that are 25% thickness or less are usually not considered to need operative management. Those that are over 25% to 50% thickness are considered to need operative intervention. All the other choices are indications for surgical intervention, whether it be a tenotomy or a tenodesis.

An "hourglass" biceps tendon (Answer A) is one in which the intra-articular portion has hypertrophied to a point that it is not able to slide into the bicipital groove when the arm is flexed. When this occurs, the tendon

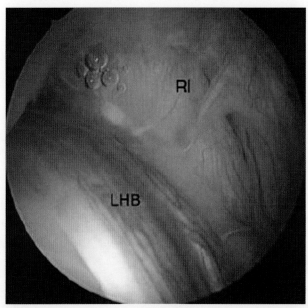

Figure 2–28 Arthroscopic view of left inflamed biceps tendon ("lipstick biceps"). LHB, long head of the biceps; RI, rotator interval.

bunches up in the joint and gets pinched between the humeral head and the glenoid, giving an appearance of an hourglass on arthroscopy when pinched. This causes a block to shoulder flexion of over 10 degrees. Surgical intervention will fix this problem.

A subscapularis tear with subluxation of the biceps tendon (Answer C), an isolated medial biceps tendon subluxation (Answer D), and an inflamed biceps tendon on arthroscopy (Answer E) all have high success rates when treated surgically. A "lipstick" biceps is so named because the inflammation causes the tendon to turn red, appearing as if there was lipstick applied to it (see Fig. 2–28).

If the patient were elderly, what would be the preferred surgical intervention?

A.   Biceps tenotomy
B.   Biceps tenodesis
C.   Reconstruction of the transverse humeral ligament
D.   Physical therapy, rest, NSAIDs, cryotherapy, and corticosteroid injections
E.   Biceps repair

Discussion
The correct answer is (A). Both biceps tenotomy and tenodesis (Answer B) have high success in alleviating symptoms and in patient satisfaction. Biceps tenotomy

has a higher incidence of a Popeye sign, cramping with extensive arm flexion, and pain in the bicipital groove. However, a change in arm aesthetics with a Popeye sign is less likely to matter to an elderly patient. The cramping with extensive arm flexion usually only occurs in patients less than 40 years old, and the pain in the bicipital groove does not translate into decreased function or patient satisfaction as compared to tenodesis. These three factors, however, might make the increased difficulty of performing a tenodesis worth it for a younger patient and some active, healthy, elderly individuals.

Reconstruction of the transverse humeral ligament (Answer C) is not a surgery that is performed nor is a biceps repair (Answer E). Conservative treatment (Answer D) is not a surgical intervention, so it is an incorrect answer to this question.

If on physical examination there was a loss of deltoid contour visible at the anterior border or the middle deltoid, what pathology is likely present?

A.   Massive rotator cuff tear with deltoid rupture
B.   Isolated massive rotator cuff tear
C.   Anterior shoulder dislocation
D.   AC joint dislocation
E.   AC joint osteoarthritis

Discussion
The correct answer is (A). With a massive rotator cuff tear, there can be superior translation of the humeral head that causes the humeral head to articulate with the acromion around the insertion of the anterior part of the middle deltoid. The humeral head can then erode the deltoid insertion off of the acromion, causing deltoid rupture and a visible defect on physical examination. If this is not identified and repaired early, functional outcomes are usually terrible.

Which of the following is not a predictor for less-favorable outcomes after rotator cuff repair surgery?

A.   Diabetes
B.   Age
C.   Worker's compensation status
D.   Supraspinatus muscle atrophy
E.   Infraspinatus muscle fatty degeneration

Discussion
The correct answer is (A). No study to date has shown diabetes to be a predictor of less favorable outcomes after rotator cuff repair surgery. Increasing age (Answer B), having a worker's compensation status (Answer C),

supraspinatus muscle atrophy (Answer D), and infraspinatus muscle atrophy and fatty degeneration (Answer E) have all been shown to result in both reduced tendon-bone healing and worse functional scores after rotator cuff repair surgery. Supraspinatus muscle fatty degeneration has been shown to have worse healing but has not been shown to result in lower clinical outcomes.

How long does it take for bone–tendon healing to occur?

A.   0 to 2 weeks
B.   2 to 4 weeks
C.   4 to 8 weeks
D.   8 to 12 weeks
E.   12 to 16 weeks

Discussion

The correct answer is (D). The terminal tendon of the rotator cuff (RC) is relatively avascular, unable to heal itself, and gets more avascular as people age. Because of this, most vascularity that helps to heal the RC in a repair comes from the holes drilled in the greater tuberosity. This also means that the healing process is slow after repair and is likely to take between 8 and 12 weeks for the tendon to heal to the greater tuberosity, which requires limited passive and no active ROM postoperatively. For a repair with a latissimus dorsi transfer, which will be discussed below, the patient should be braced and immobilized for 6 weeks at 45 degrees abduction and 30 degrees external rotation.

Objectives: Did you learn...?

- Clinically diagnose biceps tendonitis based on history and physical examination?
- Treat biceps tendonitis both conservatively and surgically?
- Decide between biceps tenotomy and tenodesis?

CASE 11

Dr. Gautam Malhotra

A 33-year-old male presents to the ED after a fall during a soccer game. He reports significant right shoulder pain and limited ROM. An x-ray taken in the ED is shown below (Fig. 2–29).

What is the next most appropriate step?

A.   Obtain an axillary view x-ray
B.   Recommend sling immobilization and no soccer for 1 week
C.   Recommend initiating gentle ROM and PT for a shoulder contusion

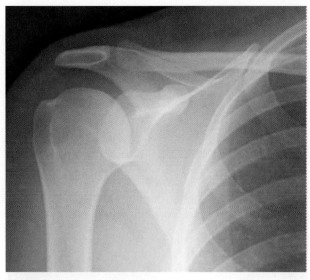

Figure 2–29

D.   Obtain an MRI to evaluate for a rotator cuff tear
E.   Obtain an MR arthrogram to evaluate for a labral tear

Discussion

The correct answer is (A). The ED image shown in Figure 2–29 includes only an AP view of the right shoulder. In the setting of an acute injury and pain, technicians may be hesitant to obtain additional views. A single view, however, is insufficient to diagnose either a fracture, as orthogonal views are required, or a shoulder dislocation which is best seen on an axillary view (see Fig. 2–30). Answers B and C are inappropriate as a diagnosis has not been established yet and a dislocation or fracture must be conclusively ruled out. Answers D and E may be options that are exercised in the clinic but do not represent the next step in the management of this patient.

Traumatic anterior instability is a common shoulder problem with an estimated incidence of 1.7%. This term encompasses both frank dislocations that require a manual reduction as well as incomplete subluxations that spontaneously reduce. It is particularly common in the young and athletic population, and it is significantly more common than other forms of instability including posterior or multidirectional instability. Understanding the natural history of anterior instability is important, as it serves as a guide to treatment. Young patients have a very high risk of recurrence; patients <20 years old have a 90% recurrence risk, between 20 and 40 years old have a 60% recurrence risk, and >40 years old have a

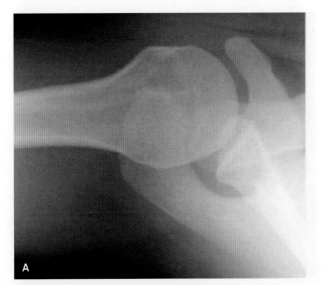 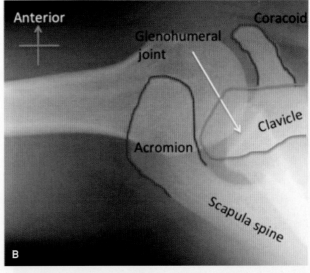

Figure 2-30 **A:** Axillary view. **B:** Axillary view with annotations.

10% risk. Recurrent events are a predictor for arthritis and necessitate aggressive treatment, particularly in the young patient.

On evaluation, a thorough history and physical should be performed. Eliciting the mechanism and position of the arm at the time of dislocation can be helpful in determining the direction of primary instability. Anterior dislocations usually occur with the arm in an abducted and externally rotated position. If the patient presents with a nonreduced anteriorly dislocated shoulder, the arm is usually held in adduction and internal rotation; abduction of the arm is particularly limited. Prior to a reduction attempt, a thorough neurovascular examination must be performed paying close attention to the axillary nerve.

Generally speaking, treatment for first-time dislocators after the initial reduction involves conservative treatment in the form of physical therapy focusing on ROM and strengthening of the dynamic shoulder stabilizers. Some authors advocate a short duration of immobilization prior to initiating PT, although recent studies have failed to demonstrate any benefit to immobilization in either an externally or internally rotated position. After a single dislocation event, the need for surgery is often dictated by associated injuries. Glenoid bone loss >20%, a Hill-Sacks lesion >20% to 40%, a displaced fracture, an irreducible shoulder, or a large cuff tear in a young patient may be indicators for surgery. Recurrent instability after conservative management is considered a failure of treatment and is also an indication for surgery.

Additional Questions

A 19-year-old woman presents to your clinic after a single dislocation episode that occurred during a motor vehicle accident. Her shoulder was reduced on the field.

What is the likelihood that she will have a successful outcome with nonoperative treatment?

A. 20%
B. 40%
C. 60%
D. 80%
E. 95%

Discussion

The answer is (A). It has been shown that traumatic dislocations in young patients have a high rate of recurrence. Patients with hyperlaxity who dislocate without a large traumatic event have a higher success rate with nonoperative treatment. Nevertheless, nonoperative treatment is still the initial modality of choice in this patient.

A 22-year-old, recreational basketball player dislocates his shoulder during a game. A reduction is performed on the field and he comes to see you in clinic 1 week later.

What will his MR arthrogram most likely show?

A. Labral tear
B. Rotator cuff tear
C. Biceps tendon subluxation
D. Hill–Sacks lesion
E. ALPSA lesion

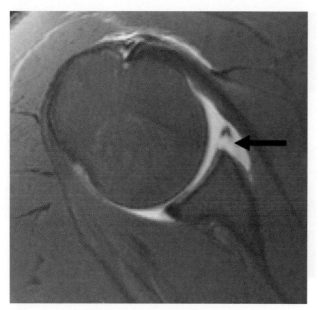

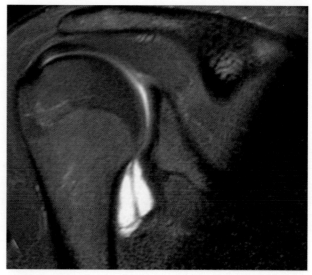

Figure 2–32

Figure 2–31 MRA demonstrating an anterior labral tear.

Discussion

The correct answer is (A). In a young patient, the most likely injury associated with a glenohumeral dislocation is a labral tear (see Fig. 2–31). In an older patient, >40 years old, a rotator cuff tear is more likely. Other possible associated injuries include:

- Bony Bankart
- Hill–Sachs
- Humeral avulsion of the glenohumeral ligament (HAGL)
- Glenoid labral articular defect (GLAD)
- Anterior labral periosteal sleeve avulsion (ALPSA)
- Fracture
- Axillary nerve injury (estimated to occur 5% of the time)

These all are less common than a labral tear. Each of these injuries need to be identified and treated appropriately at the time of surgery to ensure a satisfactory outcome.

A 24-year-old, male athlete sustains an anterior shoulder dislocation. His MRI is shown in Figure 2–32.

Which of the following ligaments is injured?

A. Anterior band of the inferior glenohumeral ligament
B. Posterior band of the inferior glenohumeral ligament
C. Superior glenohumeral ligament
D. Coracohumeral ligament
E. Middle glenohumeral ligament

Discussion

The correct answer is (A). The MRI demonstrates an HAGL lesion. The MR arthrogram shows fluid extending down the medial humerus and is indicative of an HAGL. Most commonly, with an anterior dislocation, the anterior band of the inferior glenohumeral ligament is torn. With a posterior dislocation, the posterior band is torn creating a reverse HAGL. The ligament tends to tear off the humeral side. These are important injuries to identify as arthroscopic labral repair and capsular shift may be unsuccessful without concomitant repair of the HAGL lesion. Many authors advocate an open approach to repair an HAGL lesion.

A sophomore, high school wide receiver presents to your clinic at the beginning of his football season. He reports a dislocation event after being tackled; his shoulder was "put back in place" by the on-field athletic trainer. A CT scan taken in the hospital today is shown (Fig. 2–33). He has been recruited by numerous colleges, plans to play at a division 1 school, and is very eager to return to the field.

What is the best treatment option for this patient?

A. Bracing, PT, and return to play this season once patient can tolerate sports specific drills
B. Bracing, PT, and sit out for the remainder of the season

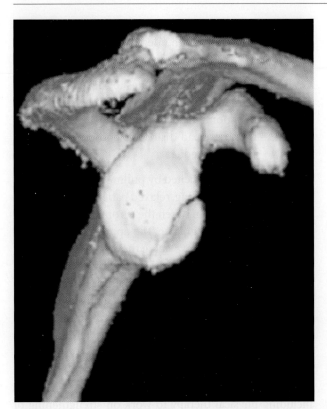

Figure 2–33

C. Latarjet procedure
D. Magnuson–Stack procedure
E. ORIF of anterior glenoid

Discussion

The correct answer is (E). A large bony fragment (>20%) makes the failure rate with nonoperative treatment (Answers A, B) unacceptably high. This question is meant to illustrate the challenges associated with treating an in-season athlete and highlighting the indications for surgery after a first time dislocation event. Typically, early in a season, providers will initiate an aggressive PT program and try and return athletes to the field within a few weeks so that they can play out the remainder of the season. Towards the end of the season, when there is insufficient time to rehab a patient, one may choose early surgery so that the patient has maximal time to recover prior to the next season. In this case, even though the patient is extremely motivated to return to the field and has only sustained a single dislocation event, the large bony Bankart lesion behooves surgical treatment. The best option for him would be to have early surgery and have a maximal amount of time to prepare for his senior season. A Latarjet procedure (Answer C) is used for patients

with recurrent anterior instability and significant glenoid bone loss, and the Magnuson–Stack procedure (Answer D) is a largely historic procedure that was used for recurrent anterior instability.

Objectives: Did you learn...?

- The common presentation of a patient with shoulder instability?
- The concomitant injuries that frequently occur with a shoulder dislocation?
- The treatment options for first time dislocators?
- The challenges associated with treating an in-season athlete?

CASE 12

Dr. Gautam Malhotra

A 28-year-old, recreational athlete presents to your clinic with shoulder pain and a history of multiple subluxations in the past. He describes a recent frank dislocation that had to be "popped" back in place on the field. His imaging is shown below (Fig. 2–34).

What treatment is most appropriate?

A. Capsulolabral repair
B. Latarjet
C. Remplissage
D. Remplissage and Bankart procedures
E. Putti–Platt procedure

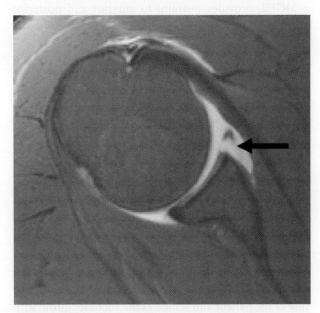

Figure 2–34

Discussion

The correct answer is (A). The question describes a young, athletic patient with a history of multiple instability events, and as such, he is very prone to subsequent instability events. Although the initial treatment involves physical therapy, it is likely that this patient will require surgical stabilization. The image demonstrates a located shoulder with a small Hill–Sachs lesion and no significant glenoid bone loss, making capsulolabral repair the appropriate treatment option. For a patient with a failed capsulolabral repair or significant anterior bone loss (>20%), a Latarjet procedure is employed. A Remplissage (Answer C) is indicated for a large Hill–Sachs lesion, which is not seen on the image provided. A Putti–Platt procedure (Answer E) involves a vest-over-pants imbrication with the goal of shortening the subscapularis and anterior capsule. This procedure was historically used for anterior instability but has been replaced by more modern techniques as it causes a significant restriction of external rotation.

Following a single, traumatic, anterior dislocation, several factors may contribute to a patient developing recurrent anterior instability. The most common of these is an anteroinferior capsulolabral avulsion. Other contributing factors include glenoid bone loss (which may be in the form of an identifiable fragment or attritional loss), a Hill–Sachs lesion, generalized hyperlaxity, younger age, and damage to static shoulder stabilizers. These include:

- Anterior band of IGHL—provides restraint to anterior and inferior subluxation with the arm in 90 degrees of abduction and external rotation (late cocking phase)
- MGHL provides restraint to anterior and posterior subluxation with arm in 45 degrees of abduction and external rotation
- SGHL provides restraint to inferior subluxation with arm at the side

On evaluation, a thorough history and physical examination should be performed. Understanding the patient's functional demands and the activities and positions that are associated with instability events will be helpful in guiding treatment and formulating a rehab strategy. The physical examination begins with a visual examination followed by range of motion, strength testing, and a thorough neurovascular examination; these are usually unremarkable. Specific tests and signs include the load and shift test, sulcus sign, and apprehension/relocation test. The load and shift test is performed in both the standing and supine position. The examiner stands to the side of the patient and stabilizes the shoulder girdle with one hand while grasping and pushing the humeral head anteriorly and posteriorly with the other hand. A grade is assigned to the degree of humeral head translation.

Grade 0—minimal translation

Grade 1—humeral head translates to the glenoid rim

Grade 2—humeral head translates over the glenoid rim but spontaneously reduces

Grade 3—humeral head dislocates and does not spontaneously reduce

The sulcus sign is elicited by pulling straight down on the humerus of a standing, relaxed patient. A positive test is marked by a divot between the acromion and humeral head that is 2 cm or greater. The apprehension–relocation test is performed by placing the arm in 90 degrees of abduction and external rotation; passive external rotation beyond this associated with pain or a sensation of impending dislocation is indicative of a positive test. The examiner's second hand is then placed anteriorly and used to push the humeral head posteriorly; this describes the relocation test, and patients will report an alleviation of the sensation of impending dislocation.

Treatment usually begins with conservative measures including physical therapy to work on strengthening of the dynamic shoulder stabilizers and activity modification to avoid proactive positions. Patients will frequently require surgical treatment, particularly those with a history of significant trauma. Broadly speaking, there are two surgical options: those that deal primarily with soft tissue and those that involve bony reconstruction of the anterior glenoid. The type of surgical treatment employed is based on the degree of glenoid bone loss. For bone loss <15%, a standard arthroscopic capsulolabral repair can be utilized. For bone loss >25%, a bony stabilization procedure is necessary. In the 15% to 25% range, opinions vary, and one must exercise clinical judgment. Specific treatment options are further discussed in Table 2–1.

Additional Questions

An 18-year-old male with a history of recurrent anterior instability is seeking surgical treatment after having failed a course of extensive PT. His examination demonstrates a Grade 2 load and shift test and positive sulcus sign. His MRA is shown in Fig. 2–35.

What is the best treatment option?

A. Putti–Platt procedure
B. Bristow coracoid transfer
C. Meyer–Burgdorff procedure
D. Isolated Bankart repair
E. Bankart repair with capsular shift

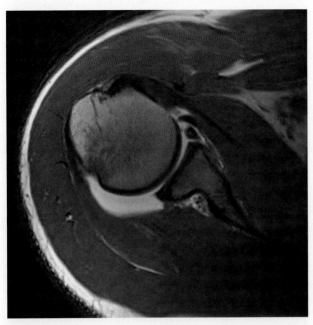

Figure 2–35

Discussion

The correct answer is (E). The question stem describes recurrent anterior instability that has failed conservative treatment and hence necessitates surgical intervention. Several surgical procedures have been described for anterior instability. In the absence of significant bone loss, the most common procedure utilized is an arthroscopic Bankart repair and capsular shift. The image provided does not demonstrate any significant bone loss, making this the correct answer. An isolated Bankart repair (Answer D) will restore the bumper effect that an intact labrum provides but will not restore the sling effect of the normal anterior capsule. A Bristow procedure (Answer B) would be appropriate in the setting of significant anterior glenoid bone loss. The other procedures represent nonanatomic procedures that are largely historical.

The various procedures described for anterior instability are listed in Table 2–4.

Table 2–4   DESCRIBED PROCEDURES FOR SHOULDER INSTABILITY

Procedure	Description
Putti–Platt[a]	Vest-over-pants imbrication with the goal of shortening the subscapularis and anterior capsule. Leads to over-constraint and stiffness
Magnuson–Stack[a]	Subscapularis transfer to a more lateral position. Leads to over-constraint and stiffness
Weber[a]	Humeral rotational osteotomy
Meyer–Burgdorff[a]	Glenoid anteverting osteotomy
Boyd–Sisk[a]	Transfer of biceps laterally and posteriorly
Arthroscopic Bankart repair	Bone anchors and sutures are used to reattach the anterior labrum to the glenoid
Open Bankart repair	Largely being replaced by arthroscopic techniques, however, may be used in the setting of large associated Hill–Sachs lesions or HAGL lesions
Capsular shift	Frequently done in conjunction with a Bankart repair. Together these are referred to as a capsulolabral repair
Du-Toit	A Bankart repair using staples instead of suture—uncommonly used secondary to a high complication rate
Bristow coracoid transfer	Used for anterior glenoid bone loss. Transfer of coracoid bone and strap muscles for a sling effect. The coracoid is transferred and fixed perpendicular to the base of the anterior glenoid
Latarjet	Compared to the Bristow a larger piece of coracoid is transferred and placed parallel to the anterior glenoid. This procedure is generally favored over the Bristow
Bone graft	Bone graft to the anterior glenoid is often employed in revision situations with significant anterior glenoid bone loss. The inner table of the iliac crest has a contour that matches the anterior glenoid with the concave inner table facing laterally and the cancellous bone sitting on the glenoid rim
Glenoid ORIF	If a large anterior glenoid fragment is evident as may be the case after a single acute dislocation event re-fixating with anchors or screws can often restore anterior stability

[a]Historic procedures that have been replaced by more "anatomic" reconstructions.

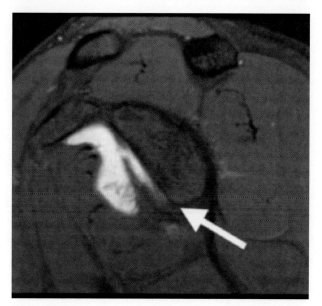

Figure 2–36

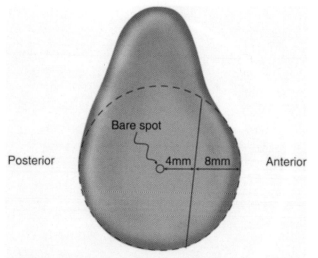

Figure 2–37 Sagittal depiction of the glenoid. Bone loss of 8 mm in the AP direction corresponds to approximately 35% and will likely require bony reconstruction. (Reproduced with permission from Piasecki DP, Verma NN, Romeo AA, et al. Glenoid Bone Deficiency in Recurrent Anterior Shoulder Instability: Diagnosis and Management. *JAAOS* 2009;17(8):482–493.)

A 22-year-old male with a history of multiple shoulder dislocations was treated with an arthroscopic Bankart repair 9 months ago. Over the last 3 months, he has tried returning to sports but reports continued anterior subluxation events. Revision surgery has been recommended, and he comes to you for a second opinion. His CT scan is shown above (Fig. 2–36).

What is the most appropriate treatment option?

A. Continue with physical therapy and focus on dynamic stabilizer strengthening
B. Latarjet procedure
C. ORIF of bony fragment
D. Repair of Hill–Sachs lesion
E. Boyd–Sisk procedure

Discussion

The correct answer is (B). In patients who have undergone a capsulolabral repair for instability and continue to be symptomatic, it is important to carefully assess the degree of glenoid bone loss. This is best done with a 3D CT scan. When viewing sagittal images, the inferior two-thirds of the glenoid should be a perfect circle. Bony defects can be appreciated by loss of this circle with bone missing from the 230 to 430 position. This may result in the glenoid taking on the classic inverted pear-shaped configuration that is associated with recurrent anterior instability (see Fig. 2–37). The average circle diameter is 24 mm and the average bone loss associated with a pear-shaped glenoid is 35% or 7.5 mm off the anterior rim. The critical amount of bone loss that

destabilizes the shoulder is between 15% and 25% hence bone loss at or above this level must be treated with a bony procedure rather than capsulolabral repair.

Answer A is incorrect as additional PT after a year is not going to make a difference especially given the degree of bone loss. Answer C is incorrect as no fixable bony fragment is seen. Answer D is incorrect as no significant Hill–Sachs lesion is seen on imaging; however, a Hill-Sachs lesion, if present, would contribute to ongoing instability. A Boyd–Sisk (Answer E) procedure was historically described for anterior instability but is no longer used.

Objectives: Did you learn…?

- The physical examination findings associated with anterior instability?
- The current and historical surgical procedures used to treat anterior instability and the indications for their use?
- How to quantify and treat glenoid bone defects?

CASE 13

Dr. Gautam Malhotra

A 19-year-old, collegiate offensive lineman presents to your clinic with vague shoulder pain that has been ongoing throughout his sophomore season. He managed to play out the season but was having significant discomfort during practice sessions and games.

On examination, he has intact strength and range of motion. He has a negative impingement sign and negative O'Brien's test. His pain is reproduced with adduction, internal rotation and a posteriorly directed force.

What is the most likely diagnosis?

A. PASTA lesion
B. Rotator cuff tear
C. Multidirectional instability
D. Posterior instability
E. Bankart lesion

Discussion

The correct answer is (D). Offensive linemen are continuously subjected to posteriorly directed forces with their arms outstretched and adducted; this places them at an increased risk for developing posterior instability. The test in the question stem describes a jerk test which is helpful in making the diagnosis of posterior instability. While the other answer choices represent possible injuries in a young athlete, the question stem does not specifically support them.

Glenohumeral instability is estimated to occur with an incidence of 2% of these 2–5% represent cases of posterior instability. Similarly, only 4% of all shoulder dislocations are posterior dislocations. These may be classified as traumatic or atraumatic. The traumatic form is more common and is often caused by a single traumatic event, classically a seizure or electrocution; the atraumatic form is usually the result of multiple, smaller traumas, classically seen in an offensive lineman. Atraumatic instability should raise the suspicion for an underlying collagen disease or bony abnormality such as excessive glenoid retroversion.

It is important to understand the normal shoulder stabilizers when discussing posterior instability. These are classified as either static or dynamic stabilizers.

Static stabilizers include:

- Bony congruency, glenoid version, and humeral version
- The labrum increases the depth of the glenoid by 50% and increases its surface area and articulation with the humeral head
- The glenohumeral ligaments act as stabilizers at the end range of motion.
  - The superior glenohumeral ligament (SGHL) and coracohumeral ligament resist posterior subluxation with the arm in flexion, adduction and internal rotation.
  - Tightening of the axillary pouch and the posterior band of the inferior glenohumeral ligament (IGHL)

are the main restraint to posterior subluxation when the arm is abducted.

- The posterior capsule is also a restraint, although it is the thinnest and weakest portion of the capsule at <1 mm thick.
- The rotator interval and its constituents (subscapularis, supraspinatus, coracoid, biceps, and humerus) provide resistance to inferior and posterior instability in the adducted and externally rotated position.

Dynamic stabilizers include:

- Rotator cuff (particularly the subscapularis), biceps, deltoid, serratus anterior, latissimus dorsi, trapezius, and the scapulothoracic complex

In posterior instability, some combination of these stabilizers are damaged or not fully functional.

It is important to obtain a thorough history from patients to appreciate their injury pattern and elicit provocative activities so as to characterize the primary direction of instability. Classically, in posterior instability, patients will have pain or apprehension when placed in adduction, flexion, and internal rotation ("at risk" position). On examination, patients generally show preserved range of motion and strength. Specific tests include the load and shift test, jerk test, and posterior stress test. The load and shift test is performed and graded in a manner similar to that described in cases 11–12 with the exception that the humeral head is being displaced posteriorly. The jerk test is performed with the patient seated. An axial force is applied to the arm in 90 degrees of abduction and internal rotation. The patient's arm is horizontally adducted while an axial load is maintained, and a jerk is appreciated as the humeral head slides off the glenoid. This is usually painful. The posterior stress test or apprehension test describes a posteriorly directed force applied to the arm in the "at risk" position. This will elicit pain or a sensation of instability.

Imaging should include x-rays, which may demonstrate posterior glenoid bone loss or an impaction fracture on the anterior-superior humeral head (Fig. 2–38). CT images with 3D reconstructions can be very useful when assessing the extent of glenoid bone loss and evaluating glenoid and humeral version. Normal glenoid version is from −2 to −8 degrees of retroversion, and this may be increased in posterior instability. MRI can also be useful when assessing the posterior labrum (Fig. 2–39).

Conservative treatment is often successful; it involves physical therapy with a focus on strengthening

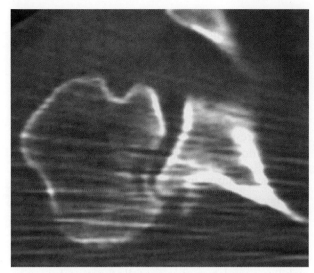

Figure 2–38 Radiographs showing a posterior shoulder dislocation.

the dynamic stabilizers (particularly the posterior deltoid, periscapular muscles, and external rotators), activity modification, and biofeedback. This is successful 65% to 80% of the time. Surgical treatment involves arthroscopic or open posterior labral repair and poster-inferior capsular shift for cases with no bony abnormalities or defects. In cases of glenoid retroversion >20 degrees, an opening wedge osteotomy may be used. In cases of normal version with posterior bone loss, bone grafting along the posterior glenoid rim may be necessary.

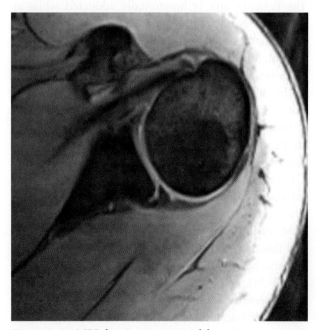

Figure 2–39 MRI showing a posterior labrum tear.

Additional Questions

An acute, posterior shoulder dislocation should be suspected in a patient with the shoulder locked in what position?

A. External rotation
B. Internal rotation
C. Abduction
D. Extension
E. Adduction

Discussion

The correct answer is (B). Posterior dislocations are significantly less common than anterior dislocations so one must maintain a high index of suspicion for these injuries. Posterior dislocations tend to occur during seizures and electrocution. Patients present with pain and a shoulder locked in internal rotation.

All of these are considered a static stabilizer of the shoulder except?

A. Labrum
B. IGHL
C. Coracohumeral ligament
D. Capsule
E. Supraspinatus

Discussion

The correct answer is (E). All of the above are shoulder stabilizers although only the supraspinatus is considered a dynamic stabilizer.

The superior glenohumeral ligament is responsible for resisting which of the following?

A. Posterior glenohumeral subluxation while the arm is in extension, adduction, and IR.
B. Anterior glenohumeral subluxation while the arm is in flexion, abduction, and ER.
C. Inferior glenohumeral subluxation while the arm is in flexion, adduction, and neutral rotation.
D. Anterior glenohumeral subluxation while the arm is in extension, adduction, and ER.
E. Posterior glenohumeral subluxation while the arm is in flexion, adduction, and IR.

Discussion

The correct answer is (E). In flexion, adduction, and internal rotation the posterior glenohumeral ligament is taut and acts like a sling preventing the humeral head from subluxing posteriorly. In posterior instability, this structure is often stretched or torn. The other answers are distractors.

A 30-year-old, basketball player presents to your clinic after an acute shoulder injury. He has significant pain and his shoulder is abducted at 130 degrees. He is unable to lower his arm.

Radiographs will most likely show that his glenohumeral joint has dislocated in what direction?

A. Posterior
B. Anterior
C. Inferior
D. Medial
E. Lateral

Discussion

The correct answer is (C). This patient has an inferior shoulder dislocation (luxatio erecta) as seen in Figure 2–40. This is a very rare type of dislocation, which represents 0.5% of all dislocations. It carries the greatest risk of having an associated neurovascular injury, with the axillary nerve being the most frequently injured structure. Patients present with the shoulder locked overhead in full abduction. Closed reduction is generally successful and a subsequent MRI may be needed to assess for soft tissue injuries.

Objectives: Did you learn…?

- To recognize the clinical presentation and physical examination findings associated with posterior GH instability?

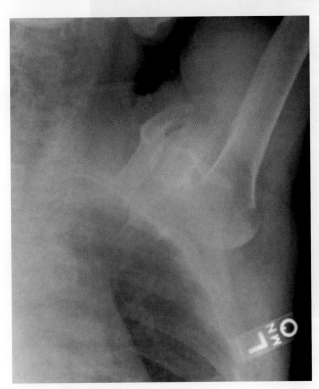

Figure 2–40 Luxatio erecta.

- The different treatment options for this condition?
- What the dynamic and static stabilizers of the shoulder are?

CASE 14

Dr. Gautam Malhotra

A 17-year-old gymnast presents to clinic with right shoulder pain. She denies any specific injury but reports increasing shoulder pain over the last 6 months. On examination, she has generalized hyperlaxity of her joints. Her bilateral shoulders demonstrate a positive sulcus sign, and her right shoulder is painful when placed in an internally rotated and flexed position as well as when placed in an abducted and externally rotated position.

What would be the most appropriate initial treatment?

A. Physical therapy
B. Cortisone injection
C. Cortisone injection + physical therapy
D. Shoulder immobilizer
E. Arthroscopic capsular shift

Discussion

The correct answer is (A). This patient's presentation is consistent with generalized hyperlaxity and multidirectional shoulder instability (MDI) in the right shoulder. It is important to differentiate these terms, as hyperlaxity implies that the patient does not have symptoms of pain or instability and does not require any treatment. Patients with hyperlaxity, however, are predisposed to developing symptomatic shoulder instability, which does require treatment. The initial treatment is usually physical therapy. There is little role for a cortisone injection (Answers B, C) in a young patient with instability. Shoulder immobilization (Answer D) may be recommended by some providers although there is no evidence to support this. Surgical treatment (Answer E) is not the initial treatment.

MDI can be defined as symptomatic shoulder instability in 2 or more directions with or without associated hyperlaxity. It is most commonly seen in overhead athletes, specifically swimmers, throwers, volleyball players and gymnasts, and is usually diagnosed in the second or third decade. It is uncommon in older individuals. Both generalized hyperlaxity and cumulative microtrauma are thought to be contributing factors.

Patients usually present with insidious onset of pain and symptoms that are recreated in specific positions. It is important to elicit what positions or activities are most uncomfortable, as this will clue the provider into the direction of primary instability. Physical examination will demonstrate a positive sulcus sign, load and shift as well as apprehension and relocation tests. The most high yield imaging modality is an MRA which may demonstrate a large patulous capsule and may show associated injuries such as a labral tear.

Treatment is initially conservative in the form of physical therapy. The goal is to strengthen the dynamic stabilizers of the shoulder and periscapular muscles, which often exhibit dyskinesia in multidirectional instability (MDI). This is most successful in patients who do not have a history of a specific traumatic event. Surgical treatment most often involves arthroscopic labral repair and capsular plication. The plication is done starting from the direction of primary instability and working from inferior to superior; the magnitude of plication is subjectively measured at the time of surgery.

Additional Questions

A 17-year-old, male, volleyball player presents to your office with shoulder pain and instability. He underwent a thermal plication at an outside hospital 2 months ago and reports that, in addition to continued instability, his shoulder feels weaker than it previously did.

What muscle and nerve is most likely affected?

A. Deltoid, axillary
B. Teres minor, axillary
C. Subscapular, nerve to subscapularis
D. Supraspinatus, nerve to supraspinatus
E. Teres major, axillary

Discussion

The correct answer is (B). Thermal plication was previously considered a viable treatment option for a patulous capsule, although more recent studies have demonstrated that it is no longer an acceptable option. One of the known complications of thermal plication is damage to the teres minor branch of the axial nerve. Cadaver studies have demonstrated that the nerve runs just 12.4 mm below the glenoid rim at the 6 o'clock position and runs 2.5 mm deep to capsule (see Fig. 2–41). Adduction and external rotation tends to move the nerve further away from the capsule into a less dangerous position. Denervation of the deltoid (Answer A) is also a possible complication, although it is less common than denervation of the teres minor. The subscapular nerve (Answer C) and supraspinatus nerve (Answer D) are generally not in the surgical field. The teres major (Answer E) is innervated by the subscapular nerve, not the axillary nerve.

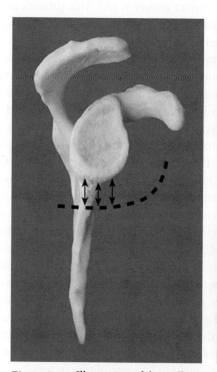 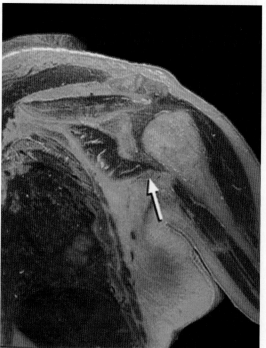

Figure 2–41 Illustration of the axillary nerve course about the shoulder. (Reproduced with permission from Price MR, Tillett ED, Acland RD, et al. Determining the Relationship of the Axillary Nerve to the Shoulder Joint Capsule from an Arthroscopic Perspective. *J Bone Joint Surg Am*, 2004 Oct; 86 (10): 2135–2142.)

A competitive high school swimmer complains of increasing left shoulder pain during practice since the beginning of his senior season. Examination reveals a positive anterior and posterior load and shift test, apprehension test, and a 2 cm sulcus sign. He has been treated with a dynamic stabilizer-strengthening program and activity modification, but he continues to be symptomatic.

The next step in management should be?

A. Immobilization in a brace for 6 weeks
B. Arthroscopic anterior and posterior capsular plication and labral repair
C. Arthroscopic rotator interval closure
D. Arthroscopic thermal capsular plication and rotator interval closure
E. Cortisone injection and continued PT

Discussion

The correct answer is (B). In a young, symptomatic athlete, if conservative treatment fails, the next step involves anterior and posterior capsular plication and labral repair if required. Immobilization (Answer A) is commonly employed postoperatively but is not used as an independent treatment modality. The role of either medial to lateral or superior to inferior rotator interval closure (Answer C) has been debated. It is sometimes utilized as an additional procedure if a shoulder continues to demonstrate instability even after capsular plication. This is usually an intraoperative decision. One of the negatives of rotator interval closure is that it restricts external rotation with the arm by the side. Thermal plication (Answer D) is no longer used and there is little role for a cortisone injection (Answer E) in a young athlete with MDI.

A 23-year-old female comes to your clinic with her mother. She recounts a history of seeing multiple orthopaedic providers with a variety of complaints and receiving little relief from their treatments. Today, her main complaint is a history of recurrent shoulder dislocations. She is voluntarily able to dislocate her shoulder anteriorly in clinic and demonstrates this several times. She reports that she has been able to do this for as long as she can remember. She has developed discomfort in this shoulder recently and is now seeking treatment options.

The next step should include?

A. Physical therapy
B. Psycological evaluation
C. Diagnostic arthroscopy

D. Cortisone injection
E. Temporary shoulder immobilization

Discussion

The correct answer is (B). When evaluating patients with instability, it is important to address the issue of voluntary control. There is a well-described subset of patients who use voluntary dislocation as a means of gaining attention. These patients are best managed with a psychological examination, as surgical treatment will quite likely fail. Two other types of nonpsychiatric voluntary dislocation have been described. The muscular type where selective activation of muscles results in a dislocation and the positional type where assuming a provocative position will result in a dislocation. The muscular type is best treated with biofeedback techniques whereas the positional type will do well with surgery.

Which of the following describes a patient with MDI who would most benefit from surgical stabilization?

A. A 17-year-old girl who is able to voluntarily dislocate her shoulder and readily demonstrated this in clinic
B. A 19-year-old swimmer who has had increasing shoulder pain over the last 6 months and examination consistent with MDI
C. A 22-year-old, professional football player with long standing complaints of shoulder instability seen in the preseason
D. An 18-year-old, late-season, collegiate football player with long standing complaints of shoulder subluxations and a recent frank dislocation
E. A 22-year-old male with a diagnosis of Marfan's syndrome shoulder pain and instability

Discussion

The correct answer is (D). Answer A describes a patient who can voluntarily dislocate her shoulder and does so repeatedly in clinic. Voluntary dislocators must be thoroughly evaluated to ensure that there is no psychological component to their dislocations. A patient who is dislocating for secondary gain will do very poorly with surgery. Answer B describes a patient with MDI without any specific trauma. It would be most appropriate to start with physical therapy in this patient. Answer C represents a pre-season athlete with no specific trauma. Pre- and early season athletes with chronic complaints, without concerning radiographic abnormalities, may benefit from rehab and return to play as soon as possible in the same season. Should they continue to be symptomatic, surgery or further PT would be appropriate in the immediate postseason. Answer D is the most appropriate surgical candidate presented. This patient, at the end of his season, will not have enough rehab time to allow him to return to the field this season. Early surgery may be appropriate to allow the patient a maximum amount of rehab time prior to the next season. Patients with connective tissue disorders (Answer E) tend to have poorer outcomes with surgical intervention.

Objectives: Did you learn...?

* To appreciate the difference between hyperlaxity and instability?
* The common presentation of MDI?
* To appreciate the commonly used treatment options?

CASE 15

Dr. Gautam Malhotra

A 17-year-old, football player with a history of multiple, left shoulder dislocations and an attempted arthroscopic repair presents to your clinic with continued right shoulder pain and instability. He has been unable to return to competition and comes to see you for a second opinion. A CT image is shown below (Fig. 2–42).

What injury should have been addressed during his index procedure?

A. Hill–Sachs lesion
B. PASTA lesion
C. ALPSA lesion
D. Bursal-sided rotator cuff tear
E. Articular-sided rotator cuff tear

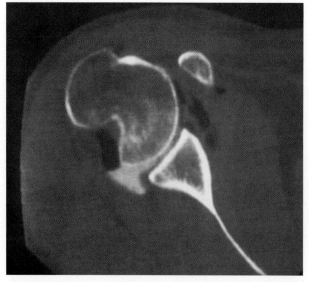

Figure 2–42

Discussion

The correct answer is (A). The imaging demonstrates an axial CT scan with a large Hill–Sachs lesion. The lesion involves a large component of the humeral head (>40%) and as such is likely clinically significant. As the humerus is rotated externally the Hill–Sachs lesion is brought closer to the anterior rim of the glenoid and eventually engages the glenoid. Patients may perceive this as a painful click or locking episode. Lesions that involve 40% of the humeral head should be repaired to adequately address instability. The other answer choices all represent injuries that may be associated with a shoulder dislocation, although the large Hill–Sachs lesion is most responsible for his ongoing instability.

Hill–Sachs lesions are compression fractures of the posterosuperolateral humeral head that occur when the head comes in contact with the glenoid during an acute anterior dislocation or after recurrent instability events. The relative incidence of these lesions is high, and it approaches 100% in patients with recurrent instability. It is important to understand that these lesions are bipolar—there is anterior glenoid damage in addition to the Hill–Sachs lesion; both of these must be addressed to optimize outcome. Lesions can be classified as engaging or nonengaging. Engaging lesions are oriented such that the long axis of the lesion is parallel to the anterior glenoid rim in the position of athletic function, i.e., abduction and external rotation. Engaging lesions tend to be more symptomatic, and instability may be associated with a sensation of catching or locking.

Physicians should obtain a complete set of x-rays. Special views include the modified Westpoint axillary (Fig. 2–43B) to evaluate for glenoid loss and the stryker notch view (Fig. 2–43A) to evaluate the Hill–Sachs lesion. This view brings the posterolateral defect into direct visualization. 3D CT imaging is also very useful for evaluating glenoid bone loss and estimating the size of the Hill–Sachs lesion.

As with most instability situations, treatment begins with conservative treatment in the form of PT, focusing on dynamic stabilizer strengthening. Should patients fail a course of PT, surgery is the next step. This will involve a labral repair, possible glenoid bony augmentation, and capsular shift (as is typical for most instability cases). The provider must also decide whether or not the Hill–Sachs lesion is clinically significant and whether it needs to be addressed surgically. Lesions that involve:

* <20% of the humeral head are considered to be clinically insignificant.
* 20% to 40% may be significant.

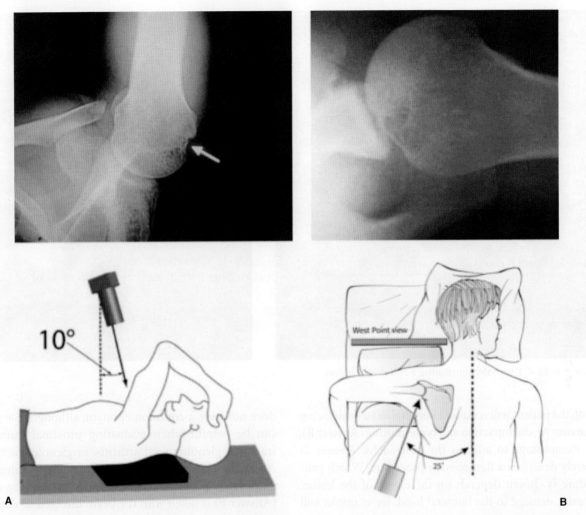

Figure 2–43 **A:** Stryker notch view. **B:** West point axillary view. (From Bucholz RW and Heckman JD. *Rockwood and Green's Fractures in Adults 7e.* Philadelphia: Wolters Kluwer, 2009.)

- >40% are significant and contribute to recurrent instability.

In addition, "engaging lesions" are considered to be clinically significant and warrant treatment. Surgical options include: humeral head bone augmentation with disimpaction and bone grafting or allograft, Remplissage procedure, or humeral head resurfacing. The most commonly used procedure is the Remplissage procedure, which involves filling in the humeral defect with a portion of the infraspinatus tendon. This is often done using an arthroscopic technique with suture through the infraspinatus tendon and a bone anchor placed directly in the defect.

Additional Questions

A 34-year-old female with recurrent anterior dislocations and a prior anterior arthroscopic capsulolabral repair presents to your clinic with continued insta-

bility episodes and pain. Her imaging demonstrates about 10% of bone loss on the anterior glenoid and a Hill–Sachs lesion that measures 40% of her humeral head.

Treatment options could include all of the following except

A. Humeral head resurfacing
B. Disimpaction and bone grafting of the humeral head defect
C. Remplissage
D. Filling in the bony defect with rotator cuff tendon
E. Latarjet procedure

Discussion

The correct answer is (E). A Hill–Sachs lesion (Fig. 2–44) that involves 40% of the humeral head is likely to be symptomatic. In addition to a labral repair and capsular

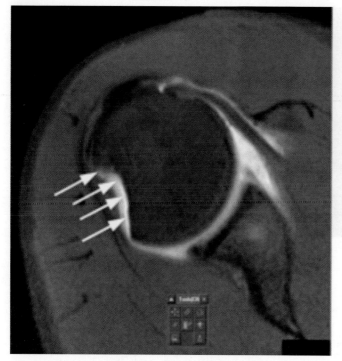

Figure 2–44 CT scan demonstrating a Hill–Sachs lesion.

shift, the patient will require: a humeral head resurfacing (Answer A), disimpaction and bone grafting (Answer B), or Remplissage to address the Hill–Sachs. Answer D merely describes a Remplissage procedure. Which procedure is chosen depends on the extent of the lesion. Greater damage to the humeral head, for example, will make resurfacing a more attractive option. A Latarjet procedure (Answer E) is indicated for glenoid bone loss >20% and is probably unnecessary here.

The best view to visualize a Hill–Sachs lesion on radiographs is?

A. With the patients hand above his head and the x-ray beam directed 10 degrees cephalad
B. With the patients hand by their side and the x-ray beam directed 10 degrees cephalad
C. An AP view with the arm in 40 degrees of external rotation
D. An axillary view
E. A serendipity view

Discussion

The correct answer is (A). This describes the stryker notch view, which is the best way to visualize the posterolateral humeral head where a Hill–Sachs lesion is most commonly located. Answer B describes a Zanca view, which is used to visualize the AC joint. Answer C

does not have a common eponym, although this view can be helpful when evaluating proximal humerus fractures, glenohumeral arthritis, or glenoid fractures. An axillary view (Answer D) is useful when evaluating anterior or posterior dislocation. A serendipity view (Answer E) is taken with the beam directed 40 degrees cephalad aiming at the clavicle; it is used to visualize the SC joint and the clavicle.

CASE 16

Dr. Gautam Malhotra

A 56-year-old male presents to your clinic 2 months after a polytrauma MVA. He was in the ICU, intubated for a week after his initial injury, and has trouble recounting the details of his hospitalization. He does recall being diagnosed with a frozen shoulder. He is currently at a rehabilitation facility and has noticed improvement in his shoulder although still reports soreness and significantly limited ROM.

The next step in management should be?

A. X-ray
B. MRA
C. Cortisone injection
D. Rotator cuff strengthening program
E. Continue PT

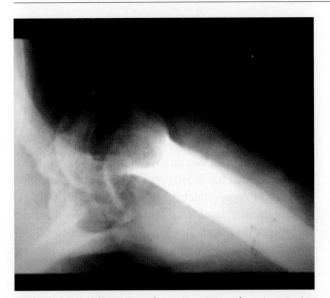

Figure 2–45 Axillary view demonstrating a chronic anterior shoulder dislocation.

Discussion

The correct answer is (A). The first step in management of this patient is obtaining a complete set of x-rays to rule out a missed shoulder dislocation (as seen in Fig. 2–45). Answers C to E describe various treatment modalities, but these cannot be instituted without a firm diagnosis. An MRA (Answer B) is most commonly used when a labral tear is suspected, but an x-ray would be the first imaging modality utilized.

Chronic shoulder dislocations are relatively uncommon injuries but represent a significant challenge even for the experienced provider. There are varying opinions on what duration of time a shoulder needs to be dislocated to be termed "chronic." Three to four weeks is a commonly accepted timeframe, although any dislocation that is not identified and treated at the time of injury can be defined as chronic. This most frequently occurs in a polytrauma patient where other, more life-threatening injuries, may cause a provider to overlook the shoulder. Treating chronic, glenohumeral dislocations can be very challenging, so the most important goal is preventing the problem by minimizing the risk of missing an acute dislocation. This is most easily done with a complete set of x-rays on any patient with a suspected shoulder injury. Obtaining an axillary view or Vallpeau view is essential as these views will most clearly demonstrate the position of the humeral head with respect to the glenoid. An AP and even a scapular Y view are insufficient to diagnose a shoulder dislocation, and

an inability to obtain a Grashey view should clue the provider into a possible dislocation.

These patients frequently present with a visible asymmetry when examined with their shirts off. This may not be apparent in overweight or muscular patients. Patients will have limited range of motion (ROM); classically chronic anterior dislocations present with limited forward flexion, abduction and internal rotation, and chronic posterior dislocations with limited external rotation. However, unlike in acute dislocations, the ROM is often within a functional range, particularly if the shoulder has been dislocated for a prolonged period of time. In these situations pain tends to be fairly minimal as well. Muscle strength may or may not be preserved.

As previously mentioned, x-rays are of critical importance. A CT scan is often useful to further define bony abnormalities and an MRI can help detect associated soft tissue conditions.

There are several pathoanatomic changes that are noted with chronic dislocations. These include: osteoporosis softening of articular cartilage, soft tissue contractures, adhesions that may involve neurovascular structures, rotator cuff tears (particularly the subscapularis with anterior dislocation), glenoid bone deficiency, and a humeral head impression fracture. The degree of these changes to some extent depends on the duration of dislocation. All of these need to be taken into account when formulating a treatment plan.

Treating chronic dislocations can be challenging. It is important to evaluate each patient individually and take into consideration the direction and duration of dislocation, size of the humeral head impression fracture, degree or glenoid bone loss, status of articular cartilage, and most importantly their functional limitations and baseline level of activity.

Nonoperative treatment may be appropriate for low demand patients as many can regain a functional ROM with minimal pain and sufficient strength after physical therapy. Closed reduction may be considered if the dislocation is <4 weeks old and it is felt that the reduction will be stable. A large glenoid defect or a large humeral head impression fracture, which are predictors if instability, are relative contraindications to this. Open reduction is frequently necessary in younger and high demand patients. In this situation, stability must also be addressed at the time of reduction. Generally speaking, the head impression fractures involving >20% of the humeral head will require an additional procedure to fill the defect to confer stability.

The stabilization procedure for anterior dislocations could involve: capsulolabral repair, disimpaction of the humeral head and bone grafting, size-matched allograft replacement when the remaining cartilage is healthy, or infraspinatus transfer with or without the greater tuberosity (to fill the humeral head defect) using a dual anterior and posterior approach. Similar options exist for posterior dislocations although the transfer would involve a subscapularis/lesser tuberosity transfer, which can be done entirely from an anterior approach.

Additional Questions

A 27-year-old banker with a seizure disorder presents to your clinic with shoulder pain and stiffness for 1.5 months since his last seizure. His X-ray is shown below (Fig. 2–46).

Which of the following is not an appropriate treatment option for this patient?

A. Open reduction and immobilization if stable
B. Open reduction and subscapularis transfer
C. Open reduction and greater tuberosity transfer
D. Open reduction and humeral head disimpaction and bone grafting
E. Open reduction and size-matched allograft transfer

Discussion

The correct answer is (C). The image demonstrates a chronically dislocated posterior glenohumeral dislocation. At 1.5 months, a dislocation closed reduction is unlikely to be successful. Each of the answer choices shows an acceptable treatment option depending on the stability of the reduction and the size of the humeral head impaction fracture except for Answer C, open reduction and greater tuberosity transfer. This would be used for posterior defects that would be seen with anterior dislocations.

A 35-year-old male has an 8-week-old chronic, anterior dislocation that has failed conservative management. At the time of open reduction, it is noted that his humeral head continues to sublux anteriorly. The surgeon decides to proceed with a greater tuberosity transfer to fill this defect and create a more stable glenohumeral complex.

What was likely the size the humeral defect?

A. 5%
B. 15%
C. 30%
D. 60%
E. 70%

Discussion

The correct answer is (C) (see Fig. 2–47). Humeral head impaction fractures involving less than 20% of the humeral head (Answers A, B) are often stable after open reduction and can do well with just a soft tissue procedure. Impaction fracture involving 20% to 40% (Answer C) frequently require an additional procedure to address the bony defect which may include disimpaction and bone grafting, allograft reconstruction, or infraspinatus/greater tuberosity transfer. Glenoid bone

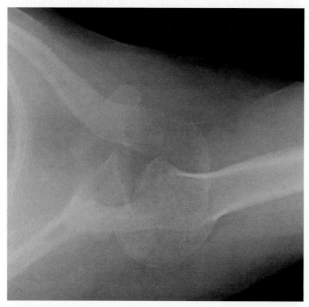

Figure 2–46

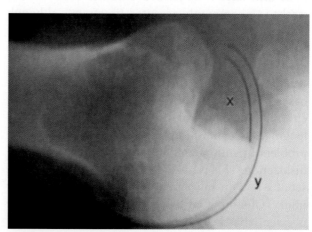

Figure 2–47 The size of the humeral head defect can be calculated by dividing the arc of impaction (x) by the total articular surface arc (y).

grafting may be needed as well, particularly if the gle-noid bone loss is >20% to 25%.

Humeral head defects >40% (Answers D, E) fre-quently require a large allograft or prosthetic recon-struction. If a prosthetic option is chosen, some authors recommend placing the prosthetic glenoid component in 10 to 15 degrees of retroversion for an anterior dislo-cation and doing the opposite for a posterior dislocation.

Objectives: Did you learn...?

- To recognize the common presentation of a patient with a chronic dislocation?
- To recognize the pathoanatomic changes associated with a chronic dislocation?
- The various treatment options and indications for their use?

CASE 17

Dr. Anna Cohen-Rosenblum

A 61-year-old, right-hand-dominant female presents with 5 years of gradually worsening right shoulder pain. The pain is worse at night and she is finding it gradually more difficult to perform certain activities such as combing her hair, putting on a coat, and reach-ing for objects on high shelves. Past medical history includes hypertension and hyperlipidemia, both well controlled with medication. Physical examination reveals that the right shoulder appears flatter in con-tour compared with the contralateral side. She has dif-fuse tenderness to palpation about the right shoulder glenohumeral joint; range of motion of the shoulder decreased in external rotation; and 5/5 strength in the rotator cuff muscles. Imaging is shown in Figures 2–48 and 2–49.

Based on the information and imaging, what is the most likely diagnosis?

A. Traumatic rotator cuff tear
B. Osteoarthritis of the glenohumeral joint
C. Cuff tear arthropathy
D. Degenerative labral tear

Discussion

The correct answer is (B). The patient's chronic pain, difficulty with external rotation, flattened appearance, combined with the imaging showing narrowed joint space, subchondral sclerosis, and osteophytes at the infe-rior aspect of the humeral head lead to the diagnosis of glenohumeral osteoarthritis. In addition, the patient has

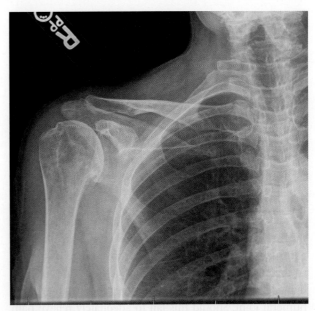

Figure 2–48

no signs of cuff deficit on examination and no history of trauma, so Answer A is incorrect. Cuff tear arthropathy (Answer C) would also be less likely given her lack of weakness combined with imaging showing typical signs of osteoarthritis without a high-riding humeral head as would be characteristic of a massive cuff tear with result-ing arthropathy. Finally, Answer D is incorrect because, even though it is probable a person her age would have a labral tear, it would manifest more as mechanical symp-toms and/or instability.

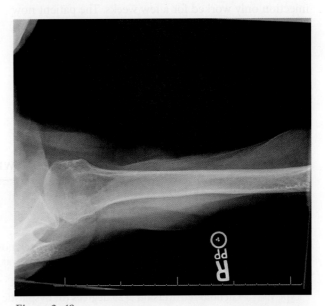

Figure 2–49

The patient says she has been taking ibuprofen daily with little to no relief. Based on the diagnosis, what would you recommend at this point?

A. Physical therapy to strengthen the rotator cuff muscles, corticosteroid injection into the subacromial space.
B. Total shoulder arthroplasty
C. Physical therapy to improve shoulder range of motion and corticosteroid injection into the glenohumeral joint
D. Reverse total shoulder arthroplasty

Discussion

The correct answer is (C). Conservative management is the first step in treating glenohumeral osteoarthritis, which consists of physical therapy to improve range of motion so the patient is better able to complete activities of daily living (ADLs) and corticosteroid injection into the glenohumeral joint. Should this fail to adequately relieve pain, the next choice would be B, total shoulder arthroplasty. Answer D is incorrect not only because the first step is conservative management, but also because the patient's rotator cuff is intact, and reverse total shoulder arthroplasty is indicated for glenohumeral arthritis with cuff deficiency and an intact deltoid. Finally, Answer A would be more appropriate for a patient with a rotator cuff tear and subacromial bursitis, as opposed to this patient whose pathology is focused on the glenohumeral joint.

Eight months later, the patient has completed a course of physical therapy and undergone two corticosteroid injections into the glenohumeral joint. The first injection relieved her pain for about 3 months, but her second injection only worked for a few weeks. The patient now says the pain and disability have returned to levels prior to the injections. You decide to proceed with operative treatment with a total shoulder arthroplasty (TSA).

What is the next step in preoperative planning?

A. CT of the right shoulder to evaluate glenoid bone stock and glenoid version

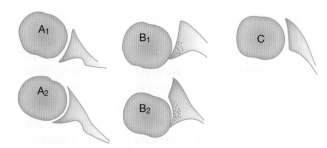

Figure 2-50 Reproduced with permission from Walch G, et al. Morphologic Study of the Glenoid in Primary Glenohumeral Osteoarthritis. *Journal of Arthroplasty* 1999;14(6):756–760.

B. MRI of the right shoulder to evaluate the rotator cuff
C. MR-arthrogram of the right shoulder to evaluate for labral tears
D. X-ray of the left shoulder to evaluate for contralateral glenohumeral osteoarthritis

Discussion

The correct answer is (A). CT would aid in preoperative planning by determining glenoid bone stock and glenoid version and is therefore the best choice. Glenoid bone stock is especially important as there must be sufficient bone stock in order to be able to place the glenoid component. The Walch classification (Table 2–5, Fig. 2–50) describes the progression of glenoid wear found in glenohumeral arthritis. "B" is incorrect because, although an intact rotator cuff is a requirement for TSA, it is assumed at this point the status of the cuff has been evaluated, and the exact nature of rotator cuff morphology is not necessary for preoperative planning. "C" is incorrect since the quality of the labrum has no effect on pre-operative planning for TSA. "D" is incorrect because osteoarthritis in the contralateral shoulder is not an important factor in preoperative planning, however, in the case of rheumatoid arthritis clinical function of other extremities does have an effect on operative decision making.

The patient undergoes a total shoulder arthroplasty via deltopectoral approach. At her 2-week postoperative

Table 2–5 WALCH CLASSIFICATION OF GLENOID WEAR

Type A	Concentric wear, no subluxation, well centered A1-minor erosion A2-deeper, central erosion
Type B	Biconcave glenoid, asymmetric glenoid wear, posterior subluxation of humeral head B1-narrowed posterior joint space, subchondral sclerosis B2-posterior wear with biconcave glenoid
Type C	Glenoid retroversion >25 degrees (of dysplastic origin), ± posterior subluxation of humeral head

From Walch G, et al. Morphologic Study of the Glenoid in Primary Glenohumeral Osteoarthritis. *Journal of Arthroplasty* 1999;14(6):756–760.

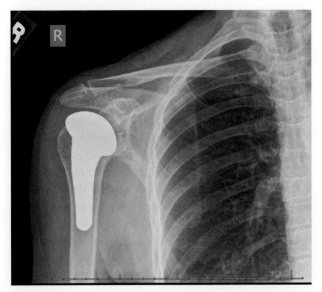

Figure 2–51

visit, the incision is healing well and her pain is controlled with 1 to 2 tablets of hydrocodone-acetaminophen daily. You give her a prescription for physical therapy. Four weeks later, the patient returns to clinic complaining of an increase in shoulder pain as well as weakness for the past 3 days, especially when getting dressed. She does not recall any traumatic event. On examination her incision remains clean, dry, and intact; there is a positive finding of weakness when resistance is applied to the arm in an adducted and internally rotated position behind the back. X-rays are shown in Figure 2–51.

What is the most likely explanation?

A. Loosening of the humeral component
B. Infection of the shoulder joint with *P. acnes*
C. Tearing of the subscapularis tendon
D. Axillary nerve palsy from intraoperative injury

Discussion

The correct answer is (C). During the deltopectoral approach, the subscapularis tendon is detached from the anterior humerus so the humeral head may be exposed. The tendon is reattached after placement of the components, and there is a postoperative risk of repair failure, especially during rehabilitation. Precautions to avoid in rehabilitation include limiting external rotation of the shoulder and avoiding such movements as pushing out of a chair. Pendulum exercises and passive range of motion supervised by physical therapy are advised, and active range of motion of the elbow, wrist, and hand should be encouraged to avoid stiffness. Choice "A" is incorrect because the patient's symptoms are more consistent with

subscapularis tear, and there is no radiographic evidence of loosening. Choice "B" is incorrect because infection is more associated with loosening. Choice "D" is incorrect because axillary nerve palsy would likely present as weakness with shoulder abduction and/or sensory changes in the skin around the deltoid.

Objectives: Did you learn...?

• Recognize the clinical presentation of glenohumeral osteoarthritis?
• Treat a patient with glenohumeral osteoarthritis?
• Manage a patient after total shoulder arthroplasty?

CASE 18

Dr. Anna Cohen-Rosenblum

A 55-year-old female with a history of rheumatoid arthritis diagnosed at age 40 presents to your clinic complaining of 3 years of right shoulder pain acutely worsening over the past week to the point that she is unable to reach for objects from high shelves and needs help getting dressed in the morning. She also notes recent intermittent fevers and severe pain in her left hand and decreased range of motion of the fingers. She participated in a 6-week course of physical therapy last year prescribed by her rheumatologist which provided no relief. She receives an injection of a TNF-alpha inhibitor every 8 weeks. Physical examination reveals tenderness to palpation, swelling and warmth about the left shoulder with decreased range of motion throughout. Her left hand is neurovascularly intact with ulnar deviation of the fingers and severe limitation of range of motion. Imaging of the right shoulder is shown in Figure 2–52.

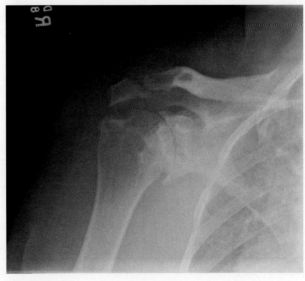

Figure 2–52

What is the most appropriate next step in diagnosis/ treatment?

A. MRI of the right shoulder
B. In-office injection of the subacromial space with corticosteroids
C. Physical therapy prescription for rotator cuff strengthening and improvement of shoulder range of motion
D. CBC, CRP, ESR, and aspiration of the glenohumeral joint with fluid culture and cell count

Discussion

The correct answer is (D). In a patient with rheumatoid arthritis, the most likely diagnosis is inflammatory arthropathy involving the shoulder, however, the presence of fevers and acutely worsening pain with swelling and warmth on physical examination necessitates a workup for septic arthritis. MRI of the shoulder (Answer A) might be indicated in the future if there is question about rotator cuff integrity in the setting of a decision to perform a total shoulder arthroplasty, but not at the time of initial diagnosis. Subacromial steroid injection (Answer B) would not be indicated in a patient in whom septic arthritis is suspected. Physical therapy (Answer C) would be helpful for conservative management of inflammatory arthritis but is not the best choice for initial diagnosis.

Aspiration of the right glenohumeral joint reveals approximately 20 cc of turbid fluid, which is sent for analysis. Gram stain reveals PMNs but no organisms, and cell count WBC 20,000, 65% polymorphonuclear leukocytes, positive for cholesterol crystals.

What is the most likely diagnosis?

A. Infection of the shoulder joint with *P. acnes*
B. Rheumatoid arthritis
C. Chondrocalcinosis
D. Osteoarthritis

Discussion

The correct answer is (B). While there are some similarities between the synovial fluid of septic arthritis (Choice A),

including turbid quality and an increased volume of fluid in the joint, the cell count in septic arthritis is generally much higher (>50,000 WBCs) and may have organisms present on gram stain. Also, while infection with *P. acnes* may have synovial fluid with a lower number of WBCs on analysis than is generally found with infection by other organisms and may not show organisms on gram stain (see Case 20), it is more likely found in the presence of orthopaedic implants or after shoulder surgery. Answer C is incorrect because it would be characterized by calcium pyrophosphate crystals in the synovial fluid, not cholesterol crystals which can be present in rheumatoid arthritis. Answer D is incorrect because the synovial fluid of arthritis is generally not turbid and has a much lower cell count (<2,000 WBCs). See Table 2–6 for more details about diagnosis based on synovial fluid analysis.

The patient's synovial fluid aspirate is held for 3 weeks with no growth. You diagnose her with rheumatoid arthritis of the shoulder.

What is the most appropriate next step in treatment?

A. Right total shoulder arthroplasty
B. Right shoulder hemiarthroplasty
C. Referral to a colleague for evaluation of her left hand deformity
D. Right shoulder arthrodesis

Discussion

The correct answer is (C). It is important in patients with rheumatoid arthritis to address other sources of pain that might impede the postoperative rehabilitation process. This patient will be unable to use her right, dominant hand as effectively after shoulder surgery, and will be far more reliant on her left hand in the postoperative period. Since she has severe pain and deformity of the left hand, she should be evaluated by a hand surgeon to determine whether this issue might be addressed prior to her undergoing an operation on her shoulder. Choice A is incorrect not only because the left hand should be evaluated first, but because imaging of her right shoulder reveals severe erosion as well as osteopenia of the glenoid,

Table 2–6

	WBC/Diff	Glucose	Protein
Septic arthritis	>100,000/mL, >75% neutrophils	<50% serum glucose	Increased
Osteoarthritis	<2,000/mL, <25% neutrophils	Same as serum glucose	Normal
Rheumatoid arthritis	15–20,000/mL, 60–70% neutrophils	<25% serum glucose	Normal/increased

Reprinted with permission from Chen A, Joseph T, Zuckerman J. Rheumatoid arthritis of the shoulder. *JAAOS* 2003;11:12–24.

which is a contraindication to total shoulder arthroplasty due to placement of the glenoid component. Choice B is incorrect only because of the timing with this patient; it is actually the most appropriate operative choice given her poor glenoid bone stock and relatively younger age. Choice D is incorrect as arthrodesis is more appropriate for patients with failed total shoulder arthroplasty, and end-stage rheumatoid arthritis (arthritis mutilans) complicated by septic arthritis.

The patient returns to your clinic in 5 months complaining of continued right shoulder pain. She has since undergone multiple MCP joint reconstructions in the left hand and is recovering well with decreased pain and increased range of motion compared with prior to surgery. You decide to treat the patient with a cemented hemiarthroplasty of the right shoulder.

For which complication is she at a greater risk compared with the general population?

A. Chronic regional pain syndrome
B. Loosening of the humeral component
C. Radial nerve palsy
D. Postoperative infection

Discussion
The correct answer is (D). Patients with rheumatoid arthritis are more susceptible to postoperative infections than the general population undergoing surgery. This patient is especially at risk given her use of a TNF-alpha inhibitor, which is a potent immunosuppressant. In general, it is advisable to avoid the use of such medications within 2 weeks of surgery. Choices A, B, and C are incorrect because, while they are all possible complications after hemiarthroplasty of the shoulder, this patient is at no higher risk of developing them than the general population.

Objectives: Did you learn...?

• Recognize the clinical and radiographic presentation of glenohumeral rheumatoid arthritis?
• Surgically treat a patient with glenohumeral rheumatoid arthritis?
• Perioperatively manage a patient with glenohumeral rheumatoid arthritis?

CASE 19

Dr. Anna Cohen-Rosenblum

A 45-year-old, left-hand-dominant male with a history of Crohn's disease presents to your clinic complaining

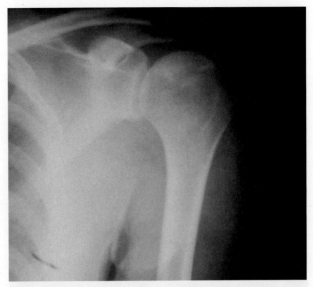
Figure 2–53

of left shoulder pain for the past 2 months. He is unable to localize the pain but says it is worse with overhead motion and radiates to his elbow. He was diagnosed with Crohn's at age 20 and his symptoms are currently under fairly good control with etanercept, but he has had multiple flares in the past treated with courses of IV and PO steroids. He notes a history of traumatic left shoulder dislocation while playing high-school football but denies any subsequent dislocations or shoulder pain prior to 2 months ago. Physical examination is significant for pain with active abduction and forward flexion of the left shoulder. Imaging is shown in Figure 2–53.

What is the most appropriate next step?

A. MRI of the left shoulder
B. CT of the left shoulder
C. PET scan
D. Diagnostic and therapeutic corticosteroid injection of the glenohumeral joint

Discussion
The correct answer is (A). In a patient with IBD and a history of steroid use, avascular necrosis (AVN) should be at the top of the differential diagnosis. Other risk factors for AVN of the humeral head include a history of trauma, chemo/radiation, Caisson disease, sickle cell disease, alcohol abuse, SLE, pregnancy, and tobacco use. The patient has x-rays with sclerotic changes suspicious for AVN, therefore MRI is the best next step for this patient. CT of the left shoulder (Answer B) would not show any of the bony edema that characterizes early

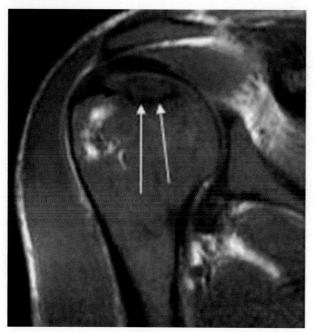

Figure 2–54

Table 2–7 FICAT CLASSIFICATION OF OSTEONECROSIS

Stage I	X-ray: no change MRI: bone marrow edema Bone scan: increased uptake
Stage II	X-ray: mixed sclerosis/osteopenia MRI: bone marrow edema Bone scan: increased uptake
Stage III	X-ray: crescent sign, no head collapse MRI: bone marrow edema
Stage IV	X-ray: Collapse of head with joint space narrowing MRI: bone marrow edema, collapse

Data from Harreld K, et al. Osteonecrosis of the Humeral Head. *JAAOS* 2009;17(6):345–355 (specifically in figure 2) and Lavernia C, Sierra R and Grieco F. Osteonecrosis of the Femoral Head. *JAAOS* 1999;7:250–261.

AVN. PET scans (Answer C) can also be used to identify early AVN but have been shown to be less accurate than MRI. D is incorrect because AVN is a higher likelihood for this patient than glenohumeral arthritis or a labral tear and therefore should be investigated first with MRI.

MRI of the right shoulder is shown in Figure 2–54. What is the diagnosis?

A. Stage I AVN of the humeral head
B. Stage II AVN of the humeral head
C. Stage III AVN of the humeral head
D. Stage IV AVN of the humeral head

Discussion

The correct answer is (B). The MRI shows bony edema consistent with avascular necrosis of the humeral head, which combined with the sclerotic radiographic changes shown in Figure 2–54, classify him as stage II in the Ficat classification. Although the Ficat classification was designed for AVN of the femoral head, it is also commonly used to classify AVN of the humeral head. Table 2–7 shows the Ficat classification stages I to IV. Different modifications of the Ficat classification exist as well, including the Steinberg and Cruess. Choices C and D are incorrect because they all are characterized by radiographic changes of varying degrees (such as osteolytic lesions, subchondral collapse, and osteoarthritis), which this patient does not have.

The patient returns to clinic to go over his MRI results. You tell him that he likely has avascular necrosis of his

left humeral head. After you explain to him what AVN is and the nature of the disease process, you start to discuss treatment options.

What are you going to recommend for the patient at this point?

A. Refer him back to his gastroenterologist for improved control over his Crohn's disease
B. Naproxen 500 mg BID taken with food
C. A short taper of PO steroids
D. Prescription for a 6-week course of physical therapy

Discussion

The correct answer is (D). As discussed in the second question, the patient is Ficat stage II and therefore conservative management must be the initial approach. In this case, the most appropriate conservative management consists of physical therapy to preserve shoulder strength and ROM and to maintain his ability to perform ADLs. Choice A is incorrect because AVN is not directly linked to the severity of Crohn's disease or any other disease process. Choice B is incorrect as the patient is unable to take NSAIDs due to his inflammatory bowel disease and the increased risk of GI bleed. Choice C is incorrect because, as with Choice A, controlling a Crohn's flare will not directly lead to improvement in the symptoms of AVN, and also it has been hypothesized that corticosteroid use over time may contribute to the risk for developing AVN.

The patient returns to you 3 months later. He participated in physical therapy and says that while he initially noticed moderate improvement in his pain, after approximately 1 month the pain has returned and he also notices decreased range of motion. Physical examination is significant for decreased range of motion compared with your examination of 3 months ago.

What is the most appropriate treatment for this patient?

A. Left shoulder hemiarthroplasty
B. Left total shoulder arthroplasty
C. Core decompression of the left humeral head
D. Left reverse total shoulder arthroplasty

Discussion

The correct answer is (C). Core decompression via insertion of pins into the area affected by AVN is thought to improve symptoms in patients with Ficat stage I or II by reducing bone marrow pressure and encouraging new vasculature to form. Patients are managed postoperatively in a sling for a few days and can perform shoulder range of motion as tolerated. Choice A would be more appropriate in a more advanced stage of AVN and/or if conservative treatment and core decompression have failed to relieve pain. Choices B and D are incorrect as they would be reserved for the elderly patient with advanced AVN characterized by concurrent osteoarthritic changes, with or without rotator cuff function.

Objectives: Did you learn…?

• Understand the etiology of osteonecrosis of the humeral head?
• Recognize the clinical presentation of osteonecrosis of the humeral head?
• Manage a patient with osteonecrosis of the humeral head?

CASE 20

Dr. Anna Cohen-Rosenblum

A 72-year-old, right-hand-dominant male with a history of type 2 diabetes, hypertension, and coronary artery disease presents to clinic for a second opinion regarding worsening left shoulder pain 8 months after undergoing a left total shoulder arthroplasty. He had an uncomplicated procedure and has had no major postoperative complications thus far; however, he has never been completely pain free since his procedure. He denies any recent trauma, fevers, chills, or drainage from the incision site. On examination, the incision sites are clean, dry, and intact, and he has mild tenderness to palpation diffusely over the left shoulder as well as decreased range of motion. Imaging is shown in Figure 2–55.

What is the most appropriate next step in his management?

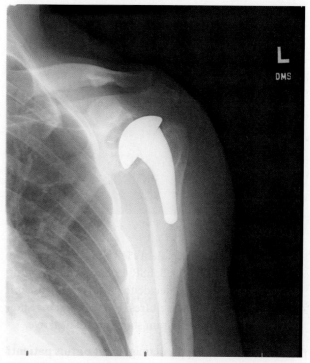

Figure 2–55

A. Schedule the patient for soonest available irrigation and debridement of left shoulder
B. MRI with contrast to evaluate for infection
C. CT arthrogram of the left shoulder to evaluate for loosening
D. Referral to physical therapy

Discussion

The correct answer is (C). This patient's story of acutely worsening pain without known trauma and with a history of orthopaedic implants is suspicious for infection. Risk factors for infection include rheumatoid arthritis, diabetes mellitus, systemic lupus erythematosus, malignancy, immunosuppression, etc. The first step in this diagnosis would be CT arthrogram of the shoulder to evaluate for loosening as sign of infection. A is incorrect as, although infection is on the differential, it has not yet definitively been diagnosed and therefore an immediate irrigation and debridement would not be indicated. MRI (Choice B) might be helpful in identifying a joint effusion or bony edema/signal intensity but would not provide as useful information as synovial fluid would at this point. Choice D is incorrect because the patient must be worked up for infection before deciding on conservative management only. As a side note, aspiration of the glenohumeral joint would be more appropriate for cases in which bacteremic seeding of a joint is suspected.

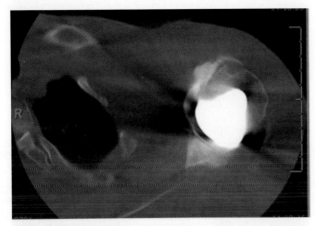
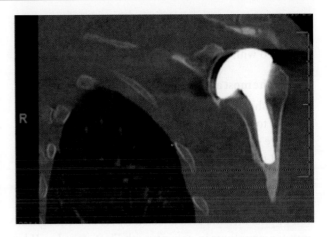

Figure 2–56

CT arthrograms of the patient's left shoulder are shown in Figure 2–56. CRP is <3, ESR 45. The patient continues to have pain, so you decide to perform arthroscopic biopsy to obtain tissue cultures. Frozen sections show <5 PMNs per hpf, and Gram stains are all negative.

What is the next step in management of this patient?

A. Referral to pain clinic for management of his chronic pain
B. Hold cultures for 3 weeks and await final report
C. Request tissue culture medium be changed to chocolate agar
D. Immediate conversion to open with washout of right shoulder and explanation of components

Discussion

The correct answer is (B). Figure shows contrast under the glenoid component. Given the patient's normal inflammatory markers and frozen sections combined with continued pain and loosening on CT, infection with *P. acnes* (an organism that is very difficult to isolate) should be investigated by holding any cultures for at least 2 weeks to see if it will eventually grow. Chocolate agar (Choice C) is mainly used for growing species such as *H. influenzae* and *Neisseria meningitidis* not *P. acnes*. A is incorrect since the patient's cell count and frozen sections are clearly abnormal, therefore referral to pain clinic would not be appropriate. However, Choice D would be too aggressive an approach given that no organisms have been isolated, frozen sections show <5 PMNs per hpf, and the patient has relatively normal inflammatory markers.

After 17 days, *P. acnes* is isolated from the culture medium.

What is the most appropriate treatment for *P. acnes* infection in a patient with a total shoulder arthroplasty?

A. Resection arthroplasty with implantation of antibiotic cement spacer
B. Resection arthroplasty with component exchange
C. Chronic suppression with antibiotic therapy
D. Resection arthroplasty with right shoulder arthrodesis

Discussion

The correct answer is (A). The patient should be treated for his infection by removing his current implants and placing an antibiotic spacer. He should also be referred to infectious diseases clinic for recommendations for antibiotic therapy. Choice B is incorrect since it would involve placement of hardware into an infected area. Choice C would be more appropriate if the patient had failed treatment with a spacer. Choice D would not be indicated at this time, and would be reserved for cases of infection that were unresponsive to long-term antibiotic treatment and caused severe pain and limited functionality in the patient.

The patient undergoes resection arthroplasty with antibiotic cement spacer and a 6-week course of IV antibiotics. He returns to clinic 4 months later with improved pain, CRP <3, however, on examination he has a positive belly press sign and increased external rotation compared with the contralateral shoulder. Imaging is shown in Figure 2–57.

What will likely be the definitive management of his infection?

A. Maintenance of antibiotic cement spacer
B. Explanation of antibiotic cement spacer with total shoulder arthroplasty
C. Additional 6 weeks of antibiotic therapy followed by rechecking CRP
D. Explanation of antibiotic cement spacer with reverse total shoulder arthroplasty

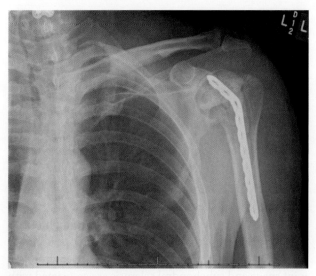

Figure 2–57

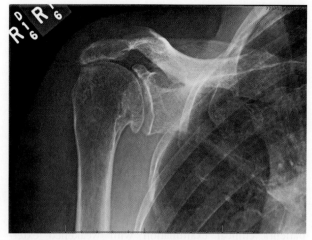

Figure 2–58

Discussion

The correct answer is (D). The patient has completed his course of antibiotics and his spacer and is now an appropriate candidate for explanation of the cement spacer with revision shoulder arthroplasty, therefore Choices A and C are incorrect. The patient's clinical examination findings point to rotator cuff tear (specifically subscapularis) which has occurred in the interval between his obtaining his initial total shoulder arthroplasty and his current examination. Therefore, total shoulder arthroplasty (Choice B) is contraindicated, and the patient should have a reverse total shoulder arthroplasty.

Objectives: Did you learn...?

• Recognize the clinical presentation of a patient with infection after total shoulder arthroplasty?

• Initiate appropriate work-up of a patient with a suspected infected total shoulder arthroplasty?

• Treat a patient with infected total shoulder arthroplasty?

CASE 21

Dr. Anna Cohen-Rosenblum

A 70-year-old, right-hand-dominant female presents to clinic complaining of 4 years of gradually worsening chronic right shoulder pain and stiffness. She says the pain is worse at night and with any range of motion, denies a history of trauma, pain in other extremities, or numbness or tingling of the right upper extremity. She notes that her mother suffered from rheumatoid arthritis that affected her shoulder. Physical examination reveals decreased muscle bulk over the right supra- and infraspinatus fossae

compared to the contralateral side, limited active and passive ROM, marked weakness with external rotation, and 4+/5 strength with shoulder abduction. X-rays of the right shoulder are shown in Figures 2–58 and 2–59.

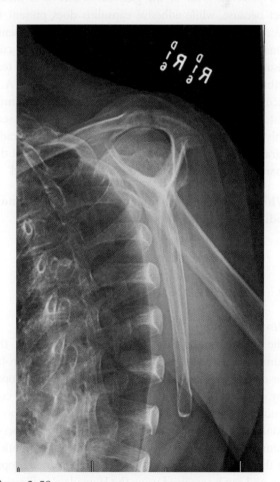

Figure 2–59

What is the most likely diagnosis?

A. Rheumatoid arthritis involving the right glenohumeral joint.
B. Frozen shoulder (adhesive capsulitis)
C. Rotator cuff tear arthropathy
D. Osteoarthritis involving the left glenohumeral joint

Discussion

The correct answer is (C). Rotator cuff tear arthropathy consists of a combination of rotator cuff insufficiency, glenohumeral joint degenerative changes, and superior humeral head migration. It is more common in women and also more often found on the dominant side. The patient's clinical examination with weakened external rotation and muscle atrophy signaling incompetent supra- and infraspinatus muscles point to rotator cuff insufficiency, and her plain films reveal narrowed glenohumeral joint space as well as superior migration of the humeral head. Choice D is incorrect because, while radiographs would show narrowing of the glenohumeral joint space, they would also likely show numerous osteophytes and posterior wear of the glenoid. Choice B is incorrect because, while adhesive capsulitis does present as decreased active and passive range of motion, the patient's constellation of symptoms pointing towards rotator cuff insufficiency along with the radiographs make cuff tear arthropathy the more likely choice. Finally, Choice A is incorrect because even though she has a positive family history of rheumatoid arthritis, it is less likely to present only in a single joint. Also, rheumatoid arthritis on radiography appears more as an erosive process without the characteristic superior migration of the humeral head.

Which of the patient's radiographic findings is most indicative of chronic rotator cuff insufficiency?

A. Superior migration of the humeral head
B. Narrowed glenohumeral joint space
C. Subchondral sclerosis
D. Osteopenia of the proximal humerus

Discussion

The correct answer is (A). Superior migration of the humeral head would be most indicative of chronic rotator cuff insufficiency associated with cuff tear arthropathy, as it is a direct result of the inability of the rotator cuff tendons to help maintain the humerus in its normal position. Acetabularization of the undersurface of the acromion is commonly associated with superior migration of the humeral head found in rotator cuff tear arthropathy, and can be assessed using the Hamada classification,

Table 2–8   HAMADA CLASSIFICATION

Grade 1	Acromiohumeral interval >6 mm
Grade 2	Acromiohumeral interval ≤5 mm
Grade 3	Grade 2 plus acromial acetabularization
Grade 4	Grade 3 plus glenohumeral joint space narrowing
Grade 5	Humeral head collapse

Kappe T, Cakir B, Reichel H, Elsharkawi M. Reliability of radiologic classification for cuff tear arthropathy. *J Shoulder Elbow Surg.* 2011;20:543–547.

which is based on measurements of the acromiohumeral interval on radiography (Table 2–8). Choices B and C are incorrect because, while narrowed glenohumeral joint space and subchondral sclerosis are associated with rotator cuff arthropathy on radiographs, they indicate degenerative joint changes rather than chronic rotator cuff insufficiency. Choice D is incorrect because it is not a specific sign of rotator cuff arthropathy.

What is the most appropriate treatment for the patient at this time?

A. Serial corticosteroid injections into the glenohumeral joint
B. Arthroscopic lavage of the glenohumeral joint
C. Arthroplasty of the glenohumeral joint
D. Physical therapy and PO nonsteroidal anti-inflammatories

Discussion

The correct answer is (D). First-line treatment for rotator cuff tear arthropathy is conservative management with physical therapy and NSAIDs. Glenohumeral steroid injections (Choice A) may partially relieve pain, but serial injections alone are not the most appropriate, initial course. Arthroscopic joint lavage (Choice B) has been tried in the past as treatment for rotator cuff tear arthropathy but it is not currently very common to perform and would definitely not be a first-line treatment. Choice C is incorrect because arthroplasty of the glenohumeral joint is a common treatment for rotator cuff tear arthropathy, it would only be indicated if the patient failed conservative management.

You send the patient to physical therapy and advise her to take ibuprofen as needed for pain. She returns to clinic in 3 months saying her pain and range of motion have not improved, and she would like to pursue operative treatment.

What is the preferred treatment for this patient?

A. Arthroscopic rotator cuff repair
B. Total shoulder arthroplasty with pectoralis tendon transfer
C. Reverse total shoulder arthroplasty with latissimus dorsi tendon transfer
D. Hemiarthroplasty of the glenohumeral joint

Discussion

The correct answer is (C). This patient has failed conservative management and continues to have pain and loss of function; therefore arthroplasty of the glenohumeral joint is now indicated. Reverse total shoulder in particular (as opposed to total shoulder arthroplasty) is indicated for this patient because of her rotator cuff insufficiency. The reverse construct will help increase the efficiency of her deltoid muscle at glenohumeral abduction, since her supraspinatus and infraspinatus are clearly atrophied and nonfunctional. Latissimus transfer is also indicated due to the patient's weakness with external rotation. Choice B is incorrect since total shoulder arthroplasty does not account for rotator cuff insufficiency and would likely lead to superior migration of the humeral prosthesis. Choice A is incorrect as the patient's rotator cuff is likely irreparable by this time, and it would not address the degenerative changes of her glenohumeral joint. Hemiarthroplasty (Choice D) is incorrect because it is not as successful as a reverse total shoulder in improving range of motion and carries the risk of humeral head subluxation.

Objectives: Did you learn...?

- Recognize the clinical presentation of a patient with rotator cuff arthropathy?
- Identify signs of rotator cuff arthropathy on imaging?
- Treat a patient with rotator cuff arthropathy?

CASE 22

Dr. Anna Cohen-Rosenblum

A 28-year-old, male, left hand-dominant, factory worker, and avid weight lifter presents to clinic complaining of 1 month history of right shoulder pain that is worse when lifting weights. He also notices the pain occasionally while driving to and from work. He does not have any other medical issues and denies any history of trauma to the right upper extremity. Physical examination reveals medial rotation of the inferior border of the right scapula when the patient raises his left arm in forward flexion (Fig. 2–60). He has 5/5 strength in forward flexion, external rotation, and

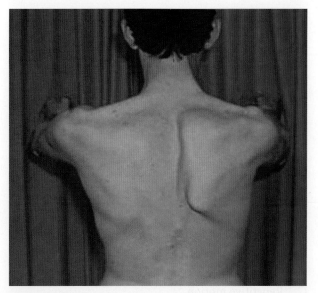

Figure 2–60

shoulder abduction and no asymmetry in shoulder shrug. Radiography reveals no abnormalities.

The patient's abnormal physical examination finding is most likely due to an abnormality involving which nerve and the muscle it innervates?

A. Spinal accessory nerve/trapezius
B. Long thoracic nerve/serratus anterior
C. Dorsal scapular nerve/rhomboid major
D. Thoracodorsal nerve/latissimus dorsi

Discussion

The correct answer is (B). The patient has evidence of medial scapular winging on physical examination, which is caused by injury to the long thoracic nerve and dysfunction of the serratus anterior muscle. This is the most common cause of scapular winging. Lateral scapular winging, which is most commonly due to injury to the spinal accessory nerve and dysfunction of the trapezius muscle (Choice A), would present as lateral rotation of the inferior border of the scapula and may combine with difficulty to shrug (Fig. 2–61). Rhomboid palsy due to dorsal scapular nerve injury (Choice C) is a less common cause of lateral winging. Latissimus dorsi palsy (Choice D) is not involved in either medial or lateral scapular winging. Table 2–9 outlines the most common causes of scapular winging.

What is the most likely etiology of this patient's pain and deformity?

A. Blunt trauma
B. Penetrating trauma

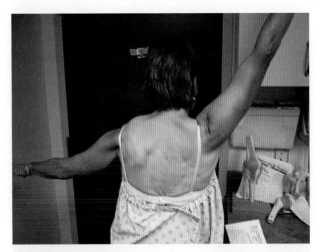

Figure 2-61

C.   Repetitive motion

D.   Guillain–Barré syndrome

Discussion

The correct answer is (C). With a hobby of weight lifting and working at a factory, repetitive motion is the most likely cause of a stretch injury to the long thoracic nerve resulting in serratus anterior palsy. The long thoracic nerve may also be damaged due to positioning during various procedures involving the chest wall. Guillain–Barré syndrome (Choice D) is another possible cause of serratus anterior palsy, but is much less common and therefore less likely to be the cause of this particular patient's nerve injury. Choices A and B are more likely to be the cause of spinal accessory nerve injury and resultant lateral winging.

What is the most appropriate next step for this patient with medial scapular winging?

A.   Electromyography of the bilateral upper extremities

B.   MRI of the right shoulder without contrast

C.   Arthroscopic decompression of the suprascapular nerve

D.   Scapular bracing to stabilize the scapula against the thorax

Discussion

The correct answer is (A). The patient's long thoracic nerve should be evaluated using electromyography (EMG) to obtain a baseline assessment of any extant nerve injury. Other initial interventions may include NSAIDs, activity modification avoiding elevation of the arm above shoulder level, and physical therapy to strengthen the rotator cuff muscles and scapular stabilizers. Scapular bracing (Choice D) is another option for conservative management of scapular winging but is often uncomfortable and difficult to enforce in terms of patient compliance. MRI (Choice B) is not indicated at this time as it would not contribute to any clinical decision-making. Entrapment of the suprascapular nerve (Choice C) would lead to atrophy of the infraspinatus and/or supraspinatus muscles, not scapular winging.

The patient undergoes an EMG showing conduction abnormalities of the long thoracic nerve. Physical therapy, stopping weight lifting, and scapular bracing do not relieve his pain. It is now approximately 1 year since his initial diagnosis.

What is the most appropriate intervention at this time?

A.   Scapulothoracic fusion

B.   Eden–Lange dynamic muscle transfer

C.   Latissimus dorsi tendon transfer

D.   Pectoralis major tendon transfer

Discussion

The correct answer is (D). Medial scapular winging and pain that does not respond to conservative management is

Table 2–9   ETIOLOGY OF SCAPULAR WINGING

Medial winging	**Trauma:** injury to long thoracic nerve (serratus anterior palsy) from MVA, collision sports, upper extremity overuse **Compression** of LTN by middle scalene muscle, between clavicle and second rib, at inferior angle of scapula **Iatrogenic:** intraoperative positioning, injury during ACDF, mastectomy, thoracostomy tube, etc. Transient brachial neuritis, Guillain–Barré , SLE, Arnold–Chiari malformation
Lateral winging	**Trauma:** injury to spinal accessory nerve (trapezius palsy) or to dorsoscapular nerve (rhomboid palsy) from falls, MVA, blunt trauma in football/hockey, penetrating trauma **Compression** of DSN by middle scalene muscle, C5 radiculopathy **Iatrogenic:** cervical lymph node biopsy

From Meininger A, Figurerres B, Goldberg B. Scapular winging: an update. *JAAOS.* 2011;19(8):453–462.

an indication for operative intervention with transfer of the sternal head of the pectoralis major muscle to the inferior border of the scapula to replace the function of the serratus anterior. Eden–Lange dynamic muscle transfer (Choice B) involves lateralization of the rhomboid muscles as well as the levator scapulae at their insertions on the scapula to act in place of the trapezius and would be indicated for lateral scapular winging caused by injury to the spinal accessory nerve. Scapulothoracic fusion (Choice A) would only be indicated if the patient continued to have pain and deformity following dynamic muscle transfer. Latissimus dorsi transfer (Choice C), while a type of dynamic muscle transfer, is not indicated for scapular winging but would be more appropriate for cases of massive rotator cuff tear.

Objectives: Did you learn...?

- Recognize the clinical presentation of a patient with scapular winging?
- Distinguish between medial and lateral scapular winging?
- Treat a patient with scapular winging?

CASE 23

Dr. Anna Cohen-Rosenblum

A 47-year-old, right-hand-dominant male presents to your clinic complaining of right shoulder weakness for the past 2 months. He denies any history of trauma but notes sudden onset of pain 2 months ago that lasted approximately 2 weeks and then subsided without any intervention and was followed by shoulder weakness. He works as a lawyer and has been going through a divorce for the past year. Physical examination reveals no tenderness to palpation about the shoulder. He has decreased sensation over the lateral aspect of the shoulder, decreased muscle bulk over the left shoulder compared with the contralateral side, and weakness with left shoulder abduction. He is distally neurovascularly intact. The patient had already been referred for an x-ray and MRI by his primary care doctor that are shown in Figures 2–62 and 2–63.

Injury to what structure is most likely responsible for his symptoms?

A. Suprascapular nerve
B. Dorsal scapular nerve
C. Axillary nerve
D. Posterior cord of the brachial plexus

Discussion

The correct answer is (C). The patient's decreased sensation over the deltoid, deltoid muscle atrophy on

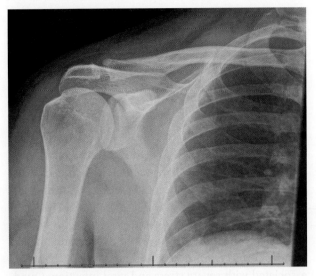

Figure 2–62

examination, and MRI with atrophy of the teres minor points to axillary nerve dysfunction. Suprascapular nerve injury (Choice A) would result in atrophy of the infraspinatus and or infraspinatus muscles, leading to weakness with external rotation and/or forward flexion. Dorsal scapular nerve injury (Choice B) would result in weakness of the rhomboid muscles and levator scapulae. While injury to the posterior cord of the brachial plexus (Choice D) would result in symptoms of axillary nerve palsy, they would also involve dysfunction of the radial nerve, which also comes off the posterior cord.

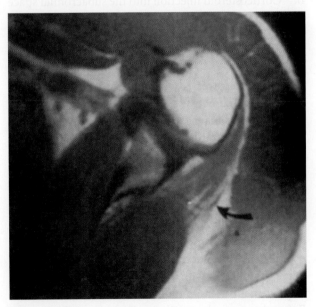

Figure 2–63

What is the most likely etiology of this patient's nerve dysfunction?

A. Quadrilateral space syndrome
B. Parsonage Turner syndrome
C. Mass effect
D. Blunt trauma

Discussion

The correct answer is (B). Parsonage Turner syndrome (brachial neuritis) is characterized by acute brachial neuropathy which can affect different nerves of the brachial plexus. In this patient, it is the most likely explanation for his atraumatic deltoid paralysis with axillary nerve palsy in a time of severe stress. The cause of Parsonage Turner Syndrome is unknown, but it has been associated with severe stress and viral infection. Quadrilateral space syndrome (Choice A) involves entrapment of the axillary nerve as it passes through the quadrilateral space, would present as chronic dull pain, and is usually not associated with decreased sensation. While Choices C and D can both be a cause of axillary nerve injury, the patient has no history of trauma and there are no masses on his MRI.

You send the patient for an EMG which shows decreased conduction through the axillary nerve and denervation of the deltoid and teres minor muscles.

What is the most appropriate management for the patient at this time?

A. Physical therapy
B. Corticosteroid injection into the subacromial space
C. Operative exploration of the axillary nerve
D. Referral to neurology for further workup

Discussion

The correct answer is (A). Physical therapy focusing on passive- and active-assisted range of motion is the cornerstone of management of Parsonage Turner syndrome. Corticosteroid injection into the subacromial space (Choice B) will not help with his decreased range of motion and weakness. Choice C would be appropriate if the patient's axillary nerve injury was traumatic, with operative nerve exploration occurring approximately 3 weeks after injury with EMG findings demonstrating loss of conduction/denervation. Operative exploration could also be considered in cases of atraumatic axillary nerve dysfunction with no evidence of clinical or EMG improvement after 6 months of conservative treatment. Referral to neurology (Choice D) is not necessary for

management of Parsonage Turner syndrome, which is a type of peripheral neuropathy.

What is the most likely outcome of this patient's condition at 1 year after the onset of symptoms if treated conservatively?

A. Complete recovery
B. Progressively improving symptoms
C. Progressively worsening symptoms
D. Loss of function of the left upper extremity

Discussion

The correct answer is (B). At 1 year after onset of symptoms, the patient is most likely to be in the recovery process but with ongoing weakness and/or pain. However, by 3 years most patients have fully recovered with conservative management alone. Should symptoms be progressively worsening at 1 year (Choice C), alternate explanations must be considered.

Objectives: Did you learn...?

• Recognize the clinical presentation of a patient with axillary neuropathy?
• Understand the etiology of axillary neuropathy?
• Treat a patient with axillary neuropathy?

CASE 24

Dr. Anna Cohen-Rosenblum

A 21-year-old, right-hand-dominant, male, college swimmer presents to clinic complaining of gradually worsening right shoulder pain for the past 6 months. He notes that his times at swim meets have been slowing with the onset of the pain but that he is still able to swim through the pain. Physical examination reveals: decreased muscle bulk over the infraspinatus fossa of the right shoulder compared with the contralateral side (shown in Fig. 2–64), full active range of motion, strength 4/5 for external rotation but otherwise normal strength, mild pain with cross-body adduction of the right shoulder, and mild tenderness to palpation over the AC joint. Imaging is shown in Figure 2–65.

Based on the information obtained thus far, what is the patient's most likely diagnosis?

A. Rotator cuff tendinitis
B. Adhesive capsulitis
C. Acromioclavicular joint arthritis
D. Suprascapular neuropathy

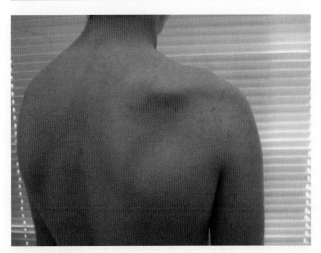

Figure 2–64

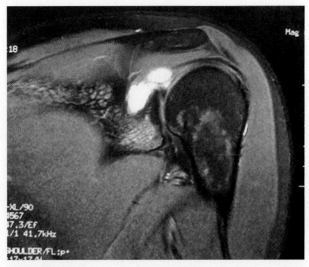

Figure 2–66

Discussion

The correct answer is (D). This patient's atrophy of the infraspinatus muscle leading to weakness with external rotation and with preserved strength in the other rotator cuff muscles is likely due to neuropathic process of the suprascapular nerve at a point along its course off the upper trunk of the brachial plexus on its way to innervate the supraspinatus and infraspinatus muscles. Choice A is incorrect as rotator cuff tendinitis would not present with muscle atrophy. AC joint arthritis (Choice C), while often presenting with tenderness to palpation over the AC joint and pain with cross body adduction, is also not usually associated with infraspinatus atrophy and would likely present with narrowed joint space or AC joint osteophytes on plain films,

unlike this patient. Choice B is incorrect as the patient has full active range of motion, while adhesive capsulitis would more likely present as decreased active and passive range of motion.

You send the patient for an MRI, which is shown in Figure 2–66.

Based on the clinical examination and imaging, what is the most likely etiology of the patient's symptoms?

A. Suprascapular nerve entrapment at the spinoglenoid notch by the spinoglenoid ligament
B. Suprascapular nerve entrapment at the suprascapular notch due to scapular body fracture
C. Suprascapular nerve entrapment at the spinoglenoid notch by a paralabral cyst
D. Suprascapular nerve entrapment at the suprascapular notch by the transverse scapular ligament

Discussion

The correct answer is (C). The patient's clinical examination findings of isolated weakness in external rotation and atrophy of the infraspinatus muscle point to suprascapular nerve entrapment at a location past the exit point for the branch to the supraspinatus muscle. Also, MRI reveals a posterior labral tear with a paralabral cyst that is compressing the suprascapular nerve at the spinoglenoid notch. Choice A, while fitting with the patient's clinical examination, does not fit with the MRI showing paralabral cyst. Choices B and D are incorrect because entrapment of the suprascapular nerve at the suprascapular notch by scapular body fracture or by the transverse scapular ligament (more common) would lead to weak-

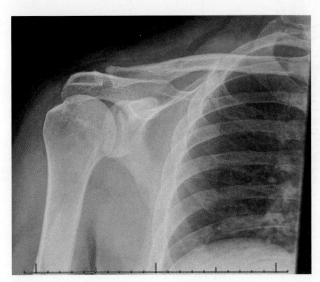

Figure 2–65

ness/atrophy in both supraspinatus and infraspinatus muscles as the suprascapular notch is proximal to the nerve branch point to the supraspinatus muscle.

What nerve is innervated by the same spinal nerves as the suprascapular nerve?

A. Axillary nerve
B. Musculocutaneous nerve
C. Dorsal scapular nerve
D. Radial nerve

Discussion

The correct answer is (A). The suprascapular nerve branches off the upper trunk of the brachial plexus and consists of fibers from C5 to C6 spinal nerves. The axillary nerve is a terminal branch from the posterior cord of the brachial plexus and also consists of fibers from C5 to C6. The musculocutaneous nerve (Choice B) is a terminal branch from the lateral cord and consists of fibers from C5 to C7. The dorsal scapular nerve (Choice C) branches off the C5 nerve root and consists of fibers from C5. The radial nerve (Choice D) is a terminal branch from the posterior cord and consists of fibers from C5 to T1. See Figure 2–67 for a diagram of the brachial plexus.

What is the most appropriate treatment at this time?

A. Physical therapy and NSAIDs
B. Arthroscopic decompression of the paralabral cyst and labral repair
C. EMG of bilateral upper extremities
D. Open decompression of the spinoglenoid and suprascapular notches

Discussion

The correct answer is (B). The patient has a clear etiology for his suprascapular nerve decompression in the paralabral cyst with symptoms that have lasted for 6 months resulting in atrophy of the infraspinatus muscle. Given that he is a college-level athlete and likely wants to improve his athletic performance, surgical decompression of the suprascapular nerve at the spinoglenoid notch is indicated at this time, which can best be accomplished arthroscopically along with labral repair. Choice D is incorrect as the patient does not require decompression of the nerve at the suprascapular notch, since he shows no sign of weakness/atrophy of the supraspinatus muscle. Choice A would be appropriate for a patient with symptoms of suprascapular nerve compression for less than 6 months of duration, without atrophy, and without

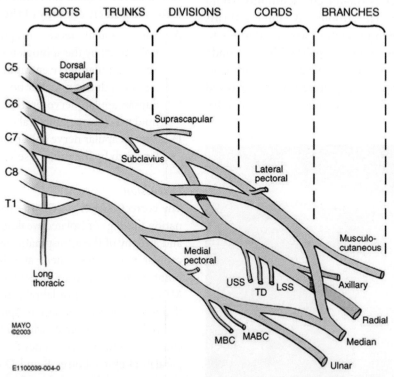

Figure 2–67 Reproduced with permission from Moran S, Steinmann S, and Shin A. Brachial plexus injuries: Mechanism, patterns of injury, and physical diagnosis. *Hand Clin* 2005;21:13–24 (Fig 2A).

any compressive mass on MRI. Choice C could aid in establishing a baseline for treatment and could localize nerve entrapment sites in a patient whom the location of suprascapular nerve entrapment was unclear but is not the most appropriate treatment for this particular patient.

Objectives: Did you learn...?

- Recognize the clinical presentation of suprascapular neuropathy?
- Distinguish between suprascapular neuropathy at the suprascapular and spinoglenoid notch?
- Treat a patient with suprascapular neuropathy?

CASE 25

Dr. Robert J. Stewart

A 29-year-old, right-hand-dominant male presented to the Emergency Department with right shoulder pain after falling while riding his mountain bike. He reports that he "flew over his handle bars." The patient was wearing a helmet and denies loss of consciousness. He denies numbness or tingling in the left, upper extremity. He notes increased swelling and pain over the clavicle. On examination, the patient's skin is tenting over the distal end of the clavicle, and he has tenderness to palpation over the coracoclavicular interspace. He is diagnosed with an acromioclavicular (AC) joint separation and is unable to reduce the injury in the ED.

What is the mechanism of this injury?

A. Hyperabduction and external rotation of the arm combined with retraction of the scapula
B. Anterior and inferior displacement of the scapula
C. Inferior displacement of the scapula in relation to the clavicle
D. Lateral translation of the acromion in relation to the clavicle
E. Medial displacement of the clavicle in relation to the acromion

Discussion

The correct answer is (C). The mechanism of an AC joint separation is inferior displacement of the scapula in relation to the clavicle. AC joint separation can occur from direct or indirect mechanisms. Direct injuries result from a direct force to the acromion with the shoulder adducted. The acromion moves inferiorly and medially and the clavicle remains stabilized by the sternoclavicular ligaments. This is the mechanism of most AC joint separations and is usually caused by a fall onto the superolateral portion of the shoulder. The force applied during this type of injury results in a systematic failure of the stabilizing ligaments. The failure of the acromioclavicular (AC) ligaments and capsule is followed by failure of the coracoclavicular (CC) ligaments and deltotrapezial fascia. The indirect mechanism results in the same injury, but due to a fall on an outstretched arm or elbow with a superiorly direct force. Hyperabduction and external rotation of the arm combined with retraction of the scapula is thought to be the mechanism for the exceedingly rare Type VI AC joint dislocation. Anterior and inferior displacement of the scapula from a force applied to the acromion is thought to be the mechanism of the relatively rare Type IV AC joint dislocation. Lateral translation of the acromion in relation to the clavicle and medial displacement of the clavicle are not described as mechanisms of AC joint separations.

What structure provides the most resistance to AC joint compression?

A. Conoid ligament
B. Trapezoid ligament
C. AC ligaments
D. Coracoacromial (CA) ligament
E. Deltotrapezial fascia

Discussion

The correct answer is (B). The AC joint is a diarthrodial joint that has both static and dynamic stabilizers. The trapezoid and conoid ligaments comprise the CC ligaments. The trapezoid ligament is a static stabilizer, which attaches more lateral than the conoid ligament on the undersurface of the clavicle and provides resistance to AC joint compression. The conoid ligament inserts more medially on the undersurface of the clavicle providing approximately 60% of the restraint to anterior and superior displacement and rotation of the clavicle. The AC ligaments (Answer C) are static stabilizers that reinforce the joint capsule and predominately control horizontal motion (anterior and posterior) of the clavicle. The coracoacromial (CA) ligament is used in CC ligament reconstruction and does not play a significant role in AC joint stability. The deltotrapezial fascia is a dynamic stabilizer of the AC joint and must be considered when AC joint reconstruction is performed.

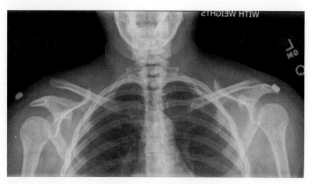

Figure 2–68

A radiograph of the patient is shown in Figure 2–68. Based on the information obtained thus far, what is the most likely classification of this injury?

A. Type II
B. Type III
C. Type IV
D. Type V
E. Type VI

Discussion

The correct answer is (D). Based on the amount of distance between the coracoid process and the clavicle (CC interspace); the fact that the distal clavicle is tenting the skin and that the joint is irreducible, this AC joint separation can best be classified as a type V. The remaining answer choices are incorrect based on the information provided in Table 2–10 describes the Rockwood classification of AC joint injuries.

What is the most appropriate way to manage this patient's injury?

A. Sling immobilization and early range of motion
B. Sling immobilization for 7 to 10 days until pain resolves
C. Figure-of-eight sling for immobilization for 7 to 10 days until pain resolves
D. Open reduction, ligamentous repair, coracoclavicular ligament repair supplementation, and repair of the deltoid and trapezial fascia
E. Open Mumford procedure

Discussion

The correct answer is (D). Type IV, V, and VI injuries all require surgical intervention. Answer E is a distal clavicle resection. Because this injury is unstable, this procedure would likely accentuate the instability.

Type I injuries can usually be treated with a simple sling for 7 to 10 days or until pain has subsided. Type II injuries can require as long as 2 weeks of immobilization to achieve resolution of symptoms. When pain has subsided, passive- and active-assisted range of motion and strengthening exercises are instituted. Contact sports and heavy lifting should be avoided for 2 to 3 months. There is controversy regarding treatment of Type III injuries. Most studies support nonsurgical management. However, discrepancies exist when managing young patients who frequently engage in activities that place high demands on the shoulder. A rigorous rehabilitation program should be undertaken when nonsurgically managing type III injuries because this may have an impact on the outcome.

Table 2–10   CHARACTERIZATION OF ACROMIOCLAVICULAR JOINT INJURIES BY THE ROCKWOOD CLASSIFICATION[a]

Type	AC Ligaments	CC Ligaments	Deltopectoral Fascia	Radiographic CC Distance Increase	Radiographic AC Appearance	AC Joint Reducible
I	Sprained	Intact	Intact	Normal (1.1–1.3 cm)	Normal	N/A
II	Disrupted	Sprained	Intact	<25%	Widened	Yes
III	Disrupted	Disrupted	Disrupted	25–100%	Widened	Yes
IV	Disrupted	Disrupted	Disrupted	Increased	Posterior clavicle displacement	No
V	Disrupted	Disrupted	Disrupted	100–300%	N/A	No
VI	Disrupted	Intact	Disrupted	Decreased	N/A	No

[a]The type of AC injury can be discerned on the pattern of ligament injury, AC joint position on radiographs, and whether the AC joint can be reduced on physical examination. (From Simovitch R, Sanders B, Ozbaydar M, Lavery K, Warner JJP. Acromioclavicular joint injuries: diagnosis and management. *J Am Acad Orthop Surg* 2009;17:207–219.)

AC, acromioclavicular; CC, coracoclavicular; N/A, not applicable.

There are several different ways to surgically manage AC joint separations. All have the same goal of obtaining and retaining anatomic reduction. There are three main groups of surgical techniques: primary fixation, fixation between the coracoid process and the clavicle, and ligament reconstruction. Some of these techniques can be combined, such as hook plate fixation with ligament reconstruction. Primary fixation with Kirschner wires has been abandoned due to risk of pin migration. Fixation with hook-plates, which is more commonly performed in Europe, can be performed. The plate must be removed at 8 weeks. Fixation between the coracoid process and the clavicle can be performed using a screw, synthetic loops (i.e., 6-mm PTFE surgical tape). Ligament reconstruction can be performed with the Weaver and Dunn procedure or some of its modifications in which the CA ligament is detached from the acromion and is then transferred to the clavicle. Alternative techniques for ligament reconstruction use semitendinosus tendon autograft or anterior tibialis tendon allograft with different fixation methods to the coracoid process and clavicle.

Objectives: Did you learn...?

- Recognize the mechanism of AC joint separations?
- Recognize different types of AC joint separations?
- Appropriately treat a patient with AC joint separation based on the type of injury while considering the individual?

CASE 26

Dr. Robert J. Stewart

A patient is brought to the emergency room trauma bay after a motor vehicle collision. During the initial trauma evaluation, a deformity and swelling is noted over the medial aspect of the right clavicle. She has noticeable venous congestion over her right neck and is complaining of numbness and tingling in the right, upper extremity. She is unable to move her right arm because of severe pain and is supporting it across her trunk with her left arm.

Based on the information provided, what is the most likely diagnosis?

A. Bilateral sternoclavicular dislocation
B. Right posterior sternoclavicular joint dislocation
C. Right anterior sternoclavicular dislocation
D. Right acromioclavicular dislocation
E. Right pneumothorax

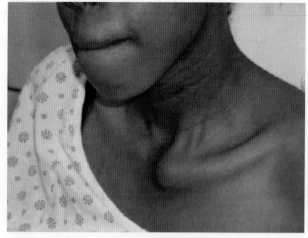

Figure 2–69

Discussion

The correct answer is (B). Sternoclavicular (SC) joint dislocations are rare and posterior dislocations are much less common than anterior. The patient will be in severe pain that is increased with any movement, particularly when the shoulders are pressed together by a lateral force or placed in a supine position. The injured arm will usually be supported by the uninjured arm. The head may be tilted toward the side of the dislocation. With an anterior dislocation of the SC joint, the medial end of the clavicle might be visibly prominent and palpable anteriorly to the sternum (Fig. 2–69).

The corner of the sternum might be easily palpated in a posterior dislocation. Swelling may obscure the ability to distinguish an anterior and posterior SC joint dislocation. Bilateral dislocations are extremely rare. Because of this patient's symptoms of venous congestion with numbness and tingling, it is likely she suffered a posterior SC joint dislocation. A right acromioclavicular dislocation would present with pain and deformity over the lateral aspect of the clavicle. A pneumothorax is a complication of a posterior SC joint dislocation.

A PA view of the chest is the only radiograph available. What additional view would be most beneficial?

A. Lateral view of the chest
B. Swimmer's view
C. Stryker notch view
D. Serendipity view

Discussion

The correct answer is (D). A serendipity view is a 40-degree cephalic-tilt view (Fig. 2–70). This provides a true caudocephalic view of both the SC joint and the medial clavicles.

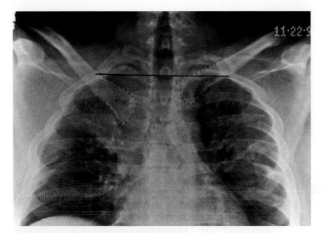

Figure 2–70

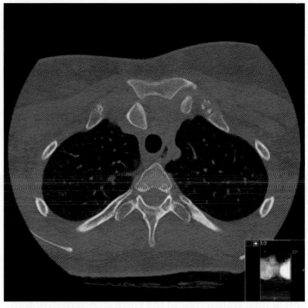

Figure 2–71

The serendipity view is usually the front line radiograph obtained, however, computed tomography (CT) is the best technique to study the SC joint. Other radiographic views of the SC joint include the Heinig view and the Hobbs view. The lateral view of the chest cannot be used to interpret SC joint dislocations because of the overlap of the medial clavicles with the first rib and the sternum. A swimmer's view is used for increased visualization of the subaxial cervical spine. The stryker notch view is used for evaluating Hill-Sachs lesions of the humeral head after glenohumeral dislocations.

What is the most common cause of a posterior sternoclavicular joint dislocation?

A. Athletic injury

B. Fall from excessive height onto outstretched arm

C. Industrial accident

D. Motor vehicle accident (MVA)

E. Atraumatic instability

Discussion

The correct answer is (D). MVA accounts for 40% of SC joint dislocations. Athletic injuries account for 21%. The remaining 39% include falls and industrial accidents. Instability of the SC joint can be classified according to different factors. It can be traumatic or atraumatic; structural or nonstructural; acute, recurrent, or persistent. Causes of atraumatic, structural instability of the SC joint include: Ehlers Danlos syndrome, abnormal clavicular shape, degenerative osteoarthritis, inflammatory arthritis, infection, or sternoclavicular hyperostosis syndrome. Answer E is incorrect because atraumatic instability is not the most common cause of posterior dislocations. SC joint dislocations can occur from direct or indirect force. Direct force only results in posterior

dislocation and is when a force is applied directly to the anteromedial aspect of the clavicle. Indirect is when a compressive force is applied to the anterolateral or posterolateral aspect of the shoulder, resulting in an anterior or posterior dislocation, respectively. Most SC joint dislocations are caused by indirect force.

A CT scan of the chest is obtained and shown in Figure 2–71. What is the next best step in managing this patient?

A. Attempting a closed reduction after assuring that a thoracic or cardiothoracic surgeon is available if complications occur

B. Open reduction with assistance from a thoracic surgeon

C. MRI to assess for soft tissue and neurovascular injuries in the mediastinum

D. Conservative management with a figure-of-eight sling

Discussion

The correct answer is (A). Both anterior and posterior SC joint dislocations that are diagnosed within 7 to 10 days of injury should be initially treated with closed reduction. The caveat is that with posterior dislocations in which there is suspicion of mediastinal involvement, a surgeon with more mediastinal expertise should be consulted. Note that anterior SC joint dislocations are inherently more unstable after closed reduction than posterior dislocations. Open reduction should only be attempted after closed reduction attempts have failed. MRI is not necessary at this point in the case. A CT scan is the preferred imaging modality in the acute setting. A figure-of-eight sling can be used after reduction to promote healing.

Which of the following basic surgical techniques is the most commonly performed for an unreduced SC joint after closed reduction has been attempted?

A. Plate and screw fixation
B. Kirschner wires
C. Steinmann pins
D. Cannulated screw fixation
E. Resecting the medial clavicle

Discussion

The correct answer is (E). Adults over the age of 23 should undergo open reduction if closed reduction has failed. If the costoclavicular ligament is intact after reduction, the clavicle medial to the ligaments should be excised. If the ligaments are disrupted, the clavicle must be stabilized to the first rib. Answers A and D are incorrect because these techniques have very limited reports of use and require hardware removal. Answers B and C are essentially contraindicated because of reported incidences of migration and serious complications, including death. If the patient is younger than 23 years old, they can likely be treated nonoperatively because the remodeling provided by the open physes will eliminate most of the bone deformity or displacement. The clavicle is the first bone to ossify (at 5 weeks of gestation), but the medial epiphysis is the last to fuse (at 23–25 years).

Objectives: Did you learn...?

• Understand that SC joint injuries are rare?
• Recognize the different mechanism of anterior and posterior SC joint dislocations?
• Describe the most appropriate radiographic view for SC joint pathology?
• Understand the different treatment options for anterior and posterior SC joint dislocations?
• Understand the important complications that can be associated with posterior SC joint dislocations and the importance for a multi-disciplinary approach when indicated?

CASE 27

Dr. Robert J. Stewart

A 55-year-old, right-hand-dominant female presents with right shoulder pain for 6 months. She localizes the pain over the anterior and superior aspect of her shoulder. The pain is worsened when she is cleaning her contralateral axilla, while showering, and fastening or unhooking her bra. The pain sometimes radiates down her arm. She has taken ibuprofen with some improvement, and she has undergone a course of physical therapy (PT) that did not relieve symptoms. She is continuing her home exercise program (HEP). On examination, the patient is tender over the acromioclavicular (AC) joint. Her range of motion (ROM) is normal, but with increased pain. She has a negative Sperling test and a positive cross-body adduction test. She has a negative Hawkins sign and Neer test. She also has a positive O'Brien's test when in supination.

Based on the information given thus far, what is the most likely diagnosis?

A. Cervical radiculopathy
B. Glenohumeral arthritis
C. SLAP tear
D. Acromioclavicular joint arthritis
E. Subacromial impingement

Discussion

The correct answer is (D). The acromioclavicular (AC) joint is a small, diarthrodial joint with a fibrocartilage disk separating the two articular surfaces. This disk is thought to begin degenerating in the second decade of life and undergoes rapid degeneration until it is no longer functional beyond the fourth decade. Because the AC joint has a small contact area experiencing large loads, it is a frequent source of clinical symptoms. Symptoms are most often due to primary osteoarthritis, post-traumatic arthritis, or distal clavicle osteolysis. The patient had a negative Sperling test and lack of neurological pain (Answer A). The patient has normal ROM, a negative O'Brien's test in pronation, and a negative Neer and Hawkin's test (Answers B, C, and E).

Which radiographic view is the most accurate view to evaluate suspected AC joint pathology?

A. Anteroposterior view
B. Stress view
C. Axillary lateral view
D. Zanca view
E. Stryker notch view

Discussion

The correct answer is (D). The Zanca view is an AP radiograph obtained by angling the x-ray beam 10 to 15 degrees

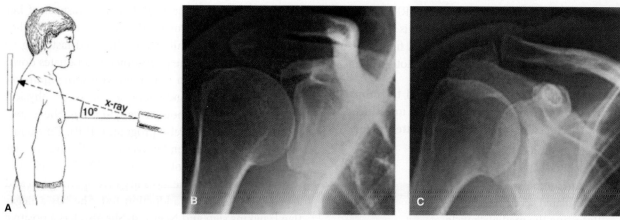

Figure 2–72 **A:** Zanca view projection. **B:** AP view of the shoulder that overpenetrates and does not show AC joint well. **C:** Zanca view demonstrates better ACJ detail. (Reproduced with permission from Shaffer BS: Painful conditions of the acromioclavicular joint. *J Am Acad Orthop Surg* 1999;7:176–188.)

superiorly and decreasing the kilovoltage (Fig. 2–72A–C). The AP and axillary views should be routinely obtained for investigation of shoulder pathology, but are not the most accurate for AC joint pathology. Stress views have been used in the past to help differentiate type II from type III AC joint instability injuries but are not helpful or indicated in AC joint osteoarthritis. A stryker notch view is used for evaluation of Hill–Sachs lesions of the humeral head after a glenohumeral dislocation.

What AC joint structure(s) is predominantly responsible for maintaining anteroposterior (AP) stability?

A. Coracoacromial ligament
B. Acromioclavicular ligaments
C. Conoid ligament
D. Trapezoid ligament
E. Coracohumeral ligament

Discussion

The correct answer is (B). The AC joint capsular ligaments (acromioclavicular ligaments) are predominantly responsible for maintaining stability in the AP plane. The coracoacromial ligament does not play a significant role in AC joint stability. The conoid and trapezoid ligaments primarily resist superior and axial translation. The coracohumeral ligament plays a role in glenohumeral stability, not AC joint stability.

What is the most appropriate next step in treating this patient with AC joint arthritis?

A. Injection with local anesthetic and corticosteroid
B. Order more PT focusing on strengthening and stretching of shoulder girdle

C. Recommend activity modification, anti-inflammatory medications, and plan to follow-up with patient in 6 weeks
D. Arthroscopic Mumford procedure
E. Open distal clavicle resection

Discussion

The correct answer is (A). Based on the information provided, the patient has continued pain but does not have loss of function. This (and the fact that she has failed other nonoperative measures including anti-inflammatory medication and PT) would make an intra-articular injection the most appropriate next step. Injections can be used both diagnostically and therapeutically. Answers B and C are incorrect because the patient has already undergone these treatments and is currently undergoing a HEP with activity modification. Indications for operative management of AC joint osteoarthritis include continued pain and loss of function despite a full course of nonoperative treatment. This patient does not have loss of function.

All of the following are advantages of arthroscopy when compared to open distal clavicle resection, EXCEPT?

A. Accelerated recovery
B. Ability to preserve AC ligaments, joint capsule, and deltotrapezial fascia
C. Ability to treat concomitant intra-articular glenohumeral lesions
D. Ability to treat concomitant subacromial lesions
E. Demonstrates significant improvement in VAS pain scores and SF-36 quality of life scores

Discussion

The correct answer is (E). Both open and arthroscopic techniques demonstrate improved VAS pain scores and SF-36 quality of life scores. Answers A, B, C, and D are all advantages of the arthroscopic technique for distal clavicle resection over the open technique.

Objectives: Did you learn...?

• Recognize the clinical presentation of acromioclavicular arthritis?

• Differentiate between primary osteoarthritis, post-traumatic arthritis, and distal clavicle osteolysis?

• Treat a patient with AC joint arthritis?

• Recognize the advantages of arthroscopic versus open distal clavicle resection?

CASE 28

Dr. Robert J. Stewart

A 65-year-old, right-hand-dominant female presents to clinic for evaluation of her right chest. She used to work as a manual laborer in the scrap metal business. She is particularly concerned about the bulging, but the pain is also becoming severe. She has tried ibuprofen without relief. On physical examination, she is afebrile with tenderness and a palpable bony protuberance over the right sternoclavicular joint that is asymmetrical when compared with the contralateral side. She has increased pain with forward flexion and abduction of the right shoulder.

Based on the information provided, the most likely diagnosis for the condition described is:

A. Condensing osteitis of the sternoclavicular joint
B. Sternoclaivcular joint rheumatoid arthritis
C. Pseudogout of the sternoclavicular joint
D. Sternoclavicular joint osteoarthritis
E. Sternoclavicular septic arthritis

Discussion

The correct answer is (D). Sternoclavicular (SC) joint osteoarthritis is the most common condition affecting this joint. Moderate to severe degenerative changes may be asymptomatic and present in over 50% of individuals over 60 years of age. Postmenopausal women, patients with chronic SC joint instability, and manual laborers are at higher risk of developing SC joint osteoarthritis. Condensing osteitis is rare and characterized by aseptic enlargement and sclerosis of the medial end of the clavicle with obliteration of the medullary cavity. Rheumatoid arthritis (RA) is incorrect because there is

no mention of RA in her history. It has been reported that 30% of people with RA have SC joint involvement. Crystal-deposition arthropathy has been described in the SC joint, but is uncommon. Septic arthritis of the SC joint is uncommon and associated with underlying disease or risk factors including RA, sepsis, infected subclavian lines, alcoholism, HIV, renal dialysis, and intravenous drug use (IVDU). It is important to take a careful history when dealing with complaints of the SC joint because many conditions are systemic.

Plain radiographs and a computed tomography (CT) scan are obtained. Neither shows signs of neoplasm or metastatic disease. The CT is shown in Figure 2–73. Which of the following treatment options is most likely to result in symptom relief for this patient?

A. Rest, anti-inflammatory medication, and moist heat
B. Intra-articular corticosteroid injection under computed tomography (CT) guidance
C. Rest, activity modification, anti-inflammatory medication, and intra-articular corticosteroid injection
D. Medial clavicle resection
E. PT alone

Discussion

The correct answer is (C). Nonoperative treatment of SC joint osteoarthritis is the mainstay of initial treatment, and most symptomatic patients will respond to these nonsurgical treatments. The other conservative treatment options listed are incorrect in this case because they would be less likely to result in symptom relief. Answer D is incorrect because conservative measures should be attempted for at least 6 months before operative treatment is considered. When performing intra-articular injections under CT guidance, the clinician

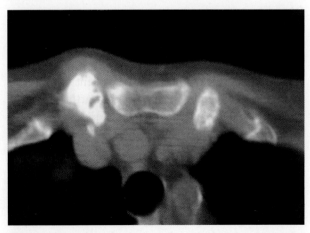

Figure 2–73

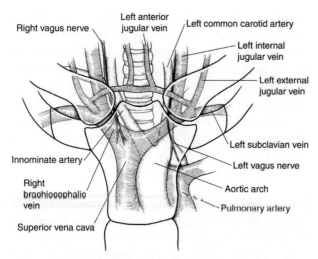

Figure 2–74 Reproduced with permission from Higginbotham TO, Kuhn JE. Atraumatic disorders of the sternoclavicular joint. *J Am Acad Orthop Surg* 2005;13(2):138–145.

should have clear knowledge of the surrounding anatomy. Figure 2–74 demonstrates the relationships of the surrounding anatomy.

Upon further questioning, the patient admits to having a history of diabetes mellitus and IVDU. Lab results show the following: WBC = 7.1, CRP = <3, ESR = 11. On closer inspection, pitting on her fingernails is noted.

What additional laboratory or physical examination finding should be pursued to rule-out a potential condition affecting her SC joint?

A. Positive rheumatoid factor (RF)
B. Presence of antinuclear antibodies (ANA)
C. Human leukocyte antigen B27 (HLA-B27)
D. Palmoplantar pustulosis
E. Positively birefringent crystals

Discussion

The correct answer is (C). Less common pathologic processes can cause SC joint symptoms similar to this case. The treatment will vary greatly depending on the underlying disease process. Because the patient is found to have pitting of the finger nails, psoriatic arthritis should be considered as an underlying disease. Seronegative spondyloarthropathies can involve the SC joint, especially psoriatic arthritis. The SC joint has been reported to be involved in 90% of patients with severe psoriatic arthropathy. Detection of HLA-B27 is usually diagnostic for seronegative spondyloarthropathies. RF and ANA are not likely to help in this case. Answer D is a physical examination finding that can be found in association SC joint osteoarthritis. Palmoplantar pustulosis with SC

joint arthritis is a rare constellation of findings that is known by different names including sternocostoclavicular hyperostosis, intersternocostoclavicular ossification, pustulotic arthroosteitis, and SAPHO syndrome. Answer E is diagnostic of pseudogout. Other rare conditions that can affect the SC joint are condensing osteitis and Friedrich's disease (aseptic necrosis of the medial clavicle).

Nonoperative management is usually sufficient for most etiologies of SC joint pain, however, the medical management and associated conditions can vary significantly. For this case, important aspects of the history would be whether the patient had any previous blood work done, a family history of seronegative spondyloarthropathies, and does she have a history of other joint pain, fevers, chills, or dermatologic conditions.

The patient is diagnosed with primary osteoarthritis of the SC joint and failed to improve after 6 months of nonsurgical treatment. The pain is quite severe and debilitating. Resection of the medial clavicle is recommended for this patient.

What structure(s) is preserved to help prevent instability postoperatively?

A. Intra-articular disk
B. Intra-articular disk ligament
C. Interclavicular ligament
D. Costoclavicular ligament

Discussion

The correct answer is (D). It is imperative that the costoclavicular ligament be preserved to maintain postoperative stabilization. It has been reported that patients who undergo medial clavicle resection arthroplasty without an intact costoclavicular ligament do poorly. Answers A and B are incorrect because these terms are used interchangeably. The structure can be a source of persistent pain when left in the joint and is usually degenerative at the age of this patient. The interclavicular ligament is usually ligated during the procedure. Figure 2–75 depicts the ligamentous structures of the SC joint.

Objectives: Did you learn...?

• Identify SC joint osteoarthritis?
• Understand the nonoperative management of SC joint osteoarthritis?
• Appreciate the danger of doing procedures involving the SC joint?
• Consider and evaluate for other conditions associated with SC joint symptoms?
• Understand the operative treatment of SC joint osteoarthritis and the important structures to preserve?

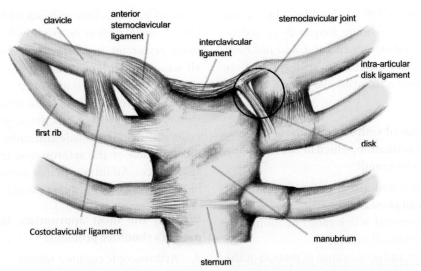

Figure 2–75 SC joint anatomy and ligaments with the intra-articular ligament circled in black. (From Martetschlager F, Warth RJ, Millett PJ. Instability and degenerative arthritis of the sternoclavicular joint: A current concepts review. *Am J Sports Med* 2013;42(4):999–1007.)

CASE 29

Dr. Robert J. Stewart

A 57-year-old, right-hand-dominant female presents with left shoulder pain and stiffness for the last 3 months. She has a history of diabetes, hypothyroidism, and breast cancer. She reports having difficulty sleeping on her left side. She localizes her pain over the deltoid insertion. The stiffness has become worse. The pain has been improving over the last 3 weeks but is exacerbated by extreme left shoulder motion. She is having difficulty dressing and combing her hair. She works as a statistical analyst and sits at a desk most of the day. On physical examination, she has normal strength with left shoulder abduction and external rotation, a negative cross-body adduction test, and no pain with a supinated O'Brien's test. An x-ray is obtained and shown in Figure 2–76.

Of the following, what is the most likely diagnosis of this patient?

A. Rotator cuff tear
B. Calcific tendinitis
C. Acromioclavicular joint arthritis
D. Adhesive capsulitis
E. Glenohumeral joint arthritis

Discussion

The correct answer is (D). Adhesive capsulitis (AC) is a specific pathologic entity that produces subsynovial chronic inflammation resulting in capsular thickening, fibrosis, and adherence of the capsule to itself and the anatomic neck of the humerus. The thickened and stiff capsule causes pain and a restraint to motion. This is called primary, or idiopathic, AC. The remaining answer choices are incorrect and can result in symptoms similar to those of AC (i.e., loss of shoulder motion and pain), but their underlying etiology is different. It is important to recognize that all these conditions can cause a stiff

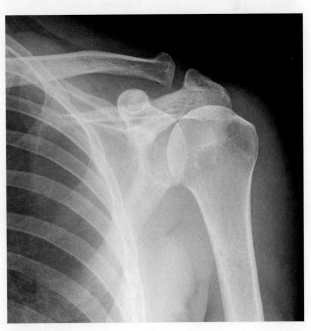

Figure 2–76

and painful shoulder (a "frozen shoulder") but is not necessarily AC. AC occurs more frequently in sedentary females in the non-dominant hand, and has been associated with diabetes mellitus, thyroid dysfunction, breast cancer treatment, cardiovascular disease and cerebrovascular disease.

The patient is diagnosed with stage 3 adhesive capsulitis. On physical examination, which of the following is the most likely to be found?

A. Decreased passive and active range of motion of the shoulder in all planes
B. Decreased passive and active range of motion of the shoulder in external rotation
C. Pain with passive and active range of motion of the shoulder
D. Pain with resisted forward flexion of the arm
E. Pain with external rotation of the arm

Discussion

The correct answer is (A). A "frozen shoulder" results from a known intrinsic, extrinsic, or systemic cause that may result in a global or partial loss of shoulder motion. However, adhesive capsulitis (AC) is idiopathic and always results in a global loss of passive and active

range of motion. Answer B would likely result from a known cause, such as an excessively tight anterior soft-tissue repair for instability. Answers C, D, and E are all associated with pain during motion. This would be expected in the early stages of AC, but due to patient's reported decreasing pain, these answer choices can be eliminated. Table 2–11 lists the stages of AC. The diagnosis and staging is made clinically. The table provides a description of the arthroscopic and histopathologic appearances. An intra-articular anesthetic injection can be used to distinguish stages 1 and 2.

What is the most appropriate treatment for this patient's shoulder problem?

A. Arthroscopic capsular release
B. Physical therapy (PT) with a home exercise program (HEP)
C. Intra-articular corticosteroid injection
D. Manipulation under anesthesia (MUA)
E. Aggressive physical therapy working on strengthening and range of motion

Discussion

The correct answer is (B). Regardless of the stage, initial nonoperative treatment is appropriate for adhesive

Table 2–11   STAGES OF ADHESIVE CAPSULITIS

	Symptoms	Signs	Arthroscopic Appearance	Biopsy Appearance
Stage 1	Pain referred to the deltoid insertion	Capsular pain on deep palpation	Fibrous synovial inflammatory reaction	Rare inflammatory cell infiltrate
	Pain at night	Empty end feel at extremes of motion	No adhesions or capsular contracture	Hypervascular, hypertrophic synovitis
		Full motion under anesthesia		Normal capsular tissue
Stage 2	Severe night pain	Motion restricted in forward flexion, abduction, internal and external rotation	Christmas tree synovitis	Hypertrophic, hypervascular synovitis
	Stiffness	Some motion loss under anesthesia	Some loss of axillary fold	Perivascular, subsynovial capsular scar
Stage 3	Profound stiffness	Significant loss of motion	Complete loss of axillary fold	Hypercellular, collagenous tissue with a thin synovial layer
	Pain only at the end of range of motion	Tethering at ends of motion	Minimal synovitis	Similar features to other fibrosing conditions
		No improvement under anesthesia		
Stage 4	Profound stiffness	Significant motion loss	Fully mature adhesions	Not reported
	Pain minimal	Gradual improvement in motion	Identification of intra-articular structures difficult	

capsulitis. The natural course has been described as self-limited and improves over a 24-month period. However, there are no true natural history studies in the literature without intervention given. The reported outcomes of minimally treated patients vary considerably, therefore patients should be treated focusing on recovery of motion and decreasing pain. PT with HEP is the mainstay of treatment. PT does not need to be aggressive and strengthening exercises are not necessary. Nonsteroidal anti-inflammatory drugs in addition to oral and intra-articular steroid injections are often combined with PT. Intra-articular corticosteroid injections appear to provide early pain relief, but this has not been shown to change the long-term outcome.

More aggressive treatments include MUA and arthroscopic or open capsular release, however, no specific indication guidelines exist. MUA and surgical treatment should not be considered when the patient is experiencing severe pain in addition to loss of motion because this may represent the inflammatory stage of the disease and could exacerbate the motion loss by increasing capsular injury. Answer D is incorrect because MUA would be utilized only after PT has failed. Some recommend an MUA prior to or as an adjunct to capsular release. The technique of MUA is critical to ensure the inferior capsule is released from the humerus without the complications of humeral fracture or rupture of the subscapularis. Arthroscopic capsular release has supplanted MUA at many institutions. Open capsular release can be considered if arthroscopic release is not successful or if aberrant anatomy prevents visualization of the appropriate structures arthroscopically. Other, less investigated forms of treatment include suprascapular nerve blocks, hydrodilation, and extracorporeal shockwave therapy.

After 12 months of being compliant with her home exercise program and undergoing multiple steroid injections, the patient continues to have difficulty with her range of motion and is not happy with her shoulder function. She is inquiring about other treatment options.

When taking into account surgical options for this patient, arthroscopic release of the anterosuperior capsular region and the rotator interval will most likely result in what improved motion?

A. Abducted external rotation of the arm
B. Adducted internal rotation
C. Adducted external rotation
D. Abduction in neutral rotation
E. Forward flexion in the scapular plane

Discussion

The correct answer is (C). The limitation of external rotation of the adducted shoulder is associated with contracture of the anterosuperior capsular and rotator interval. Release of this area would increase adducted external rotation. Releasing the anteroinferior capsule would increase abducted external rotation. Adducted internal rotation range of motion would be increased with posterior capsule release. Abduction in neutral position and forward flexion can be increased with MUA. The outcomes are generally good with arthroscopic treatment of AC, but close follow-up is required. A long recovery and rehabilitation period can be expected.

Objectives: Did you learn...?

- Recognize a patient with adhesive capsulitis based on history and physical examination findings?
- Understand the basic pathogenesis of adhesive capsulitis?
- Appropriately stage adhesive capsulitis based on history and physical examination findings?
- Treat adhesive capsulitis appropriately with either conservative or operative approaches?
- Understand the outcome and prognosis of adhesive capsulitis?

CASE 30

Dr. Robert J. Stewart

A 44-year-old, right-hand-dominant male with well-controlled diabetes and hypertension presents to clinic with left shoulder pain. The patient denies a history of trauma or injury. He localizes his pain over the superolateral aspect of the shoulder, and it radiates to the deltoid insertion. He has experienced pain over the past few months, but it has progressively become more severe over the past several days. He has difficulty sleeping and with range of motion because of severe pain. While examining the patient, he has a warm and tender left shoulder, and while performing a range of motion evaluation, the patient notes that he has a sensation of "catching." He has a positive Hawkins sign, negative drop arm test, and pain with a cross body adduction test. A radiograph of the left shoulder is shown in Figure 2–77.

What is the most likely diagnosis?

A. Rotator cuff arthropathy
B. Septic arthritis

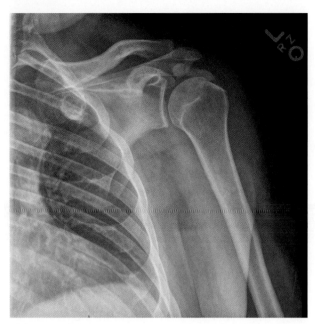

Figure 2–77

C. Acromioclavicular (AC) joint osteoarthritis
D. Calcifying tendinitis
E. Glenohumeral (GH) joint osteoarthritis

Discussion

The correct answer is (D). Calcific tendonitis (CT) is a condition characterized by the buildup of calcium hydroxyapatite crystals within tendons. It typically occurs around synovial joints and has been reported in the hip, paraspinal muscles, hand, and foot. It most frequently occurs around the shoulder in patients who are 30 to 50 years old. No one over the age of 71 has been recorded having this condition. Degenerative calcification and reactive calcification have both been proposed as mechanisms for the deposition of calcium. Although the etiology is not understood, most believe that it is a reactive mechanism involving an active, cell-mediated process in a viable tendon. The cell-mediated process has been divided into three distinct phases: precalcific, calcific, and postcalcific. Depending on the stage, imaging, and physical examination characteristics can differ. The calcific stage can be further classified into three phases: formative, resting, and resorption. Rotator cuff arthropathy is seen in older patients with chronic, massive, rotator cuff tears and glenohumeral osteoarthritis. Septic arthritis can look similar to CT, but this patient has had a history of shoulder pain without fever or other risk factors for infection. Answers C and E are incorrect

because there are no signs of osteoarthritis of the AC or GH joint on radiograph or physical examination.

What can be said about the phase of this patient's shoulder pathology?

A. The calcium is most likely being deposited
B. The calcium deposit is mostly likely undergoing resorption
C. The tenocytes are likely undergoing metaplasia
D. The tenocytes are likely becoming ischemic and losing vascularity
E. The musculotendinous junction is the area most likely causing the patient's pain

Discussion

The correct answer is (B). In calcific tendonitis (CT), calcium must be deposited for it to be resorbed. Patients presenting during the resorptive phase of the calcific stage will have this type of acute, inflammatory shoulder syndrome that this patient most closely represents. This hyperalgic syndrome will typically last 2 weeks. This is very different from the formative and resting phase, when calcium crystals are being deposited and isolated in the tendon. These phases can last for 2 to 3 years and may be associated with intermittent or constant symptoms. The resorptive and formative phases are important to distinguish for treatment purposes. It should be noted that whereas other musculoskeletal diseases progress from an acute to chronic phase, CT will progress from a chronic phase followed by an acute phase. Answer C is incorrect because this may be happening in the precalcific stage, which is not the patient's current stage. Answer D is incorrect because this is one theory of how the calcific stage is prompted. Answer E is incorrect because calcification at the musculotendinous junction is considered degenerative or dystrophic calcification, which will typically occur in older patients.

Which structure is most likely to be affected on the basis of the information obtained thus far, including the radiograph Figure 2–77?

A. Deltoid
B. Infraspinatus
C. Supraspinatus
D. Teres minor
E. Subscapularis

Discussion

The correct answer is (C). Calcific tendonitis (CT) is most often localized in the supraspinatus tendon. Radiographic views should include a true AP in internal and external rotation, axillary, and scapular-Y to evaluate for calcium deposits in the tendons of the rotator cuff. There are no reports of the deltoid muscle being involved in CT. Radiographs also help to distinguish resorptive and formative phases. Two radiographic types have been described: Type I (associated with the resorptive phase and acute pain) is a deposit that is fluffy or fleecy in appearance with a poorly defined periphery. Type II (associated with the formative phase and chronic pain) has discrete, homogeneous deposits that have a well-defined periphery.

How should this patient be initially managed?

A. Therapeutic ultrasound
B. Extracorporeal shock wave therapy (ESWT)
C. Needle aspiration and lavage
D. Arthroscopic calcium deposit decompression
E. Combined needle aspiration followed by ESWT

Discussion

The correct answer is (C). When managing calcific tendonitis (CT), it is important to distinguish between the formative and resorptive phases for proper treatment. Conservative measures (i.e., physical therapy, moist heat, nonsteroidal anti-inflammatory drugs, sling) should be attempted in all cases if the symptoms are not severe. Needle aspiration with lavage is often successful during the acute, resorptive phase because the consistency of the calcification tends to be creamy or toothpastelike. Therapeutic ultrasound has been utilized by physical therapists, but no long-term benefit has been found. ESWT is being utilized with encouraging results, however, more investigation is needed to identify long-term outcomes and safety concerns. Arthroscopic or open surgical intervention is very rarely indicated in the resorptive phase. Surgery is typically only indicated after 6 to 12 months of failed conservative treatment, during the formative phase, and progressive symptoms that are negatively impacting daily activities.

What is the most likely outcome of this patient after being treated?

A. Will require repeat needle aspiration and lavage
B. Decreased pain and resolution of symptoms
C. Will likely require arthroscopic surgery
D. Decreased range of motion and increased pain

Discussion

The correct answer is (B). The most likely outcome for this patient is decreased pain and resolution of

symptoms with supportive care provided. Most cases of calcific tendonitis (CT) are self-limiting, and the role of the clinician is to control pain and maintain function until recovery occurs. During the resorptive phase, natural mechanisms usually succeed in removing the deposit. Rarely will repeated needle aspiration be necessary. Surgery is very rarely indicated for the resorptive phase of CT, particularly after needle aspiration and lavage have been performed. The patient is likely to experience increased range of motion and less pain with continued supportive measures if necessary.

Objectives: Did you learn...?

- Recognize and diagnose a patient with calcific tendonitis?
- Realize that the etiology of calcific tendonitis is not known?
- Recognize that patients may present while in the resorptive phase or formative phase of calcific tendonitis and treatments will differ for each?
- Recognize that the chronic phase of calcific tendonitis occurs prior to the acute phase?
- Recognize the different conservative and operative treatment options available for calcific tendonitis and when to implement them?
- Appreciate that the outcome of calcific tendonitis is typically favorable with conservative measures?

CASE 31

Dr. Robert J. Stewart

A 29-year-old, left-hand-dominant male presents to clinic complaining of left arm and shoulder pain for the last three days. The patient is an avid weight-lifter and was doing the bench press when his arm began to bother him. He has been using ice and resting with mild relief but has not been able to use his left arm for anything more than carrying light-weight objects. He is also having difficulty with simple activities such as putting on his shirt. On physical examination, the patient has ecchymosis and a prominent cord-like structure on the anterior left axilla. He has significant weakness with left shoulder adduction and internal rotation. He has a negative Hawkins sign and a negative Yergason sign.

Based on the information obtained thus far, which of the following is the most likely diagnosis?

A. Rotator cuff tear
B. Pectoralis major muscle rupture
C. Ruptured biceps tendon

D. Poland syndrome

E. Pectoralis minor muscle rupture

Discussion

The correct answer is (B). A pectoralis major muscle (PMM) tear or rupture usually occurs in weight-lifters while performing the bench press, but it can occur during any activity in which the arm is extended and externally rotated while under maximal contraction (eccentric loading force). Patients often present with pain, swelling, ecchymosis, weakness and loss of the axillary fold in the acute setting. In the chronic setting, the swelling and ecchymosis have typically subsided. They may report an audible pop or a tearing sensation. On examination, there can be an apparent continuous muscle or tendon that is mistaken for an intact PMM tendon, but this represents the fascia of the PMM that is continuous with the fascia of both the brachium and the medial antebrachial septum. This continuous fascia will examine as a cord-like structure as shown in Figure 2–78.

The sternocostal portion of the muscle is injured more often than the clavicular. A rotator cuff tear and biceps tendon injury are unlikely given the mechanism of injury and physical examination findings. In addition, this patient is young for a rotator cuff tear. Poland syndrome is the congenital absence of the PMM. Pectoralis minor muscle rupture is scarcely reported and would not have the same history and physical examination findings.

Radiographs were normal. What is the most appropriate next step in management?

A. Ultrasound

B. Computed tomography (CT)

C. Magnetic resonance imaging (MRI)

D. Radiographs of humerus

E. Radiographs of the contralateral shoulder

Discussion

The correct answer is (C). Although pectoralis major muscle (PMM) injuries are primarily diagnosed clinically, MRI is the imaging modality of choice to evaluate a PMM tendon injury. The extent and location of the injury can many times be assessed with MRI. The Tietjen's classification system can be used for PMM injuries. Type I is a contusion or sprain. Type II is a partial tear. Type III injuries are complete tears and further classified by anatomic location: III-A (muscle origin), III-B (muscle belly), III-C (musculotendinous junction), III-D (tendinous insertion). Further subclassification were suggested including III-E (bony avulsion from the insertion) and II-F (muscle tendon substance rupture). Type II and Type III injuries have been reported at rates of 9% and 91%, respectively. Among complete tears, type III-D has been reported as the most common (65%). Ultrasound is a reasonable alternative to MRI, particularly if its use means avoiding delay of surgical repair. Ultrasound is much more user-dependent. CT will not allow adequate soft tissue evaluation. Further radiographic evaluation is incorrect because a radiograph of the injured shoulder has already been obtained. The radiographic findings are often normal, but the clinician should look for bony avulsions. The characteristic findings on radiographs are soft tissue swelling and absence of the PMM shadow.

After evaluating the MRI, the patient is diagnosed with a complete rupture of the pectoralis major tendon (Fig. 2–79). What is the recommended first step in management?

A. Sling immobilization in adducted and internally rotated position, cold compression, analgesics, and plan for surgical repair in 4 to 8 weeks

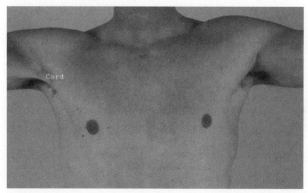

Figure 2–78

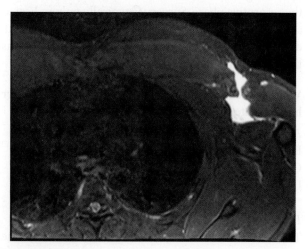

Figure 2–79

B. Cold compression, analgesics, and follow-up for surgical discussion

C. Shoulder immobilizer, cold compression, analgesics, follow-up as an outpatient in 1 to 2 weeks for transition to range of motion (ROM) exercises

D. Active ROM exercises until follow-up for outpatient surgery in 1 week to avoid loss of strength and range of motion postoperatively

E. Take immediately to the operating room for repair

Discussion

The correct answer is (A). Regardless of how the injury is definitively treated (nonoperative or operative), the first step should be rest, ice, compression, and pain control. Surgery is indicated for all young, active patients. If the patient was able to injure the pectoralis major muscle (PMM), then they likely utilize the muscle and should have it repaired. There is no consensus on the timing of when to repair PMM injuries; however, it would make sense to delay for ecchymosis and swelling to subside. Some believe the ideal timing for the surgery is between 4 and 8 weeks after injury. Others feel that chronicity does not affect outcome of repair even when performed 13 years after injury. Nonoperative treatment is reserved for elderly patients, suspected partial or muscle belly ruptures, and for low-demand patients. Answers B and D would risk further retraction of the tendon into the muscle belly. Answer C represents an initial nonoperative management protocol and is inappropriate for this patient.

All of the following are reported complications of operative management of a pectoralis major muscle injury, EXCEPT?

A. Re-rupture of the pectoralis major tendon

B. Numbness in the distribution of C6

C. Postoperative infection

D. Heterotopic ossification

E. Hematoma

Discussion

The correct answer is (B). Numbness in the distribution of C6 has not been reported in pectoralis major muscle (PMM) injuries, and the more likely injury in the case of surgical treatment for a PMM rupture is disruption of lateral or medial pectoral nerves. The incidence of re-rupture of the tendon has been reported as high as 7.7%. Answer C is incorrect because postoperative infection is considered one of the most concerning postoperative complications following PMM tendon repair because

of the location. The axillary area lends itself to higher bacterial burden with an increased infectious risk. Heterotopic ossification and hematoma have both been reported as complications.

Objectives: Did you learn ...?

- Diagnose a pectoralis major muscle injury?
- Understand which imaging modalities are available for the evaluation of a pectoralis major rupture?
- Distinguish when to conservatively manage or surgically repair a pectoralis major injury?
- Understand the initial management of a pectoralis major injury?
- Understand some of the complications that may be associated with pectoralis major injuries?

CASE 32

Dr. Robert J. Stewart

A 50-year-old, right-hand-dominant female presents to clinic with posterior right shoulder pain and sometimes a loud noise while using her right upper extremity for overhead activities. Her pain is concentrated over the superomedial border of her scapula, but she also says her pain is underneath her shoulder blade. What is most bothersome is the fact that she is unable to brush her hair because of the discomfort she experiences. She reports that it started as only noise several years prior, but over the last several months she has developed debilitating pain with overhead activities. She works as a salon hair stylist and denies a history of trauma to her right upper extremity.

Which of the following is the most likely diagnosis?

A. Impingement syndrome

B. Rotator cuff tendinitis

C. Suprascapular nerve entrapment

D. Supraspinatus muscle tear

E. Scapulothoracic bursitis

Discussion

The correct answer is (E). Scapulothoracic bursitis is commonly known as snapping scapula syndrome. This syndrome can be classified on the basis of the cause, which can result in either scapulothoracic crepitus or scapulothoracic bursitis. However, these can many times be indistinguishable in clinical practice because mechanical crepitus can lead to symptomatic bursitis, and conversely, symptomatic bursitis can lead to mechanical crepitus. The woman in this case likely developed bursitis from her mechanical crepitus because she was experiencing a noise without pain for several years. Scapulothoracic crepitus has been found in 31% of 100 normal asymptomatic people. Patients with scapulothoracic bursitis have often experienced symptoms for a long period of time, and these symptoms can range from mild, intermittent discomfort to notable functional disability. Common complaints are that symptoms are causing a decrease in athletic performance or pain with overhead activities. When obtaining the patient's history, it is important to know their hand dominance, occupation, and activity level. Impingement syndrome, rotator cuff tendinitis, and a supraspinatus tear are less likely in this case given the history of a loud noise prior to the pain and the location of the pain. Answer C is incorrect because the patient is not complaining of weakness.

When examining a patient with suspected scapulothoracic bursitis it is not only important to evaluate bilateral scapula, but also crucial to closely examine which of the following?

A. Cervical and thoracic spine
B. Lumbar spine
C. Ipsilateral sternoclavicular range of motion
D. Biceps brachii motor strength

Discussion

The correct answer is (A). When examining patients with scapulothoracic bursitis, it is important to examine the cervical and thoracic spine for fixed or postural kyphosis that may contribute to scapulothoracic incongruity. Evaluation of the cervical spine should also be performed to rule out referred pain. Inspection of each scapula should include looking for asymmetry, winging, or audible snapping. It is important to specifically test muscle strength of the trapezius, rhomboid, levator scapulae, serratus anterior, and latissimus dorsi muscles. Weakness in any of these can cause imbalances leading to a pathologic state. The lumbar spine should not affect scapulothoracic bursitis. The ipsilateral sternoclavicular joint and biceps brachii muscle should be evaluated, but this is not critical to the diagnosis of scapulothoracic bursitis.

The patient's symptoms fail to improve after 6 months of conservative management, including activity modification, physical therapy (PT), nonsteroidal anti-inflammatory drugs, and ultrasound guided injections. The injections provided short-term relief. Radiographs and a three-dimensional CT scan were obtained. The patient had an anterior "horn-like" projection at the

superomedial angle of the scapula. Surgical intervention is planned using a modified mini-open approach with arthroscopy-assisted bursectomy. Portals are placed 3 cm medial to the medial scapular border.

Which structure(s) are avoided with this portal placement?

A. Long thoracic nerve
B. Suprascapular nerve
C. Dorsal scapular artery and nerve
D. Transverse cervical artery
E. Spinal accessory nerve

Discussion

The correct answer is (C). The dorsal scapular artery and nerve travel beneath the rhomboid minor and major muscles approximately 1 to 2 cm medial to the medial scapular border. Portal placement should therefore be located approximately 3 cm medial to the medial scapular border (Fig. 2–80).

Answer A is incorrect because the long thoracic nerve is rarely endangered unless dissection is carried lateral. The suprascapular nerve can be endangered if a portal is placed superior to the scapular spine. The deep branch of the transverse cervical artery becomes the dorsal scapular artery. The spinal accessory nerve travels with the superficial branch of the transverse cervical artery, and its branches are at risk if a portal is placed superior to the scapular spine. Scapulothoracic bursitis

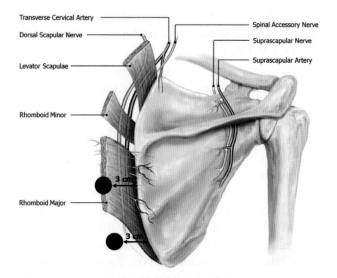

Figure 2–80 Reproduced with permission from Warth, RJ, Spiegl UJ, Millet PJ. Scapulothoracic bursitis and snapping scapula syndrome: a critical review of current evidence. *Am J Sports Med* 2014 Mar 24. [Epub ahead of print]

is usually managed nonoperatively. Nonoperative treatment includes activity modification, NSAIDs, PT, and corticosteroid injections. If symptoms are recalcitrant to conservative management or associated with an osseous or soft tissue mass, surgical intervention is indicated. Arthroscopic, open, or a combined operative approach can be performed. Arthroscopy is more technically demanding, but it does not require postoperative immobilization because the rhomboids and levator scapulae are not transected and reattached to the scapula after partial scapula resection is performed.

As mentioned, radiographs and a CT were obtained. If an osseous lesion is suspected, the threshold to obtain three-dimensional imaging should remain low. MRI can be used to identify soft tissue lesions and to help prevent misdiagnoses and unnecessary surgical intervention. Ultrasound has been used to identify inflamed bursal tissue, although it is more commonly used for diagnostic and therapeutic injections. Electromyogram can sometimes be necessary for patients with imbalances in the periscapular musculature and asymmetry.

A superomedial scapular resection as well as bursectomy is performed. While dissecting laterally, the suprascapular notch becomes visible in the operative field. What structure runs superficial to the transverse scapular ligament?

A. Suprascapular nerve
B. Transverse cervical artery
C. Spinal accessory nerve
D. Suprascapular artery
E. Long thoracic nerve

Discussion
The correct answer is (D). The suprascapular artery runs superficial to the transverse scapular ligament. The suprascapular nerve travels deep to the ligament. Answers B, C, and E are not closely associated with the transverse scapular ligament.

What is the ideal patient position for both injections and operative treatment of scapulothoracic bursitis?

A. Prone with affected arm in 90 degrees of abduction and internally rotated
B. Prone with affected arm in extension and internal rotation
C. Lateral decubitus with affected arm adducted and externally rotated
D. Prone with affected arm adducted and externally rotated

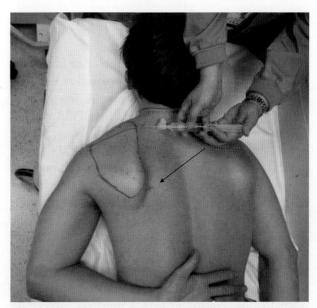

Figure 2–81 (From Lazar MA, Kwon YW, Rokito AS. Current concepts review: snapping scapula syndrome. *J Bone Joint Surg Am.* 2009;91:2251–2262.)

Discussion
The correct answer is (B). The so-called chicken-wing position is utilized to elevate the medial border of the scapula to gain access to both the superior and inferior bursa (Fig. 2–81).

Answers A, C, and D are incorrect because none of these positions would help to elevate the medial border of the scapula. The scapulothoracic articulation is unique because it does not rely on hyaline cartilage, but rather muscle layers and interposing bursal tissue to achieve smooth motion. Symptoms can result from overuse and inflammation of this bursal tissue or can be caused by bony abnormality. Periscapular bursae include infraserratus, supraserratus, and scapulotrapezial bursa. Symptoms over the superomedial scapula area could be caused by the infraserratus or supraserratus bursae. Occasionally, patients will have symptoms localized to the medial border of the scapula at the level of scapular spine, which can be attributed to inflammation of the scapulotrapezial bursa.

Objectives: Did you learn …?

- Diagnose scapulothoracic bursitis?
- Recognize the different names for scapulothoracic bursitis and that crepitus can lead to bursitis and vice-versa?
- Understand how to conservatively and surgically manage scapulothoracic bursitis?
- Understand common complications associated with performing surgery for scapulothoracic bursitis?

CASE 33

Dr. Joseph Cohen

A 42-year-old female presents to the office for follow up after sustaining a minimally displaced radial head fracture 3 months prior. She states she was initially treated in long-arm splint by the ER and did not follow up with an orthopaedic surgeon until now. Per her report, she removed the splint 4 weeks after the injury, but did not move her elbow due to pain. She now has no pain but is unable to reach that hand to her face or head. The remaining history is significant for previous ulnar nerve surgery for which she is unable to provide details. On physical examination, her upper extremity is normal except for limited flexion/extension, measured to be 80 to 50 degrees by goniometer. In addition, she has a well-healed surgical incision about the medial elbow, consistent with a previous surgery on her ulnar nerve. Her images are shown (Figs. 2–82 to 2–84).

What is the diagnosis?

A. Early post-traumatic intrinsic joint contracture
B. Late post-traumatic extrinsic joint contracture
C. Late combined post-traumatic joint contracture
D. Early combined post-traumatic joint contracture

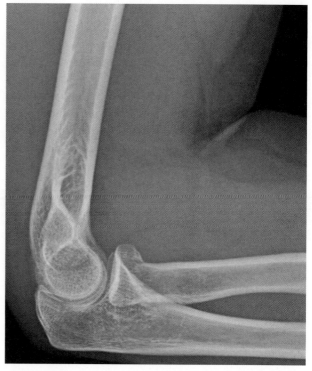

Figure 2–83

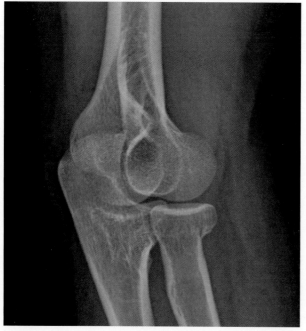

Figure 2–82

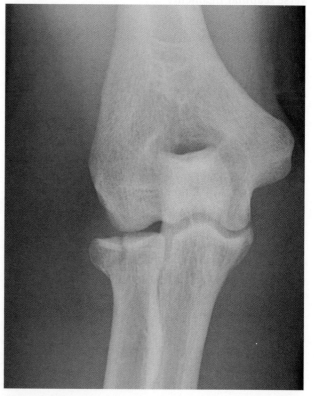

Figure 2–84

Discussion

The correct answer is (A). Classification of post-traumatic elbow stiffness allows for better understanding of the disease and allows the clinician to treat the underlying cause of the joint contracture. Intrinsic causes include: any problem within the joint such as incongruency, loose bodies, or severe osteoarthritis. Extrinsic causes include capsular tightness, muscle contracture, heterotopic ossification, and skin contractures. Early is defined as within 6 months of the injury while late is considered to be greater than 6 months after the injury. Patients that present in the early time frame have a significantly better chance at having a good result both from nonoperative and operative treatment.

What is the preferred first line of treatment at this time?

A. Manipulation under anesthesia, followed by physical therapy two times per week
B. Arthroscopic capsular release and limited debridement, followed by physical therapy two times per week
C. Daily supervised physical therapy with static or dynamic progressive splinting
D. Open capsular release, followed by a splint in extension for 14 days

Discussion

The correct answer is (C). Daily, supervised physical therapy should be the first line of treatment in most cases. Major gains in elbow motion are made within the first 3 to 6 months after initiating treatment, however, patients can continue to progress up to a year from the injury. If the contracture is from a tight capsule alone, it is unusual that operative management will be required.

If surgical intervention is warranted, which of the following would be the best option?

A. Total elbow arthroplasty
B. Fascial interpositional arthroplasty
C. Open osteocapsular release followed by supervised physical therapy
D. Arthroscopic osteocapsular debridement and a home exercise program
E. Arthrodesis

Discussion

The correct answer is (C). Open osteocapsular release would be the best option for this patient. Arthroscopic treatment is ideal for stiffness secondary to capsular contracture, however, given the history of ulnar nerve decompression and or transposition, arthroscopic treatment is contra-indicated.

Which of the following structures needs to be prophylactically addressed when surgically treating patients with a limitation of elbow flexion of 90 to 100 degrees?

A. Ulnar nerve
B. Anterior bundle of the MCL
C. Posterior band of the MCL
D. Fascia of the flexor pronator mass
E. Medial intermuscular septum

Discussion

The correct answer is (A). Prophylactic treatment of the ulnar nerve should be done before the osteocapsular release in order to prevent undo compression on the nerve as a result of the increased flexion. Anatomic studies have shown that the cubital tunnel significantly decreases in size with a corresponding increase in the pressure seen within the ulnar nerve with flexion greater than 90 degrees.

Objectives: Did you learn...?

• The common causes and differential for a patient with a stiff elbow?
• Nonoperative treatment and the indications for surgical management?
• Keys to achieving adequate patient satisfaction?

CASE 34

Dr. Joseph Cohen

A 32-year-old male presented to the emergency department 1 hour after sustaining a fall while skateboarding. The patient complained of pain in the elbow with swelling and deformity present. He denied numbness or tingling.

Examination reveals deformity about the elbow with no open lesions or skin tenting. He has a palpable radial and ulnar pulse and is neurologically intact. His images are shown (Figs. 2–85 to 2–88).

What is the diagnosis and direction of displacement?

A. Monteggia fracture dislocation, posterolateral displacement of the forearm about the humerus
B. Simple elbow dislocation, posterolateral displacement of the forearm about the humerus
C. Transolecranon complex elbow dislocation
D. Simple elbow dislocation, posteromedial displacement of the forearm about the humerus

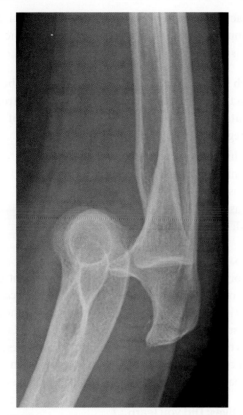

Figure 2–85

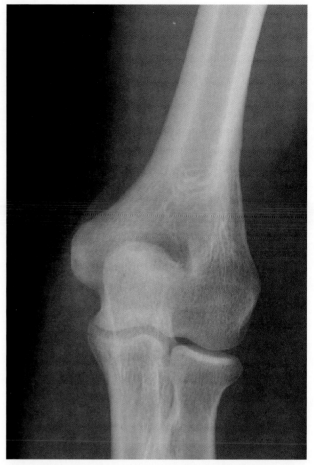

Figure 2–87

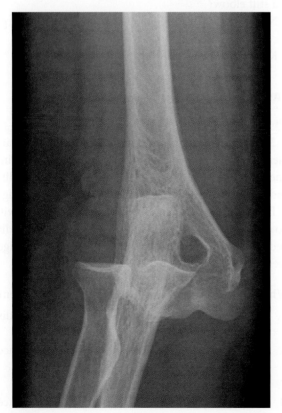

Figure 2–86

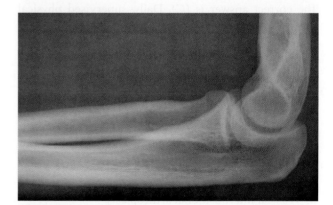

Figure 2–88

Discussion

The correct answer is (B). This is the most common type of elbow dislocation, and often does not cause any osseous injury. Posterolateral and posteromedial dislocation account for approximately 90% of dislocations.

Adequate pre- and post-reduction films are necessary to evaluate for fracture, which would change the classification to a complex injury.

What are the next best steps in management?

A. Repeat x-rays, followed by reduction of the joint, repeat neurovascular examination, and splinting of the elbow in 110 degrees of flexion
B. Reduction of the joint followed by splinting in 90 degrees of flexion and postreduction x-rays
C. Reduction of the joint, followed by examination of the joint to evaluate re-dislocation in extension, repeat neurovascular examination, and splinting of the elbow in 90 degrees of flexion and postreduction films
D. Reduction of the joint in the operating room followed by ligament reconstruction

Discussion

The correct answer is (C). All patients with an elbow dislocation should be reduced on an urgent basis. It is important to document the neurovascular examination both pre- and post-reduction. Once reduced, the elbow should be taken through a range of motion to evaluate if and when the elbow subluxes or redislocates. This will allow for improved ability to rehab the patient safely. Adequate postreduction films are necessary to evaluate the concentricity of the joint, as well as to further look for fractures not seen on the injury films.

Which static stabilizer of the elbow typically fails first?

A. Radial head
B. Lateral ulnar collateral ligament (LUCL)
C. Ulnar collateral ligament (UCL)
D. Anterior and posterior capsular disruption

Discussion

The correct answer is (B). LUCL is the first structure that is disrupted in posterolateral elbow dislocations. The rotational force is then transferred to the anterior and posterior capsule, and finally the UCL if there is enough force.

In which of the following situations is surgery to restore stability indicated?

A. If the elbow requires flexion beyond 50 to 60 degrees to remain reduced
B. In all posteromedial elbow dislocations

C. When the elbow redislocates in 30 degrees of extension immediately after reduction
D. If the patient has a contralateral forearm fracture

Discussion

The correct answer is (A). Surgery is rarely indicated for acute simple elbow dislocations. When the elbow requires flexion beyond 50 to 60 degrees to remain reduced, it indicates that both the collateral ligaments and the secondary stabilizers are disrupted. The MCL is the primary stabilizer of the ulnohumeral joint, whereas the LUCL primarily keeps the ulna from subluxing posteriorly and the radial head from rotating away from the humerus in supination. With more unstable elbows, there is an increased likelihood that the secondary stabilizers (the flexor-pronator mass and extensor origins) are disrupted. Repair can be of one or both of the collateral ligaments. Typically, the LUCL is repaired first and the stability of the elbow is examined for need to repair the UCL.

Objectives: Did you learn…?

• Common mechanisms of injury and classification?
• Diagnosis and acute management/reduction techniques?
• Be able to identify a stable versus unstable elbow?
• Definitive treatment and long-term expectations?

CASE 35

Dr. Joseph Cohen

A 54-year-old male presented to the ED with left elbow pain after sustaining an injury in a low speed motor vehicle accident. He denied any other injuries. On examination, he had no open injuries and was neurovascularly intact. He had gross deformity about the elbow. His images are below (Figs. 2–89 to 2–92).

What is the diagnosis?

A. Posterolateral simple elbow dislocation
B. Posterolateral complex elbow dislocation
C. Posteromedial complex elbow dislocation
D. Posteromedial simple elbow dislocation

Discussion

The correct answer is (C). Posteromedial complex elbow dislocation. This injury is proposed to result from axial load combined with posteromedial rotation, varus force, and elbow flexion. This is opposed to the more

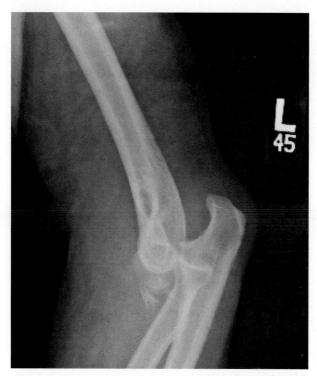

Figure 2–89 Pre- and post-reduction films showing complex elbow dislocation, coronoid fracture.

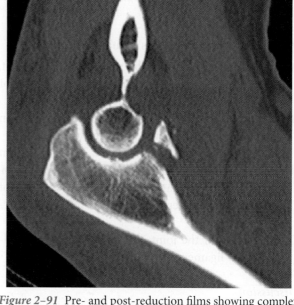

Figure 2–91 Pre- and post-reduction films showing complex elbow dislocation, coronoid fracture.

frequently seen posterolateral dislocation. There is a fracture of the coronoid, which is typical for this type of injury.

Which structure is most commonly fractured in a posteromedial elbow dislocation?

A. Coronoid
B. Radial head
C. Olecranon
D. Capitellum
E. Supracondylar distal humerus

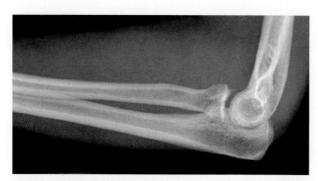

Figure 2–90 Pre- and post-reduction films showing complex elbow dislocation, coronoid fracture.

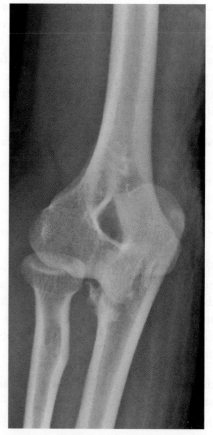

Figure 2–92 Pre- and post-reduction films showing complex elbow dislocation, coronoid fracture.

O'Driscoll Coronoid Fracture Classification

Fracture	Subtype	Description
Tip	1	≤2 mm of coronoid height
	2	>2 mm of coronoid height
Anteromedial	1	Anteromedial rim
	2	Anteromedial rim and tip
	3	Anteromedial rim and sublime tubercle (± tip)
Basal	1	Coronoid body and base
	2	Transolecranon basal coronoid fracture

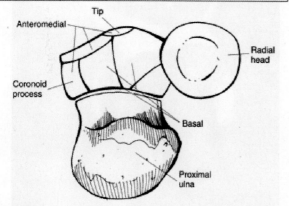

Figure 2–93 Reproduced with permission from Tashjian RZ and Katarincic JA. Complex Elbow Instability. *J Am* 2006;14(5):278–286.

Discussion

The correct answer is (A). Coronoid process fracture (see Fig. 2–93). The medial trochlea is thought to fracture the anteromedial facet of the coronoid allowing the elbow to dislocate. The lateral collateral ligament (LCL) ligamentous complex is also torn with this type of injury however the radial head often remains intact. This is in contrast to posterolateral elbow dislocations in which the radial head is the most commonly fractured bone, followed by the coronoid.

Although the radial head in this case is intact, which of the following would be the preferred treatment for a 5-part radial head fracture in conjunction with an elbow dislocation?

A. Radial head resection
B. ORIF with small interfragmentary screws
C. ORIF with radial head plate and screws
D. Radial head arthroplasty
E. Nonoperative

Discussion

The correct answer is (D). Radial head arthroplasty has been shown to allow for the best patient outcomes for comminuted radial head fractures compared to ORIF or radial head resection.

Which of the follow structures is the most important restraint to valgus and posteromedial rotatory force?

A. Anterior bundle of the MCL
B. Posterior bundle of the MCL
C. LUCL complex
D. Radial head
E. Flexor pronator mass

Discussion

The correct answer is (A). Anterior bundle of the MCL is of prime importance in elbow stability. It originates from the anteroinferior aspect of the medial epicondyle and inserts on the sublime tubercle at the base of the coronoid. The LCL functions as an important restraint to varus and posterolateral rotator instability. The radial head and the flexor pronator mass are secondary stabilizers of the elbow. In the setting of a disrupted anterior bundle of the MCL, the radial head serves as the most important stabilizer.

What is the preferred method of treatment at this time?

A. Treat the injury as you would a simple dislocation since there is no radial head injury
B. Treat the injury as you would a simple dislocation since the coronoid fracture is too small too fix
C. Open reduction internal fixation of the coronoid
D. Surgically repair the LCL without fixing the coronoid
E. Open reduction internal fixation of the coronoid and repair of the LCL

Discussion

The correct answer is (E). Open reduction internal fixation of the coronoid and repair of the LCL. The steps most commonly involved in surgical repair of fracture dislocations about the elbow include fixation of the osseous elements first, followed by inspection of the ligaments. Frequently, the LCL is avulsed from the lateral epicondyle. The stability of the elbow is then documented and need for repair of the MCL is determined upon the basis of the degree of stability. It is thought that an elbow that is stable from 30 degrees of flexion to full flexion does not require MCL repair.

Objectives: Did you learn...?

• Be able to recognize a fracture dislocation about the elbow and predict degree of instability?

- Understand the treatment algorithm for stabilization?
- Understand the goals of treatment and the long-term outcomes?

CASE 36

Dr. Joseph Cohen

A 46-year-old male presents to the clinic for evaluation regarding right elbow pain. He states he sustained an elbow dislocation 1 year ago. He reports that there were no fractures associated with the injury. His main complaint is pain along the outer part of his elbow with range of motion and a persistent "popping" feeling with certain movements. He is unable to do a pushup due to the pain.

There is a positive lateral pivot shift of the elbow but does not open medially with isolated valgus stress. MRI is shown (Figs. 2–94 and 2–95).

What is the most likely diagnosis?

A. Posterolateral rotatory instability (PLRI)
B. Lateral epicondyle fracture
C. Medial collateral ligament (MCL)
D. Isolated injury to the lateral ulnar collateral ligament (LUCL)

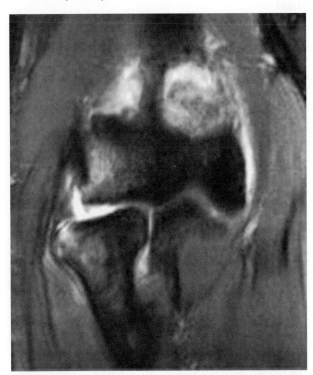

Figure 2–94

Discussion

The correct answer is (A). Posterolateral instability. Patients with this condition nearly always have a history

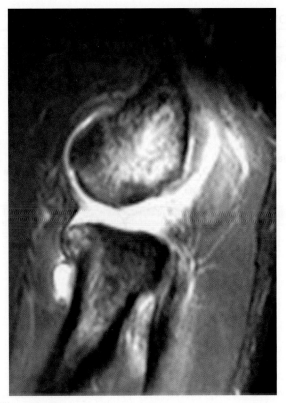

Figure 2–95

of one or more elbow dislocations. Lateral pain and recurrent mechanical symptoms (clicking, popping, subluxations) are common complaints. They also notice worsening with certain activities; such as push-ups, using the arm to stand from a chair etc. PLRI is thought to occur to due failure of multiple stabilizers, not just the LUCL in isolation.

What other condition can present in a similar fashion?

A. Valgus instability
B. Lateral epicondylitis
C. Extensor carpi radialis brevis avulsion
D. Capitellar osteochondritis dissecans (OCD) lesion

Discussion

The correct answer is (A). Valgus instability can be difficult to distinguish from PLRI. Physical examination is critical to differentiate the two. In PLRI, the most sensitive physical examination maneuver is the lateral pivot shift. With the patient lying supine, a valgus stress is applied to the elbow while simultaneously flexing it. This reproduces the patient's symptoms. In the case of valgus instability, the anterior band of the MCL should be isolated when examined. This is best done with the shoulder internally rotated, the forearm in pronation, and the elbow flexed to 30 degrees. A valgus stress is

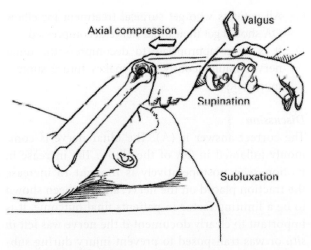

Figure 2–96 Reproduced with permission from Morrey BF. Acute and Chronic Instability of the Elbow. *JAAOS* 1996;4(3):117–128.

then placed on the elbow (see Fig. 2–96). Pain or joint opening may be indicative of MCL incompetence.

Which of the following is the most appropriate method of surgical management?

A. Acute LUCL reconstruction in all simple elbow dislocations
B. Acute direct repair of the LUCL in all simple elbow dislocations
C. Direct repair or reconstruction with palmaris autograft of the LUCL in patients with symptomatic PLRI
D. Radial head arthroplasty with a large head to increase lateral stability

Discussion
The correct answer is (C). Direct repair or reconstruction of the LUCL. Surgery is indicated to restore the lateral ligamentous stabilizers when there is recurrent, symptomatic instability. Acute repair is not necessary most of the time as the ligament frequently scars in. Only when there is symptomatic instability is surgery warranted.

What is the most common complication following surgical reconstruction of the LUCL?

A. Infection
B. PIN neuropraxia
C. Recurrent instability
D. Greater than 30-degree flexion contracture

Discussion
The correct answer is (C). Persistent instability is the main concern after surgical treatment. Patients with degenerative arthritis and radial head excision are less likely to have a satisfactory outcome. PIN neuropraxia and infection are potential complications but are not as prevalent as recurrent instability. A small flexion contracture does frequently occur, but this is typically not severe enough to produce any functional limitations.

Objectives: Did you learn...?
- Identify the relevant anatomy and pathoanatomy that are involved in elbow instability?
- Physically examine a patient for classic posterolateral instability?
- Understand the potential treatment options?

CASE 37

Dr. Joseph Cohen

A 53-year-old, left-hand-dominant male presents to your office for evaluation regarding his elbow pain. He states that for the past 5 years he has had pain in his left elbow. It seems to be worsening over the past 6 months. He states he works as a mechanic and the pain is limiting the amount of time he can spend working. He takes anti-inflammatories with some relief. His images are shown (Figs. 2–97 and 2–98).

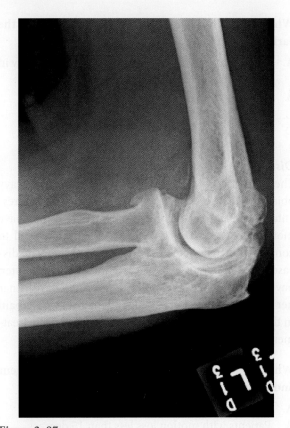

Figure 2–97

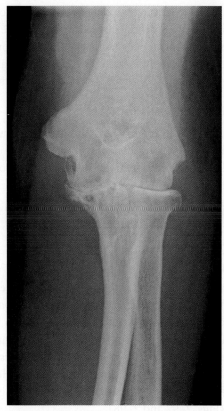

Figure 2–98

Which of the following symptoms is common in the early stages of osteoarthritis (OA)?

A. Pain when carrying heavy objects with the elbow in extension
B. Pain at mid-arc range of motion
C. Motion loss greater than 30 degrees
D. Ulnar neuritis

Discussion

The correct answer is (A). Pain when carrying heavy objects with the elbow in extension is a classic presentation for patients with early disease. They also have motion loss less than 15 degrees and respond well to conservative treatments. Patients with intermediate disease have moderate pain at the ends of motion, often have loss of extension >30 degrees and have ulnar nerve symptoms. Patients with end-stage OA have pain in the mid-arc of motion, have failed conservative treatment and have motion loss greater than 30 degrees.

When is simultaneous osteocapsular debridement and ulnar nerve decompression warranted?

A. Ulnar neuritis and flexion less than 100
B. Patients with motion loss less than 15 degrees

C. All patients who get surgical treatment for elbow OA should get their ulnar nerve decompressed
D. It is never appropriate to decompress the ulnar nerve simultaneously as it makes future surgery more risky

Discussion

The correct answer is (A). The ulnar nerve is commonly inflamed in OA of the elbow. The increase in motion seen postoperatively is thought to increase the traction placed on the nerve, and has been shown to be a limiting factor in patients final outcome. It is important to clearly document if the nerve was left *in situ* or was transposed to prevent injury during subsequent surgery.

Which of the following is predictive of postoperative motion following arthroscopic osteocapsular debridement?

A. Preoperative motion
B. Intraoperative motion
C. Motion seen at 2 weeks postoperative
D. Amount of preoperative pain based on the visual analog scale (VAS)
E. Degree of joint space narrowing

Discussion

The correct answer is (B). It has been shown that the amount of motion achieved after completion of the soft tissue and bony release correlates the most with final outcome.

What is the most common complication of total elbow arthroplasty in a younger population?

A. Infection
B. Triceps avulsion
C. Aseptic/mechanical loosening
D. PIN neuropraxia
E. Ulnar nerve neuropraxia

Discussion

The correct answer is (C). Aseptic or mechanical loosening is the most common cause of failure in the younger, more active population. The estimated incidence of implant loosening is between 7% and 15%. Although the newer, semi-constrained prosthesis has significantly lower rates of loosening than the fully constrained implant, mechanical failure is still of primary concern. Infection occurs between 5% and 8% of the time, and triceps insufficiency is from 3% to 8%.

What restrictions would the patient have to adhere to if he wished to proceed with total elbow arthroplasty?

A. Cannot extend beyond 30 degrees
B. 10 lb life-long weight limit
C. Must take daily prophylactic antibiotics for 10 years postoperatively
D. Would be unable to pronate and supinate

Discussion

The correct answer is (B). Patients are advised to lift no more than 10 lb for a single lift and no more than 2 to 5 lb for repetitive lifting for the duration of their life. Despite this precaution, there is still a high rate of revision for aseptic loosening.

Objectives: Did you learn…?

- Identify etiology and natural history of osteoarthritis of the elbow?
- Identify indications for selecting different treatment options?
- Recognize common complications seen with total elbow replacement?

CASE 38

Dr. Joseph Cohen

A 78-year-old female with a history of rheumatoid arthritis for the past 20 years presents to the office for an evaluation of her bilateral elbows. She initially presented with symptoms in her hands and wrists and has been poorly compliant with her antirheumatic medication.

She has received multiple corticosteroid injections into her elbows over the past 3 years, but she no longer gets relief. Her images are shown (Figs. 2–99 to 2–102).

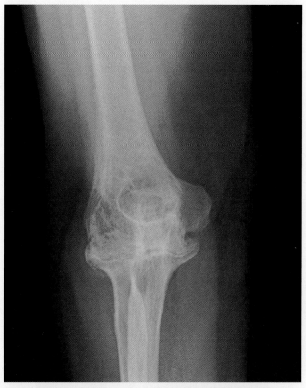

Figure 2–100

Approximately what percentage of patients with rheumatoid arthritis develop elbow involvement within 5 years?

A. 10%
B. 5%
C. 75%
D. 60%
E. 40%

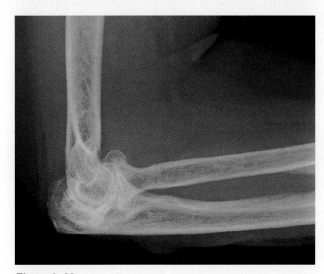

Figure 2–99

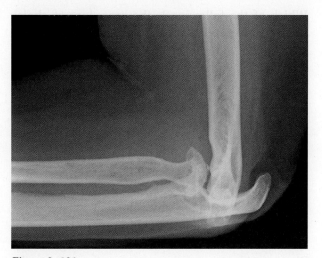

Figure 2–101

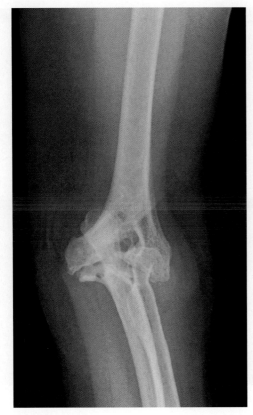

Figure 2–102

Discussion

The correct answer is (E). Between 20% and 50% of patients with rheumatoid arthritis will develop elbow arthritis. Isolated presentation of the elbow is rare and only occurs about 5% of the time. Care should be given to provide the best treatment for the entire upper extremity when evaluating and treating a patient with rheumatoid arthritis.

Which of the following is the procedure of choice when treating an advanced, debilitating rheumatoid elbow?

A. Elbow arthrodesis
B. Open synovectomy
C. Radial head excision
D. Arthroscopic synovectomy
E. Semi-constrained total elbow

Discussion

The correct answer is (E). Semi-constrained total elbow is the definitive procedure of choice when treating an elbow with extensive articular damage and subluxation or ankylosis of the joint (see Fig. 2–103). Rheumatoid patients place a lower demand on the

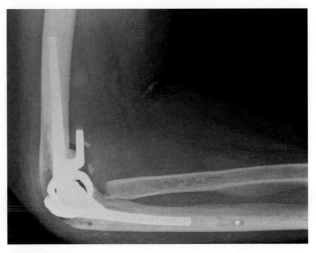

Figure 2–103

prosthesis than patients with primary osteoarthritis (OA), and thus have a lower incidence of mechanical loosening. Due to the ligamentous laxity, prosthetic instability is the complication that most commonly inhibits success.

Which of the following antirheumatic drugs should be continued prior to surgery?

A. Methotrexate
B. Sulfasalazine
C. Infliximab
D. Adalimumab
E. Etanercept

Discussion

The correct answer is (A). Methotrexate is the only agent that should be continued throughout the operative period. In general, biologic agents such as TNF antagonists (Infliximab, adalumimab, etanercept) should be withheld for 1 week pre-op and restarted 10 to 14 days postoperatively. The goal is to reduce the risk of infection and optimize wound healing. Routine consultation with the patient's rheumatologist is recommended before undergoing any surgical procedure.

Objectives: Did you learn...?

- Identify etiology and natural history of rheumatoid arthritis affecting the elbows?
- Become familiar with the variety of medical treatment options commonly used?
- Recognize the potential surgical options including their outcomes and complications?

CASE 39

Dr. Joseph Cohen

A 20-year-old male presents to the office with right elbow pain. He states he fell 5 years ago and was told he broke his elbow but was treated without surgery. He has since developed worsening pain in his elbow with pain present throughout his entire arc of motion. The pain is more severe in the morning and at night, and he reports frequent swelling of his elbow. He is active and has not yet had any formal treatment. His x-rays can be seen in Figures 2–104 and 2–105.

Initial management includes which of the following?

A. Arthroscopic debridement
B. Corticosteroid injection and physical therapy
C. Hinged elbow brace
D. Total elbow arthroplasty
E. Radial head resection

Discussion

The correct answer is (B). Young active patients with post-traumatic arthritis are challenging, and achieving an elbow equal to that of the normal contralateral arm is unlikely. Treatment should consist of conservative measures until the level of pain or patient loss of function requires more aggressive treatment. Arthroscopic debridement works better for patients with pain at the extremes of motion rather than throughout the entire arc. Total elbow is a poor option at this point given the age and activity level of the patient.

For a young patient with elbow arthritis and pain only at extremes of motion, what would be the most appropriate surgical intervention?

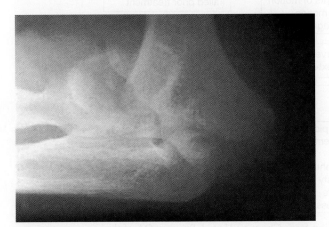

Figure 2–104

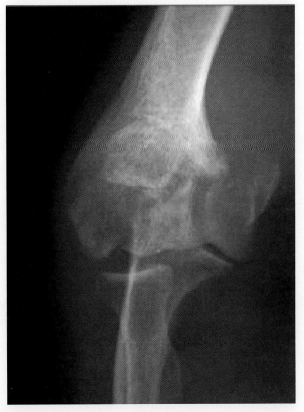

Figure 2–105

A. Radial head replacement
B. Radial head resection
C. Arthroscopic osteocapsular debridement
D. Distal humerus osteotomy
E. Fascial interpositional arthroplasty

Discussion

The correct answer is (C). Pain at terminal motion is a symptom that is present in the early stages of arthritis. It is often due to periarticular osteophytes and capsular contracture with relative sparing of the articular surface. Radial head replacement and partial ulnohumeral arthroplasty is a viable option with arthritis isolated to one compartment. Fascial interposition arthroplasty is more appropriate for a patient with end stage arthritis with destruction of the majority of the articular bearing surface.

For a young patient with elbow arthritis and pain throughout the arc of motion, which of the following would be the best surgical option?

A. Arthroscopic debridement
B. Microfracture
C. Open osteocapsular debridement

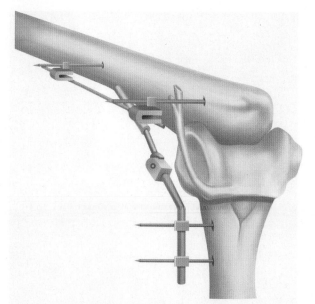

Figure 2-106 Reproduced with permission from Cheung EV, et al. Primary OA of the Elbow: Current Treatment Options. *JAAOS* 2008;16(2):77–87.

D. Fascial interposition arthroplasty
E. Total elbow arthroplasty

Discussion

The correct answer is (D). Fascial interposition arthroplasty (Fig. 2–106) has shown to produce reliable pain relief in young patients in which a total elbow would not be appropriate. It typically involves resurfacing the bearing surface with either autograft or allograft. Although most patients see improvement with this procedure, it

is still seen as a salvage procedure with one of its main benefits being that it does not compromise subsequent procedures. Figure 2–107 shows a decision-making algorithm for treatment based on the current stage of elbow osteoarthritis.

Objectives: Did you learn...?

- Understand the primary goals of treatment for a young patient with posttraumatic elbow arthritis?
- Be able to differentiate patients that have pain at terminal motion versus pain throughout the arc of motion?
- Understand indications and outcomes of the surgical options?

CASE 40

Dr. Joseph Cohen

A 16-year-old male baseball player presents to your office for evaluation of his worsening right elbow pain. He denies acute injury or inciting event. The pain is located on the posteromedial aspect of his elbow and is exacerbated by throwing. It has been present for the past 6 months, but it has been more severe over the past 3 months.

On examination, he has tenderness to palpation over his olecranon and pain with terminal elbow extension. He has no evidence of varus or valgus instability. No pain with resisted wrist flexion. His images are shown (Figs. 2–108 to 2–110).

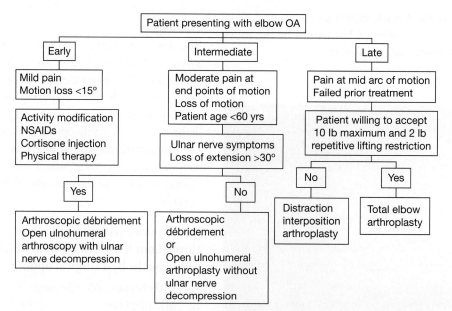

Figure 2-107 Reproduced with permission from Cheung EV, et al. Primary OA of the Elbow: Current Treatment Options. *JAAOS* 2008;16(2):77–87.

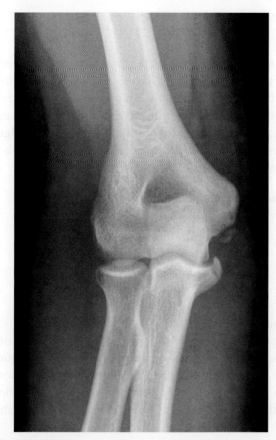

Figure 2–108

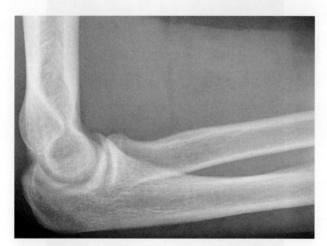

Figure 2–109

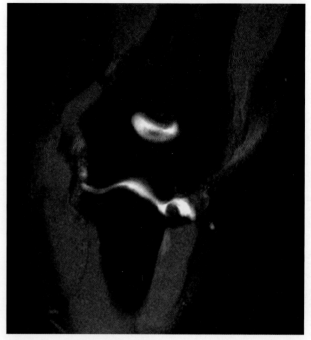

Figure 2–110

What is the diagnosis?

A. Valgus extension overload
B. Medial epicondylitis
C. Osteochondritis dissecans (OCD)
D. Olecranon stress fracture
E. Medial collateral ligament (MCL) rupture

Discussion

The correct answer is (A). This syndrome occurs most commonly in competitive pitchers, with pain that is worse in the deceleration phase and at terminal extension. The resulting chronic stress results in chondrolysis, osteophyte formation, and attenuation of the MCL. Medial epicondylitis is also common in pitchers, but the pathology is limited to the flexor pronator mass. Pain is over the medial epicondyle and is worse with wrist and forearm flexion. OCD lesions are most common in the capitellum, often present with mechanical symptoms. Olecranon stress fractures result from repetitive abutment into the olecranon fossa. This is a plausible answer, however, the MRI findings are not consistent. MCL rupture is typically acute and is not seen on the MRI shown.

What would be the most appropriate initial treatment?

A. Arthroscopic osteocapsular debridement
B. MCL debridement and reconstruction
C. Rest, physical therapy, and modification of pitching biomechanics
D. Cortisone injection
E. Open olecranon debridement

Discussion

The correct answer is (C). A nonoperative protocol that consists of 2 to 4 weeks of rest, NSAIDs, physical therapy, and biomechanics coaching is the primary treatment of choice. Only once nonoperative treatment has failed for 3 to 6 months should you proceed with surgical intervention. Surgical intervention is also warranted with acute ruptures of the ulnar collateral ligament (UCL). Cortisone injections are contraindicated as further ligamentous attenuation could occur.

What neurologic syndrome is commonly found in a patient with valgus extension overload?

A. Intersection syndrome
B. Carpal tunnel syndrome
C. Cubital tunnel syndrome
D. Radial tunnel syndrome

Discussion

The correct answer is (C). The increased traction and stress placed on the medial elbow not only effects the osseous and ligamentous structures, but also can lead to ulnar neuropathy. In addition, compression can occur from osteophytes, synovitis, or thickened intermuscular septum. Nonoperative treatment is recommended and typically does not require any different treatment than that of valgus extension overload alone.

Ten months after olecranon debridement the patient still complains of pain and "laxity" of his elbow, which structure is likely damaged?

A. Flexor pronator mass
B. Annular ligament
C. Anterior bundle of the MCL
D. Transverse ligament
E. Oblique bundle

Discussion

The correct answer is (C). Care must be taken when performing osseous debridement of the posteromedial olecranon to not remove the attachment site of the MCL as this would result in further destabilization of the elbow. The MCL complex consists of the anterior bundle (which is the most important for valgus stability), the posterior bundle, and the transverse ligament (also known as the oblique ligament).

Objectives: Did you learn...?

• Understand the pathoanatomy and typical clinical presentation?
• Learn the differential diagnoses when evaluating a patient with medial elbow pain?
• Understand the radiographic findings seen in patients with valgus overload?
• Identify indications for operative intervention?

CASE 41

Dr. Min Lu

A 14-year-old baseball pitcher presents to the office with left throwing elbow pain for the past two months when he throws or lifts weights. Examination reveals lateral joint line tenderness with no detectable effusion and full range of motion without crepitation. Moving valgus stress test does not elicit pain. His elbow radiograph is shown below (Fig. 2–111).

What is the next most appropriate treatment?

A. Elbow arthroscopy, debridement of the lesion
B. Arthroscopic drilling of the lesion
C. Ulnar collateral ligament repair
D. Corticosteroid injection of the elbow
E. Cessation of throwing activities

Discussion

The correct answer is (E). This patient has osteochondritis dissecans (OCD) of the capitellum. He has not undergone any conservative treatment. Stable, nondisplaced lesions can heal spontaneously with rest and discontinuation of throwing. Surgical treatment is reserved for unstable

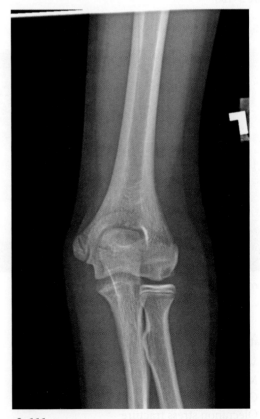

Figure 2–111

lesions or loose bodies. This patient's examination is not consistent with an ulnar collateral ligament (UCL) injury. Little league elbow is another commonly encountered diagnosis in this patient population, but like UCL injuries, manifests with medial sided pain after throwing.

Besides baseball, what other sport is this condition most commonly seen with?

A. Football linemen
B. Rugby players
C. Rowers
D. Gymnasts
E. Swimmers

Discussion

The correct answer is (D). The exact etiology and natural history of osteochondritis dissecans of the capitellum is poorly understood. It is mainly encountered in adolescent age groups, although with earlier youth sports participation, it is now seen in younger athletes as well. It most commonly develops in female gymnasts as well as in the throwing elbow of male pitchers, as both of these sports involve repetitive loading of the elbow joint.

Which of the following findings differentiates Panner's disease from osteochondritis dissecans of the capitellum?

A. Site of involvement within the elbow
B. Extent of capitellar involvement
C. Symptoms may resolve with conservative management
D. Collateral ligament instability

Discussion

The correct answer is (B). Panner's disease is a separate disorder of the immature capitellum that must be distinguished from OCD. Panner's disease usually arises in patients younger than 10 years of age, whereas OCD lesions of the capitellum typically arise after age 11. Both disorders involve the capitellum, causing lateral joint tenderness. Whereas OCD of the capitellum represents a focal injury of the cartilage and subchondral bone, Panner's disease is idiopathic chondrosis and fragmentation of the entire capitellum. Both conditions can resolve with conservative treatment and are not dependent on collateral ligament instability.

What is the suspected etiology of capitellar osteochondritis dissecans?

A. Nutritional deficiency
B. Infection
C. Traumatic and vascular
D. Congenital
E. Malignancy

Discussion

The correct answer is (C). While the exact etiology of OCD lesions of the capitellum is poorly understood, trauma and ischemia are suspected to play a significant role. OCD occurs in overhead throwing athletes and female gymnasts, supporting the theory that repetitive trauma serves as an inciting event. The capitellum receives its blood supply from posterior end-arteries that traverse the growth plate, without metaphyseal collateral contribution. This tenuous vascular anatomy implicates an ischemic contribution to OCD. Several case studies have reported on familial or hereditary predisposition to OCD; however, the condition is not present at birth.

The patient undergoes conservative management consisting of rest, anti-inflammatory medications, and physical therapy. After six months, he is still not able to return to play and has progressively worsening symptoms with attempted throwing. He has a moderate elbow effusion as well as a 20-degree flexion contracture. An elbow MRI arthrogram is obtained and shown (Fig. 2–112). He elects to proceed with elbow arthroscopy. Intraoperative arthroscopic images are shown (Figs. 2–113 and 2–114).

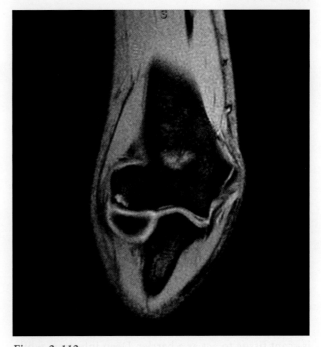

Figure 2–112

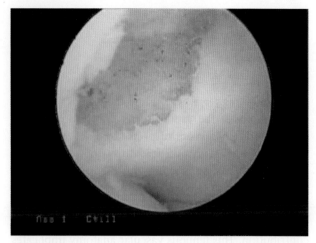

Figure 2–113

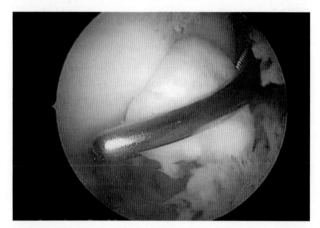

Figure 2–114

being the most serious postoperative complication, is relatively rare (0.8%). In one series, the rate of transient neurological injuries was found to be 2%. These result from compression, local anesthetic injection, and direct trauma. A thorough understanding of the neurovascular anatomy of the elbow is crucial to achieve proper portal placement. Loss of elbow motion was reported in approximately 1% of cases and is usually minor (less than 20 degrees).

Objectives: Did you learn...?

- Recognize the clinical and radiographic presentation of elbow osteochondritis dissecans?
- Formulate a differential diagnosis for pediatric sports elbow injuries?
- Treat elbow osteochondritis dissecans?

CASE 42

Dr. Min Lu

A 21-year-old, right-hand-dominant, collegiate pitcher presents to the office with elbow pain and loss of velocity and control over the last 6 weeks. Examination reveals tenderness along the medial aspect of the elbow, negative Tinel sign, and pain with valgus stress through the mid-arc of motion. He has no pain with wrist range of motion or forearm pronation and supination. Imaging study is shown below (Fig. 2–115).

Which of the following is the most commonly reported complication of elbow arthroscopy?

A. Contracture
B. Compartment syndrome
C. Septic joint
D. Neuropraxia
E. Vessel injury

Discussion

The correct answer is (D). The overall reported rate of transient and permanent complications after elbow arthroscopy is around 10% and is much higher than the rate after knee and shoulder arthroscopy (1–2%). The overall most commonly reported complication is prolonged drainage or erythema around portal sites. The lateral portal sites are susceptible to this issue as the joint is relatively subcutaneous in this area, and there is scant tissue to act as a barrier. Deep infection, while

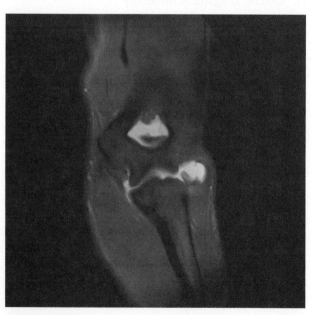

Figure 2–115

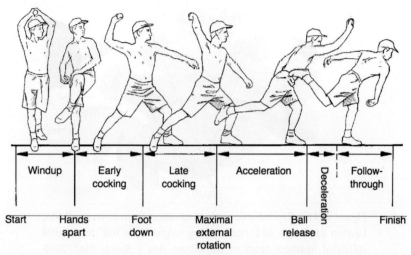

Figure 2-116 Phases of throwing: The greatest valgus stress at the elbow occurs during the late cocking and early acceleration phases of throwing. (Reproduced with permission from Chen FS, Rokito AS, Jobe FW. Medial elbow problems in the overhead-throwing athlete. *J Am Acad Orthop Surg.* 2001;9(2):99–113.)

What anatomic structure is the primary cause of the patient's symptoms?

A. Ulnar collateral ligament
B. Ulnar nerve
C. Common flexor origin
D. Olecranon osteophytes
E. Biceps tendon

Discussion

The correct answer is (A). This patient has pain with mid-flexion valgus stress suggesting an injury to his ulnar collateral ligament. Throwing athletes can have multiple causes for pain at the medial elbow, which can be elucidated by history and physical examination. This patient has a negative Tinel sign and no numbness, tingling or weakness to suggest ulnar nerve injury. Likewise, the flexor pronator mass may become irritated in pitchers, but it is not the primary cause of this patient's symptoms. His pain is not at terminal extension, and therefore olecranon osteophytes or valgus extension overload would not seem to be the cause. He does not have any findings suggestive of biceps tendon pathology.

During which phase of throwing is the ulnar collateral ligament most likely to be injured?

A. Wind up
B. Early cocking
C. Late cocking
D. Ball release
E. Deceleration

Discussion

The correct answer is (C). The late cocking and early acceleration phase of overhead throwing places the greatest amount of valgus stress on the elbow (see Fig. 2–116). At this point, the elbow is in mid flexion while the forearm lags behind the upper arm, producing a valgus moment at the elbow. The anterior band of the ulnar collateral ligament is the primary restraint to valgus stress between 30 and 120 degrees of flexion. The wind up phase does not place any stress on the elbow. In early cocking, the rotator cuff and deltoid are active and susceptible to injury. Ball release occurs after acceleration as the forearm is brought forward. At this point, the valgus stresses on the UCL are dissipated. Finally, in deceleration, the posterior compartment of the elbow and elbow flexors are subject to stress to prevent hyperextension.

Which of the following is the most sensitive physical examination finding for ulnar collateral ligament injury?

A. Lateral pivot shift test
B. Pain with resisted wrist flexion
C. Static valgus stress test
D. Palpable medial ligamentous laxity
E. Moving valgus stress test

Discussion

The correct answer is (E). The lateral pivot shift test is used to assess the lateral ulnar collateral ligament and suggests posterolateral rotatory instability. Pain with resisted wrist flexion indicates inflammation at the common

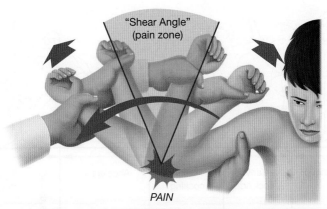

Figure 2-117 Reproduced with permission from O'Driscoll SW, Lawton RL, Smith AM. The "moving valgus stress test" for medial collateral ligament tears of the elbow. *Am J Sports Med.* 2005 Feb;33(2):231–9.

flexor origin, and is suggestive of medial epicondylitis. The moving valgus stress test is highly sensitive (100%) and specific (75%) for ulnar collateral ligament injury, as it reproduces the stresses and elbow positions present during throwing. Pain with static valgus testing is not as accurate as the moving valgus stress test (sensitivity 65%, specificity 50%) as it does not test an arc of motion that pitchers experience. Palpable ligamentous laxity is poorly sensitive (19%) but highly specific (100%).

The moving valgus stress test is performed with the patient upright and the shoulder abducted 90 degrees (Fig. 2–117). With the elbow flexed, a valgus stress is applied to the elbow until the shoulder reaches full external rotation. While a constant valgus torque is maintained, the elbow is quickly extended to 30 degrees.

The patient undergoes conservative treatment consisting of rest and physical therapy, followed by a progressive throwing program. However, he is unable to return to throwing after 3 months. He elects for ulnar collateral ligament reconstruction.

What types of outcomes have been seen with ulnar collateral ligament reconstruction with professional pitchers?

A. High rates of persistent elbow pain and retirement from sport
B. Loss of velocity and performance
C. High rate of return to play at a similar level
D. 30% rate of revision surgery

Discussion

The correct answer is (C). Studies in Major League Baseball have shown that over 80% of pitchers returned

to the major leagues at a mean 20 months after UCL reconstruction, while over 97% return to major and minor leagues combined. Meanwhile, the revision rate for surgery is approximately 4%. Pitch velocity and common performance measurements do not seem to differ from pre-injury levels.

What is the most common surgical complication seen with ulnar collateral ligament reconstruction?

A. Postoperative stiffness requiring reoperation
B. Ulnar neuropathy
C. Superficial infection
D. Tenderness at graft harvest site
E. Permanent cutaneous sensory deficit

Discussion

The correct answer is (B). The overall complication rate after ulnar collateral ligament reconstruction is 10% (range 3–25%). Ulnar neuropathy is the most commonly reported complication after ulnar collateral ligament reconstruction ranging from 2% to 21%. In one study, performance of obligatory ulnar nerve transposition led to 75% excellent results and 14% with ulnar neuropathy. Without obligatory nerve transposition, that study found 89% excellent results and 6% rate of ulnar neuropathy. Studies report a 1% rate of stiffness requiring reoperation. Cutaneous nerve injuries after Tommy John surgery tend to be transient neuropraxias as opposed to permanent deficits. Infection and graft site tenderness are not as common complications as ulnar neuropathy.

Objectives: Did you learn...?

• Identify and evaluate patients with ulnar collateral ligament instability?

- Comprehend anatomic and biomechanical considerations for medial elbow instability?
- Understand the role for surgery and the outcomes of ulnar collateral ligament reconstruction?

CASE 43

Dr. Min Lu

A 9-year-old, baseball pitcher presents to the office with 4 weeks of elbow pain of his throwing arm. He denies locking or catching symptoms. Examination reveals tenderness to palpation about the medial elbow, normal range of motion, and no instability with moving valgus stress. Radiographs are normal.

What is the most likely underlying pathology in this condition?

A. Microtraumatic vascular insufficiency of the capitellum
B. Medial epicondylar apophysitis
C. Idiopathic osteochondrosis of the capitellum
D. Ulnar collateral ligament disruption
E. Olecranon apophysitis and osteochondrosis

Discussion

The correct answer is (B). This patient has little league elbow which results from repetitive valgus stress in skeletally immature athletes. In this condition, chronic traction from the flexor-pronator mass leads to medial epicondylar apophysitis. Injuries in this age group result from medial tensile or lateral compressive overload. Osteochondritis dissecans (Answer A) usually affects adolescents older than age 13 years, and typically manifests as pain in the lateral compartment. Likewise, Panner's disease (Answer C) also affects the capitellum and presents with lateral pain. Ulnar collateral ligament injuries are uncommon in skeletally immature athletes. Posterior compartment injuries (Answer E) are also uncommon and typically present with pain on terminal extension.

What is the most appropriate initial management for the patient in the question above?

A. Epicondylar debridement
B. Open reduction internal fixation
C. Rest, cessation of throwing activities
D. MRI
E. Corticosteroid injection

Discussion

The correct answer is (C). Conservative management is the mainstay of initial treatment for little league elbow.

This consists of 2 to 4 weeks of rest and oral anti-inflammatories, followed by focused stretching and strengthening exercises. Athletes may return to throwing at 6 weeks if symptom free. Symptoms may persist after inadequate periods of rest and immobilization. Surgery, MRI, or injections are not routinely warranted as the first line of treatment in this condition.

Which of the following is not a risk factor for developing arm pain in young pitchers?

A. High number of innings pitched
B. High number of pitches per game
C. Staying in games after pitching, at other positions besides pitcher or catcher
D. Pitching with arm fatigue
E. Taller, heavier athletes

Discussion

The correct answer is (C). Multiple studies have looked at risk factors for shoulder and elbow injuries among adolescent pitchers. The 10-year-cumulative risk for an adolescent pitcher developing a serious injury is 5%. Studies have consistently found that arm overuse is a risk factor for joint injuries, and preventative strategies have focused on limiting pitch counts and avoiding pitching with arm fatigue. Taller, heavier athletes appear to be at higher risk as well as pitchers who throw with greater velocity. Inconsistent reports have been published regarding the link between breaking pitches and arm injury. Data seems to indicate that pitchers may remain in games and play other positions beside catcher without significantly increased risk for shoulder or elbow injury.

What is the most common radiographic finding with little league elbow?

A. Fragmentation and separation of the capitellum
B. Olecranon osteophytes
C. Loose body
D. Medial epicondyle fracture
E. Fragmentation and separation of the medial epicondyle

Discussion

The correct answer is (E). Fragmentation and separation of the capitellum can be seen with osteochondritis dissecans or Panner's disease, with the distinguishing factor being the amount of capitellar involvement. Osteochondritis dissecans involves a focal articular defect, whereas Panner's disease involves the entire capitellum. Olecranon osteophytes are encountered with valgus

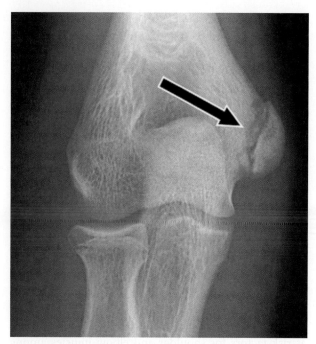

Figure 2–118 Medial epicondylar separation seen in little league elbow.

extension overload. Loose bodies may be seen in later stages of osteochondritis dissecans. Medial epicondyle avulsion fracture is a rare cause of acute elbow pain in skeletally immature athletes and is treated according to amount of displacement. Fragmentation and separation of the medial epicondyle is the characteristic radiographic finding of little league elbow (see Fig. 2–118). Previous studies have found separation or widening of the physis in over 50% of players while fragmentation occurred in roughly 20%.

Objectives: Did you learn...?

- Recognize chronic overuse injuries in adolescent athletes?
- Manage a patient with little league elbow?
- Counsel pediatric athletes on risk factors for arm injury?

CASE 44

Dr. Min Lu

A 45-year-old, male laborer presents with elbow pain after an injury at work. He was carrying a heavy object, felt it slip, and hyperextended his elbow. He felt a pop and immediate pain in his antecubital fossa. He is neurovascularly intact distally with weakness at the elbow. He has ecchymosis and swelling at the elbow. Hook test is inconclusive.

What is the next most appropriate step in treatment?

A. Sling immobilization until asymptomatic with follow-up examination
B. Physical therapy to focus on elbow range of motion and strengthening
C. Elbow arthroscopy
D. Open exploration of the antecubital fossa
E. Elbow MRI

Discussion

The correct answer is (E). This patient has a suspected distal biceps tendon rupture. He has the classic presentation of an eccentric overload injury along with a pop and pain in the antecubital fossa. However, his examination is inconclusive for complete versus partial tendon tear. The hook test is performed by asking the patient to actively flex the elbow to 90 degrees and fully supinating the forearm (see Fig. 2–119). The examiner then attempts to hook their index finger under the lateral edge of the tendon and palpate a cordlike structure representing the biceps tendon. This test has been shown to be both highly sensitive and specific (up to 100%), but it is inconclusive in this case. An MRI is warranted to assess the integrity of the distal biceps tendon, to distinguish between complete versus partial rupture (Fig. 2–120). This could alter management as the optimal treatment of partial tendon ruptures is not entirely clear. There is relative urgency to doing this, as early surgical intervention after injury is preferred to facilitate primary repair.

What is the most significant strength deficit resulting from nonoperative treatment of a distal biceps tendon injury?

A. Elbow flexion
B. Elbow extension
C. Forearm pronation
D. Forearm supination
E. Shoulder forward flexion

Discussion

The correct answer is (D). By its anatomic insertion on the radial tuberosity, the biceps brachii serves as both an elbow flexor and supinator of the forearm. There is a greater percentage loss of supination strength as the brachialis serves as the primary elbow flexor. Nesterenko et al. showed that patients with a unilateral biceps rupture lost 37% flexion strength and 46% supination strength. Different reports exist regarding the effect of biceps injury on elbow endurance. Given the functional

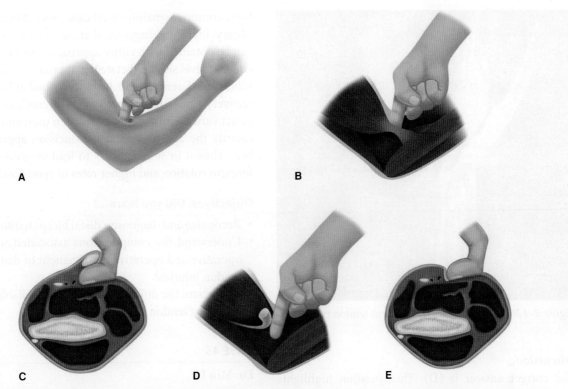

Figure 2–119 Figures demonstrating the hook test. **(A–C)** The patient actively supinates with the elbow flexed 90 degrees. An intact hook test allows the examiner to hook their index finger under the intact biceps tendon from the lateral side. **(D–E)** With an abnormal hook test, there is no cord-like structure under which to hook a finger. (Reproduced with permission from Sutton KM, Dodds SD, Ahmad CS, Sethi PM. Surgical treatment of distal biceps rupture. *J Am Acad Orthop Surg.* 2010 Mar;18(3):139–48.)

deficits associated with nonoperative treatment of complete ruptures, conservative treatment is reserved for only low demand or medically infirm patients in these cases.

What is the most common nerve injury encountered after operative treatment of distal biceps tendon ruptures?

A. Median
B. Radial
C. Musculocutaneous
D. Lateral antebrachial cutaneous
E. Posterior interosseous

Discussion

The correct answer is (D). Lateral antebrachial cutaneous neuropraxia is the most common complication of distal biceps tendon repair. It is reported in up to 26% of cases. This is usually the result of excessive retraction and can be avoided with adequate exposure and toe-ing in of the retractors. The nerve pierces the fascia between the biceps and brachialis at the antecubital fossa and runs in the subcutaneous tissues parallel to the cephalic

vein. Injury to the radial sensory (6%) and posterior interosseous (4%) nerves has also been reported, although more rare. Pronation of the forearm protects the posterior interosseous nerve. These nerve injuries after distal biceps tendon repair are usually self-limited complications. Other general complications include superficial infection, symptomatic heterotopic ossification, and re-rupture.

Which of the following statements is true regarding one versus two-incision technique for repair of acute distal biceps tendon ruptures?

A. The single incision approach affords a significantly faster recovery time
B. The single incision approach is associated with lower biomechanical strength and higher fixation failure rates
C. The two incision approach is shown to have lower rates of heterotopic ossification
D. The single incision approach is associated with higher rates of neurologic complications, whereas the two incision approach is associated with increased rates of proximal radioulnar joint synostosis

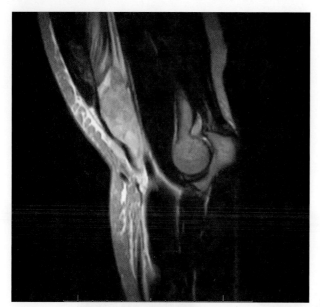

Figure 2–120 MRI depicting distal biceps tendon rupture.

Discussion

The correct answer is (D). This question highlights some controversies surrounding the optimal approach for treatment of distal biceps tendon ruptures. Historically, distal biceps tendon injuries were repaired through a single anterior extensile approach. Due to a high rate of neurologic complications, the Boyd Anderson dual incision technique was developed, and this was further modified to address the complication of radioulnar synostosis (Fig. 2–121). Given that distal bicep tendon injuries are relatively rare, the literature on this topic comprises mainly small case series. Most contemporary literature suggests that satisfactory outcomes can be obtained with either approach, and that surgeon comfort level should dictate the approach used. No significant differences have been described in regards to recovery time. The biomechanical strength of the construct varies with the type of fixation used and not necessarily the approach. The two-incision approach has been shown in some studies to lead to greater loss of forearm rotation and higher rates of synostosis.

Objectives: Did you learn...?

- Recognize and diagnose a distal biceps tendon injury?
- Understand the complications associated with nonoperative and operative management of distal biceps tendon injuries?
- Appreciate the different approaches available for distal biceps tendon repair?

CASE 45

Dr. Min Lu

A 23-year-old, semi-professional football linebacker presents with left elbow pain after a game. He extended his arm while falling to the ground and felt a pop and immediate pain in the posterior aspect of his arm. On examination, he is distally neurovascularly intact with swelling and palpable deformity about the posterior aspect of the elbow. He has difficulty extending his arm with 3/5 strength. His elbow lateral x-ray is shown below (Fig. 2–122).

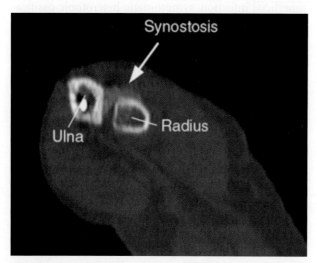

Figure 2–121 CT shows one complication of distal biceps repair: proximal radioulnar joint synostosis.

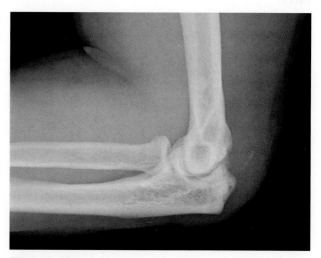

Figure 2–122

What is the most likely diagnosis?

A. Calcific tendonitis
B. Osteochondral defect
C. Distal triceps tendon rupture
D. Distal biceps tendon rupture
E. Elbow dislocation

Discussion

The correct answer is (C). The patient's injury mechanism, physical examination, and imaging findings are most consistent with an acute distal triceps tendon rupture. Triceps tendon ruptures are very rare and among the least commonly reported sports tendon injuries (<1% of all tendon injuries). Most injuries are associated with weightlifting or football due to the training regimens, potential for anabolic steroid use, and violent forces exerted. The mechanism for injury is a sudden, eccentric load applied to the contracting muscle such as from weightlifting or a fall onto an outstretched hand. Penetrating trauma or direct blows may also cause tendon injury as can higher energy mechanisms such as motor vehicle accidents. The lateral elbow radiograph shows flecks of avulsed bone from the olecranon insertion of the triceps, which is almost always pathognomonic for triceps tendon rupture. This finding should not be mistaken for calcific tendonitis with the given clinical history. It is also not consistent with an intra-articular loose body.

What is the next most appropriate step in management?

A. Sling for comfort
B. Splint immobilization in 30 degrees of flexion
C. Functional elbow brace
D. Surgical exploration and tendon repair
E. MRI

Discussion

The correct answer is (E). Although the diagnosis is most consistent with a distal triceps tendon rupture, this patient has 3/5 motor strength. An MRI must be obtained in this instance to assess the location and degree of tendon involvement (see Fig. 2–123). Physical examination and strength grading can be difficult and inconsistent in the acute setting, even leading to some missed diagnoses. Partial ruptures may present with profound strength deficits, whereas complete ruptures may exhibit little or no strength deficit due to compensation from an intact lateral triceps expansion or the anconeus. This makes an MRI essential

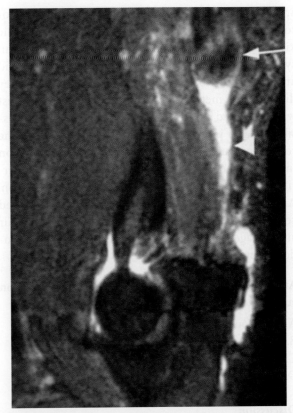

Figure 2-123 MRI depiction of retracted triceps tendon (*white arrow*) and fluid filled gap (*arrowhead*).

for accurate diagnosis and preoperative planning. In general, tears <50% can be managed conservatively with satisfactory results. Partial tears >50% are managed on an individualized basis. They can be managed nonsurgically in sedentary or medically infirm individuals, with repair indicated for active or younger individuals. Complete tears are usually best treated surgically.

Which of the following is not a risk factor for distal triceps tendon rupture?

A. Anabolic steroid use
B. Female gender
C. Chronic kidney disease
D. Local corticosteroid injections
E. Rheumatoid arthritis

Discussion

The correct answer is (B). There is a 2:1 male predominance in all age groups for distal triceps tendon rupture. Local corticosteroid injection and olecranon bursitis are elbow site–specific risk factors for tendon injury. Other systemic risk factors for this condition are numerous and include anabolic steroid use, fluoroquinolone use, metabolic bone disease, chronic kidney disease, insulin-dependent diabetes, Marfan syndrome, osteogenesis imperfecta, and rheumatoid arthritis. It has been postulated that chronic kidney disease and metabolic bone diseases that manifest with increased parathyroid hormone levels could possibly lead to increased osteoclastic activity and bone resorption, ultimately weakening the bone–tendon interface. Rheumatoid conditions and olecranon bursitis lead to synovitis with weakening of the tendon. Anabolic steroids, as well as oral or locally injected corticosteroids, are thought to impair tendon repair and collagen distribution and thus predispose to tendon injury.

At what anatomic location do distal triceps tendon ruptures occur in most cases?

A. Osseous insertion
B. Tendon midsubstance
C. Myotendinous junction
D. Muscle belly

Discussion

The correct answer is (A). Most cases of complete tendon rupture are found to be avulsions at the tendo-osseous junction. Ruptures at the myotendinous junction and within the muscle belly have been reported but are less common. The location of the tear can play a role in management. Tears within the muscle belly are likely to heal with scar tissue and with similar outcomes regardless of what type of treatment is rendered. Recent studies have looked at the anatomy of the triceps insertion in order to develop more anatomic repair techniques. These have found that the footprint is a wide area (466 mm^2), which encompasses the entire olecranon, as well as medial and lateral borders of the proximal ulna. Previous repair techniques including transosseous tunnel repair and suture anchor techniques have not sought to replicate this anatomic insertion. The clinical significance of anatomic footprint restoration is not yet known.

Objectives: Did you learn...?

- Diagnose and work up a triceps tendon injury?
- Identify risk factors associated with triceps tendon injuries?
- Determine indications for operative management?
- Understand anatomic considerations in triceps tendon rupture?

CASE 46

Dr. Min Lu

A 45-year-old, right-hand-dominant, male plumber presents with elbow pain of insidious onset. He denies any injury or trauma. He has lateral elbow pain with repetitive movements of the wrist at work. Examination of the shoulder and wrist is normal. He has tenderness to palpation about the elbow at the lateral epicondyle. His symptoms are reproduced with resisted wrist extension. Radiographs are normal.

What is the structure primarily affected by this condition?

A. Lateral ulnar collateral ligament
B. Extensor carpi radialis brevis
C. Extensor carpi radialis longus
D. Extensor digitorum communis
E. Extensor carpi ulnaris

Discussion

The correct answer is (B). This patient has lateral epicondylitis or tennis elbow, the most common cause for elbow pain presenting to an orthopaedic surgeon's office. The condition most frequently develops during the fourth or fifth decade of life. The prevalence in the general population is 1% to 3%, and it is more commonly encountered in strenuous labor occupations. It affects males and females equally and presents more frequently in the dominant upper extremity. It is a very common ailment in tennis players, with up to 50% developing this condition at some point during life. The most commonly cited location of pathology is the proximal extensor carpi radialis brevis origin, although Nirschl and colleagues have reported 35% to 50% involvement of the extensor digitorum communis as well. Radiographs are typically normal.

What is the most commonly encountered histology within the affected tendon upon surgical treatment?

A. Acute inflammation
B. Calcium hydroxyapatite deposition
C. Angiofibroblastic tendinosis
D. Chondroblastic proliferation
E. Osteoblastic proliferation

Discussion

The correct answer is (C). The characteristic presentation of lateral epicondylitis consists of repetitive microtearing of the tendon origin followed by repair attempts (Fig. 2–124). The typical histopathology of the involved

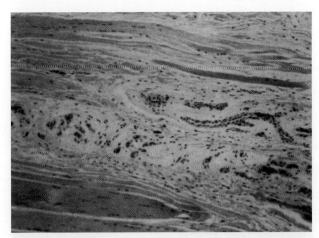

Figure 2–124 Figure showing focal hyaline degeneration and vascular proliferation in the proximal extensor carpi radialis brevis. (Regan W, Wold LE, Coonrad R, Morrey BF. Microscopic histopathology of chronic refractory lateral epicondylitis. *Am J Sports Med.* 1992;20(6):746–749.)

tendon shows angiofibroblastic tendinosis with neovascularization, disordered collagen deposition and mucoid degeneration. Notably, acute inflammation is usually not encountered. Calcium hydroxyapatite deposition is seen with calcific tendonitis, not lateral epicondylitis. Chondroblastic and osteoblastic proliferation are also not characteristic for this disorder.

The patient has had symptoms for four weeks with no significant treatment to date. What is the most appropriate initial treatment?

A. MRI of the elbow
B. Splint immobilization of the elbow
C. Corticosteroid injection
D. Anti-inflammatory medication and physical therapy exercises
E. Arthroscopic or open tendon debridement

Discussion

The correct answer is (D). The patient has had symptoms of relatively short duration and has had no significant treatment to date. Rest, anti-inflammatory pain medication, and physical therapy are simple measures used to alleviate pain and promote natural tendon healing. Recent attention has focused in particular on eccentric strengthening of forearm muscles in order to induce hypertrophy of the muscle–tendon unit and reduce tension on the tendon itself. While MRI, injections, or surgery might be indicated for recalcitrant disease, they are not used as a first line treatment. A variety of orthotic devices have been prescribed for lateral epicondylitis

including forearm bands and cock-up wrist splints, with the goal being to reduce tension on the common extensor origin. While conflicting data exists on these devices, rigid immobilization of the elbow is not generally advocated.

Which of the following is a favorable prognostic indicator for success of nonoperative treatment in lateral epicondylitis?

A. Dominant arm involved
B. Manual laborer
C. Poor coping mechanisms
D. High baseline pain level
E. Short duration of symptoms at presentation

Discussion

The correct answer is (E). Previous literature shows that most patients with lateral epicondylitis improve with conservative management. Approximately 80% of patients report symptomatic improvement at 1 year, and only 4% to 11% of patients seeking medical attention for this condition require eventual surgery. Negative prognostic indicators for successful conservative treatment include: involvement of dominant arm, manual laborer, high baseline pain level, extended duration of symptoms, and poor coping mechanisms.

The patient returns after 6 weeks of physical therapy exercises and anti-inflammatory medications with continued pain and weakness of grip strength. In counseling him on the risks and benefits of injections for lateral epicondylitis, which of the following statements is correct?

A. Botulinum toxin injection has been shown to reduce pain and improve strength at long-term follow-up
B. Glucocorticoid, botulinum toxin, and blood product injection have all consistently been shown to be favorable to placebo in terms of pain relief and improved function
C. Injections are relatively safe second-line treatments with unproven long-term benefit
D. Injections are a risk-free treatment option for patients wishing to avoid surgical intervention

Discussion

The correct answer is (C). The literature varies widely on the efficacy of various injection therapies. Glucocorticoids have been in use for the longest period of time historically. Studies have shown initial pain relief (<6 weeks), followed by diminished benefit at long-term follow-up. Botulinum toxin injections have been shown to reduce pain but also exhibit weakness of finger and wrist extension strength. Finally, the data on platelet-rich plasma and autologous whole blood is mixed in comparing these injections to saline or local anesthetic. Large-scale systematic reviews and meta-analyses generally agree that the safety profile of these injections is reasonable for a second-line treatment option prior to surgery. However, injections are not risk free and can lead to infection, skin depigmentation, fat atrophy, and extensor tendon rupture.

Objectives: Did you learn...?

- Understand the anatomy and pathology of lateral epicondylitis?
- Review conservative treatment strategies for lateral epicondylitis?
- Counsel patients on the efficacy of various injection therapies?

CASE 47

Dr. Min Lu

A 44-year-old, right-hand-dominant female is in the office with persistent lateral elbow pain of 2 years duration. She has pain at the lateral aspect of her elbow, as well as a deep aching pain that radiates down the dorsal aspect of her forearm. She has tried NSAIDs, physical therapy, bracing, and multiple injections to her lateral epicondyle without relief. On examination, she is neurovascularly intact distally with tenderness over the lateral epicondyle as well as in the proximal portion of her forearm. She has pain with resisted wrist extension, resisted long finger extension, and resisted supination. She has weakness of her finger extensors.

In addition to her extensor carpi radialis brevis, what other anatomic structure is most likely affected?

A. Extensor digitorum communis to the long finger
B. Extensor indicis proprius
C. Extensor carpi radialis longus
D. Radial nerve
E. Ulnar nerve

Discussion

The correct answer is (D). The patient has an atypical presentation of lateral epicondylitis, and it is important to rule out associated conditions such as radial tunnel syndrome. Radial tunnel syndrome is a compression neuropathy of the radial nerve, which unlike carpal tun-

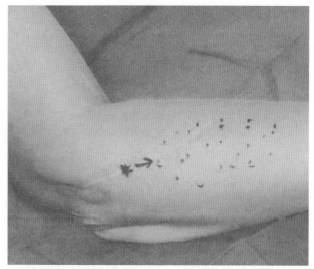

Figure 2–125 Markings depicting typical area of dysesthesia for posterior cutaneous nerve of the forearm neuroma. (Reproduced with permission from Dellon AL, Kim J, Ducic I. Painful neuroma of the posterior cutaneous nerve of the forearm after surgery for lateral humeral epicondylitis. *J Hand Surg Am.* 2004 May;29(3):387–90.)

nel and cubital tunnel syndromes, does not lend itself to quick and easy pattern recognition (Fig. 2–125). It can coexist with lateral epicondylitis in few cases, making diagnosis more difficult. Patients can have variable involvement of the dorsal sensory radial nerve and the posterior interosseous nerve. Symptomatology typically involves aching pain in the dorsal forearm, as well as tenderness to palpation distal to the typical site at the lateral epicondyle. Provocative tests such as pain with resisted long finger extension and resisted pronation/supination are described, although sensitivity and specificity of these tests is not well described. Nerve conduction studies are unreliable in diagnosis. Local anesthetic injection at the site of radial nerve compression has been described as a highly specific diagnostic modality.

The patient opts for open debridement of the extensor carpi radialis brevis origin, as well as radial tunnel decompression. Postoperatively, she develops pain and catching in her elbow when pushing up out of a chair.

What structure is at risk and may have been injured in this case?

A. Annular ligament
B. Lateral ulnar collateral ligament
C. Radial nerve
D. Extensor carpi radialis brevis
E. Extensor digitorum communis

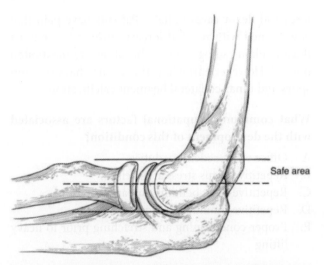

Figure 2-126 Safe zone for debridement to avoid the lateral ulnar collateral ligament. (Reproduced with permission from Calfee RP, Patel A, DaSilva MF, Akelman E. Management of lateral epicondylitis: current concepts. *J Am Acad Orthop Surg.* 2008 Jan;16(1):19–29.)

Discussion

The correct answer is (B). Surgical management of lateral epicondylitis is recommended when pain and dysfunction persist after 6 to 12 months of conservative treatment. The extensor carpi radialis brevis may be released open, percutaneously, or arthroscopically. Specific open debridement techniques vary but generally involve a 2 to 3 cm incision centered distal to the lateral epicondyle. Using sharp dissection, the degenerative tissue within the extensor carpi radialis brevis is debrided, the underlying bone is decorticated, and the tendon is reattached to the bone. With excessive debridement, the lateral ulnar collateral ligament may be compromised resulting in iatrogenic posterolateral rotatory instability. Keeping debridement anterior to the equator of the radial head prevents destabilization of the elbow (Fig. 2–126).

Neuroma formation is another potential complication of open epicondylar debridement. What nerve does this usually affect?

A. Radial
B. Posterior interosseous
C. Median
D. Lateral antebrachial cutaneous
E. Posterior antebrachial cutaneous

Discussion

The correct answer is (E). Painful neuroma is one possible cause of persistent pain after lateral epicondylar

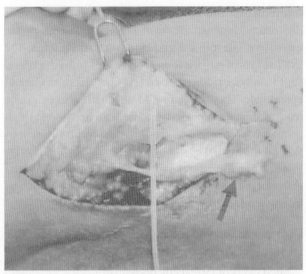

Figure 2-127 Intraoperative photo of a posterior cutaneous nerve of the forearm neuroma. (Reproduced with permission from Dellon AL, Kim J, Ducic I. Painful neuroma of the posterior cutaneous nerve of the forearm after surgery for lateral humeral epicondylitis. *J Hand Surg Am.* 2004 May;29(3):387–90.)

debridement. The posterior antebrachial cutaneous nerve (Fig. 2–127) is at risk with any approach to the lateral elbow. It branches from the radial nerve in the upper third of the humerus and travels in the subcutaneous tissue in the posterolateral aspect of the upper arm toward the elbow. At the elbow it is 1.5 cm anterior to the lateral epicondyle. Dellon et al. reported on a series of nine consecutive patients treated for this complication after lateral epicondylar debridement. Patients reported cutaneous dysesthesia distal and posterior to the incision. The diagnosis was made preoperatively by using a local anesthetic block to obtain symptomatic relief. Subsequently, the neuromas were excised and the proximal nerve stumps were buried within muscle.

Which other structure shares a proximal attachment with the extensor carpi radialis brevis?

A. Palmaris longus
B. Pronator teres
C. Brachioradialis
D. Extensor digiti minimi
E. Extensor pollicis longus

Discussion

The correct answer is (D). This is a pure anatomy question regarding the common extensor origin. The muscles originating from the lateral epicondyle include the common extensor tendon, which includes the extensor digitorum longus, extensor digitorum communis, extensor digiti minimi, and extensor carpi ulnaris. The extensor carpi radialis longus originates from the lateral supracondylar ridge and by a few fibers from the lateral epicondyle. The supinator and anconeus also originate from the lateral epicondyle. The palmaris longus and pronator teres originate from the common flexor tendon on the medial epicondyle. The brachioradialis originates from the lateral supracondylar ridge, while the extensor pollicis longus originates from the ulna and interosseous membrane.

Objectives: Did you learn...?

• Discuss treatment options for refractory or complicated cases of lateral epicondylitis?
• Recognize complications associated with surgical treatment for lateral epicondylitis?

CASE 48

Dr. Min Lu

A 55-year-old, right-hand-dominant male presents to the office complaining of medial-sided, right elbow pain for the past year. He denies any numbness or paresthesias. He complains of pain primarily at the medial epicondyle. He has seen a couple of other doctors for this problem and has had physical therapy, bracing, and corticosteroid injections which gave him short-lived relief. He is an avid golfer. On physical examination, he is neurovascularly intact distally with full elbow range of motion. He has tenderness at the medial epicondyle and pain with resisted wrist flexion. He has no instability with valgus stress.

What is the most likely diagnosis?

A. Ulnar nerve entrapment
B. Ulnar collateral ligament tear
C. Valgus extension overload
D. Medial epicondylitis
E. Elbow osteoarthritis

Discussion

The correct answer is (D). This patient has medial epicondylitis or golfer's elbow. This entity is 7 to 20 times less common than its lateral counterpart. It occurs during the fourth and fifth decades of life, with equal male to female prevalence rates. The condition is characterized by medial elbow pain of insidious onset. Tenderness is distal to the medial epicondyle in the pronator

teres and flexor carpi radialis. Patients have pain that is worsened with resisted forearm pronation or wrist flexion. Plain radiographs of the elbow are most often normal. However, throwing athletes may have traction spurs and ulnar collateral ligament calcification.

What common occupational factors are associated with the development of this condition?

A. Office work, sedentary duties
B. Repetitive varus stress at the elbow
C. Repetitive wrist bending, forearm rotation
D. Repetitive shoulder abduction
E. Proper conditioning and stretching prior to heavy lifting

Discussion

The correct answer is (C). Medial epicondylitis occurs in 0.4% to 0.6% of the working age population. Although termed golfer's elbow, it is commonly found in baseball pitchers as well as a variety of sports and occupations which create valgus stresses at the elbow. Golf, rowing, baseball (pitching), javelin and tennis (serving) are commonly cited recreational activities associated with this condition. It also tends to be found in manual laborers. In a large, longitudinal study, self-reported physical exposures involving repetitive and prolonged wrist bending and forearm rotation were associated with medial epicondylitis. Repetitive bending/straightening of the elbow may also be associated with disease occurrence. Proper conditioning and stretching are protective, not a risk factor for medial epicondylitis. Varus stress and shoulder abduction are not risk factors for this condition.

Which of the following tendons does not share a proximal origin with the flexor-pronator mass?

A. Flexor pollicis longus
B. Pronator teres
C. Flexor carpi radialis
D. Palmaris longus
E. Flexor carpi ulnaris

Discussion

The correct answer is (A). The flexor pollicis longus originates from the volar surface of the radius and adjacent interosseous membrane, not the common flexor-pronator mass. In addition to answer Choices B, C, D, and E, the flexor digitorum superficialis is the other muscle that shares the common flexor tendon origin. All of the common flexor muscles are innervated by the median nerve, except for flexor carpi ulnaris which is innervated by the ulnar nerve.

The patient presented above undergoes further conservative treatment but develops web space atrophy and diminished sensation of his ring and small finger. He elects to proceed with surgery.

In addition to common flexor tendon debridement, what other procedure must be considered for this patient?

A. Tendon transfer
B. Neuroma excision
C. Carpal tunnel release
D. Ulnar nerve transposition
E. Ulnar collateral ligament repair

Discussion

The correct answer is (D). This patient has medial epicondylitis with concomitant ulnar neuropathy. Ulnar nerve symptoms are associated with medial epicondylitis in 23% to 60% of cases according to reports. In these cases, ulnar nerve release or transposition must be considered in the same sitting. Results of medial epicondylitis surgery are generally more guarded when ulnar nerve symptoms are present.

What nerve is prone to injury with surgical treatment for medial epicondylitis?

A. Median
B. Anterior interosseous
C. Medial antebrachial cutaneous
D. Radial
E. Posterior antebrachial cutaneous

Discussion

The correct answer is (C). The medial antebrachial cutaneous nerve arises from the medial cord of the brachial plexus in most cases (nearly 80%). It travels parallel to the course of the median and ulnar nerves in the upper arm and divides into anterior and posterior branches above the elbow. Due to its variable location, the posterior branch is more commonly reported to be injured in the literature. Injury of the medial antebrachial cutaneous nerve is thought to be underreported as it does not affect the hand and patients may be minimally symptomatic.

Objectives: Did you learn...?

- Diagnose medial epicondylitis?
- Recognize occupational and activity related risk factors for medial epicondylitis?
- Understand nerve conditions related to medial epicondylitis?

BIBLIOGRAPHY

Case 1

Boyer M. *AAOS Comprehensive Orthopaedic Review 2*. Rosemont, IL: American Academy of Orthopaedic Surgeons, Copyright; 2014:921–923.

Boyer M. *AAOS Comprehensive Orthopaedic Review 2*. Rosemont, IL: American Academy of Orthopaedic Surgeons, Copyright; 2014:913.

Tennent TD, Beach WR, Meyers JF. A review of the special tests associated with shoulder examination. Part I: the rotator cuff tests. *Am J Sports Med.* 2003;31(1):154–160.

Case 2

Burkhart SS, Esch JC, Jolson RS. The rotator crescent and rotator cable: an anatomic description of the shoulder's "suspension bridge". *Arthroscopy.* 1993;9(6):611–616.

Burkhart SS, Danaceau SM, Pearce CE Jr. Arthroscopic rotator cuff repair: analysis of results by tear size and by repair technique-margin convergence versus direct tendon-to-bone repair. *Arthroscopy.* 2001;17(9):905–912.

Burkhart SS, Lo IK. Arthroscopic rotator cuff repair. *J Am Acad Orthop Surg.* 2006;14(6):333–346.

Case 3

Burk DL Jr, Karasick D, Kurtz AB, et al. Rotator cuff tears: prospective comparison of MR imaging with arthrography, sonography, and surgery. *AJR Am J Roentgenol.* 1989;153(1):87–92.

Yamakado K. Histopathology of residual tendon in high-grade articular-sided partial-thickness rotator cuff tears (PASTA lesions). *Arthroscopy.* 2012;28(4):474–480.

Yamaguchi K, Tetro AM, Blam O, Evanoff BA, Teefey SA, Middleton WD. Natural history of asymptomatic rotator cuff tears: a longitudinal analysis of asymptomatic tears detected sonographically. *J Shoulder Elbow Surg.* 2001;10(3):199–203.

Case 4

Hawkins RH, Dunlop R. Nonoperative treatment of rotator cuff tears. *Clin Orthop Relat Res.* 1995;(321):178–188.

Hawkins RJ, Misamore GW, Hobeika PE. Surgery for full-thickness rotator-cuff tears. *J Bone Joint Surg Am.* 1985;67(9):1349–1355.

Case 5

Cofield RH, Parvizi J, Hoffmeyer PJ, Lanzer WL, Ilstrup DM, Rowland CM. Surgical repair of chronic rotator cuff tears. *J Bone Joint Surg Am.* 2001;83-A(1):71–77.

Gerber C, Hersche O, Farron A. Isolated Rupture of the Subscapularis Tendon. Results of Operative Repair. *J Bone Joint Surg Am.* 1996;78(7):1015–1023.

Lo IK, Burkhart SS. The comma sign: an arthroscopic guide to the torn subscapularis tendon. *Arthroscopy.* 2003;19(3):334–337.

Lyons RP, Green A. Subscapularis tendon tears. *Am Acad Orthop Surg.* 2005;13(5):353–363.

Pappou IP, Schmidt CC, Jarrett CD, Steen BM, Frankle MA. AAOS appropriate use criteria: optimizing the management of full-thickness rotator cuff tears. *J Am Acad Orthop Surg.* 2013;21(12):772–775.

Wolff AB, Sethi P, Sutton KM, Covey AS, Magit DP, Medvecky M. Partial-thickness rotator cuff tears. *J Am Acad Orthop Surg.* 2006;14(13):715–725.

Case 6

Burkhart SS, Lo IK. Arthroscopic rotator cuff repair. *J Am Acad Orthop Surg.* 2006;14(6):333–346.

Gerber C, Pennington SD, Nyffeler RW. Reverse total shoulder arthroplasty. *J Am Acad Orthop Surg.* 2009;17(5): 284–295.

Goutallier D, Postel JM, Bernageau J, Lavau L, Voisin MC. Fatty muscle degeneration in cuff ruptures. Pre- and postoperative evaluation by CT scan. *Clin Orthop Relat Res.* 1994; (304):78–83.

Ecklund KJ, Lee TQ, Tibone J, Gupta R. Rotator cuff tear arthropathy. *J Am Acad Orthop Surg.* 2007;15(6):340–349.

Kuzel BR, Grindel S, Papandrea R, Ziegler D. Fatty infiltration and rotator cuff atrophy. *J Am Acad Orthop Surg.* 2013; 21(10):613–623.

Omid R, Lee B. Tendon transfers for irreparable rotator cuff tears. *J Am Acad Orthop Surg.* 2013;21(8):492–501.

Case 7

Edwards SL, Lee JA, Bell JE, et al. Nonoperative treatment of superior labrum anterior posterior tears improvements in pain, function, and quality of life. *Am J Sports Med.* 2010;38(7):1456–1461.

Nam EK, Snyder SJ. Clinical sports medicine update. The diagnosis and treatment of superior labrum, anterior and posterior (SLAP) lesions. *Am J Sports Med.* 2003;31(5): 798–810.

Snyder SJ, Karzel RP, Del Pizzo W, Ferkel RD, Friedman MJ. SLAP lesions of the shoulder. *Arthroscopy.* 1990;6(4):274–279.

Tennent TD, Beach WR, Meyers JF. A review of the special tests associated with shoulder examination. Part II: laxity, instability, and superior labral anterior and posterior (SLAP) lesions. *Am J Sports Med.* 2003;31(2):301–307.

Case 8

Boileau P, Parratte S, Chuinard C, Roussanne Y, Shia D, Bicknell R. Arthroscopic treatment of isolated type ii slap lesions biceps tenodesis as an alternative to reinsertion. *Am J Sports Med.* 2009;37(5):929–936.

Flannigan B, Kursunoglu-Brahme S, Snyder S, Karzel R, Del Pizzo W, Resnick D. MR arthrography of the shoulder: comparison with conventional MR imaging. *AJR Am J Roentgenol.* 1990;155(4):829–932.

Mileski RA, Snyder SJ. Superior labral lesions in the shoulder: pathoanatomy and surgical management. *J Am Acad Orthop Surg.* 1998;6(2):121–131.

Williams MM, Snyder SJ, Buford D Jr. The Buford complex—the "cord-like" middle glenohumeral ligament and absent anterosuperior labrum complex: a normal anatomic capsulolabral variant. *Arthroscopy.* 1994;10(3):241–247.

Case 9

Hottya GA, Tirman PF, Bost FW, Montgomery WH, Wolf EM, Genant HK. Tear of the posterior shoulder stabilizers after posterior dislocation: MR imaging and MR arthrographic findings with arthroscopic correlation. *AJR Am J Roentgenol.* 1998;171(3):763–768.

Gerber C, Ganz R. Clinical assessment of instability of the shoulder. With special reference to anterior and posterior drawer tests. *J Bone Joint Surg Br.* 1984;66(4):551–556.

Millett PJ, Clavert P, Hatch GF 3rd, Warner JJ. Recurrent posterior shoulder instability. *J Am Acad Orthop Surg.* 2006; 14(8):464–476.

Rouleau DM, Hebert-Davies J, Robinson CM. Acute traumatic posterior shoulder dislocation. *J Am Acad Orthop Surg.* 2014; 22(3):145–152.

Case 10

Ahrens PM, Boileau P. The long head of biceps and associated tendinopathy. *J Bone Joint Surg Br.* 2007;89(8): 1001–1009.

Nho SJ, Strauss EJ, Lenart BA, et al. Long head of the biceps tendinopathy: diagnosis and management. *J Am Acad Orthop Surg.* 2010;18(11):645–656.

Post M, Benca P. Primary tendinitis of the long head of the biceps. *Clin Orthop Relat Res.* 1989;(246):117–125.

Case 11

Bui-Mansfield LT, Taylor DC, Uhorchak JM, Tenuta JJ. Humeral avulsions of the glenohumeral ligament: imaging features and a review of the literature. *AJR Am J Roentgenol.* 2002;179(3):649–655.

Clough TM, Bale RS. Bilateral posterior shoulder dislocation: the importance of the axillary radiographic view. *Eur J Emerg Med.* 2001;8(2):161–163.

Robinson CM, Howes J, Murdoch H, Will E, Graham C. Functional outcome and risk of recurrent instability after primary traumatic anterior shoulder dislocation in young patients. *J Bone Joint Surg Am.* 2006;88(11):2326–2326.

Case 12

Haltom JD, Gary WM. *Bankart repair and capsule shift.Management of the Unstable Shoulder: Arthroscopic and Open Repair.* Thorofare, NJ: SLACK Inc; 2011.

Koo SS, Burkhart SS, Ochoa E. Arthroscopic double-pulley remplissage technique for engaging Hill-Sachs lesions in anterior shoulder instability repairs. *Arthroscopy.* 2009; 25(11):1343–1348.

Lafosse L, Lejeune E, Bouchard A, Kakuda C, Gobezie R, Kochhar T. The arthroscopic Latarjet procedure for the treatment of anterior shoulder instability. *Arthroscopy*. 2007; 23(11):1242.e1–e5.

Case 13

Boardman ND, Debski RE, Warner JJ, et al. Tensile properties of the superior glenohumeral and coracohumeral ligaments. *J Shoulder Elbow Surg*. 1996;5(4):249–254.

Groh GI, Wirth MA, Rockwood CA Jr. Results of treatment of luxatio erecta (inferior shoulder dislocation). *J Shoulder Elbow Surg*. 2010;19(3):423–426.

Halder AM, Halder CG, Zhao KD, O'Driscoll SW, Morrey BF, An KN. Dynamic inferior stabilizers of the shoulder joint. *Clin Biomech (Bristol, Avon)*. 2001;16(2):138–143.

Kim SH, Park JC, Park JS, Oh I. Painful jerk test A predictor of success in nonoperative treatment of posteroinferior instability of the shoulder. *Am J Sports Med*. 2004;32(8):1849–1855.

Lippitt S, Matsen F. Mechanisms of glenohumeral joint stability. *Clin Orthop Relat Res*. 1993;(291):20–28.

Case 14

Ball CM, Steger T, Galatz LM, Yamaguchi K. The posterior branch of the axillary nerve: an anatomic study. *J Bone Joint Surg Am*. 2003;85-A(8):1497–1501.

Mallon WJ, Speer KP. Multidirectional instability: current concepts. *J Shoulder Elbow Surg*. 1995;4(1 Pt 1):54–64.

Rowe CR, Pierce DS, Clark JG. Voluntary dislocation of the shoulder. *J Bone Joint Surg Am*. 1973;55(3):445–460.

Wolf EM, Eakin CL. Arthroscopic capsular plication for posterior shoulder instability. *Arthroscopy*. 1998;14(2):153–163.

Case 15

Ito H, Takayama A, Shirai Y. Radiographic evaluation of the Hill-Sachs lesion in patients with recurrent anterior shoulder instability. *J Shoulder Elbow Surg*. 2000;9(6):495–497.

Lafosse L, Boyle S, Gutierrez-Aramberri M, Shah A, Meller R. Arthroscopic latarjet procedure. *Orthop Clin North Am*. 2010;41(3):393–405.

Case 16

Rowe CR, Zarins B. Chronic unreduced dislocations of the shoulder. *J Bone Joint Surg Am*. 1982;64(4):494–505.

Case 17

Izquierdo R, Voloshin I, Edwards S, et al. Treatment of glenohumeral osteoarthritis. *J Am Acad Orthop Surg*. 2010; 18(6):375–382.

Miller SL, Hazrati Y, Klepps S, Chiang A, Flatow EL. Loss of subscapularis function after total shoulder replacement: a seldom recognized problem. *J Shoulder Elbow Surg*. 2003;12(1):29–34.

Case 18

Boyd AD Jr, Thomas WH, Scott RD, Sledge CB, Thornhill TS. Total shoulder arthroplasty versus hemiarthroplasty: indications for glenoid resurfacing. *J Arthroplasty*. 1990; 5(4):329–336.

Majithia V1, Geraci SA. Rheumatoid arthritis: diagnosis and management. *Am J Med*. 2007;120(11):936–939.

Case 19

Kay SP, Amstutz HC. Shoulder hemiarthroplasty at UCLA. *Clin Orthop Relat Res*. 1988;(228):42–48.

Mont MA, Maar DC, Urquhart MW, Lennox D, Hungerford DS. Avascular necrosis of the humeral head treated by core decompression. A retrospective review. *J Bone Joint Surg Br*. 1993;75(5):785–788.

Case 20

Bohsali KI, Wirth MA, Rockwood CA Jr. Complications of total shoulder arthroplasty. *J Bone Joint Surg Am*. 2006; 88(10):2279–2292.

Cofield RH, Edgerton BC. Total shoulder arthroplasty: complications and revision surgery. *Instr Course Lect*. 1990; 39:449–462.

Petersen SA, Hawkins RJ. Revision of failed total shoulder arthroplasty. *Orthop Clin North Am*. 1998;29(3):519–533.

Sperling JW, Kozak TK, Hanssen AD, Cofield RH. Infection after shoulder arthroplasty. *Clin Orthop Relat Res*. 2001; (382):206–216.

Case 21

Kappe T, Cakir B, Reichel H, Elsharkawi M. Reliability of radiologic classification for cuff tear arthropathy. *J Shoulder Elbow Surg*. 2011;20:543–547.

Tabaraee E, Feeley BT. Rotator cuff arthropathy. *Basic Principles and Operative Management of the Rotator Cuff*; 2012: 331.

Worland RL. Rotator cuff arthropathy. *J Bone Joint Surg Am*. 2000;82-A(11):1670–1671.

Case 22

Iceton J, Harris WR. Treatment of winged scapula by pectoralis major transfer. *J Bone Joint Surg Br*. 1987;69(1):108–110.

Post M. Pectoralis major transfer for winging of the scapula. *J Shoulder Elbow Surg*. 1995;4(1 Pt 1):1–9.

Meininger A, Figurerres B, Goldberg B. Scapular winging: an update. *JAAOS*. 2011;19(8):453–462.

Case 23

Feinberg JH, Radecki J. Parsonage–Turner syndrome. *HSS J*. 2010;6(2):199–205.

Perlmutter GS. Axillary nerve injury. *Clin Orthop Relat Res*. 1999;(368):28–36.

Safran MR. Nerve injury about the shoulder in athletes, part 1 suprascapular nerve and axillary nerve. *Am J Sports Med*. 2004;32(3):803–819.

Case 24

Moore TP, Hunter RE. Suprascapular nerve entrapment. *Oper Techn Sports Med*. 1996;4(1):8–14.

Ringel SP, Treihaft M, Carry M, Fisher R, Jacobs P. Suprascapular neuropathy in pitchers. *Am J Sports Med*. 1990;18(1):80–86.

Case 25

Bishop JY, Kaeding C. Treatment of the acute traumatic acromioclavicular separation. *Sports Med Arthrosc.* 2006; 14(4):237–245.

Mouhsine E, Garofalo R, Crevoisier X, Farron A. Grade I and II acromioclavicular dislocations: results of conservative treatment. *J Shoulder Elbow Surg.* 2003;12(6):599–602.

Tossy JD, Mead NC, Sigmond HM. Acromioclavicular separations: useful and practical classification for treatment. *Clin Orthop Relat Res.* 1963;28:111–119.

Case 26

Barth E, Hagen R. Surgical treatment of dislocations of the sternoclavicular joint. *Acta Orthop Scand.* 1983;54(5):746–747.

Cope R, Riddervold HO, Shore JL, Sistrom CL. Dislocations of the sternoclavicular joint: anatomic basis, etiologies, and radiologic diagnosis. *J Orthop Trauma.* 1991;5(3):379–384.

Ferrandez L, Yubero J, Usabiaga J, No L, Martin F. Sternoclavicular dislocation. Treatment and complications. *Ital J Orthop Traumatol.* 1988;14(3):349–355.

Jougon JB, Lepront DJ, Dromer CE. Posterior dislocation of the sternoclavicular joint leading to mediastinal compression. *Ann Thorac Surg.* 1996;61(2):711–713.

Case 27

Bontempo NA, Mazzocca AD. Biomechanics and treatment of acromioclavicular and sternoclavicular joint injuries. *Br J Sports Med.* 2010;44(5):361–369.

Brooks CN, Brigham CR. *Acromioclavicular Joint Arthritis.* American Medical Association; The Guides News Letter: September/October 2005.

Salter EG Jr, Nasca RJ, Shelley BS. Anatomical observations on the acromioclavicular joint and supporting ligaments. *Am J Sports Med.* 1987;15(3):199–206.

Sellards R, Nicholson GP. Arthroscopic distal clavicle resection. *Oper Techn Sports Med.* 2004;12(1):18–26.

Case 28

Bisson LJ, Dauphin N, Marzo JM. A safe zone for resection of the medial end of the clavicle. *J Shoulder Elbow Surg.* 2003; 12(6):592–594.

Ernberg LA, Potter HG. Radiographic evaluation of the acromioclavicular and sternoclavicular joints. *Clin Sports Med.* 2003;22(2):255–275.

Kier R, Wain SL, Apple J, Martinez S. Osteoarthritis of the Sternoclavicular Joint Radiographic Features and Pathologic Correlation. *Invest Radiol.* 1986;21(3):227–233.

Case 29

Griggs SM, Ahn A, Green A. Idiopathic adhesive capsulitis. *J Bone Joint Surg.* 2000;82(10):1398–1398.

Melzer C, Wallny T, Wirth CJ, Hoffmann S. Frozen shoulder—treatment and results. *Arch Orthop Trauma Surg.* 1995; 114(2):87–91.

Neviaser RJ, Neviaser TJ. The Frozen Shoulder Diagnosis and Management. *Clin Orthop Relat Res.* 1987;(223):59–64.

Case 30

Ark JW, Flock TJ, Flatow EL, Bigliani LU. Arthroscopic treatment of calcific tendinitis of the shoulder. *Arthroscopy.* 1992;8(2):183–188.

Seil R, Litzenburger H, Kohn D, Rupp S. Arthroscopic treatment of chronically painful calcifying tendinitis of the supraspinatus tendon. *Arthroscopy.* 2006;22(5):521–527.

Uhthoff HK, Sarkar K, Maynard JA. Calcifying tendinitis: a new concept of its pathogenesis. *Clin Orthop Relat Res.* 1976;(118):164–168.

Case 31

Bak K, Cameron EA, Henderson IJ. Rupture of the pectoralis major: a meta-analysis of 112 cases. *Knee Surg Sports Traumatol Arthrosc.* 2000;8(2):113–119.

Potter BK, Lehman RA Jr, Doukas WC. Pectoralis major ruptures. *Am J Orthop (Belle Mead NJ).* 2006;35(4):189–195.

Case 32

Kuhn JE, Plancher KD, Hawkins RJ. Symptomatic scapulothoracic crepitus and bursitis. *J Am Acad Orthop Surg.* 1998; 6(5):267–273.

Lehtinen JT, Tetreault P, Warner JJ. Arthroscopic management of painful and stiff scapulothoracic articulation. *Arthroscopy.* 2003;19(4):E28.

Case 33

Pizzetti M, Fredella D, Erriquez A. Post-traumatic elbow stiffness. *The Elbow.* Vienna: Springer; 1991:195–199.

Tan V, Daluiski A, Simic P, Hotchkiss RN. Outcome of open release for post-traumatic elbow stiffness. *J Trauma.* 2006; 61(3):673–678.

Case 34

Dürig M, Müller W, Rüedi TP, Gauer EF. The operative treatment of elbow dislocation in the adult. *J Bone Joint Surg Am.* 1979;61(2):239–244.

King GJ, Morrey BF, An KN. Stabilizers of the elbow. *J Shoulder Elbow Surg.* 1993;2(3):165–174.

Case 35

Duckworth AD, Ring D, Kulijdian A, McKee MD. Unstable elbow dislocations. *J Shoulder Elbow Surg.* 2008;17(2):281–286.

Field LD, Callaway GH, O'Brien SJ, Altchek DW. Arthroscopic assessment of the medial collateral ligament complex of the elbow. *Am J Sports Med.* 1995;23(4):396–400.

Knight DJ, Rymaszewski LA, Amis AA, Miller JH. Primary replacement of the fractured radial head with a metal prosthesis. *J Bone Joint Surg Br.* 1993;75(4):572–576.

Case 36

Lee BP, Teo LH. Surgical reconstruction for posterolateral rotatory instability of the elbow. *J Shoulder Elbow Surg.* 2003;12(5):476–479.

O'Driscoll SW, Bell DF, Morrey BF. Posterolateral rotatory instability of the elbow. *J Bone Joint Surg Am.* 1991;73(3):440–446.

Case 37

Lee DH. Posttraumatic elbow arthritis and arthroplasty. *Orthop Clin North Am*. 1999;30(1):141–162.

Ogilvie-Harris DJ, Gordon R, MacKay M. Arthroscopic treatment for posterior impingement in degenerative arthritis of the elbow. *Arthroscopy*. 1995;11(4):437–443.

Sanchez-Sotelo J, Morrey BF. Total elbow arthroplasty. *J Am Acad Orthop Surg*. 2011;19(2):121–125.

Soojian MG, Kwon YW. Elbow arthritis. *Bull NYU Hosp Jt Dis*. 2007;65(1):61–71.

Case 38

Loeffler BJ, Patrick MC. Total elbow arthroplasty for rheumatoid arthritis. *Oper Tech Shoulder Elbow Surg*. 2010:379.

Case 39

Bruno RJ, Lee ML, Strauch RJ, Rosenwasser MP. Posttraumatic elbow stiffness: evaluation and management. *J Am Acad Orthop Surg*. 2002;10(2):106–116.

Froimson AI. Fascial interposition arthroplasty of the elbow. In: Morrey BF. *Master Techniques in Orthopaedic Surgery – The Elbow*. Lippincott Williams and Wilkins; 1994:329–342.

Case 40

Ahmad CS, ElAttrache NS. Valgus extension overload syndrome and stress injury of the olecranon. *Clin Sports Med*. 2004;23(4):665–676.

Dugas JR. Valgus extension overload: diagnosis and treatment. *Clin Sports Med*. 2010;29(4):645–654.

Wilson FD, Andrews JR, Blackburn TA, McCluskey G. Valgus extension overload in the pitching elbow. *Am J Sports Med*. 1983;11(2):83–88.

Case 41

Bradley JP, Petrie RS. Osteochondritis dissecans of the humeral capitellum: diagnosis and treatment. *Clin Sports Med*. 2001; 20(3):565–590.

Ruch DS, Poehling GG. Arthroscopic treatment of Panner's disease. *Clin Sports Med*. 1991;10(3):629–636.

Takahara M, Mura N, Sasaki J, Harada M, Ogino T. Classification, treatment, and outcome of osteochondritis dissecans of the humeral capitellum. *J Bone Joint Surg Am*. 2007;89(6):1205–1214.

Case 42

Makhni EC, Lee RW, Morrow ZS, Gualtieri AP, Gorroochurn P, Ahmad CS. Performance, Return to Competition, and Reinjury After Tommy John Surgery in Major League Baseball Pitchers A Review of 147 Cases. *Am J Sports Med*. 2014;42(6):1323–1332.

Rohrbough JT, Altchek DW, Hyman J, Williams RJ 3rd, Botts JD. Medial collateral ligament reconstruction of the elbow using the docking technique. *Am J Sports Med*. 2002;30(4): 541–548.

Case 43

Benjamin HJ, Briner WW Jr. Little league elbow. *Clin J Sport Med*. 2005;15(1):37–40.

Hang DW, Chao CM, Hang YS. A clinical and roentgenographic study of Little League elbow. *Am J Sports Med*. 2004;32(1):79–84.

Klingele KE, Kocher MS. Little league elbow. *Sports Med*. 2002;32(15):1005–1015.

Case 44

Savvidou OD, Papagelopoulos PJ, Mavrogenis AF, et al. Distal biceps tendon rupture. *Eur J Orthop Surg Traumatol*. 2004;14(3):155–160.

Savvidou OD, Papagelopoulos PJ, Mavrogenis AF, et al. Distal biceps tendon rupture. *Eur J Orthop Surg Traumatol*. 2006; 16(4):400.

Seiler JG 3rd, Parker LM, Chamberland PD, Sherbourne GM, Carpenter WA. The distal biceps tendon: two potential mechanisms involved in its rupture: arterial supply and mechanical impingement. *J Shoulder Elbow Surg*. 1995; 4(3):149–156.

Case 45

Mair SD, Isbell WM, Gill TJ, Schlegel TF, Hawkins RJ. Triceps tendon ruptures in professional football players. *Am J Sports Med*. 2004;32(2):431–434.

Sollender JL, Rayan GM, Barden GA. Triceps tendon rupture in weight lifters. *J Shoulder Elbow Surg*. 1998;7(2):151–153.

Case 46

Nirschl RP, Pettrone FA. Tennis elbow. The surgical treatment of lateral epicondylitis. *J Bone Joint Surg Am*. 1979; 61(6A):832–839.

Regan W, Wold LE, Coonrad R, Morrey BF. Microscopic histopathology of chronic refractory lateral epicondylitis. *Am J Sports Med*. 1992;20(6):746–749.

Struijs PA, Kerkhoffs GM, Assendelft WJ, Van Dijk CN. Conservative treatment of lateral epicondylitis brace versus physical therapy or a combination of both a randomized clinical trial. *Am J Sports Med*. 2004;32(2):462–469.

Case 47

Assendelft WJ, Hay EM, Adshead R, Bouter LM. Corticosteroid injections for lateral epicondylitis: a systematic overview. *Br J Gen Pract*. 1996;46(405):209–216.

Roles NC, Maudsley RH. Radial tunnel syndrome resistant tennis elbow as a nerve entrapment. *J Bone Joint Surg Br*. 1972;54(3):499–508.

Case 48

Descatha A, Leclerc A, Chastang JF, Roquelaure Y; Study Group on Repetitive Work. Medial epicondylitis in occupational settings: prevalence, incidence and associated risk factors. *J Occup Environ Med*. 2003;45(9):993–1001.

Jobe FW, Ciccotti MG. Lateral and medial epicondylitis of the elbow. *J Am Acad Orthop Surg*. 1994;2(1):1–8.

Masear VR, Meyer RD, Pichora DR. Surgical anatomy of the medial antebrachial cutaneous nerve. *J Hand Surg Am*. 1989;14(2 Pt 1):267–271.

Vangsness CT Jr, Jobe FW. Surgical treatment of medial epicondylitis. Results in 35 elbows. *J Bone Joint Surg Br*. 1991; 73(3):409–411.

3

Wrist

Sunil Thirkannad

CASE 1

A 14-year-old patient presents with pain in the wrist after a fall. Examination reveals tenderness over the anatomical snuff box. X-ray picture is shown below (Fig. 3–1). What is the next course of treatment?

A. Analgesia only
B. No further treatment
C. Ace wrap
D. Thumb spica splint
E. Injection to tender area

Discussion

The correct answer is (D). Injuries to the wrist with tenderness over the anatomical snuff box should raise the suspicion of a scaphoid fracture. Often, a scaphoid fracture may not be visible on initial x-ray pictures. It is prudent in such cases to suspect an "occult scaphoid fracture" and treat the patient in a splint. A repeat x-ray taken 2 to 4 weeks later can often reveal a fracture.

The same patient is seen in clinic 4 weeks later and still has persistent pain. An x-ray ordered at this time reveals the findings shown (Fig. 3–2). What is the more prudent thing to do next?

A. Continue splinting
B. Discontinue splinting and start mobilization
C. Surgery
D. Start the patient on calcium supplements
E. Steroid injection

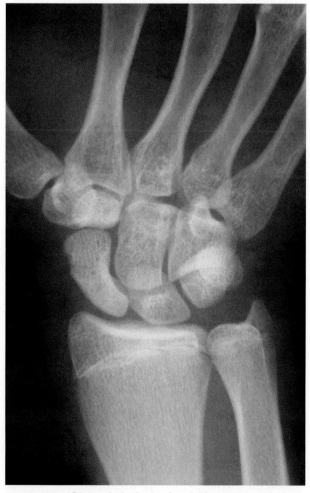

Figure 3–1 (©) Sunil Thirkannad and Christine M. Kleinert.

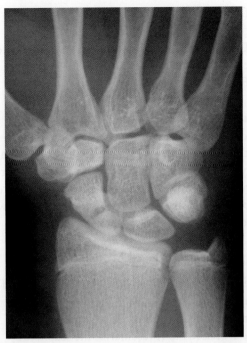

Figure 3–2 (©) Sunil Thirkannad and Christine M. Kleinert.

Discussion

The correct answer is (A). The x-ray reveals a fracture of the scaphoid. Healing rates are around 75% with nonsurgical treatment in adults compared to around 95% after surgery. However, since the patient is a 14-year-old child and has already been in a splint for 4 weeks, a prudent course would be to continue splinting for a further 2 to 4 weeks.

The patient returns 4 weeks later. What is the best method to determine whether or not the fracture has healed?

A. X-rays
B. CT scan
C. MRI
D. Ultrasound
E. Clinical examination

Discussion

The correct answer is (B). As was evident from the very first x-ray picture taken in this patient, scaphoid fractures can be difficult to detect on x-rays. Consequently, their role in determining healing of a fracture is equally unreliable. While the continued presence of a gap at the fracture site indicates a failure of healing, the corollary cannot be true. In other words, the apparent absence of a gap on x-rays does not conclusively prove healing. Often, a slight change in positioning of the wrist can effectively mask a gap and thus falsely suggest healing. CT scans of the scaphoid can reveal the actual presence

of bridging callus across the fracture site and are hence a more reliable method of determining healing.

CT scans show a persistent fracture line with no signs of healing or bridging callus across the fracture. How would you treat this problem next?

A. Scaphoid excision only
B. Scaphoid excision with four-corner fusion
C. ORIF with bone graft
D. Radioscapholunate fusion
E. Radial styloidectomy

Discussion

The correct answer is (C). ORIF of the fracture with fresh cancellous bone graft would be the best option at this stage. Headless compression screws are the preferred method of fixation of scaphoid fractures.

Objectives: Did you learn…?

- Treat occult scaphoid fractures?
- Treat scaphoid fractures in the pediatric population?
- Use CT scan to assess fracture healing?
- Treat scaphoid nonunion?

CASE 2

A patient is brought to you with history of fall on an outstretched hand several weeks ago. He was treated initially at an outlying facility in a thumb spica splint and was subsequently referred to you. An x-ray reveals the following (Fig. 3–3). What would the next prudent course be?

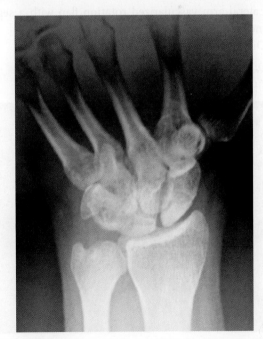

Figure 3–3 (©) Sunil Thirkannad and Christine M. Kleinert.

A. Analgesia only
B. Aspirin
C. CT scan
D. Change to an above elbow splint
E. MRI with contrast

Discussion

The correct answer is (E). The x-ray reveals a fracture of the scaphoid with sclerosis of the proximal fragment. This should raise suspicion of avascular necrosis. MRI with contrast is the best method to determine the vascular status of the scaphoid.

A contrast MRI is obtained and is as shown below. What is the next course of action?

A. Continue splinting
B. Excision of the proximal pole
C. Open reduction and internal fixation with a vascularized bone graft
D. Percutaneous pinning of the fracture with k wires
E. Radioscapholunate fusion

Discussion

The correct answer is (C). The MRI (Fig. 3–4) reveals avascularity of the proximal pole. This is best treated by open reduction and internal fixation with a vascularized bone graft.

Which of the following procedures would you choose to revascularize the scaphoid?

A. Lateral arm vascularized rotation flap with a segment of the humerus
B. Distally based radial artery fascial flap

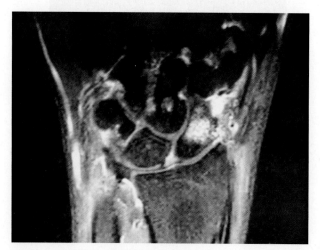

Figure 3–4 (©) Sunil Thirkannad and Christine M. Kleinert.

C. Distal radius bone graft based on the 1–2 intercompartmental supraretinacular artery
D. Distal radius bone graft based on the 5th extensor compartmental artery
E. Free phalangeal transfer

Discussion

The correct answer is (C). A distal radius bone graft based on the 1–2 intercompartmental supraretinacular artery (1–2 ICSRA) would be the best option to revascularize a scaphoid. A graft based on the 5th extensor compartmental artery would be too short and would not reach the scaphoid.

Objectives: Did you learn...?

• Identify radiographic findings of AVN of the scaphoid?
• Surgically treat scaphoid AVN?
• Use 1-2ICSRA to revascularize the scaphoid?

CASE 3

A patient is brought into the emergency room following a motor vehicle accident. He complains of severe pain in his wrist. Physical examination reveals a tender and swollen wrist. X-rays (Figs. 3–5A–B) are as follows. What is your diagnosis?

A. Normal wrist x-rays
B. Lunotriquetral coalition
C. Kienbock's disease
D. Perilunate injury
E. Tietze syndrome

Discussion

The correct answer is (D). This x-ray reveals a perilunate injury of the wrist. It is important to be aware of the various radiological parameters that reveal disruption of carpal alignment. Literature suggests that a perilunate injury is missed as much as 25% to 40% of the times.

Which radiological signs of perilunate injury can be seen on the above Figs. 3–5A–B.

A. Triangle sign
B. Break in Gilula's lines
C. Spilt teacup sign
D. Choices B and C
E. All of the above

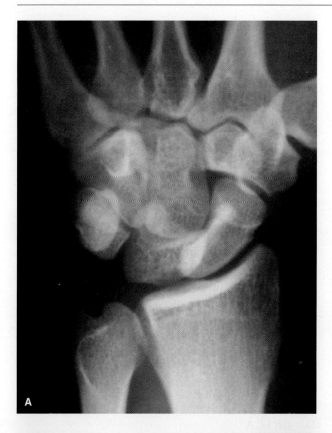

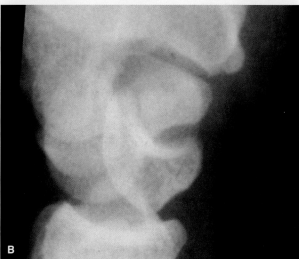

Figure 3–5 **A–B.** (©) Sunil Thirkannad and Christine M. Kleinert.

Discussion

The correct answer is (E). All three radiological signs are seen on this x-ray. Triangle sign refers to the shape of the lunate seen on the PA view. A normal, well located lunate looks like a tilted trapezium. A triangular-shaped lunate suggests that it is in a hyperflexed position. In the lateral view, a subluxated and volar-tilted lunate has the appearance of a "spilt

teacup." In the above x-ray, Gilula's first and second lines are broken.

What is the definitive treatment for the problem?

A. Proximal row carpectomy
B. Scaphoid excision and four-corner fusion
C. Closed reduction and splinting
D. Open reduction and pinning with repair of ligaments
E. Excision of lunate and replacement with a silastic prosthesis

Discussion

The correct answer is (D). Open reduction of the carpus followed by pinning is the best option. At the same sitting, all ligaments can be repaired. Closed reduction and splinting may be appropriate as an immediate measure but is not definitive. Proximal row carpectomy and partial wrist fusions are usually salvage procedures and are not indicated in the acute setting unless there are multiple comminuted fractures of the carpal bones with significant cartilage or bone loss that renders them irreparable. That does not appear to be the case here as can be determined by x-rays.

Which nerve is at greatest risk in a perilunate injury?

A. Median nerve in the carpal tunnel
B. Ulnar nerve in Guyon's canal
C. Deep motor branch of the ulnar nerve
D. Palmar cutaneous branch of the medial nerve
E. Superficial branch of the radial nerve

Discussion

The correct answer is (A). The median nerve in the carpal tunnel is at the greatest risk of injury following a perilunate injury. If the patient presents with significant numbness and tingling in the distribution of the median nerve, a carpal tunnel release needs to be performed during the initial surgery.

Objectives: Did you learn...?

• Identify radiographic findings of perilunate injury?
• Surgically manage perilunate injury?
• Identify neurovascular complications of perilunate injury?

CASE 4

A patient presents with deep-seated pain in the mid-dorsal aspect of the wrist. There is no history of

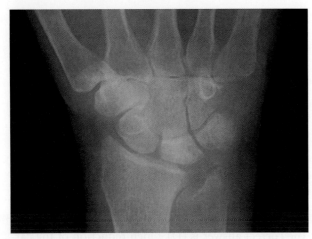

Figure 3–6 (©) Sunil Thirkannad and Christine M. Kleinert.

trauma. Examination is inconclusive except for some tenderness over the dorsal aspect of the scapholunate joint. X-ray (Fig. 3–6) is as follows. What is your diagnosis?

A. Scapholunate diastasis
B. Perilunate injury
C. Osteoid osteoma
D. Normal x-ray
E. Kienbock's disease

Discussion

The correct answer is (E). The x-ray shows a sclerotic lunate which should raise the suspicion of Kienbock's disease.

What radiological finding is commonly known to be associated with Kienbock's?

A. Type 2 lunate
B. Brachymetacarpia
C. Subperiosteal erosions of the distal phalanges
D. Ulna-negative variance
E. Bipartite ulnar styloid

Discussion

The correct answer is (D). An ulna-negative variance, wherein the distal end of the ulna is shorter than the distal end of the sigmoid notch of the radius, is known to be associated with Kienbock's disease. While the exact cause–effect relation between the two has not been established with certainty, it is hypothesized that a shorter ulna leads to increased loading at the radiolunate joint, predisposing the lunate to avascular necrosis.

What investigation would you perform to confirm the diagnosis?

A. MRI with gadolinium
B. Arthroscopic evaluation of the short radiolunate ligament
C. Arthrogram with intra-articular injection of contrast
D. Gamma imaging after injection with radioisotope tagged erythrocytes
E. CT scan with soft tissue suppression

Discussion

The correct answer is (A). MRI reveals a poor or absent enhancement of the lunate after injection with Gadolinium contrast in cases of hypo- or avascularity. Subtle subchondral fractures can also be detected by MRI and help plan a suitable treatment.

If you decide to revascularize the lunate, what would the pedicle of choice be?

A. 1–2 ICSRA
B. 4–5 ICSRA
C. 5th ECA
D. 4th ECA
E. 4th on 5th ECA

Discussion

The correct answer is (E). The pedicle that works best for revascularizing a lunate is the 4th extensor compartmental artery, further extended on the 5th extensor compartmental artery.

1–2 ICSRA will often not reach the lunate. The 4th and 5th extra compartmental arteries are also often too short by themselves to reach the lunate especially if one were to account for the expected normal range of motion for the wrist. 4–5 ICSRA does not exist.

Objectives: Did you learn…?

• Identify imaging findings of Kienbock's disease?
• Use 4th and 5th ECA to revascularize the lunate?

CASE 5

A carpenter presents with wrist pain of 8 months duration. The pain is worse when he uses a screwdriver or hammer. When asked, he points to the ulnar side of his wrist. X-ray is shown (Fig. 3–7). What is your diagnosis?

A. Tear of the ulnotriquetral ligament
B. Guyon's canal syndrome

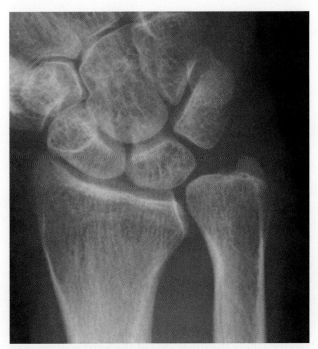

Figure 3–7 (©) Sunil Thirkannad and Christine M. Kleinert.

C. Ulnolunate impaction
D. Carpal coalition
E. Pisotriquetral arthritis

Discussion

The correct answer is (C). The x-ray reveals an ulna-positive variance with secondary cystic changes seen in the lunate. These are quite typical of ulnolunate impaction.

Which of the following clinical tests is likely to be positive in this patient?

A. Ulnar shuck test
B. Piano key sign
C. Lunotriquetral ballottement test
D. Watson's test
E. Finkelstein's test

Discussion

The correct answer is (A). In a patient with ulnolunate abutment, a sudden ulnar deviation of the wrist exaggerates the impaction between the dome of the ulna and the lunate leading to pain.

What changes would the TFCC most likely show in this wrist?

A. Avulsion from the ulnar styloid
B. Central tear
C. Normal appearance

D. Avulsion from the sigmoid notch
E. Intra ligamentous ganglion

Discussion

The correct answer is (B). Due to constant grinding of the lunate against the dome of the ulna, the intervening TFCC progressively undergoes attenuation, often leading to a central tear.

What would be the preferred treatment in this case?

A. Ulnar shortening
B. Darrach's procedure
C. Distal radioulnar joint (DRUJ) arthroplasty
D. Curettage of the lunate cyst
E. Surgical intervention does not help

Discussion

The correct answer is (A). Shortening the ulna by about 2 mm increases the gap between the lunate and dome of the ulna and helps relieve the impaction.

Objectives: Did you learn...?

• Recognize imaging fingins of ulnolunate impaction?
• Use provocative tests for ulnolunate impaction?
• Identify Pathological findings of the TFCC?
• Manage the ulnolunate impaction?

CASE 6

Which of the following is the principal stabilizer of the distal radioulnar joint?

A. Curvature of the sigmoid notch of radius
B. Pronator quadrates
C. ECU subsheath
D. Ulnolunate ligament
E. Triangular fibrocartilage complex (TFCC)

Discussion

The correct answer is (E). While all of the above structures provide some stability to the distal end of the ulna, the principal among them is the TFCC.

Which part of the TFCC provides maximum stability to the DRUJ?

A. The deep dorsal and deep volar radioulnar ligaments
B. The superficial dorsal and superficial volar radioulnar ligaments
C. The central portion of the TFCC

D. The meniscal homologue

E. None of the above

Discussion

The correct answer is (A). Although there are many structures that contribute to the stability of the DRUJ, the deep dorsal and deep volar radioulnar ligaments provide the maximum stability.

Where are the deep dorsal and deep volar radioulnar ligaments attached?

A. Tip of the ulnar styloid

B. Ulno carpal capsule

C. Extensor Carpi Ulnaris (ECU) subsheath

D. Fovea

E. Pisotriquetral ligament

Discussion

The correct answer is (D). The deep dorsal and deep volar radioulnar ligaments arise from the dorsal and volar lips of the sigmoid notch of the radius, respectively, and insert into the fovea at the base of the ulnar styloid process.

What maneuver is used during arthroscopy to judge integrity of the TFCC?

A. Needle poke test

B. Triangulation technique

C. Suction washout maneuver

D. Transillumination test

E. Trampoline test

Discussion

The correct answer is (E). Integrity of the TFCC is judged by pushing down on it with an arthroscopic probe. An intact TFCC has a taut springy feel like a "trampoline."

Objectives: Did you learn...?

• Identify the primary stabilizers of the DRUJ?

• Identify the anatomy of the TFCC?

• Arthroscopically evaluate the TFCC?

CASE 7

A carpenter presents with pain at the ulnar side of his hand associated with tingling and numbness of his small and ring fingers. Which of the following clinical signs would you expect to be positive?

A. Positive Tinel's over the Guyon's canal

B. Positive Tinel's over the carpal tunnel

C. Positive Watson's test

D. Positive Kanavel's signs

E. Positive insertional activity on EMG of the abductor pollicis brevis muscle

Discussion

The correct answer is (A).

He also complains of the small and ring fingers turning white on exposure to cold. What is your diagnosis?

A. Prieser's disease

B. Ulnar hammer syndrome

C. Saddle syndrome

D. Seymour's lesion

E. Longitudinal radioulnar dissociation

Discussion

The correct answer is (B). Ulnar hammer syndrome occurs due to repeated blows to the ulnar side of the wrist. This is typically seen in professions such as carpentry, where the ulnar side of the wrist is often used as a hammer when using tools like chisels. This leads to thrombosis of the ulnar artery and also signs of compression of the ulnar nerve in the Guyon's canal.

What investigation would provide the best information to plan further treatment?

A. Digital subtraction angiography

B. MR angiography

C. CT angiography

D. Conventional angiography

E. Doppler angiography

Discussion

The correct answer is (D). Conventional angiography provides a clear visualization of the vascular tree in the forearm, wrist, and hand. It is especially valuable as it provides the best picture of the palmar arch and digital vessels. The other forms of angiography listed above do not provide a good visualization of small vessels at the arch and beyond and hence are of little value in planning further management.

Angiography (Fig. 3–8) shows complete thrombosis of a 2 cm segment the ulnar artery, extending from the wrist to the palmar arch, with backfilling of the remainder of the arch from the radial artery. What would your management plan be?

A. Thrombolytics

B. Resection of the thrombosed segment with repair or possible interposition vein graft

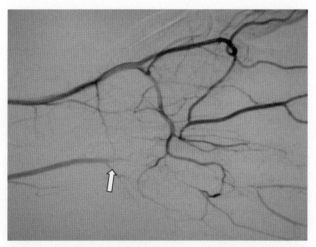

Figure 3–8 (©) Sunil Thirkannad and Christine M. Kleinert.

C. Ligation of the thrombosed ulnar artery
D. Guyon's canal decompression alone
E. Calcium channel blockers

Discussion

The correct answer is (B). Resection of the thrombosed segment with direct repair or interposition vein graft is the best option in this case. Thrombolytics are not effective if the thrombus is 2 cm long. Ligating the artery alone or Guyon's canal decompression alone are poor alternatives. Calcium channel blockers are of benefit in Raynaud's phenomenon.

Objectives: Did you learn...?

• Identify the physical examinations of ulnar neuropathy?
• Describe signs and symptoms of ulnar hammer syndrome?
• Use conventional angiography for the diagnosis of ulnar artery thrombosis?
• Treat ulnar artery thrombosis?

CASE 8

A patient presents with constant pain over the dorso-ulnar aspect of the wrist joint. The symptoms are particularly severe during pronosupination and lifting weights. Which joint is most likely to be involved?

A. Lunotriquetral joint
B. Scaphotrapeziotrapezoidal joint
C. Third carpometacarpal joint
D. Distal radioulnar joint
E. Triquetrohamate joint

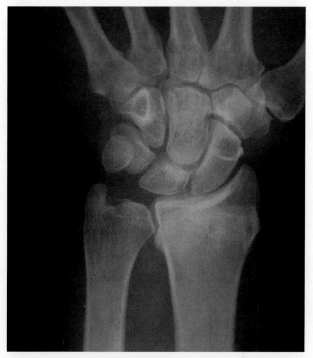

Figure 3–9 (©) Sunil Thirkannad and Christine M. Kleinert.

Discussion

The correct answer is (D).

Radiography (Fig. 3–9) reveals the following picture. What is your next recommendation?

A. Steroid injection to the DRUJ
B. Total DRUJ arthroplasty
C. Observation with no further treatment at this stage
D. Darrach's procedure
E. Long arm splint for 6 weeks

Discussion

The correct answer is (A). The x-ray picture reveals early osteoarthritis of the DRUJ with a small osteophyte. However, the presence of constant pain precludes mere observation; while on the other hand, surgical intervention would not be the first choice of treatment. Splinting for 6 weeks is unlikely to help in the case of osteoarthritis. Given this scenario, a steroid injection is the best option.

The patient goes through a sufficient period of conservative management but has persistent symptoms. You are now contemplating surgical intervention. Which would be indicated in this patient?

A. Darrach's procedure
B. Total DRUJ arthroplasty

C. Trimming the osteophyte
D. Hemiarthroplasty of the ulnar head
E. Wafer's procedure

Discussion

The correct answer is (C).

The patient returns several years later with a completely eroded DRUJ. He is in constant pain and wants relief. He mentions that he is currently a construction worker. Treatment options that you would offer the patient would include which of the following?

A. Place the patient on a permanent one-hand status
B. Darrach's procedure with no restrictions on activity
C. Conversion to a one-bone forearm
D. Total DRUJ arthroplasty if the patient agrees to a lifelong limitation of 25 lb
E. Both B and D

Discussion

The correct answer is (E). If the patient wants to return to heavy duty as a construction worker, a Darrach's procedure would be preferred. However, if a change of job is possible and the patient agrees to a lifelong limitation of 25 lb, one can consider total DRUJ arthroplasty. Permanently restricting the patient to one-hand status or conversion to a one-bone forearm are extremes that would not be indicated.

Objectives: Did you learn...?

• Identify physical examination findigns of DRUJ arthritis?
• Identify radiographic findgins of DRUJ arthritis?
• Surgically manage DRUJ arthritis?

CASE 9

A patient with long-standing rheumatoid arthritis presents with a painful dorsal prominence of the ulnar head. Which clinical sign would you expect to see in her?

A. Piano key sign
B. Accordion sign
C. Wartenberg's sign
D. Von Jackson's sign
E. Froment's sign

Discussion

The correct answer is (A). Chronic instability of the DRUJ with dorsal subluxation of the ulnar head is a common problem in patients with long-standing rheumatoid arthritis. The unstable ulnar head can be pushed back into the sigmoid notch but typically springs back, much like a piano key.

What long-term complication could you expect in this patient?

A. Carpal tunnel syndrome
B. Kienbock's disease
C. Carpal boss formation
D. Zigzag deformity of the wrist
E. Rupture of long extensors of the fingers

Discussion

The correct answer is (E). Long-standing DRUJ instability typically leads to a dorsally displaced head of ulna. Over time this is known to cause attritional rupture of the long extensor tendons. The problem characteristically affects the extensors of the small finger first and progresses in an ulnar to radial direction.

Surgical management in the above patient in addition to repair of the tendons may also include:

A. Darrach's procedure
B. Radial styloidectomy
C. Removal of Lister's tubercle
D. Carpal tunnel release
E. Radial tunnel decompression of the posterior interosseous nerve

Discussion

The correct answer is (A). The head of the ulna is chronically displaced and often misshapen in these cases. It is hence quite common to perform a Darrach's procedure along with tendon repair. While it is possible that any of the other procedures listed above may also be needed in a patient with rheumatoid arthritis, their indications are unique and separate from chronic rupture of finger extensors.

The treatment algorithm for surgical repair of the attritional extensor tendon rupture should include:

A. Primary repair of the extensor tendons
B. Tenodesis or transfer to extensor tendon slips of adjacent digits
C. Free tendon grafts
D. Transfer of flexor digitorum superficialis (FDS) of the ring finger to extensors
E. All of the above

Discussion

The correct answer is (E). Attritional tendon ruptures lead to significantly frayed and retracted tendon ends that may or may not be amenable to primary tendon repair. Consequently, a treatment algorithm in such cases needs to include all forms of reconstruction including tendon transfers and free tendon grafts. The rupture is very longstanding; the extensor muscles may be very atrophic, necessitating transfer of FDS of the ring finger to animate finger extensors.

Objectives: Did you learn...?

- Identify the piano key sign?
- Identify complications of rheumatoid arthritis?
- Treat a chronically displaced head of ulna with the Darrach's procedure?
- Do the Algorithm of attritional tendon rupture repair?

CASE 10

A patient presents with history of feeling a sudden "pop" while exercising followed by pain in the ulnar side of the wrist 4 months ago. Examination reveals antero-posterior mobility of the ulna on stressing the DRUJ in neutral rotation. What is the significance of this finding?

A. The joint is unstable
B. The joint is normal
C. Some laxity of the DRUJ can be expected in neutral rotation
D. No clinical significance can be attributed to this finding whatsoever
E. There is an associated midcarpal instability

Discussion

The correct answer is (C). Some laxity of the DRUJ can be expected in neutral rotation. Whether this is normal or pathological depends on the extent of laxity and is best determined by comparing it to the opposite, uninjured side.

Further examination reveals that the DRUJ shows abnormal laxity on stressing in a fully pronated position. Which structures have to be incompetent for this to occur?

A. TFCC
B. Radioscaphocapitate ligament
C. Ligament of Testut
D. A and B
E. B and C

Discussion

The correct answer is (A). The TFCC plays an important role in stabilizing the DRUJ. The other two structures have no role in stabilizing this joint.

Given that the joint was unstable in a fully pronated position, which part of the TFCC is most likely injured?

A. Central part
B. Deep dorsal radioulnar ligament
C. Deep volar radioulnar ligament
D. Meniscal homologue
E. None of the above

Discussion

The correct answer is (B). The deep dorsal radioulnar ligament provides stability to the DRUJ in a fully pronated position. In contrast, the deep volar radioulnar ligament stabilizes it in a fully supinated wrist. The central part of the TFCC is a relatively thinner structure spanning the above two ligaments and acts more as a buffer between the dome of the ulna and the carpal bones, notably the lunate and triquetrum. It has a very minimal role in providing stability to the DRUJ. The meniscal homologue is a localized shelf-like projection seen sometimes between the ulna and carpus and once again plays a very minimal role in stabilizing the DRUJ.

You take the patient for surgical correction and successfully reconstruct the dorsal radioulnar ligament. Following that, you decide to place the patient in a long arm splint. Which position would you choose "not" to place the forearm in?

A. Full pronation
B. Full supination
C. Neutral
D. Position of the forearm does not matter as it is a reconstruction and not a repair
E. Semi supinated

Discussion

The correct answer is (A). After reconstructing the dorsal radioulnar ligament, the forearm needs to be placed either in neutral or a supinated position. A fully pronated forearm places maximum tension on dorsal structures. Consequently, if the forearm were to be immobilized in this position, there is risk of the reconstructed ligament healing in a "stretched" position leading to persistent laxity.

Objectives: Did you learn…?

• Physically examine for DRUJ instability?
• Identify the role of the TFCC in DRUJ instability?
• Care for DRUJ repair postoperatively?

CASE 11

A patient presents to your clinic with ulnar-sided wrist pain. X-ray is as shown in Figure 3–10. What is your diagnosis?

A. Fracture of the triquetrum
B. Osteochondroma
C. Chondrocalcinosis
D. Pisotriquetral arthritis
E. Ectopic ossification

Discussion

The correct answer is (D). The findings in the radiographs are consistent with pisotriquetral arthritis.

What sort of bone is the pisiform?

A. Atavistic bone
B. Sesamoid bone
C. Pseudo-membranous bone

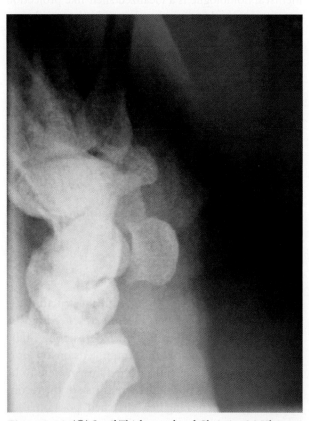

Figure 3–10 (©) Sunil Thirkannad and Christine M. Kleinert.

D. Migratory bone
E. Midcarpal bone

Discussion

The correct answer is (B).

In which tendon would you find the pisiform?

A. Flexor carpi radialis
B. Flexor carpi ulnaris
C. Flexor pisiformis brevis
D. Palmaris brevis
E. Abductor digitorum longus

Discussion

The correct answer is (B). The pisiform is located within the flexor carpi ulnaris tendon. There are no muscles named either the flexor pisiformis brevis or abductor digitorum longus.

Which of the following ligaments is "not" a distal extension of the FCU-pisiform complex?

A. Pisotriquetral ligament
B. Piso-hamate ligament
C. Piso 5th metacarpal ligament
D. Piso-scaphoid ligament
E. All of the above are part of the FCU-pisiform complex

Discussion

The correct answer is (D).

Objectives: Did you learn…?

• Identify radiographic findings of pisotriquetral arthritis?
• Identify the osteology of the pisiform?
• Describe the anatomy of the pisiform?

CASE 12

A 68-year-old farmer presents to your clinic with pain in his wrist. He mentions that it started as an intermittent discomfort about 1 year ago but has progressively worsened to the point where he cannot perform his daily activities without experiencing considerable pain. During examination, you decide to perform the Watson's test. How would you do this?

A. Start by holding the wrist in ulnar deviation and move it into radial deviation while simultaneously applying a dorsally directed force to the scaphoid tubercle
B. Start by holding the wrist in radial deviation and move it into ulnar deviation while simultaneously

applying a volarly directed force to the scapholunate region

C. Twist the wrist in a pronosupinatory maneuver while simultaneously applying a traction force

D. Flex and extend the wrist while simultaneously applying a compressive force toward the radius

E. Apply axial pressure along the thumb while simultaneously twisting it along its long axis in a grinding manner

Discussion

The correct answer is (A).

Which joint are you testing for by performing a Watson's test?

A. Midcarpal joint

B. Lunotriquetral joint

C. Scaphotrapeziotrapezoidal joint

D. Scaphocapitate joint

E. Scapholunate joint

Discussion

The correct answer is (E).

X-ray (Fig. 3–11) taken at the time of the visit is as shown. The radiologist reports this as SLAC wrist. What does SLAC stand for?

A. Scapholunate arthritic condition

B. Scaphoid laxity and collapse

C. Scapholunate–advanced collapse

D. Severe lunate arthritic collapse

E. None of the above

Discussion

The correct answer is (C).

Which of the following procedures would be a reasonable option for this patient?

A. Proximal row carpectomy

B. Scaphoid excision and four-corner fusion

C. Scaphoid excision and replacement with a silastic scaphoid prosthesis

D. Radio carpal interposition arthroplasty with fascia lata

Discussion

The correct answer is (B). The patient has a severe SLAC wrist with involvement of the midcarpal joint. Loss of cartilage over the proximal pole of the capitate precludes a proximal row carpectomy. By the same token, interposition arthroplasty at the radio carpal joint alone fails to address the midcarpal problem. The use of a silastic prosthesis for the scaphoid has been abandoned due to very high rates of failure.

Objectives: Did you learn…?

• Properly perform the Watson's test?

• Identify a SLAC wrist and treat it?

CASE 13

A patient presents with a history of chronic wrist pain of 6 years duration. He stated that he sustained a fall 9 years ago. Immediately after injury, he did not seek any medical attention, thinking that he had merely sprained his wrist. An x-ray taken at this visit is shown (Fig. 3–12). What does he have?

A. SNAC wrist

B. SLAC wrist

C. Prieser's disease

D. Snack wrist

E. Slack wrist

Discussion

The correct answer is (A).

What does SNAC stand for?

A. Scapho-navicular arthritic changes

B. Severe navicular arthitic changes

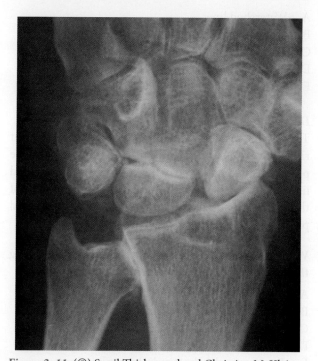

Figure 3–11 (©) Sunil Thirkannad and Christine M. Kleinert.

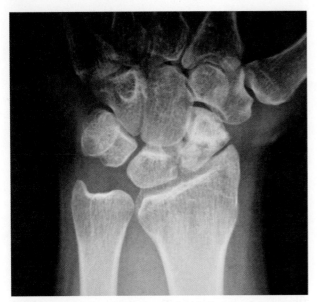

Figure 3–12 (©) Sunil Thirkannad and Christine M. Kleinert.

C. Scaphoid nonunion with advanced collapse
D. Scaphoid nonunion with arthritis changes
E. None of the above

Discussion
The correct answer is (C).

What treatment options can be considered in general for a patient with SNAC wrist?

A. Scaphoid excision with four-corner fusion
B. Proximal row carpectomy
C. Total wrist arthroplasty
D. Total wrist fusion
E. All of the above

Discussion
The correct answer is (E). Any of the above-mentioned procedures can be considered for a patient with SNAC wrist. The specific procedure chosen depends on the amount of midcarpal and radio carpal (especially radiolunate) involvement, as well as the patient's level of physical activity participation.

You choose to perform a scaphoid excision with four-corner fusion. Which four bones are fused in this procedure?

A. Trapezium, trapezoid, capitate, and hamate
B. Pisiform, triquetrum, trapezium, and trapezoid
C. Capitate, hamate, triquetrum, and pisiform
D. Lunate, capitate, trapezium, and trapezoid
E. Lunate, triquetrum, capitate, and hamate

Discussion
The correct answer is (E).

Objectives: Did you learn...?
• Identify radiographic findings of SNAC wrist?
• Define the concept and treatment of SNAC wrist?
• Identify the mechanis of four-corner fusion?

CASE 14

A patient presents after a fall on an outstretched hand. X-rays reveal a distal radius and ulnar styloid fracture. You decide to perform open reduction and internal fixation with a volar plate and screws. Which segment of the distal radius is considered to be the keystone in fixing these fractures?

A. Radial styloid
B. Lister's tubercle
C. The volar ulnar part of the lunate fossa
D. The dorsal half of the sigmoid notch
E. Scaphoid fossa

Discussion
The correct answer is (C).

While placing the plate, you remember hearing that the plate needs to be placed proximal to a certain landmark line. What is this line called?

A. Watershed line
B. Cardinal line
C. Translational line
D. Tectonic line
E. Finish line

Discussion
The correct answer is (A). The watershed line is a faint ridge corresponding roughly to the distal border of the pronator quadratus and its aponeurosis. It is shaped like an asymmetric double curve with the ulnar part of the curve extending a little more distal than the radial part.

What complication are you likely to avoid by placing the plate proximal to the watershed line?

A. Dorsal penetration of screws
B. Attritional rupture of flexor pollicis longus
C. Rotational malalignment of fracture fragments
D. Screw penetration through the sigmoid notch
E. Damage to the short radiolunate ligament

Discussion

The correct answer is (B). Placing the plate distal to the watershed line leads to a prominence of the distal edge of the plate. Over time, the flexor pollicis longus can sustain attritional rupture due to friction against this prominent edge.

Which of the following features of an ulnar styloid fracture has been shown to definitively predispose to instability of the distal radioulnar joint?

A. Fractures involving greater than 50% of the size of the styloid
B. Fractures displaced more than 2 mm
C. Fractures with greater than 90-degree rotation of the fragment
D. All of the above
E. None of the above

Discussion

The correct answer is (E). No studies have consistently shown any feature of the ulnar styloid fracture that can successfully predict instability of the distal radioulnar joint.

Objectives: Did you learn...?

- Perform the proper technique for open reduction and internal fixation of distal radius fractures?
- Identify complications of ORIF of distal radius fractures and how to avoid them?

CASE 15

A 19-year-old female patient presents with progressive aching pains in her wrist. She does not recollect any injury to her wrist. An x-ray (Fig. 3–13) is as shown. What do you think she has?

A. Radial club hand
B. Madelung's deformity
C. Malunited distal radius fracture
D. Achondroplasia
E. Fibrous dysplasia

Discussion

The correct answer is (B).

What is the purported cause of a Madelung's deformity?

A. Injury to the volar ulnar corner of the distal radial epiphysis
B. Injury to the volar radial corner of the distal radial epiphysis

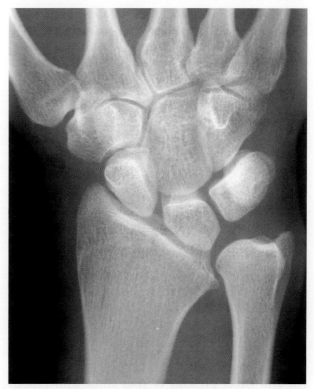

Figure 3–13 (©) Sunil Thirkannad and Christine M. Kleinert.

C. Injury to the dorsal ulnar corner of the distal radial epiphysis
D. Injury to the dorsal radial corner of the distal radial epiphysis
E. None of the above

Discussion

The correct answer is (A).

What structure has been implicated in causing a proximal luxation of the lunate?

A. Radio-scaphocapitate ligament
B. Ulno-triquetral bundle
C. Cooper's ligament
D. Vicker's ligament
E. Ligament of Legue and Juvarra

Discussion

The correct answer is (D). Vicker's ligament is a thickened fibrous structure that connects the lunate to the radius. Often, a beak-like protrusion can be seen on the ulnar volar aspect of the distal radius corresponding to the point of attachment of the ligament. It has been proposed that as the ulna continues to grow, the lunate is prevented from migrating distally with growth by Vicker's ligament which tethers it to the radius thus leading to an eventual proximal luxation.

Which of the following procedures have been used in the treatment of Madelung's deformity?

A. Osteotomy and realignment of the distal radius
B. Epiphyseodesis of the ulna
C. Total replacement of the distal radioulnar joint
D. A and B
E. All of the above

Discussion
The correct answer is (E).

Objectives: Did you learn...?

- Identify Madelung's deformity on a radiograph?
- Describe the etiology of Madelung's deformity?
- Treat Madelung's deformity?

CASE 16

An avid golfer presents to your clinic with sudden onset of pain at the base of his hypothenar eminence when he accidentally struck the ground mid swing. You suspect a fracture of the hook of the hamate. Routine PA and lateral x-rays do not reveal any fracture. Which of the following views would you then ask for?

A. Notch view
B. Grip view
C. Carpal tunnel view
D. Ulnar-deviated PA view
E. Roberts view

Discussion
The correct answer is (C).

X-rays are still inconclusive. Which of the following imaging modalities is most sensitive in detecting acute fractures?

A. MRI
B. CT scan
C. CT arthrogram
D. Ultrasound scan
E. X-ray tomography

Discussion
The correct answer is (A).

A fracture of the hook of hamate is confirmed. You decide to proceed with open reduction and internal fixation with a headless screw. Which structure is at risk of injury during surgery?

A. Motor branch of median nerve
B. Deep branch of ulnar nerve
C. Nerve of Henle
D. Common digital nerve to the fourth web
E. Palmar cutaneous branch of the median nerve

Discussion
The correct answer is (B). The ulnar nerve trifurcates in the distal part of Guyon's canal into the deep motor branch, the ulnar digital nerve of the small finger, and the common digital nerve to the fourth web. The deep motor branch curves radially along the base of the hook of the hamate and is particularly vulnerable to injury during surgery.

Which of the following structures is principally inserted into the hook of the hamate?

A. Capitato-hamate ligament
B. Ligament of Testut
C. Naviculo-hamate ligament
D. Piso-hamate ligament
E. Hamato-lunate ligament

Discussion
The correct answer is (D). The piso-hamate ligament is an extension of the FCU tendon. Consequently, pain on resisted flexion of the wrist in ulnar deviation (i.e., resisted flexion of the FCU) can help confirm injury to the hook of the hamate.

Objectives: Did you learn...?

- Properly image for the diagnosis of hamate fractures?
- Use MRI in the diagnosis of hamate fractures?
- Identify complications of ORIF of hook and hamate fractures?
- Describe the anatomy of the hamate?

CASE 17

A young sportsman presents with the following injury to his thumb (Figure 3–14). What is your diagnosis?

A. Barton's fracture
B. Rolando's fracture
C. Chauffeur's fracture
D. Benton's fracture
E. None of the above

Discussion
The correct answer is (E). The lesion shown here is a Bennett's fracture dislocation.

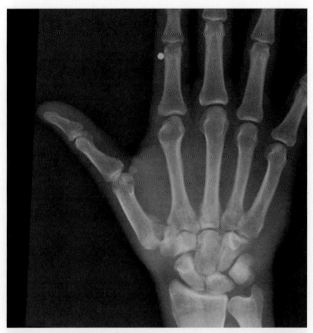

Figure 3–14 (©) Sunil Thirkannad and Christine M. Kleinert.

Which structure is responsible for stabilizing the proximal fragment in a Bennett's fracture dislocation?

A. Tip ligament
B. Beak ligament
C. Deep transverse ligament
D. Ligament of Testut
E. Triscaphe ligament

Discussion
The correct answer is (B).

Which two muscles are mainly responsible for the deformity seen here?

A. Abductor pollicis brevis and first dorsal interosseous
B. Abductor pollicis longus and first dorsal interosseous
C. First dorsal interosseous and adductor pollicis
D. Abductor pollicis longus and adductor pollicis
E. Abductor pollicis longus and extensor pollicis brevis

Discussion
The correct answer is (D). The abductor pollicis longus (APL) exerts a proximal pull on the distal fragment causing it to migrate proximally while the adductor pollicis causes it to adduct, resulting in the characteristic deformity.

Which of the following is not part of management of an acute Bennett's fracture?

A. Closed reduction and splinting
B. Open reduction and pinning of the first metacarpal to the trapezium
C. Open reduction and release of the insertion of the abductor pollicis longus
D. Closed reduction and pinning of the first metacarpal to the second metacarpal
E. Open reduction and fixation with a screw

Discussion
The correct answer is (C). Release of the insertion of the abductor pollicis longus is not required in an acute injury. However, in chronically displaced fractures, secondary contracture of the APL may occur, necessitating this procedure.

Objectives: Did you learn...?
• Identify imaging of Bennett's fractures?
• Describe the deforming forces of Bennett's fractures?
• Manage Bennett's fractures?

CASE 18

A construction worker presents with persistent pain many years after sustaining an injury to his wrist. He indicates that he expects to continue in his present job for many more years. His x-ray is shown (Fig. 3–15). Which of the following surgical options would best suit his purpose?

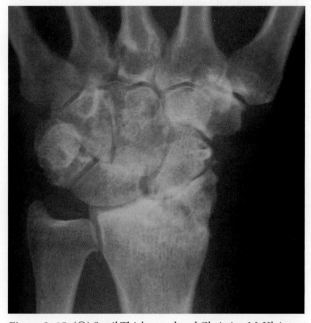

Figure 3–15 (©) Sunil Thirkannad and Christine M. Kleinert.

A. Total wrist fusion
B. Total wrist arthroplasty
C. Proximal row carpectomy
D. Scaphoid excision and four-corner fusion
E. Radio scapholunate fusion

Discussion

The correct answer is (A). The x-ray pictures reveal a malunited distal radius fracture with pan carpal arthritis involving the radio carpal and midcarpal joints. Options C, D, or E cannot be recommended in this situation. While a total wrist arthroplasty may be an option in a less demanding patient, it would not be appropriate for someone involved in heavy manual labor as a construction worker.

What is the optimal position for fusion of the wrist?

A. 10- to 20-degree flexion
B. 0- to 30-degree extension
C. 40- to 60-degree extension
D. 30- to 40-degree radial deviation
E. 30- to 40-degree ulnar deviation

Discussion

The correct answer is (B).

What joint is not included in a typical total wrist fusion?

A. Radioscaphoid joint
B. Scaphocapitate joint
C. Scaphotrapezoidal joint
D. Scapholunate joint
E. 3rd carpometacarpal joint

Discussion

The correct answer is (C).

Implant loosening over time has been commonly attributed to failure to achieve fusion across which joint?

A. Scapholunate joint
B. Lunotriquetral joint
C. Capitate-hamate
D. 3rd carpometacarpal joint
E. Luno-capitate joint

Discussion

The correct answer is (D).

Objectives: Did you learn...?

• Diagnose distal radius malunion?
• Describe proper position of wrist fusion?

• Identify the joints involved in wrist fusion?
• Identify the cause of implant loosening in wrist fusion?

CASE 19

Several months after sustaining a fall on his outstretched hand, a patient presents to your clinic with pain over the central part of his wrist. You obtain the following x-ray (Fig. 3–16). What do you see?

A. Perilunate injury
B. VISI
C. SLAC
D. DISI
E. SNAC

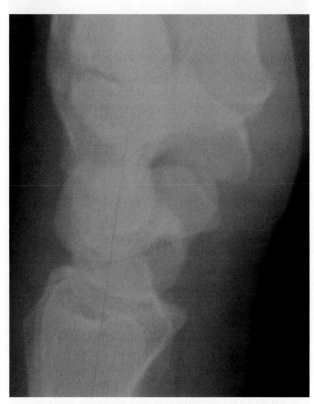

Figure 3–16 (©) Sunil Thirkannad and Christine M. Kleinert.

Discussion

The correct answer is (D).

What does DISI stand for?

A. Dorsal inter scapholunate instability
B. Dorsal intracarpal scapholunate instability
C. Dorsal intercalated segmental instability
D. Dorsal intercarpal segmental instability
E. Dorsal intercalated scapholunate instability

Discussion

The correct answer is (C).

What part of the carpus does the term intercalated refer to?

A. Capitate
B. Scapholunate joint
C. Scapholunate ligament
D. Radioscaphocapitate ligament
E. None of the above

Discussion

The correct answer is (E). The term intercalated refers to the scaphoid. This is the only bone in the carpus that bridges both the proximal and distal rows. Consequently it acts much like the crankshaft of a railway engine wheel and is hence referred to as an "intercalated" segment.

Which are the strongest parts of the scapholunate ligament?

A. Dorsal part
B. Proximal part
C. Volar part
D. A and C
E. A and B

Discussion

The correct answer is (D). The scapholunate ligament is horseshoe-shaped. The dorsal and volar parts are the thickest and strongest, while the proximal part is usually much thinner.

Objectives: Did you learn...?

• Identify the concepts and mechanics of DISI deformity?
• Describe the mechanics of the scapholunate ligament?

CASE 20

Following a long-standing injury, a sportsman presents a radiology report indicating that he has a VISI deformity. Which part of the carpus is most likely injured?

A. The capitohamate joint
B. The scaphocapitate joint
C. The radiolunate joint
D. The lunotriquetral joint
E. The pisotriquetral joint

Discussion

The correct answer is (D).

If the patient has a VISI deformity, which radiographic measurement can be affected?

A. The radiolunate angle
B. The luno-capitate angle
C. The scapholunate angle
D. The lunotriquetral interval
E. All of the above

Discussion

The correct answer is (E).

What is the normal scapholunate angle?

A. 10 to 20 degrees
B. 30 to 60 degrees
C. 60 70 degrees
D. 0 degree
E. 90 degrees

Discussion

The correct answer is (B).

What is the normal intercarpal distance in adults?

A. 1 mm
B. <3 mm
C. 3 to 5 mm
D. Differs between each set of bones

Discussion

The correct answer is (B).

Objectives: Did you learn...?

• Describe the pathoanatomy of VISI deformity?
• Identify VISI deformity from radiographs?
• Describe the normal scapholunate angle?
• Describe the intercarpal distance in adults?

CASE 21

Following an intense game of football, a player is brought to you with complaints of pain over the ulnar side of his wrist. X-rays reveal a transverse pisiform fracture. What is your treatment plan?

A. Surgery; as these fractures do not heal
B. Short arm splint
C. Steroid injection
D. Ace wrap
E. Do nothing as these fractures heal uneventfully

Discussion

The correct answer is (B). A period of splinting in a short arm splint is a reasonable initial line of treatment for a pisiform fracture.

The pisiform is classified as what type of bone?

A. Atavistic
B. Membranous
C. Rudimentary
D. Intercalated
E. Sesamoid

Discussion

The correct answer is (E).

The pisiform is located within which tendon?

A. ECU
B. FCU
C. FDP of the small finger
D. FDS of the small finger
E. Palmaris brevis

Discussion

The correct answer is (B).

Your patient fails to respond to an initial period of splinting and you decide on a surgical approach. What is the preferred surgical procedure in this case?

A. ORIF with k wires
B. ORIF with a headless screw
C. Excision of the pisiform
D. Intraosseous wiring
E. Injection of platelet-rich plasma

Discussion

The correct answer is (C). Excision of the pisiform is a frequently used procedure for chronic, intractable pain associated with pisiform fractures. It generally does not cause any measurable functional deficit.

Objectives: Did you learn...?

• Treat pisiform fractures?
• Describe the osteology of the pisiform?
• Identify anatomy and surgical treatment of pisiform fractures?

CASE 22

An elderly lady complains of pain at the base of both of her thumbs. She mentions that it is progressive and does not recollect any trauma to the region. An x-ray is shown (Fig. 3–17). What do you suspect?

A. 1st carpometacarpal (CMC) arthritis
B. Bennett's fracture
C. Pathological fracture of the base of the trapezium

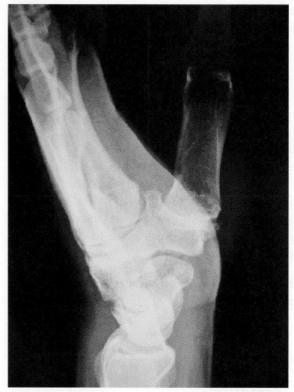

Figure 3–17 (©) Sunil Thirkannad and Christine M. Kleinert.

D. Avascular necrosis of the trapezium
E. Secondaries in the trapezium

Discussion

The correct answer is (A).

She says that she has been suffering for too long and would like to proceed with surgery. Which of the following procedures has demonstrated the best long-term results?

A. Trapezium excision alone
B. Trapeziectomy followed by interposition arthroplasty using a free tendon graft anchovy
C. Trapeziectomy followed by a sling arthroplasty using the FCR
D. Trapeziectomy followed by a sling arthroplasty using the ECRL
E. No difference has been demonstrated between any of the above procedures

Discussion

The correct answer is (E). Long-term studies have failed to demonstrate any appreciable differences between simple trapeziectomy versus any of the other procedures requiring some form of interposition or arthroplasty by ligament reconstruction. However, individual surgeons continue to perform any of the above procedures or their numerous variations based on personal preference.

You elect to perform a trapeziectomy and sling arthroplasty using part of the FCR tendon. Which structure is at direct risk of injury during dissection for this procedure?

A. Sensory branch of the radial nerve
B. Median nerve
C. Palmar cutaneous branch of the median nerve
D. Radial artery
E. All of the above

Discussion

The correct answer is (E). The sensory branches of the radial nerve pass very closely to the site of incision over the 1st CMC joint. The median nerve as well as the palmar cutaneous branch of the median nerve are closely related to the FCR tendon and are at risk if an open dissection technique is used to harvest the tendon. The radial artery crosses the anatomical snuff box and is at risk during deep dissection around the trapezium.

During surgery, you discover that the FCR tendon has undergone attritional rupture and is unavailable for ligament reconstruction. Which alternate tendon has been used in these circumstances to recreate a similar biomechanical construct?

A. EPL
B. EPB
C. ECRL
D. ECRB
E. Palmaris longus

Discussion

The correct answer is (C). The ECRL tendon also inserts to the base of the second metacarpal like the FCR. The difference lies in the fact that the FCR is volar while the ECRL is dorsal. Use of the ECRL to create a sling between the 1st and 2nd metacarpals recreates a similar biomechanical structure as would using the FCR. However, care must be taken to ensure that the ECRL tendon graft is passed deep to the radial artery prior to being delivered into the CMC joint area. Failing to do so and passing the tendon graft superficial to the radial artery can create a pincer effect on the artery and potentially lead to its occlusion and thrombosis.

Objectives: Did you learn...?
• Identify CMC arthritis from radiographs?
• Treat CMC arthritis?
• Name the structures at risk during surgical treatment?
• Identify the ligaments used for reconstruction?

CASE 23

A 30-year-old lady in her third trimester of pregnancy presents with pain at the base of her right thumb. She denies history of any trauma and mentions that it is particularly painful while turning on her car keys. What would you consider most likely to be the cause of her pain?

A. Wartenburg's syndrome
B. DeQuervain's tenosynovitis
C. 1st CMC arthritis
D. Radial artery thrombosis in the anatomical snuff box
E. Radio-scaphoid arthritis

Discussion

The correct answer is (B). DeQuervain's tenosynovitis is known to be aggravated or sometimes even precipitated by pregnancy. While all the other conditions listed above can also potentially cause pain at the base of the thumb, they are significantly less common given the age and circumstances of this particular patient.

Which extensor compartment is affected in DeQuervain's tenosynovitis?

A. 1st
B. 1st and 2nd
C. 2nd
D. 1st and 3rd
E. 2nd and 3rd

Discussion
The correct answer is (A).

What tendons are affected by DeQuervain's tenosynovitis?

A. ECRL and ECRB
B. APL and EPB
C. EPB and EPL
D. APL and APB
E. APB and EPL

Discussion
The correct answer is (B).

Following a period of conservative treatment, you decide to proceed with surgery. Intraoperatively, you open the compartment and discover two tendons. Traction on both of these tendons produces abduction of the thumb metacarpal. You do not see any other tendons in this area. What is the most likely scenario?

A. Nothing unusual. You have successfully decompressed the affected compartment
B. The EPB is most likely missing in this patient
C. The EPB has most likely ruptured in this patient
D. The EPB is most likely located within a separate subcompartment
E. The patient has a combined extensor pollicis longus et brevis

Discussion

The correct answer is (D). While responses A, B, C and are all possible, the commonest variation seen is the presence of a separate subcompartment. In fact, studies have shown that the presence of a separate subcompartment for the EPB may actually be more common than the presence of a single compartment for the APL and EPB.

Objectives: Did you learn...?

• Identify the compartment affected by DeQuervains tenosynovitis?
• Treat DeQuervains tenosynovitis?
• Identify variatons of the first compartment anatomy?

CASE 24

A 23-year-old auto mechanic presents with several months of an achy pain over the dorsum of his wrist. An x-ray is shown (Fig. 3–18). What is your diagnosis?

A. VISI deformity
B. DISI deformity
C. Osteosarcoma
D. Subluxation of the CMC joint
E. Carpal boss

Discussion

The correct answer is (E).

What further investigation would you recommend in this case?

A. MRI without contrast
B. MRI with contrast

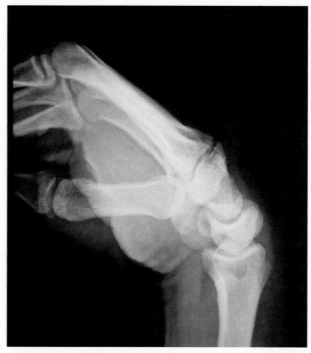

Figure 3–18 (©) Sunil Thirkannad and Christine M. Kleinert.

C. Thin slice CT scans
D. Radioisotope bone scan
E. None of the above

Discussion

The correct answer is (E).
Plain radiography is sufficient to make a diagnosis of a carpal boss.

What is a carpal boss?

A. Synonym for osteochondroma
B. Osteophytes arising from the 2nd or 3rd CMC joint
C. A malunited avulsed fracture of the ECRL tendon
D. Ectopic calcium deposits secondary to hyperparathyroidism
E. None of the above

Discussion

The correct answer is (B).

Which structures are at greater risk of rupture during surgery for a carpal boss?

A. EPL at Lister's tubercle
B. The Juncturae tendinum between the EDC tendons
C. ECRB tendon
D. ECU tendon
E. Extensor digitorum quinti tendon

Discussion

The correct answer is (C). The ECRB tendon inserts to the base of the 3rd metacarpal which is the most common site of a carpal boss. Often this tendon needs to be sharply dissected away from the metacarpal to enable excision of the osteophytes. Consequently, it is at a greater risk for potential rupture during surgery.

Objectives: Did you learn...?

- Identify a carpal boss?
- Diagnose a carpal boss?
- Identify the structures at risk during treatment of carpal boss?

CASE 25

Following a fall on his outstretched hand, a 27-year-old teacher presents with mild pain in his wrist. You obtain an x-ray which is shown (Fig. 3–19). What is your diagnosis?

A. Carpal coalition
B. Perilunate dislocation
C. DISI
D. VISI
E. None of the above

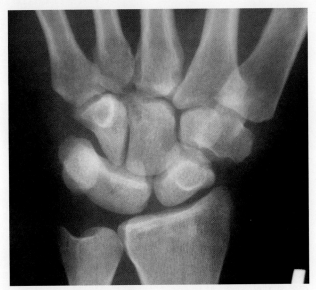

Figure 3–19 (©) Sunil Thirkannad and Christine M. Kleinert.

Discussion

The correct answer is (A).

People of which ethnicity have a high incidence of lunotriquetral coalition?

A. White Caucasians
B. Native Americans
C. Chinese Americans
D. African Americans
E. Ashkenazi Jews

Discussion

The correct answer is (D).

Which classification system is commonly used for lunotriquetral coalitions?

A. Steindler classification
B. Minnaar classification
C. Swanson classification
D. American Wrist Society classification
E. Kleinert classification

Discussion

The correct answer is (B).

Which of the following radiological features is considered to be typical of Minnaar type 1 coalition?

A. Fluted champagne glass appearance
B. Notched appearance
C. Complete coalition
D. Triangle sign
E. Signet Ring sign

Discussion

The correct answer is (A). Minnaar Type 1 refers to a fibrous/cartilaginous type of coalition. In these cases, the lunotriquetral joint is seen as a narrowed space, often slightly wider distally than proximally, giving the appearance of a fluted champagne glass.

Objectives: Did you learn...?

- Identify carpal coalition from the imaging?
- Manage carpal coalition?
- Classify Carpal coalition?

CASE 26

An active, 19-year-old gymnast complains of ulnar-sided wrist pain. She has already obtained an MRI scan which reveals ECU tendinitis. Where does this tendon principally insert?

A. Base of 4th metacarpal
B. Hamate
C. Dorsal ridge of triquetrum
D. Blends with the 4th dorsal interosseous aponeurosis
E. Base of 5th metacarpal

Discussion

The correct answer is (E).

What is the anatomical peculiarity of the ECU?

A. It receives dual nerve supply
B. It is the only extensor which also provides attachment to a lumbrical muscle
C. It contains a sesamoid bone
D. It is enclosed by a separate subsheath
E. It is the only extensor not contained within a compartment

Discussion

The correct answer is (D).

Which extensor compartment does the ECU pass through?

A. 4th
B. 5th
C. 6th
D. 7th
E. None of the above

Discussion

The correct answer is (C).

In addition to acting as a wrist extensor, what other role has been attributed to the ECU?

A. It stabilizes the ulnar head preventing dorsal subluxation
B. It enables opposition of the 5th metacarpal
C. It is responsible for rotary movements at the capitate-hamate joint
D. It augments the dorsal radio-triquetral bundle
E. It provides attachment to the TFCC

Discussion

The correct answer is (A). The ECU tendon, along with its subsheath, acts as a dorsal stabilizer of the ulnar head. It passes through a groove on the dorsoulnar aspect of the head of the ulna and is known to play a role in preventing its dorsal subluxation.

Objectives: Did you learn...?

• Recognize the anatomy of the ECU?
• Identify the role of the ECU?

CASE 27

Several years after sustaining an injury to his wrist, a firefighter presents to your clinic with chronic wrist pain. What does his x-ray (Fig. 3–20) reveal?

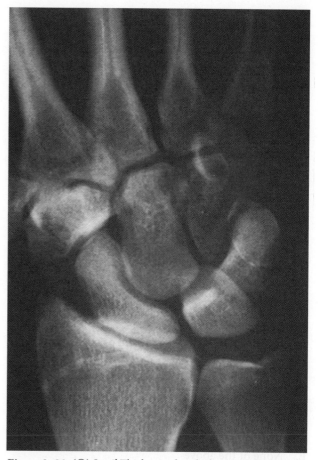

Figure 3–20 (©) Sunil Thirkannad and Christine M. Kleinert.

A. DISI
B. Carpal coalition
C. Ulnar translation
D. VISI
E. None of the above

Discussion

The correct answer is (C).

How much does the width of the lunate need to be off the radius for a diagnosis of ulnar translation to be made?

A. >30%
B. >50%
C. >25%
D. Is determined by the displacement of the scaphoid in the scaphoid fossa
E. None of the above

Discussion

The correct answer is (B).

Ulnar translation of the lunate serves as a relative contraindication for which procedure?

A. Total wrist fusion
B. Total wrist arthroplasty
C. Four-corner fusion
D. Proximal row carpectomy
E. Fascia lata interposition arthroplasty

Discussion

The correct answer is (D). Ulnar translation of the lunate indicates weakness of the radio-scaphocapitate ligament. This serves as a relative contraindication for proximal row carpectomy as the risk of the capitate also translating ulnar wards is high, leading to an unstable wrist.

Which of the following surgical procedures is indicated in correcting ulnar translation of the carpus?

A. Radioscapholunate fusion
B. Radial styloidectomy
C. Arthroscopic debridement of the TFCC
D. Ulnar shortening
E. Scaphoid excision and four-corner fusion

Discussion

The correct answer is (A).

Objectives: Did you learn...?

• Identify criteria of ulnar translation?
• Identify contraindications of proximal row carpectomy?
• Surgically manage ulnar translation of the carpus?

CASE 28

A young lady presents with chronic pain in her wrist which she describes as a deep boring type. An x-ray (Fig. 3–21) is shown. She denies any history of trauma in the past. What do you suspect?

A. Kienbock's disease
B. Osteoid osteoma
C. Preiser's disease
D. Osteopetrosis
E. Hyperparathyroidism

Discussion

The correct answer is (C).

What investigation would help confirm your diagnosis?

A. CT scan
B. Arthroscopy

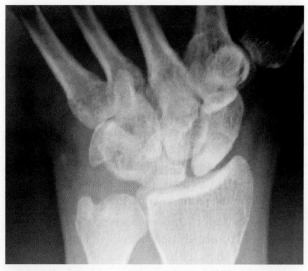

Figure 3–21 (©) Sunil Thirkannad and Christine M. Kleinert.

C. Arthrogram
D. MRI with contrast
E. Angiogram

Discussion

The correct answer is (D).

Preiser's disease is a spontaneous avascular necrosis of the scaphoid. MRI with gadolinium is the most sensitive modality to confirm this condition.

What is your preferred treatment for this condition?

A. Scaphoid excision and four-corner fusion
B. Botox injection
C. Daily application of nitroglycerine paste over the scaphoid
D. Proximal row carpectomy
E. Vascularized bone graft to the scaphoid

Discussion

The correct answer is (E).

Which pedicle is commonly used to revascularize the scaphoid?

A. 2–3 ICSRA
B. 1–2 ICSRA
C. 1st ECA
D. 2nd ECA
E. Dorsal carpal arch

Discussion

The correct answer is (B).

- Diagnose Preiser's disease?
- Identify signs and symptoms of Preiser's disease?
- Operatively manage Preiser's disease?

CASE 29

A 19-year-old girl presents to you with a painful wrist. As part of your investigations, you ask for x-rays of the wrist. Your radio technician is inexperienced and unsure of how to obtain proper views. How would you position the patient to obtain a PA view?

A. Shoulder adducted, elbow flexed to 90 degrees with forearm pronated and hand placed flat on the film

B. Shoulder abducted to 90 degrees, elbow flexed to 90 degrees with forearm neutral and hand placed flat on the film

C. Shoulder adducted, elbow flexed to 90 degrees with forearm supinated and hand placed flat on the film

D. Shoulder abducted to 90 degrees, elbow flexed to 90 degrees with forearm supinated and hand placed flat on the film

E. Shoulder abducted to 90 degrees, elbow flexed to 90 degrees with forearm pronated and hand placed flat on the film

Discussion
The correct answer is (B).

How would you position your patient for a lateral view of the wrist?

A. Shoulder adducted, elbow flexed to 90 degrees with forearm neutral and ulnar border of hand placed on the film

B. Shoulder abducted to 90 degrees, elbow flexed to 90 degrees with forearm neutral and ulnar border of hand placed on the film

C. Shoulder adducted, elbow flexed to 90 degrees with forearm supinated and ulnar border of hand placed on the film

D. Shoulder abducted to 90 degrees, elbow flexed to 90 degrees with forearm supinated and ulnar border of hand placed on the film

E. Shoulder abducted to 90 degrees, elbow flexed to 90 degrees with forearm pronated and ulnar border of hand placed on the film

Discussion
The correct answer is (A).

Whose lines are used to determine proper intercarpal alignment within the proximal and distal carpal rows?

A. Shenton's lines
B. Kleinert's lines
C. Zaidemberg's lines
D. Barton's lines
E. Gilula's lines

Discussion
The correct answer is (E). Gilula described three smooth lines drawn on a PA view. The first corresponds to the proximal articular surfaces of the scaphoid, lunate, and triquetrum. The second line is along the distal articular surfaces of the scaphoid, lunate, and triquetrum while the third line is along the proximal articular surfaces of the capitates and hamate.

How is the carpal height ratio determined on an x-ray of the wrist?

A. Ratio of the height of the lunate to the height of the capitate

B. Ratio of the height of the carpus to the height of the third metacarpal

C. Ratio of the height of the capitate to the height of the carpus

D. Both B and C

E. Ratio of the height of the lunate to the longitudinal axis of the scaphoid

Discussion
The correct answer is (D). The carpal height ratio is classically described as the ratio of the height of the carpus to the height of the third metacarpal. However, as most wrist x-rays do not include the entire third metacarpal, the ratio of the height of the capitate to the height of the carpus is accepted as an alternate method of assessing the carpal height ratio.

Objectives: Did you learn...?

- How to properly position the upper extremity for a PA view of the wrist?
- Describe the significance of Gilula's Lines?
- How to determine the carpal height ratio on x-ray?

CASE 30

You are invited by your medical school to speak to first year medical students about the anatomy of the wrist. One of the students asks you about the most

likely role of the terminal branches of the posterior interosseous nerve. What is your response?

A. They carry cutaneous nerves to the dorsum of the wrist
B. They supply proprioceptive branches to the wrist joint
C. They carry motor nerves to the 3rd and 4th dorsal interossei
D. They carry sympathetic fibers to the dorsal carpal arch artery
E. They carry sudomotor nerves to the dorsum of the wrist

Discussion

The correct answer is (B). The posterior interosseous nerve ends in a pseudoganglion over the dorsum of the carpus. Small terminal branches pass from this to the wrist joint. The general consensus is that these fibers are mainly proprioceptive in nature and may also carry deep pain sensations. Resection of the posterior interosseous nerve over the wrist joint is often carried out as a remedy for intractable wrist pain.

Another student asks you to name the weak spot over the carpus that has been implicated in lunate and perilunate dislocations. What would you say?

A. Parona's space
B. Midpalmar space
C. Poisuelli's space
D. Poirier's space
E. Carpal recess

Discussion

The correct answer is (D). The space of Poirier is a bare area over the volar aspect of the lunate that is not covered by any extrinsic or intrinsic carpal ligament. While controversy exists about the exact nomenclature of the ligaments that border this space, it is generally agreed that this is the weak spot through which volar luxations of the lunate occur.

Your old anatomy teacher tells you that he thinks there is a muscle that has a dual nerve supply in the hand but is unable to recollect its name. What would you say to him?

A. There is no muscle with a dual nerve supply in the hand
B. Flexor pollicis brevis
C. Second lumbrical
D. Palmaris brevis
E. Abductor digitorum minimus

Discussion

The correct answer is (B). The FPB has two bellies and receives supply from both the median nerve and deep branch of the ulnar nerve.

Finally, a bright, eager student asks you what the nerve of Henle is. What is your response?

A. It is a branch of the ulnar nerve that carries sympathetic fibers
B. It is an anomalous connection between the median and ulnar nerves in the wrist
C. It is a branch from the posterior interosseous nerve that provides proprioception to the carpus
D. It is an anomalous branch from the median nerve that can sometimes supply the palmaris brevis muscle
E. It is the nerve supplying the anomalous extensor digitorum manus brevis muscle

Discussion

The correct answer is (A).

Objectives: Did you learn...?

- Discuss the role of the terminal branches of the posterior interosseous nerve?
- Identify the significance of Poirier's space?
- Identify the innervation of the FPB?
- Describe the nerve of Henle?

BIBLIOGRAPHY

Case 1

Henderson B, Letts M. Operative management of pediatric scaphoid fracture nonunion. *J Pediat Orthop.* 2003;23(3): 402–406.

Mittal RL, Dargan SK. Occult scaphoid fracture: a diagnostic enigma. *J Orthop Trauma.* 1989;3(4):306–308.

Roolker W, Maas M, Broekhuizen AH. Diagnosis and treatment of scaphoid fractures, can non-union be prevented? *Arch Orthop Trauma Surg.* 1999;119(7–8):428–431.

Case 2

Boyer MI, Von Schroeder HP, Axelrod TS. Scaphoid nonunion with avascular necrosis of the proximal pole. Treatment with a vascularized borne graft from the dorsum of the distal radius. *J Hand Surg Br.* 1998;23(5): 686–690.

Steinmann SP, Bishop AT, Berger RA. Use of the 1, 2 intercompartmental supraretinacular artery as a vascularized pedicle bone graft for difficult scaphoid nonunion. *J Hand Surg Am.* 2002;27(3):391–401.

Steinmann SP, Adams JE. Scaphoid fractures and nonunions: diagnosis and treatment. *J Orthop Sci.* 2006;11(4): 424–431.

Case 3

Basar H, Başar B, Erol B, Tetik C. Isolated volar surgical approach for the treatment of perilunate and lunate dislocations. *Indian J Orthop.* 2014;48(3):301.

Boyer MI. *AAOS Comprehensive Orthopaedic Review 2.* Rosemont, IL: American Academy of Orthopaedic Surgeons, Copyright; 2014:1058.

Boyer MI. *AAOS Comprehensive Orthopaedic Review 2.* Rosemont, IL: American Academy of Orthopaedic Surgeons, Copyright; 2014:356–360.

Case 4

Bonzar M, Firrell JC, Hainer M, Mah ET, McCabe SJ. Kienböck disease and negative ulnar variance. *J Bone Joint Surg Am.* 1998;80(8):1154–1157.

Moran SL, Cooney WP, Berger RA, Bishop AT, Shin AY. The use of the 4 + 5 extensor compartmental vascularized bone graft for the treatment of Kienböck's disease. *J Hand Surg Am.* 2005;30(1):50–58.

Szabo RM, Greenspan A. Diagnosis and clinical findings of Kienbock's disease. *Hand Clin.* 1993;9(3):399–408.

Case 5

Friedman SL, Palmer AK. The ulnar impaction syndrome. *Hand Clin.* 1991;7(2):295–310.

Garcia-Elias M. Clinical examination of the ulnar-sided painful wrist. *Arthroscopic Management of Ulnar Pain.* Springer: Berlin, Heidelberg; 2012:25–44.

Köppel M, Hargreaves IC, Herbert TJ. Ulnar shortening osteotomy for ulnar carpal instability and ulnar carpal impaction. *J Hand Surg Br.* 1997;22(4):451–456.

Tomaino MM, Weiser RW. Combined arthroscopic TFCC debridement and wafer resection of the distal ulna in wrists with triangular fibrocartilage complex tears and positive ulnar variance. *J Hand Surg Am.* 2001;26(6):1047–1052.

Case 6

Atzei A. New trends in arthroscopic management of type 1-B TFCC injuries with DRUJ instability. *J Hand Surg Euro Vol.* 2009;34(5):582–591.

Boyer MI. *AAOS Comprehensive Orthopaedic Review 2.* Rosemont, IL: American Academy of Orthopaedic Surgeons, Copyright; 2014:1046.

Cannada LK. *Orthopaedic Knowledge Update 11.* Rosemont, IL: American Academy of Orthopaedic Surgeons, Copyright; 2014:435

Case 7

Ferris BL, Taylor LM Jr, Oyama K. Hypothenar hammer syndrome: proposed etiology. *J Vasc Surg.* 2000;31(1):104–113.

Pascarelli EF, Hsu YP. Understanding work-related upper extremity disorders: clinical findings in 485 computer users, musicians, and others. *J Occup Rehabil.* 2001;11(1):1–21.

Pineda CJ, Weisman MH, Bookstein JJ, Saltzstein SL. Hypothenar hammer syndrome. Form of reversible Raynaud's phenomenon. *Am J Med.* 1985;79(5):561–570.

Vayssairat M, Debure C, Cormier JM, Bruneval P, Laurian C, Juillet Y. Hypothenar hammer syndrome: seventeen cases with long-term follow-up. *J Vasc Surg.* 1987;5(6): 838–843.

Case 8

Masala S, et al. Diagnostic and therapeutic joint injections. *Seminars in Interventional Radiology.* Vol. 27. No. 2. Thieme Medical Publishers; 2010.

Tulipan DJ, Eaton RG, Eberhart RE. The Darrach procedure defended: technique redefined and long-term follow-up. *J Hand Surg Am.* 1991;16(3):438–444.

Case 9

Blue AI, Spira M, Hardy BS. Repair of extensor tendon injuries of the hand. *Am J Surg.* 1976;132(1):128–132.

Teoh LC, Yam AK. Anatomic reconstruction of the distal radioulnar ligaments: long-term results. *J Hand Surg Br.* 2005; 30(2):185–193.

Case 10

Boyer MI. *AAOS Comprehensive Orthopaedic Review 2.* Rosemont, IL: American Academy of Orthopaedic Surgeons, Copyright; 2014:1045–1046.

Ward LD, Ambrose CG, Masson MV, Levaro F. The role of the distal radioulnar ligaments, interosseous membrane, and joint capsule in distal radioulnar joint stability. *J Hand Surg Am.* 2000;25(2):341–351.

Watanabe H, Berger RA, Berglund LJ, Zobitz ME, An KN. Contribution of the interosseous membrane to distal radioulnar joint constraint. *J Hand Surg Am.* 2005;30(6): 1164–1171.

Case 11

Berger RA. The anatomy of the ligaments of the wrist and distal radioulnar joints. *Clin Orthop Relat Res.* 2001;(383): 32–40.

Carroll RE, Coyle MP Jr. Dysfunction of the pisotriquetral joint: treatment by excision of the pisiform. *J Hand Surg.* 1985;10(5):703–707.

Johnston GH, Tonkin MA. Excision of pisiform in pisotriquetral arthritis. *Clin Orthop Relat Res.* 1986;(210):137–142.

Tsai TM, Stilwell JH. Repair of chronic subluxation of the distal radioulnar joint (ulnar dorsal) using flexor carpi ulnaris tendon. *J Hand Surg Br.* 1984;9(3):289–294.

Case 12

Krakauer JD, Bishop AT, Cooney WP. Surgical treatment of scapholunate advanced collapse. *J Hand Surg Am.* 1994; 19(5):751–759.

Van Den Abbeele KL, Loh YC, Stanley JK, Trail IA. Early results of a modified Brunelli procedure for scapholunate instability. *J Hand Surg Br.* 1998;23(2):258–261.

Watson HK, Ballet FL. The SLAC wrist: scapholunate advanced collapse pattern of degenerative arthritis. *J Hand Surg Am.* 1984;9(3):358–365.

Watson HK, Weinzweig J. Physical examination of the wrist. *Hand Clin.* 1997;13(1):17–34.

Case 13

Cannada LK. *Orthopaedic Knowledge Update 11*. Rosemont, IL: American Academy of Orthopaedic Surgeons, Copyright; 2014:422, 435.

Sauerbier M, Bickert B, Tränkle M, Kluge S, Pelzer M, Germann G. [Surgical treatment possibilities of advanced carpal collapse (SNAC/SLAC wrist)]. *Unfallchirurg*. 2000; 103(7):564–571.

Wiesel SW, ed. *Operative Techniques in Orthopedic Surgery*. Philadelphia, PA: Lippincott, Williams and Wilkins, Copyright; 2011:2811.

Case 14

May MM, Lawton JN, Blazar PE. Ulnar styloid fractures associated with distal radius fractures: incidence and implications for distal radioulnar joint instability. *J Hand Surg Am*. 2002;27(6):965–971.

Orbay J. Volar plate fixation of distal radius fractures. *Hand Clin*. 2005;21(3):347–354.

Zenke Y, Sakai A, Oshige T, Moritani S, Nakamura T. The effect of an associated ulnar styloid fracture on the outcome after fixation of a fracture of the distal radius. *J Bone Joint Surg Br*. 2009;91(1):102–107.

Case 15

Cannada LK. *Orthopaedic Knowledge Update 11*. Rosemont, IL: American Academy of Orthopaedic Surgeons, Copyright; 2014:820–821.

Schmidt-Rohlfing B, Schwöbel B, Pauschert R, Niethard FU. Madelung deformity: clinical features, therapy and results. *J Pediatr Orthop B*. 2001;10(4):344–348.

Case 16

Andresen R, Radmer S, Scheufler O, Adam C, Bogusch G. [Optimization of conventional X-ray images for the detection of hook of hamate fractures]. *Rontgenpraxis*. 2005;56(2):59–65.

Andress MR, Peckar VG. Fracture of the hook of the hamate. *Br J Radiol*. 1970;43(506):141–143.

Bishop AT, Beckenbaugh RD. Fracture of the hamate hook. *J Hand Surg*. 1988;13(1):135–139.

Fredericson M, Kim BJ, Date ES, McAdams TR. Injury to the deep motor branch of the ulnar nerve during hook of hamate excision. *Orthopedics*. 2006;29(5):456.

Nisenfield FG, Neviaser RJ. Fracture of the hook of the hamate: a diagnosis easily missed. *J Trauma*. 1974;14(7):612-616.

Case 17

Boyer MI. *AAOS Comprehensive Orthopaedic Review 2*. Rosemont, IL: American Academy of Orthopaedic Surgeons, Copyright; 2014:348–349.

Thurston AJ, Dempsey SM. Bennett's fracture: a medium to long-term review. *Aust N Z J Surg*. 1993;63(2):120–123.

Case 18

Field J, Herbert TJ, Prosser R. Total wrist fusion: a functional assessment. *J Hand Surg Br*. 1996;21(4):429–433.

Louis DS, Hankin FM. Arthrodesis of the wrist: past and present. *J Hand Surg Am*. 1986;11(6):787–789.

Weiss AP, Hastings H 2nd. Wrist arthrodesis for traumatic conditions: a study of plate and local bone graft application. *J Hand Surg Am*. 1995;20(1):50–56.

Case 19

Boyer MI. *AAOS Comprehensive Orthopaedic Review 2*. Rosemont, IL: American Academy of Orthopaedic Surgeons, Copyright; 2014:358, 1057.

Boyer MI. *AAOS Comprehensive Orthopaedic Review 2*. Rosemont, IL: American Academy of Orthopaedic Surgeons, Copyright; 2014:356.

Case 20

Fischer J, Neville WT, Harrison JWK. *Traumatic Instability of the Wrist. Diagnosis, Classification, and Pathomechanics*. London: Springer; 2014.

Nakamura R, Hori M, Imamura T, Horii E, Miura T. Method for measurement and evaluation of carpal bone angles. *J Hand Surg Am*. 1989;14(2 Pt 2):412–416.

Patterson RM, Elder KW, Viegas SF, Buford WL. Carpal bone anatomy measured by computer analysis of three-dimensional reconstructions of computed tomography images. *J Hand Surg Am*. 1995;20(6):923–929.

Yeager BA, Dalinka MK. Radiology of trauma to the wrist: dislocations, fracture dislocations, and instability patterns. *Skeletal Radiol*. 1985;13(2):120–130.

Case 21

Boyer MI. *AAOS Comprehensive Orthopaedic Review 2*. Rosemont, IL: American Academy of Orthopaedic Surgeons, Copyright; 2014:1044.

Carroll RE, Coyle MP Jr. Dysfunction of the pisotriquetral joint: treatment by excision of the pisiform. *J Hand Surg*. 1985;10(5):703–707.

Case 22

Livesey JP, Norris SH, Page RE. First carpometacarpal joint arthritis: a comparison of two arthroplasty techniques. *J Hand Surg Br*. 1996;21(2):182–188.

Nylén S, Johnson A, Rosenquist AM. Trapeziectomy and Ligament Reconstruction for Osteoarthrosis of the Base of the Thumb A prospective study of 100 operations. *J Hand Surg Br*. 1993;18(5):616–619.

Van Heest AE, Kallemeier P. Thumb carpal metacarpal arthritis. *J Am Acad Orthop Surg*. 2008;16(3):140–151.

Yao J, Park MJ. Early treatment of degenerative arthritis of the thumb carpometacarpal joint. *Hand Clin*. 2008;24(3):251–261.

Case 23

Schumacher HR Jr, Dorwart BB, Korzeniowski OM. Occurrence of De Quervain's tendinitis during pregnancy. *Arch Intern Med*. 1985;145(11):2083.

Yuasa K, Kiyoshige Y. Limited surgical treatment of de Quervain's disease: decompression of only the extensor pollicisbrevissubcompartment.*JHandSurgAm*.1998;23(5): 840–843.

Case 24

Huffaker SJ, Christoforou DC, Jupiter JB. Spontaneous rupture of the extensor carpi radialis brevis in a 51-year-old man: case report. *J Hand Surg Am*. 2012;37(6): 1221–1224.

Park MJ, Namdari S, Weiss AP. The carpal boss: review of diagnosis and treatment. *J Hand Surg Am*. 2008;33(3): 446–449.

Türker T, Robertson GA, Thirkannad SM. A classification system for anomalies of the extensor pollicis longus. *Hand (NY)*. 2010;5(4):403–407.

Case 25

Alemohammad AM, Nakamura K, El-Sheneway M, Viegas SF. Incidence of carpal boss and osseous coalition: an anatomic study. *J Hand Surg Am*. 2009;34(1):1–6.

Laurencin CT, Cummings RS, Jones TR, Martin L. Fracture-dislocation of the lunotriquetral coalition. *J Natl Med Assoc*. 1998;90(12):779.

Simmons BP, McKenzie WD. Symptomatic carpal coalition. *J Hand Surg Am*. 1985;10(2):190–193.

Tsionos I, Drapé JL, Le Viet D. Bilateral pisiform-hamate coalition causing carpal tunnel syndrome and tendon attrition. *Acta Orthop Belg*. 2004;70(2):171–176.

Case 26

Boyer MI. *AAOS Comprehensive Orthopaedic Review 2*. Rosemont, IL: American Academy of Orthopaedic Surgeons, Copyright; 2014:1045.

Miller MD, ed. *Review of Orthopaedics*. 6th ed. Philadelphia, PA: WB Saunders; 2012:518.

Rockwell WB, Butler PN, Byrne BA. Extensor tendon: anatomy, injury, and reconstruction. *Plast Reconstr Surg*. 2000; 106(7):1592–1603.

Case 27

Calandruccio JH. Proximal row carpectomy. *J Am Soc Surg Hand*. 2001;1(2):112–122.

Halikis MN, Colello-Abraham K, Taleisnik J. Radiolunate fusion. The forgotten partial arthrodesis. *Clin Orthop Relat Res*. 1997;(341):30–35.

Rutgers M, Jupiter J, Ring D. Isolated posttraumatic ulnar translocation of the radiocarpal joint. *J Hand Microsurg*. 2009;1(2):108–112.

Case 28

De Smet L, Aerts P, Walraevens M, Fabry G. Avascular necrosis of the carpal scaphoid: Preiser's disease: report of 6 cases and review of the literature. *Acta Orthop Belg*. 1993;59(2):139–142.

Moran SL, Cooney WP, Shin AY. The use of vascularized grafts from the distal radius for the treatment of Preiser's disease. *J Hand Surg Am*. 2006;31(5):705–710.

Case 29

Belsole RJ. Radiography of the wrist. *Clin Orthop Relat Res*. 1986;(202):50–56.

Elsaidi G, Ruch DS, Kuzma GR, Smith BP. Dorsal wrist ligament insertions stabilize the scapholunate interval: cadaver study. *Clin Orthop Relat Res*. 2004;(425): 152–157.

Patterson RM, Elder KW, Viegas SF, Buford WL. Carpal bone anatomy measured by computer analysis of three-dimensional reconstructions of computed tomography images. *J Hand Surg Am*. 1995;20(6):923–929.

Case 30

Elgafy H, Ebraheim NA, Rezcallah AT, Yeasting RA. Posterior interosseous nerve terminal branches. *Clin Orthop Relat Res*. 2000;(376):242–251.

Homma T, Sakai T. Thenar and hypothenar muscles and their innervation by the ulnar and median nerves in the human hand. *Acta Anat (Basel)*. 1992;145(1):44–49.

McCabe SJ, Kleinert JM. The nerve of Henle. *J Hand Surg Am*. 1990;15(5):784–788.

Spinner M, Freundlich BD, Teicher J. Posterior interosseous nerve palsy as a complication of Monteggia fractures in children. *Clin Orthop Relat Res*. 1968;58: 141–146.

4

The Hand

Chaitanya S. Mudgal

CASE 1

A 28-year-old, right-hand-dominant male caught big air going off a jump while snowboarding for the first time. He landed awkwardly on his non-dominant left hand and immediately developed pain.

Radiographs were obtained at the slope side indicating multiple fractures in the hand (Fig. 4–1A and B).

He was then splinted and presented to your office on the fourth day after injury.

The most appropriate management at this time for this injury would be:

A. Short-arm splint for 6 weeks
B. Short-arm cast in intrinsic plus position for 6 weeks
C. Long-arm cast in intrinsic plus position for 6 weeks
D. Open reduction, internal fixation of all fractures

Discussion

The correct answer is (D). This patient has suffered multiple displaced metacarpal fractures in contiguous digits. The most appropriate treatment would be an open

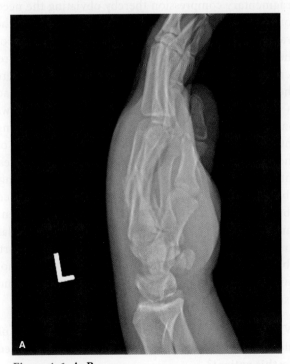

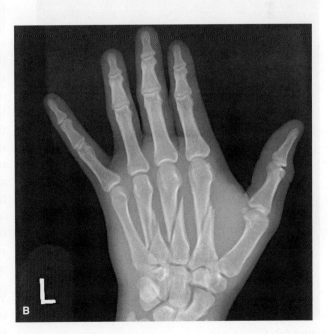

Figure 4–1 **A–B**

reduction and internal fixation in order to give the patient an earlier, rehabilitative start.

The reasons for open treatment of these contiguous fractures include which of the following?

A. Restoration of anatomy
B. Decompression of the interosseous muscles
C. Restoration of longitudinal length of metacarpals and the length–tension relationships of the intrinsic musculature
D. Restoration of the transverse arch of the hand
E. All of the above

Discussion

The correct answer is (E). The metacarpals in the hand have longitudinal arches and are arranged in the transverse arch such that the first metacarpal lies slightly volar to the second metacarpal with the apex of the arch forming at the level of the third metacarpal. In addition, the space between the metacarpals is occupied by the interossei, both the volar and dorsal. Displacement of multiple metacarpal fractures are associated with a significant degree of soft tissue swelling and are especially associated with high-energy injuries such as this one. Internal fixation of these contiguous, multiple metacarpal fractures allows for: restoration of both longitudinal

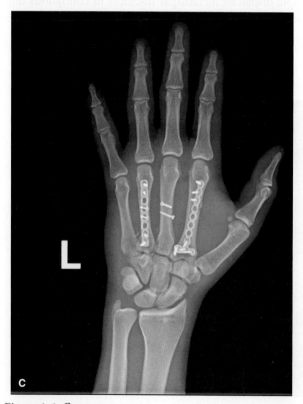

Figure 4–1 C

and transverse arches; decompression of the interosei to reduce swelling; restoration of longitudinal length and thereby the length-tension relationship of the intrinsic muscles; and restoration of the skeletal stability which allows for early rehabilitation of the hand, optimizing his functional outcome.

You notice that one of his fractures has been fixed with only interfragmentary screws while the other fractures have been fixed with plates and screws (Fig. 4–1C).

Basic requirements for fixation of a tubular bone shaft fracture in the hand using only interfragmentary screws include which of the following?

A. Length of the fracture should be more than twice the diameter of the bone at the central part of the fracture.
B. The amount of bone available around the head of the screw should be at least three times the size of the screw being utilized.
C. The screws must follow the spiral of the fracture.
D. All of the above.

Discussion

The correct answer is (D). When fixing fractures with interfragmentary screws only, it is critical that they be stable enough for early motion. Interfragmentary screws, when utilized appropriately, produce interfragmentary compression thereby obviating the need for plate neutralization. To do so, the length of the fracture should be more than twice the diameter of the bone in the middle of the fracture. Furthermore, screws should be placed in the part of the bone where the amount of bone available around the screw head is three times the size of the screw head. This allows one to exert compression from the screw head during interfragmentary compression without splitting of the bone from tightening the screw. In most instances, interfragmentary screws are suitable for either long, oblique fractures, fulfilling the criteria described above, or for spiral fractures. Therefore, interfragmentary screws, which are usually placed perpendicular to the fracture line, follow the line of the spiral. Short, oblique fractures and transverse fractures are not suited for just interfragmentary screw fixation and usually require the use of a neutralization plate.

Which of the following are possible complications of such an injury and of the surgical procedure utilized for this patient?

A. Stiffness of the interphalangeal joints
B. Problems due to soft tissue irritation from the hardware
C. Extensive tendon irritation
D. Stiffness of the metacarpophalangeal joints
E. All of the above

Discussion

The correct answer is (E). Multiple metacarpal fractures as mentioned above are high-energy injuries. Every effort should be made to fix them if they are displaced and to start early rehabilitation. Failure to do so is likely to cause stiffness of the small joints in the hand. This can occur not only due to the injury itself but from: the edema of the intrinsics; the resulting atony from the injury; the loss of the length–tension relationships of the intrinsics; as well as the stiffness that can occur from swelling, bleeding, and lack of use should these fractures be treated nonoperatively. Early rehabilitation after stable internal fixation allows for the treating surgeon to minimize all of these possibilities. Plates placed over the hand, especially the metacarpals, are known to cause difficulties with tendon irritation. It is therefore critical that, after placing the plate over the dorsal aspect of the metacarpal, every effort is made to cover the metacarpal with surrounding soft tissue, namely the interosseous fascia so as to insert a layer of soft tissue between the plate and the overlying extensor mechanism. Furthermore, plates placed very distally on the metacarpals are likely to interfere with the metacarpophalangeal joint capsule causing pain and resulting in stiffness. In some studies, problems associated with symptomatic hardware after metacarpal fracture fixation are as high as 40%. However, while tendon irritation associated with metacarpal plating remains a problem, routine removal of metacarpal plates, if asymptomatic, is not recommended.

Objectives: Did you learn...?

• Treat for multiple metacarpal fractures?
• Identify reasons for open reduction and internal fixation?
• Identify complications of open reduction and internal fixation?

CASE 2

An 18-month-old, male child comes to your office accompanied by his parents who have recently noticed that while he is using his hand, he appears unable to extend his thumb fully (Fig. 4–2A). The child is able to use his hand very well, does not appear to be in any pain, does not cry or fuss, and his sibling does not have a similar problem. Of note, the

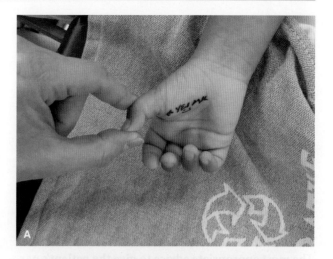

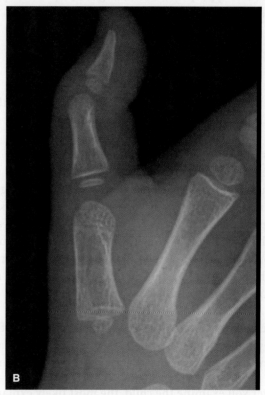

Figure 4–2 **A–B**

child was born full-term, and the mother reports that she had not seen this when the child was born. The other side remains unaffected. The x-ray is shown in Figure 4–2B.

The most likely diagnosis is:

A. Failure of development of extensive pollicis longus
B. Post-traumatic flexion contracture of the interphalangeal joint
C. Scar formation of the interphalangeal flexion crease
D. Trigger thumb
E. None of the above

Discussion

The correct answer is (D). This is a well-described and typical presentation for a trigger thumb in a child. Traditionally, trigger thumb was referred to as a congenital trigger thumb. However, there is increasing data showing that a large number of children who present with trigger thumb do not necessarily have it noted at birth. It has also been noted that developmental trigger thumb can occur in children. The exact nature of its causation remains unclear.

The parents are inquiring about treatment options and are confused about what the next step in treatment should be.

The most appropriate advice to give the patient's parents would be:

A. Nothing needs to be done
B. The child will grow out of it
C. Surgery within the next week
D. Surgery within the next month
E. Observation for 6 months, and if there is no further improvement, then consider surgery

Discussion

The correct answer is (E). Longitudinal studies on the natural history of trigger thumb suggest that most trigger thumbs that do not resolve by the age of 2 years, are likely to persist and are more likely to require surgical release. A thumb with a flexion contracture is an extremely common form of presentation, and the classical triggering with clicking and popping of the thumb in adults is not frequently noted in children.

The parents are also concerned about a swelling that they noticed over the volar aspect of the thumb, and they wonder if the child is developing a cyst in this area.

After you examine the child, the most likely explanation for the swelling would be:

A. Flexor sheath ganglion
B. Hypertrophic sesamoid
C. Notta's node
D. Subluxed metacarpophalangeal (MP) joint
E. None of the above

Discussion

The correct answer is (C). Pediatric patients with trigger thumb oftentimes will present with a localized thickening or a globular swelling over the volar aspect of the MP joint at the level of the A1 pulley. This is called a Notta's node. It

represents a thickening of the proximal pollicis longus and at the level of the A1 pulley as a response to the pulley's stenotic condition. In most circumstances, this thickening resolves with the passage of time after the A1 pulley has been released surgically. The patient and the parents need re-assurance that this is part of the entire process, does not represent a separate, pathological process, and that resolution is commonplace after A1 pulley release.

The patient returns to you at the age of 2½ years with no resolution of the thumb flexion deformity. At that stage, you elect to operatively release the A1 pulley of the thumb.

The structure which is most vulnerable to injury during the operative procedure is:

A. The flexor pollicis longus
B. The volar plate
C. The radial digital nerve
D. The ulnar digital nerve
E. All of the above

Discussion

The correct answer is (C). The radial digital nerve lies immediately subcutaneous along the MP flexion crease of the thumb. It must be noted that anatomically, when faced with the thumb in the palm up position, the flexor pollicis longus and the A1 pulley lie slightly more ulnar than would be obvious. Therefore, the incision has to be made at the MP joint flexion crease, slightly ulnar than expected. If the incision is placed a little more radial than planned, the surgeon is likely to encounter the radial digital nerve, and if not careful, the radial digital nerve which lies immediately subcutaneous is likely to get injured. The same condition applies to the adult trigger thumb release as well. During the consenting process for surgery, it is vital that patients who undergo trigger thumb release be alerted to the possibility of this occurrence, however rare.

Objectives: Did you learn...?

- Identify the clinical presentation of trigger thumb in a child?
- Treat initially for trigger thumb?
- Idenfity structures at risk during surgery?

CASE 3

A 24-year-old male sustained an injury to his right thumb while skiing. He was holding onto a ski pole when he fell going downhill. He immediately developed pain in the right thumb. He was seen at the mountainside and diagnosed to have a sprain. He presented to your office a week later because of ongoing pain and swelling in the thumb. Examination revealed a swollen metacarpophalangeal joint of the thumb, as well as swelling on the ulnar side of the metacarpophalangeal joint.

The most likely diagnosis is:

A. Sprain of the metacarpophalangeal joint
B. Volar plate injury
C. Gamekeeper's thumb
D. Extensor pollicis brevis rupture

Discussion

The correct answer is (C). This is a classic mechanism of injury, and although the description of a classic gamekeeper's thumb is a chronic injury to the ulnar collateral complex of the metacarpophalangeal joint of the thumb, in contemporary terms any injury to the ulnar collateral complex of the thumb metacarpophalangeal joint is classified as a gamekeeper's thumb. The more contemporary name for this condition is a skier's thumb, which implies an acute injury to the ulnar collateral complex of the thumb metacarpophalangeal joint. However, this injury can occur from various mechanisms of injury, skiing being one of them.

The pathoanatomy of gamekeeper's thumb consists of injuries to which of the following structures?

A. Ulnar collateral complex of the metacarpophalangeal joint of the thumb
B. Volar plate junction with the ulnar collateral complex
C. Dorsal capsule
D. All of the above

Discussion

The correct answer is (D). Although classically, the description of the injury is limited to the ulnar collateral complex of the thumb, one has to remember that the ulnar collateral complex is confluent with the volar plate at the volar ulnar corner and dorsally blends in with the dorsal capsule of the metacarpophalangeal joint. Therefore, in most circumstances an injury which spans the ulnar side of the thumb includes an injury not only to the ulnar collateral ligament itself but also to the accessory collateral ligament and its confluence with the volar plate.

If the injury extends dorsally, which occurs in most cases, the injury also includes the dorsal ulnar corner of the capsule of the metacarpophalangeal joint.

This patient had a swelling which was noted on the ulnar side of the metacarpophalangeal joint, and upon palpation it was a localized globular swelling.

This appearance is typically associated with which of the following?

A. Stener lesion
B. Rupture of the extensor pollicis brevis
C. Rupture and proximal retraction of the volar plate
D. None of the above

Discussion

The correct answer is (A). This is the typical clinical description of a Stener lesion. A Stener lesion is an injury of the ulnar collateral complex, which includes the distal avulsion from the base of the proximal phalanx as the thumb gets radial deviation force during the act of the injury. As the deviation force continues, the ulnar collateral ligament, which has now torn off the base of the proximal phalanx, continues proximal retraction and displacement, and the thumb deviates radially. The adductor aponeurosis, which is superficial to the ulnar collateral ligament, now gets interposed between the ulnar collateral ligament and the proximal phalanx base. As a result of this, the distally avulsed ulnar collateral ligament is now superficial to the adductor aponeurosis and may sometimes be rolled upon itself giving a globular appearance, which is clinically palpable on the ulnar side of the metacarpal head. Although this appearance can signify a Stener lesion, it does not always occur, and its absence does not indicate the lack of a Stener lesion.

The most appropriate treatment for this patient would be:

A. Short-arm thumb spica cast
B. Long-arm thumb spica cast
C. Open repair of the ulnar collateral complex
D. External fixation of the metacarpophalangeal joint
E. None of the above

Discussion

The correct answer is (C). This patient has a gamekeeper's thumb with a localized globular swelling over the metacarpal head on the ulnar side, indicating the presence of a Stener lesion. Given the pathoanatomy of the Stener lesion wherein the adductor aponeurosis is interposed between the ulnar collateral complex and the original proximal phalangeal attachment of the ligament, such an injury is highly unlikely to heal and almost inevitably leads to ongoing ulnar-sided instability of the metacarpophalangeal joint. Therefore, extraction of this ligament, re-positioning it deep to the adductor aponeurosis, and repairing it to the base of the proximal phalanx would be the most appropriate treatment so as to establish ulnar-sided stability of the metacarpophalangeal joint.

Objectives: Did you learn...?

- Identify clinical presentation of game keepers thumb?
- Identify the pathoanatomy of gamekeepers thumb?
- Understand the clinical description of Stener lesions?
- Treatment of Stener lesions?

CASE 4

A 54-year-old, male banker was traveling in a bus when it jerked to a sudden stop. In an effort to stop himself from falling, he held onto the overhead bar. However, he continued to fall, and in trying to hold onto the overhead bar, he noticed immediate onset of pain in his ring finger. Thereafter, he was unable to flex it fully, immediately developed pain and swelling, and presented to your office 4 days later with a swollen and painful ring finger (Fig. 4–3B). Examination revealed a swollen finger with bruising over the pulp (Fig. 4–3A). He was able to flex his proximal interphalangeal (PIP) joint to some extent, but was unable to flex his distal interphalangeal (DIP) joint. Radiographs did not show any bony injury of the finger.

The most likely diagnosis is:

A. Sprain of the DIP joint
B. Avulsion of the profundus tendon from its attachment to the base of the distal phalanx
C. Dislocation of the DIP joint
D. Fracture of the distal phalanx

Discussion

The correct answer is (B). This injury is also known as a "jersey finger" when the profundus tendon is detached from the base of the distal phalanx. Such patients usually present with a swollen digit and usually with bruising of the pulp. They also demonstrate lack of profundus function and the inability to flex the DIP joint. In this patient, the radiographs were unremarkable. Therefore, he does not have either a DIP dislocation or a fracture.

After evaluating the patient, the next step in management of this injury would be:

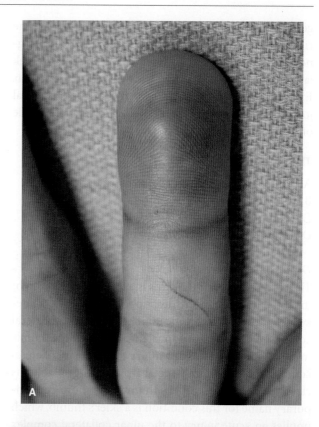

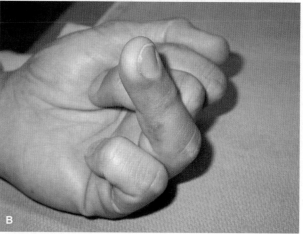

Figure 4–3 **A–B**

A. Gentle rehabilitation
B. Splinting for 3 weeks followed by a range of motion program
C. Open repair of the avulsed profundus tendon
D. Pinning of the DIP joint in 30 degrees of flexion
E. Primary arthrodesis of the DIP joint.

Discussion

The correct answer is (C)—early open repair of the avulsed profundus tendon. Profundus tendon avulsions are described by Leddy and Packer to be of three basic types. In type 1, the flexor tendon, which is avulsed, retracts into the palm at or proximal to the level of the A1 pulley. In type 2, the tendon is trapped at the level of the A3 pulley at the level of the PIP joint. In type 3, the tendon is usually retracted only minimally and usually lies at the level of the A4 pulley just proximal to the DIP joint. Other types include bony avulsions of the profundus tendon with a piece of the distal phalangeal base still attached to it. These usually tend to retract very minimally. In more complex types, the patient can also have avulsion of the tendon from the fragment of the bone that has also been avulsed, and in a more complex type, the distal phalangeal shaft itself can also fracture. The ideal time to repair these profundus avulsions is as soon as possible, and it appears that these are best done within the first week to 10 days. Thereafter, the musculotendinous unit undergoes a significant degree of myostatic shortening, and it may not be possible to restore the profundus tendon back to its attachment at the base of the distal phalanx, especially if the avulsion is a type 1.

Factors that adversely affect outcome of profundus avulsion include which of the following?

A. Type of avulsion
B. Time since injury
C. Presence of a bony fragment
D. Loss of vincular blood supply
E. All of the above

Discussion

The correct answer is (E). As mentioned above, outcomes are reported to be better in patients who undergo early repair, after which restoring the tendon to its attachment at the base of the distal phalanx can be extremely difficult. Furthermore, avulsions that retract to the level of the A1 or proximal to the A1 can do so only after the vincule, which supplies the tendon, are ruptured. This does affect tendon vascularity and nourishment and may adversely affect tendon healing to site of attachment. Therefore, delayed presentations and type 1 ruptures can have poorer outcomes. Furthermore, bony avulsions are likely to have better outcomes if there is a single large bony fragment, which can be restored back into its bed at the base of the distal phalanx. This is because bony healing remains a lot more predictable, and stable bony healing and fixation can be achieved to allow early mobilization. In most circumstances with the soft tissue the avulsion of the tendon without any bony fragment the tendon has to be re-attached to the base of the distal philanx either with the help of a pullout suture which is tied over a button on the dorsal aspect of the nail plate or with the help of mini-suture anchors. Biomechanical studies have shown that suture anchor repair has the same mechanical strength as a pullout suture.

Which of the following are likely associated complications of this injury?

A. Stiffness of the PIP joint
B. Stiffness of the DIP joint
C. Instability of the DIP joint
D. Nail plate deformity
E. All of the above

Discussion

The correct answer is (E). Avulsions of the profundus tendon which retract to the level of the A3 pulley or even further proximally, can compromise pull through of the FDS tendon and thereby affect flexion and extension of the PIP joint as well. This may leave the patient not only with loss of DIP flexion but may also compromise PIP flexion from the scarred tendon in the flexor sheath. Stiffness of the DIP from lack of flexion also remains a distinct possibility. In some circumstances, these patients can develop delayed instability of the DIP joint from imbalance of an extensor which is able to extend the distal phalanx in the absence of a flexor which would normally flex the distal phalanx. This instability can be disabling, and in most circumstances, once the patient develops instability, DIP arthrodesis remains a solution. Finally, patients who undergo repair of the profundus tendon with the help of a pullout suture should be cautioned preoperatively about the possibility of a dystrophic nail. This can occur if the pullout suture passes through the germinal matrix, in which case the patient may develop a dystrophic nail (Fig. 4–4).

Objectives: Did you learn...?

- Identify the clinical presentation of avulsion of the profundus tendon?
- Describe the factors that affect the outcome of profundus avulsion?
- Understand the complications of these injury?

CASE 5

A 30-year-old male fell while he was out for a run. He landed awkwardly on his left thenar eminence sustaining an injury to this area. There were some abrasions over the base of the thenar eminence when he presented to the office 3 days later. On examination, you noted that the abrasions were healing, and you obtained a radiograph shown in Figure 4-4.

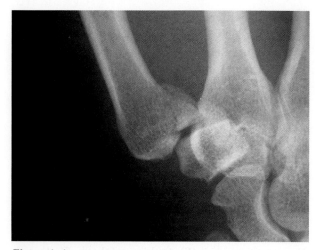

Figure 4–4

The most likely diagnosis is:

A. Bennett's fracture
B. Avulsion of the oblique ligament
C. Dislocation of the carpometacarpal (CMC) joint
D. None of the above

Discussion

The correct answer is (A). This injury, in which there is an intra-articular fracture at the base of the first metacarpal accompanied by subluxation of the metacarpal at the CMC joint, is called a Bennett's fracture-dislocation. The fragment is on the volar ulnar corner, the attachment of the volar-oblique ligament at the CMC joint. The fragment itself remains in position and is not displaced. The metacarpal shaft is displaced, causing a joint subluxation or dislocation.

The deforming forces on the metacarpal include which of the following?

A. Extensor pollicis brevis
B. Abductor pollicis longus and adductor pollicis
C. Abductor pollicis brevis
D. Extensor pollicis longus
E. All of the above

Discussion

The correct answer is (B). Although the deforming force on the base of the metacarpal is the abductor pollicis longus causing subluxation of the metacarpal base at the CMC joint, the adductor pollicis also can act as a deforming force adducting the head of the metacarpal and thereby narrowing the first web space and influencing the deformity. The abductor pollicis longus has an uncontrolled pull on the first metacarpal base. These fractures are unstable and the metacarpal base can continue to subluxate or dislocate.

The most appropriate next step in the management of this patient would be which of the following?

A. Closed reduction and cast application
B. Closed reduction and splint application
C. Closed reduction and percutaneous pin fixation
D. Open reduction, internal fixation
E. All of the above

Discussion

The correct answer is (E). In fractures that are either undisplaced or minimally displaced and the joint is not subluxed to a large extent, it is possible to perform a closed reduction and a carefully molded cast or splint may be able to hold the reduction. However, due to the instability of this injury, oftentimes it is not possible to hold this injury for the 4-week period that it would take for the fracture to heal. Therefore, the most common, appropriate step would be to splint the patient in the emergency room and advise them of the possibility for surgical fixation. The choice of surgical fixation is variable and largely surgeon-dependent. There is no data to suggest the superiority of one technique over another. The simplest technique would be to perform a closed reduction and pin it such that the fracture is allowed to heal and the joint is held in the reduced position for a period of 4 to 6 weeks in a short-arm cast. The pin is then pulled, and rehabilitation commences. Open reduction internal fixation also remains a viable option. However, it does require a much larger procedure, and in situations where the fragments are extremely small, screws may not obtain an adequate purchase. In the case shown here, the fragment was large enough that it was possible to fix internally with the help of screws.

The reduction maneuver for this fracture consists of which of the following?

A. Abduction at the CMC joint
B. Pronation of the metacarpal
C. Pressure on the base of the metacarpal
D. All of the above

Discussion

The correct answer is (D). The metacarpal is displaced such that it is migrating proximally. Therefore, length has to be restored with the help of traction. Once length is restored, the metacarpal has to be brought back into the joint by placing pressure on the metacarpal base. As explained before, the adductor pollicis can cause the head of the metacarpal to adduct into the web space. Therefore, abduction allows the metacarpal base to achieve proximity with the Bennett fragment. Finally, the metacarpal must be pronated so that the fracture surfaces are allowed to approximate each other. Therefore, the correct maneuver consists of: traction; abduction of the metacarpal; pressure at the base; pronation of the metacarpal, allowing accurate approximation of fracture surfaces; and then pinning of the joint. Pinning of the fragment is not mandatory. Simply holding the joint in the reduced position so that the fragment and the parent bone are well approximated allows the fracture to unite uneventfully and the joint to be stabilized.

Objectives: Did you learn...?

- Pinpoint the radiographic features of a Bennett's fracture?
- Determine the deforming forces on the metacarpals?
- Perform the reduction maneuvers for Bennett's fractures?

CASE 6

A 21-year-old male was involved in an altercation. During the course of this altercation, he struck a hard object after missing his opponent. He immediately developed pain over the ulnar side of his hand and was seen in the emergency room. X-rays are shown (Fig. 4–5A and B).

The most likely diagnosis is:

A. Fracture of the fifth metacarpal shaft
B. Fracture of the fifth metacarpal neck
C. Dislocation of the fifth CMC joint
D. None of the above

Discussion

The correct answer is (B). This patient has sustained a fifth metacarpal neck fracture. This fracture is also known as a "boxer's fracture." It usually occurs from impact of the ulnar side of the hand against a hard object, leading to a sudden flexion force on the fifth metacarpal neck and distal shaft that results in a fracture of the fifth metacarpal in the very distal shaft or in the neck, with dorsal angulation of the apex. Most commonly, the patient does not have malrotation but tends to have an angulatory deformity.

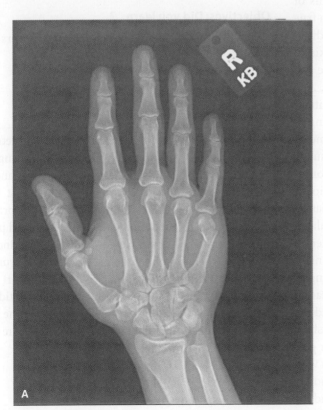
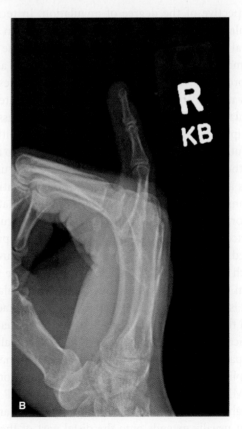

Figure 4–5 **A–B**

A decision is made to treat the patient. Which of the following factors affect the treatment of this patient?

A. Measurement of the angulation at the fracture site
B. Presence of an open wound
C. Presence of malrotation
D. All of the above

Discussion

The correct answer is (D). Association of an open wound over a fracture dictates that the fracture should be considered an open fracture unless proven otherwise. Fractures that are open should be addressed expeditiously and emergently with irrigation and debridement of the open wound. Repair of the lacerated structures, if any, and treatment of the fracture (either with closed reduction and percutaneous pin fixation or with open reduction/internal fixation depending on the location, nature of fracture, and degree of comminution) should then be addressed. Should the injury be closed, then the degree of angulation and the presence of malrotation are essential features in decision-making. If the patient presents with malrotation, which is extremely uncommon, the fracture needs to be reduced and either pinned percutaneously or fixed internally in an open manner irrespective of the degree of angulation. In terms of angulation, these fractures are best measured on a true lateral view. A line is drawn along the axis of the distal fragment, and a line is also drawn along the axis of the proximal fragment. The angle formed by these two lines depicts the angulation at the fracture site. Any angulation in excess of 30 to 40 degrees necessitates manipulative reduction followed by either splinting or percutaneous pin fixation. A common error is to measure the angulation in an oblique view, which usually gives an erroneous impression, with magnification of the angulation leading to unnecessary manipulations.

North American literature suggests that angulation in excess of 30 to 40 degrees should be manipulated closed. This is done utilizing the Jahss maneuver in which the fracture site is anesthetized with the instillation of a hematoma block, the metacarpophalangeal joint is flexed, and pressure is applied on the metacarpal head through the proximal phalanx so as to extend the metacarpal head and align it with the metacarpal shaft. The patient's hand is then immobilized in an ulnar gutter splint, holding the finger in the correct position with the MP joint flexed 80 to 90 degrees and the IP joints straight. This is called the intrinsic plus position, and the splint usually extends onto the distal part of the forearm. Angulations of less than 30 degrees do not need manipulation and can simply be splinted and followed with radiographs on a weekly basis.

The most common complication encountered after such an injury is:

A. Avascular necrosis of the metacarpal head
B. Instability of metacarpophalangeal joint
C. Malrotation
D. Angulation apex dorsal at the fracture site

Discussion

The correct answer is (D). In most circumstances, these fractures unite in the position in which they presented in if no treatment had been carried out. This is usually an apex dorsal deformity, and in rare circumstances, patients may complain of a palmar prominence of the metacarpal head, especially during power gripping activities. Despite this angulation, most patients have very satisfactory clinical outcomes with essentially full range of motion. During the recovery period, it is not uncommon for patients to have difficulty achieving complete extension of the metacarpophalangeal joint, which does resolve with the passage of time. However, angulations which are excessive may be associated with a pseudo-claw deformity.

Objectives: Did you learn...?

- Identify the radiographic features of a Boxers fracture?
- Describe complications of this injury?

CASE 7

A retired, 80-year-old, Caucasian, male obstetrician is asked to see you for a painful and swollen fingertip. Three days ago, he noticed the onset of swelling and this was followed by the development of a fluctuant swelling over the dorsal aspect of the DIP joint. His primary care doctor diagnosed him with an infection and placed him on oral antibiotics. He continues to have increasing pain. There is some redness, but he denies running any fever. Of note, he is otherwise healthy apart from being hypertensive and taking hydrochlorothiazide. He denies having any other past medical history. The clinical appearance and radiograph are shown in Figure 4–6A and B.

The mostly likely diagnosis is:

A. Acute paronychia
B. Pyoarthrosis of the DIP joint

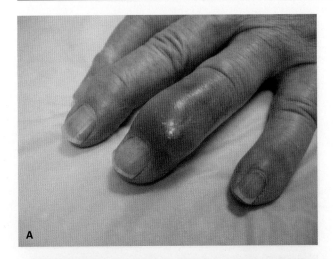

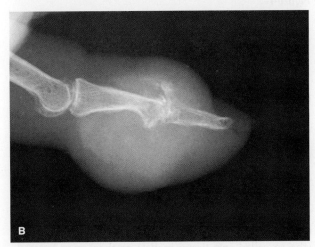

Figure 4–6 **A–B**

C. Acute tophaceous gout
D. Cellulitis
E. Cutaneous wart

Discussion
The correct answer is (C). This appearance is typical of acute tophaceous gout in a patient in this age group. There is increasing evidence to show that acute tophaceous gout of the distal interphalangeal (DIP) joint is the first form of presentation in the elderly. This is typically seen in patients over the age of 70, with a pre-existing arthritic DIP joint, and who happen to be on diuretics. Gout is a disorder of purine metabolism in which there is deposition of monosodium biurate crystals in areas which are affected by arthritis. The DIP joint is one of the most commonly affected joints in the hand and therefore appears to be particularly prone to developing symptoms of acute tophaceous gout.

The most appropriate management at this stage would be to do which of the following?

A. Stop oral antibiotics and switch to intravenous antibiotics
B. Starting the patient on oral antigout medication such as allopurinol
C. Drainage of acute tophaceous gout, confirmation of the diagnosis, and starting the patient on acute gout medication such as colchicine
D. Emergent irrigation, excision, and debridement in the operating room with fusion of the DIP joint

Discussion
The correct answer is (C). Although the appearance is fairly typical and may be considered classic, it is important to confirm the diagnosis. Inflammatory markers can be elevated in gout and the uric acid levels are not always elevated. It is therefore important to acquire a fluid sample and examine it under the microscope to see the needle-shaped, negatively birefringent, monosodium biurate crystals. The technique for asipration described by Mudgal involves the placement of two large bore needles proximal to the tophaceous area without disturbing the thin, soft tissue envelope over the tophaceous area. The large bore needles allow aspiration of the material and allow the soft tissue envelope to collapse on itself. The DIP joint is then held splinted and wrapped so as to allow egress of the material. The patient is encouraged to begin soaks on a daily basis. The holes made by the needles usually don't close for a couple days, and the saline soaks allow the material to be washed out. Gout crystals being water soluble helps in reduction of the tophus burden. After this has been done, the patient's joint is splinted and edema control is achieved with the help of elasticated wraps.

The fluid shows the presence of crystals confirming the diagnosis of gout. The patient is started on medication for his gout including colchicine and allopurinol. Eight weeks later, the patient comes in to see you, and the appearance of the digit is much better than before. However, he continues to have a painful, unstable joint, and he wonders if he can have something done so that he may be able to use the finger in a more effective fashion.

The next step in management would be which of the following?

A. QuickCast application for 8 weeks
B. Orthoplast splint application for the rest of his life

C. No active treatment required since the patient is not working

D. Arthrodesis of the DIP joint

Discussion

The correct answer is (D). The patient, albeit retired, is active and functioning. He has a painful and unstable DIP joint. Radiographs demonstrate that this joint is an extremely arthritic joint. Therefore, this joint is a non-salvageable joint and is unlikely to have any motion that is meaningful. All these criteria make him an excellent candidate for DIP arthrodesis. Multiple techniques have been described for DIP arthrodesis including the use of wires, steel wires, and headless screws. DIP arthrodesis can be done by open techniques or by percutaneous techniques. In situations where there is no obvious deformity but there is instability and the joint is collinear, percutaneous arthrodesis is indicated. A headless screw is placed from the tip of the distal phalanx, across the DIP joint and into the medullary canal of the middle phalanx. Excellent compression is generated and, since the joint has no meaningful articular cartilage, these patients go on to develop arthrodesis over the course of the next 3 to 4 months. Percutaneous arthrodesis is a well-described technique and is suitable only for patients who have an extremely arthritic and/or painful joint without a static deformity. If the deformity of the DIP joint is fixed and noncorrectable, these patients are not suitable for percutaneous arthrodesis and need to have a formal open arthrodesis, whereby the joint surfaces are resected, the joint is realigned, and then a fusion is performed.

Objectives: Did you learn...?

- Distinguish the clinical presentation of acute tophaceous gout?
- Initially treat acute tophaceous gout?
- Determine definitive treatment?

CASE 8

A 17-year-old male sustained an injury to his middle finger while catching a football. When examined by his coach on the field, it was felt to be a sprain, and he continued playing the game. After he finished the game, he was noted to have a finger bent at the distal interphalangeal joint, and he was unable to straighten it (Fig. 4–7). He was seen in the emergency room where x-ray showed no obvious fracture. He was then splinted and asked to see you in consultation.

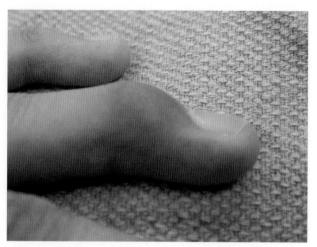

Figure 4–7

The most likely diagnosis in this situation is:

A. DIP joint dislocation

B. Flexor profundus avulsion

C. Mallet finger

D. Sprain of the DIP joint

Discussion

The correct answer is (C). This is a typical presentation of a mallet finger. A mallet finger is an injury which affects the insertion of the terminal extensor mechanism onto the base of the distal phalanx. This can present as avulsion of the tendon without a bony fragment being attached (the so-called soft tissue mallet) or there may be avulsion of a bony fragment (also known as a bony mallet). In this instance, the patient had x-rays that did not show any bony injury, so this would qualify as a soft tissue mallet.

The patient is noted to have no ability to extend his DIP joint actively; however, passive extension is full. The patient wishes to continue playing football.

The most appropriate management at this time would be which of the following?

A. Application of a tip protector splint maintaining the DIP joint at neutral and the PIP joint free

B. Closed reduction and percutaneous pin fixation of the DIP joint

C. Open repair of the extensor mechanism

D. Open repair and pinning of the DIP joint

Discussion

The correct answer is (A). A soft tissue mallet, such as this one, can be treated nonoperatively. The patient's sporting interest should not factor significantly in the decision making process. Should the patient have any degree of subluxation, which would be seen on the lateral radiograph of the finger, then the most appropriate recommendation would be to perform a closed reduction, realign the joint, and pin it. However, in this case where the lateral radiograph does not show any evidence of subluxation and there is no evidence of bony injury, such an injury can be treated effectively with a splint. There are numerous splints available for the treatment of soft tissue mallets. In the experience of this group of authors, a quick-setting, fiberglass cast application, which maintains the DIP joint at neutral and leaves the PIP joint free, is extremely effective in treating this condition. The patient and his family should be cautioned that irrespective of the duration of treatment and irrespective of the method of treatment, in most circumstances this injury heals with a slight dorsal bump and a slight droop with lack of the terminal few degrees of extension.

On the day the patient comes to see you, he is accompanied by one of his colleagues who also sustained a similar injury but whose x-rays show that he has a bony avulsion of the distal phalanx base. The size of the fragment involves about 30% to 40% of the articular surface, and there is no evidence of any joint subluxation.

The most appropriate recommendation for this patient would be which of the following?

A. Open repair of the bony avulsion
B. Closed reduction and percutaneous pin fixation of the bony avulsion
C. Treatment with a splint
D. Open repair and trans-articular pinning

Discussion

The correct answer is (C). This patient has a bony avulsion. While some investigators believe that the size of the fragment is important in the decision-making about the need for internal fixation, there is no evidence to suggest that fragment size affects the long-term outcome. However, subluxation of the joint does affect long-term outcome as it promotes early degeneration. In this particular instance, the lateral radiograph does not show any evidence of subluxation. Therefore, although this patient has a bony mallet and the fragment appears to be 35% to 40% of the articular surface, this can also be treated nonoperatively. A similar cast, as applied to the other patient, is applied on this patient as well. Most bony mallets tend to heal in a more predictable fashion and over a shorter duration of time (4 weeks), whereas soft tissue mallets tend to require

longer duration of splinting. It also appears that bony mallets tend to have a lesser droop and a smaller dorsal bump than soft tissue mallets. In both instances, the indications for internal fixation are the presence of subluxation of the joint. Patients who present early can have the subluxation reduced in the operating room, and the joint may be pinned, disregarding the size of the fragment and allowing the joint to heal in its anatomical position. However, should the subluxation not be reducible, a formal open reduction and joint reduction as well as internal fixation needs to be performed.

Objectives: Did you learn...?
*   Identify clinical presentation of Mallet finger?
*   Treat Mallet finger?

CASE 9

A 34-year-old female got into an altercation in a pub. During the course of the altercation, she struck a mirror sustaining a laceration to the dorsal aspect of her hand as shown in Figure 4–8. She presents to you now a few days out from the injury with difficulty in hand function. She is otherwise healthy, has no other medical problems, and has been in a splint to the fingertips.

The most likely cause of her dysfunction is:

A. Splint-related stiffness affecting all the joints in the hand
B. Pain inhibition leading to loss of function in the hand
C. Extensor tendon lacerations of the middle and ring fingers
D. Reflex sympathetic dystrophy
E. None of the above

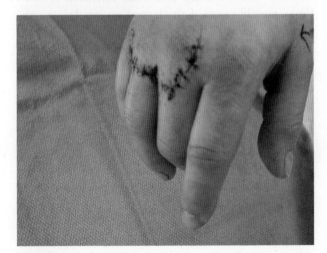

Figure 4–8

Discussion

The correct answer is (C). This patient has sustained a laceration across the dorsal aspect of the MP joint of the hand. When the hand is formed into a fist, the extensor tendons are immediately subcutaneous. It is therefore extremely common for any laceration in this area, which runs across the long axis of the extensor mechanism, to sever the extensor mechanism of the fingers partially if not completely. The appearance is fairly typical. In most circumstances, patients are unable to extend their fingers fully at the metacarpophalangeal joint. Should there be any doubt about the ability to extend the metacarpophalangeal joints, infiltration of local anesthetic in this area and an examination in the office can reveal the weakness of extension. The ability to maintain extension against resistance is also a good test, and patients who have partial injury will often times be unable to maintain extension against resistance, the so-called piano key sign.

You have made a clinical diagnosis of extensor tendon injury. The most appropriate form of management at this stage would be which of the following?

A. Short-arm cast with the metacarpophalangeal joints at neutral and the interphalangeal joints free
B. Short-arm cast to the fingertips with all joints at neutral
C. Exploration and open repair of affected structures
D. Dynamic splinting with early range of motion program

Discussion

The correct answer is (C). This patient has a clinical examination consistent with extensor tendon lacerations. It must be noted that weak extension is often times possible even if the laceration involves a substantial amount of the extensor tendon. Another reason to have weak extension is for the patient to be able to extend the digit through the juncturae. The juncturae attach to the extensor mechanism, and should there be a laceration proximal to the junctura, then the patient may still be able to demonstrate extension of the affected digit by using the extensor of the neighboring digit and pulling through the junctura. In this particular circumstance, the patient's hand needs to be explored further, and the extensor mechanism needs to be repaired.

The patient is taken to the operating room and the extensor mechanism of the middle and ring fingers are noted to be completely lacerated. After repair, the patient is called back to the office for a postoperative follow-up on the fifth day following surgery.

At this stage, the most appropriate form of postoperative rehabilitation and management would be which of the following?

A. Short-arm cast, MCP joints at neutral, and PIP joints free
B. Dynamic splinting with range of motion program
C. Short-arm splint with MCP joint at neutral, and PIP joints free
D. All of the above

Discussion

The correct answer is (D). While surgeon preferences may dictate which type of rehabilitation is performed on the patient, there is no conclusive evidence to show the superiority of one method of rehabilitation of extensor tendon injuries in this particular zone. Extensor tendon injuries are classified into zones 1 through 8 with the odd numbers lying over the distal interphalangeal (DIP), proximal interphalangeal (PIP), metacarpohalangeal (MCP) and the wrist joint, respectively, whereas the even numbers lie over the middle phalanx, proximal phalanx, metacarpals and proximal to the wrist. Extensor tendon injuries in zones 4 and 5 are commonly seen in patients who sustain punching injuries against a sharp object as described in this case. Postoperatively, after repair, these injuries can be immobilized for a period of 3 weeks before starting a range of motion program, and the immobilization can be done either in a splint or a cast. On the other hand, there is some data to suggest that early rehabilitation with dynamic splinting protocol is superior in terms of early recovery of motion.

Objectives: Did you learn...?

• Pinpoint the clinical presentation of extensor tendon laceration?
• Treat extensor tendon lacerations?
• Establish appropriate postoperative rehabilitation?

CASE 10

A 14-year-old male was playing basketball and went up for a rebound. As he reached for the ball, he immediately developed pain in his ring finger and noticed a deformity. He was unable to generate any motion. Clinical appearance and a lateral radiograph taken in the emergency room are shown in Figure 4–9A and B.

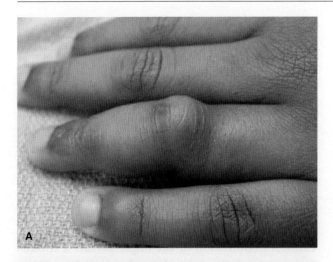

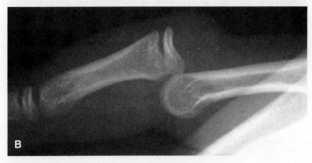

Figure 4–9 **A–B**

The correct diagnosis is:

A. Dorsal dislocation of the PIP
B. Complex PIP dislocation
C. Rupture of the flexor digitorum superficialis
D. Rupture of the volar plate
E. None of the above

Discussion

The correct answer is (A). This patient has sustained a dorsal dislocation of his PIP joint. This injury is commonly associated with ball-associated sports, namely during blocking while playing volleyball, trying to catch a football, or while playing basketball during the act of either accepting a pass or rebounding. These are the most commonly described mechanisms, but this injury can also be sustained by other mechanisms, such as a fall. During the course of dorsal dislocation of the PIP, there is inevitably an injury to the volar plate as well as both collateral ligaments. The most common dislocation is in a dorsal direction with the base of the middle phalanx lying dorsal to the head of the proximal phalanx. In some circumstances, there might be an angulatory displacement as well. Motion is usually limited secondary to the joint being dislocated as well as pain from the injury itself.

The most appropriate treatment at this time would be:

A. Closed reduction and percutaneous pin fixation
B. Open reduction and internal fixation
C. Closed reduction and assessment of stability
D. Open reduction and volar plate repair

Discussion

The correct answer is (C). In most circumstances, a simple closed dislocation of the PIP joint can be reduced closed. The stability of the joint is thereafter assessed, and again, in most circumstances, the joint is stable. It is not uncommon for the patient to be able to range the joint fully. The dislocation is best reduced closed in the emergency room. The finger is anesthetized with the help of a digital block. The MP joint is then flexed to relax the intrinsics, and with the combination of gentle traction on the fingertip as well as a milking maneuver over the dorsal aspect of the middle phalanx, it is possible to reduce the middle phalanx back into joint with the proximal phalanx. Thereafter, the patient is assessed in terms of stability and range of motion, and in most circumstances, it is possible to simply splint the patient with the joint slightly flexed for a couple of days to let the swelling and the pain settle down. Thereafter, with buddy taping to the neighboring digit, the patient may start a range of motion program. In some circumstances, the joint may be unstable at the extremes of extension. In these situations, the patient is splinted with the joint slightly flexed to about 15 to 20 degrees, and the finger is gradually straightened out to achieve full extension over the course of about 2 to 3 weeks.

The most common sequela from this injury includes which of the following?

A. Some soreness for a few months
B. Residual swelling for a few months
C. Residual stiffness for a few months
D. All of the above

Discussion

The correct answer is (D). Most simple closed dorsal dislocations of the PIP can be reduced closed, and patients start on a range of motion program, as mentioned above, within the first few days. In most circumstances, patients regain motion within the first 3 weeks. However, it is not uncommon for some degree of soreness, swelling, and terminal stiffness to persist for several months. However, it has been noted that younger patients regain motion sooner and also do not have the same degree of residual stiffness and soreness as older patients. In addition to starting a range of motion program, it is beneficial to start the patient on an edema control program. This can be done by an experienced occupational therapist. In most circumstances, the range of motion program can be done unsupervised as a home exercise program.

The same patient could also present with a similar injury with an angulatory deformity, rotary deformity, and a lateral radiograph which does not confirm dorsal dislocation.

In this situation, the most likely diagnosis is:

A. Complex dislocation of the PIP joint
B. Rupture of only one collateral complex
C. Rupture of the volar plate
D. Rupture of the flexor digitorum superficialis
E. None of the above

Discussion

The correct answer is (A). Complex dislocation of the PIP joint usually involves buttonholing of the proximal phalanx head through the dorsal extensor mechanism. In such situations, the head of the condyle of the proximal phalanx usually buttonholes in the gap between the central tendon and the lateral band, and as a result, the head of the proximal phalanx is actually trapped in the noose formed by the central tendon and the lateral band. Attempts at reducing these with a combination of traction and corrective force can actually render the dislocation irreducible on account of tightening of the soft tissues around the buttonholed head of the proximal phalanx. Should simple, gentle manipulation not reduce these in the emergency room, most of these injuries require a formal open reduction. This is usually done through a dorsal approach, and the head of the proximal phalanx is immediately obvious as having buttonholed through the gap between the central tendon and lateral band. Gently elevating the lateral band allows prompt reduction of the proximal phalanx into the joint. These injuries thereafter require repair of the extensor mechanism and pinning of the joint provisionally for 2 to 3 weeks while the extensor mechanism heals. In most circumstances, these injuries in younger patients, as described in this situation, are likely to lead to very satisfactory outcomes with near full range of motion.

Objectives: Did you learn...?

- Describe the clinical and radiographic presentation of dislocation of the PIP joint?

- Treat PIP dislocation?
- Identify sequela from this type of injury?

CASE 11

A 26-year-old female was traveling with her fiancé. At a rest stop, as she got out of the car, he accidentally shut the car door on her left ring finger. There was immediate swelling and bleeding, and after application of first aid, the finger remained swollen and the patient is now here to see you. Radiographs do not show any obvious bony abnormality.

Clinical examination of the finger reveals a swollen finger, a tender pulp, and a subungual hematoma, which occupies approximately 50% of the nail plate. The next step in management would be:

A. Drainage of the subungual hematoma
B. Removal of the nail plate and repair of the nail bed
C. Reassurance and splinting for comfort
D. Open repair, release of the eponychial fold, exploration of the sterile and germinal matrix, and replacement of the nail plate as a stent

Discussion

The correct answer is (C). As described, the patient does not have severe discomfort. In the absence of an obvious fracture, the only indication for drainage of a subungual hematoma would be for pain control where the patient has excruciating pain from a subungual hematoma. Since that is not the case, this subungual hematoma does not need to be drained. Traditional teaching has suggested that if a subungual hematoma exceeds 30% to 40% of the size of the nail plate, then the nail should be removed and the nail bed should be repaired. However, longitudinal studies have shown that removal of the nail plate and repair of the nail bed does not appear to influence nail growth positively in most patients. Therefore, in the absence of a fracture and if the nail plate is well fixed, irrespective of the size of the hematoma, not only does the hematoma not need to be drained, but the nail plate should not be removed, and the nail bed does not need repair. In this situation, the patient's finger may be splinted for comfort for a few days, elevation and icing is recommended, and range of motion is started at the earliest possibility.

At the same time that the patient injured her ring finger, the middle finger also sustained an injury. The middle finger radiographs, however, show that she has a fracture of the distal phalanx which is essentially nondisplaced and a subungual hematoma which occupies 50% of the size of the nail plate.

The most appropriate management for the middle finger would be which of the following?

A. Nail plate removal and repair of the nail bed
B. Drainage of the hematoma
C. Pinning of the distal phalanx
D. Splinting for comfort and range of motion to be started as soon as comfortable

Discussion

The correct answer is (D). Although the patient has a hematoma which occupies 50% of the nail plate, the description of this finger suggests that the fracture of the distal phalanx is completely nondisplaced. In such situations, there is no indication to remove the nail plate and repair the nail bed. A well-fixed nail plate and nondisplaced fracture of the distal phalanx essentially form a splint for the nail bed and allow the fracture and nail bed to heal in as anatomical position as possible. By removing a well fixed nail plate, the nail bed is destabilized and the support that the nail plate would afford for distal phalangeal fracture is also lost. Therefore, the nail plate is not to be removed in this situation. The patient would simply benefit from a splint and starting range of motion program as soon as the fracture gets more comfortable which is usually around 2 to 3 weeks.

During the same accident, the patient also sustained a fracture of the index finger. The index finger showed a fracture of the distal phalanx which was displaced. The fracture was at the base, and the nail plate was elevated in the proximal eponychial fold from which there was bleeding.

The most appropriate management for this injury would be which of the following?

A. Removal of the nail plate, replacement of the distal phalanx, reduction of the distal phalangeal fracture, fixation with Kirschner wire, open repair of the nail bed, and repair of the nail plate or stenting open the eponychial fold
B. Closed reduction and wire fixation
C. Splinting for comfort
D. Volar approach plate fixation of the distal phalanx

Discussion

The correct answer is (A). This digit has a displaced fracture with proximal avulsion of the nail plate from the eponychial

fold. This situation involves an injury to the germinal matrix of the nail bed and one which is unlikely to heal in the most optimal circumstances unless the distal phalanx is repositioned anatomically, fixed, and then the nail bed is repaired meticulously. To do this, the nail plate is initially removed. The laceration and the nail bed are carefully assessed. If necessary, small incisions are made in the lateral eponychial folds so that the eponychial fold can be folded back. After irrigation and debridement of the fracture site, it is reduced and carefully pinned with a wire. Then, the nail bed is repaired carefully with absorbable sutures, usually chromic catgut. The nail plate is cleaned and repositioned in the nail fold to act as a stent to keep it open in order for the new nail to grow back. The patient should be cautioned about unpredictability of nail growth, that nail growth can take 6 months to stabilize, and to understand the final outcome from a nail bed repair.

Objectives: Did you learn...?

- Idenftify indications for subungal hematoma drainage?
- Treat a distal phalanx fracture?

CASE 12

A 24-year-old, law student injured her left index finger during a volleyball game and developed immediate pain and deformity. By her description, this deformity occurred at the level of the PIP joint. Courtside, one of her colleagues immediately pulled on the finger, and she presents to your office 3 days later. Clinically, she has a swollen finger, but there is no obvious deformity. Radiographs are shown in Figure 4–10A and B.

The most likely diagnosis is which of the following?

A. Condylar fracture of the proximal phalanx
B. Fracture dislocation of the PIP joint
C. Shaft fracture of the proximal phalanx
D. Bony avulsion of the flexor digitorum superficialis

Discussion

The correct answer is (A). Radiographs show a unicondylar fracture of the proximal phalanx, in this case involving the ulnar condyle. The condyle is displaced, and there appears to be an articular stepoff. The patient's description of the injury and deformity are consistent with what could have occurred at the time of the injury, and the displacement at the time of injury may have been more significant than that being noted on the radiographs at this time.

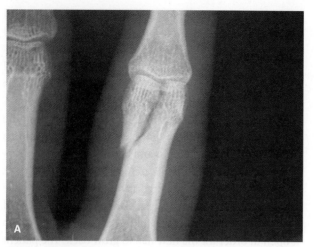

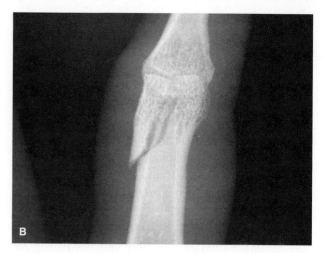

Figure 4–10 **A–B**

The most appropriate form of treatment at this time would be which of the following?

A. Closed reduction and buddy taping to the middle finger

B. Closed reduction and placement of the index finger in a volar splint allowing the patient DIP motion

C. Closed reduction and percutaneous pin fixation of the proximal phalanx

D. Open reduction and internal fixation of the proximal phalanx

E. Either C or D

Discussion

The correct answer is (E). This is an unstable injury as evidenced by the patient's description of the deformity at the time of injury and by the radiographs seen in the office. The fracture is displaced and is an intra-articular fracture. There is an articular stepoff. Furthermore, it is an oblique fracture. All of these features indicate that this is an unstable injury, and treatment by closed means is unlikely to be successful. In fractures that are completely nondisplaced, closed nonoperative treatment remains an option. However, in this instance where there is articular stepoff and displacement has occurred, it is vital to restore the length of the fragment, and more critically restore articular congruity especially in this young person. Closed reduction and percutaneous fixation as shown in the postoperative radiographs can be effective if perfect reduction of the joint is achieved (Fig. 4–10C to E). Failure to achieve perfect joint reduction by closed means necessitates an open reduction and treatment with either pins or screws.

Should open reduction and internal fixation of this joint be performed, which of the following are likely complications?

A. Dysvascularity of the displaced condyle

B. Stiffness of the proximal interphalangeal joint

C. Stiffness of the DIP

D. Both A and B

E. All of the above

Discussion

The correct answer is (C). Irrespective of which treatment is utilized in this instance, it is almost always safe to allow the patient gentle range of motion of the DIP joint. Therefore, stiffness of the DIP joint is usually not a concern in these injuries. However, during open reduction internal fixation of this injury it is vital to maintain the attachment of the collateral ligament to the fractured proximal phalanx condyle. The vascularity of the head of the proximal phalanx is achieved through this attachment of the collateral complex. Therefore, any injudicious handling of this soft tissue attachment of the proximal phalangeal fragment, in an attempt to restore perfect radiographic anatomy, will inevitably lead to dysvascularity of this fragment and avascular necrosis with passage of time. Despite judicious handling of this fragment, it is not uncommon for the patient with this injury after open reduction internal fixation to develop stiffness of the PIP joint. Therefore, every attempt is made to achieve radiographic perfection without disturbing the soft tissue envelope by using percutaneous pinning techniques to achieve radiographic anatomical perfection, especially at the joint.

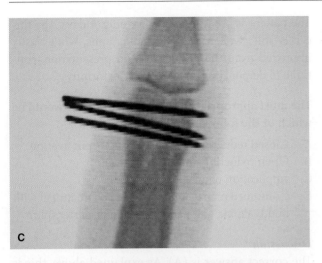

C

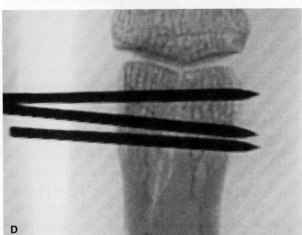

D

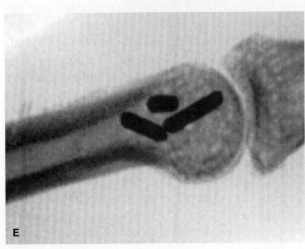

E

Figure 4–10 **C–E**

Objectives: Did you learn...?

- Describe the radiographic features of condylar fracture of the proximal phalanx?
- Treat these fractures?

- Pinpoint complications of open reduction and internal fixation of these fractures?

CASE 13

A 56-year-old homemaker fell down the steps of her basement injuring her left ring finger. She was seen at an outside facility with significant deformity of the ring finger. There were no open wounds. There was severe pain and limited motion. Radiographs are shown in Figures 4–11A and B.

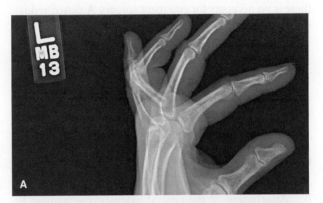

A

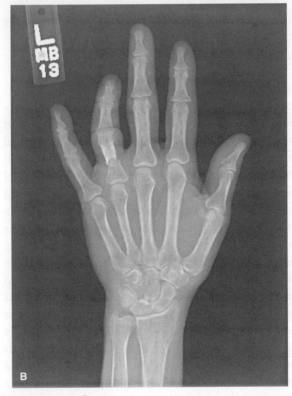

B

Figure 4–11 **A–B**

The most appropriate treatment at this time would be which of the following?

A. Emergent open reduction and internal fixation of the ring finger

B. Emergent closed reduction and splinting

C. Emergent closed reduction and percutaneous pin fixation

D. Application of an external fixator to restore length

Discussion

The correct answer is (B). This patient has essentially a closed but significantly displaced, angulated fracture of the proximal shaft of the ring finger's proximal phalanx. There is no open wound and the digit is well perfused. Therefore, there is no necessity for emergent surgery. A closed reduction, which can be performed in the emergency room, would be appropriate initial treatment.

The deformity seen in Figure 4–11A and B shows angulation of the digit with apex of the deformity volar.

The causation of the deformity includes which of the following?

A. Deforming force from the fall

B. Attachment of the central extensor mechanism to the base of the middle phalanx

C. Flexion of the base of the proximal phalanx by the attachment of the intrinsics

D. All of the above

Discussion

The correct answer is (D). In most instances, these fractures are caused by fall on the outstretched hand. In these, the deforming force is the extension that is applied to the proximal phalanx as the base of the proximal phalanx is held fixed due to the metacarpophalangeal joint, which takes the impact. Typically, after fracturing the shaft of the proximal phalanx, the deformity is apex volar. The central tendon of the extensor, which attaches to the base of the middle phalanx, exerts a deforming force on the distal fragment, and the interossei which attach to the base of the proximal phalanx tend to flex the proximal fragment. Therefore, the apex of this deformity is volar. In situations where the patient has an open wound with this deformity, the wound is usually volar. The attachment of the flexor digitorum superficialis to the base of the middle phalanx is distal to the attachment of the central tendon and therefore is not a deforming force for this particular fracture.

The patient is seen in your office after 4 days. The finger is still swollen and the radiographs, while vastly improved from the radiographs on presentation, continue to demonstrate an apex volar deformity.

The most appropriate treatment at this time would be which of the following?

A. Closed reduction and percutaneous pin fixation

B. Open reduction and plate fixation

C. Application of an external fixator

D. Continued management with closed treatment with buddy taping and hand-based ulnar gutter splint

Discussion

The correct answer is (A). As explained above, this is a significant injury with a large deformity at the time of presentation. The patient does have some residual deformity, and it is very likely that with passage of time and as the fracture heals, the deforming forces described above will not be sufficiently neutralized by a splint. Furthermore, as swelling reduces, the ability of the splint to control deforming forces is likely to be significantly suboptimal. Therefore, this fracture is best treated by closed reduction and percutaneous pin fixation. These pins may be placed across the head of the metacarpal into the base of the proximal phalanx and within the proximal phalangeal medullary cavity. This is the so-called Eaton–Belsky technique. Alternatively, after closed reduction, pins may be placed from the condyles of the proximal phalanx into the medullary canal so as to achieve the same effect without going across the metacarpophalangeal joint. These pins are usually maintained for a period of 3 to 4 weeks before being pulled out, and range of motion is instituted.

The most likely complication after this fracture is likely to be which of the following?

A. Stiffness of the PIP and DIP joints

B. Difficulty with excursion of the FDS and the FDP

C. Reflex sympathetic dystrophy affecting the ring finger

D. Complex regional pain syndrome affecting the ring finger

E. Complex regional pain syndrome

F. Both A and B

Discussion

The correct answer is (E). Displaced fractures of the proximal phalanx which have an apex volar deformity and have this degree of displacement are likely to be associated with some degree of deformity due to the surrounding soft tissue trauma to the floor of the flexor sheath which is the proximal phalanx. Patients who have this injury should be cautioned at the time of the initial consultation that the flexor tendons may get adherent to the periosteum of the proximal phalanx in the floor of the flexor sheath at the site of the fracture during the course of immobilization as the fracture is healing. Therefore, a small but definite number of patients who have this degree of displacement and deformity despite adequate rehabilitative exercises are likely to need a localized flexor tenolysis to free up the flexor tendons, which tend to get "spot welded" at the site of the fracture. This localized tenolysis which is best performed through a volar approach after releasing the A1 pulley is uniformly successful in restoring range of motion. However, cautioning the patient at the time of the initial consultation is critical in the management.

Objectives: Did you learn...?

- Treat angulated fractures of the proximal phalanx?
- Describe complications of this injury?

CASE 14

A 22-year-old male was climbing a tree when he lost his hold and fell out onto an outstretched left upper limb. He presented to the emergency room with a small wound over the volar aspect of his left palm, minimal clinical deformity, difficulty with moving his index finger and with severe pain. Clinical appearance and radiographs are shown in Figure 4–12A to E.

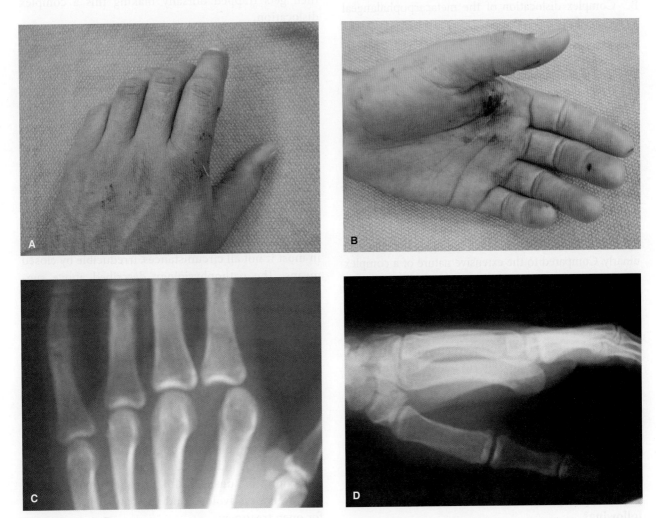

Figure 4–12 **A–D**

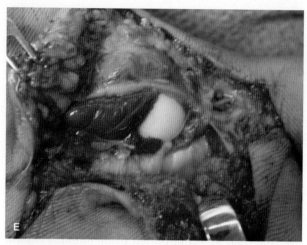

Figure 4–12 **E**

The most likely diagnosis is:

A. Sprain of the index finger metacarpophalangeal joint
B. Complex dislocation of the metacarpophalangeal joint of the index finger
C. Subluxation of the metacarpophalangeal joint of the index finger
D. Laceration of flexor tendons of the index finger
E. Contusion of index finger

Discussion

The correct answer is (B). The patient has an open wound over the index finger metacarpophalangeal volar aspect. He also has a minimal deformity of the left index finger. This appearance is classic in complex dislocations of the metacarpophalangeal joint of the index finger. These subluxations present with a much greater deformity with the index finger usually pointing dorsally and ulnarly. Compared to the extensive nature of a complex dislocation, counter-intuitively a subluxation, which is a much less significant injury, appears to have a much greater degree of deformity. The patient's radiographs also show in the PA view that the degree of deformity is minimal. However, the metacarpal and the index of proximal phalanx are not collinear unlike the other three digits, which is the first clue to suggest that this joint is dislocated. Careful assessment of the lateral view shows the base of the proximal phalanx of the index finger lying dorsal to the metacarpal head of the index finger. This finding confirms the presence of a complex dislocation.

The components of complexity of an index metacarpophalangeal joint dislocation include which of the following?

A. Injury to the volar plate
B. Buttonholing of the metacarpal head between the flexor tendons and the lumbrical
C. Dorsal entrapment of the volar plate
D. All of the above

Discussion

The correct answer is (D). During the injury, as hyperextension of the metacarpophalangeal joint occurs, the volar plate, which is attached to the base of the proximal phalanx and the volar aspect of the neck of the metacarpal, is avulsed from its proximal attachment. As the deforming force continues, the collateral ligaments are also torn and the metacarpal head is now free to be displaced volarly as the proximal phalanx gets displaced dorsally. The metacarpal head then displaces volarly in the space between the lumbrical and the flexor tendons with the lumbrical lying radial and the flexor tendons lying ulnar. The volar plate then gets trapped dorsally making this a complex dislocation.

The most appropriate treatment of a complex dislocation at this time is which of the following?

A. Sustained longitudinal traction with flexion
B. Gentle traction with a milking over the base of the proximal phalanx as the finger is flexed slowly
C. Placement of the digit in finger traps for 20 minutes followed by attempt at reduction
D. Primary open reduction of the metacarpophalangeal joint

Discussion

The correct answer is (D). Complex dislocations are, in most if not all circumstances, irreducible by closed means. The pathophysiology described above suggests that the head of the metacarpal is trapped in a so-called "noose," which is formed by the lumbrical on one side, the flexor tendons on the other side, and by the distal and dorsal entrapment of the volar plate. The noose is completed by the deep transverse metacarpal ligament. Therefore, the metacarpal head is essentially trapped within these four structures. Any attempt at closed reduction by providing traction, almost inevitably tightens this "noose" making a closed manipulative reduction impossible. Therefore, if a single judicious and gentle attempt at closed reduction is unsuccessful, further manipulative trauma is best avoided and the patient is scheduled for open treatment.

Open reduction of the metacarpophalangeal joint dislocation of the index finger can be attempted by:

A. Volar approach
B. Dorsal approach
C. Either approach

Discussion

The correct answer is (C). Open reduction of a dislocated MP joint of the index finger has been described using both volar as well as dorsal approaches. The volar approach has been traditionally described. However, it places the radial digital nerve of the index finger at risk. This is contiguous with the lumbrical and is tented over the head of the metacarpal which inevitably lies below the open wound as seen in this patient's palm. Therefore, any incisions made in this area have to be made carefully so as to avoid an iatrogenic injury to the index radial digital nerve. To facilitate reduction, it is usually necessary to release the A1 pulley thereby creating some degree of slack within the flexor tendons, which are then retracted and the volar plate is then extracted from behind the metacarpal head allowing the phalanx to be reduced upon the metacarpal head. Proponents of the dorsal approach suggest simple splitting of the extensor mechanism between the EDC and EIP, approaching the base of the phalanx dorsally. This allows direct visualization of the dorsally displaced volar plate, which is then split longitudinally, thereby allowing for a safer reduction of the phalanx on the metacarpal head. The dorsal technique does not endanger the radial digital nerve of the index finger.

Objectives: Did you learn...?

- Identify the clinical and radiographic appearance of MCP joint dislocation?
- Describe the pathoanatomy of the injury?
- Select surgical approaches for open reduction and internal fixation?
- Treat these injuries?

CASE 15

A 54-year-old female comes to your office with a chief complaint of a painful left palm. When further questioned, she mentioned that she has difficulty moving her finger first thing in the morning and occasionally finds that the finger catches, and she has difficulty opening the palm. Review of systems is negative and the patient reports that she is in otherwise good health. This has been going on the past 6 to 8 weeks.

The mostly likely diagnosis is:

A. Osteoarthritis of PIP and DIP
B. Trigger finger
C. Carpal tunnel syndrome
D. Work-related pain in the left hand
E. None of the above

Discussion

The correct answer is (B). Trigger fingers are commonly seen in patients over the age of 35 to 40 years. There is no data to show that it is related to hand dominance. However, the ring finger appears to be the most commonly affected. Symptoms can vary, and trigger fingers have been classified into different types. Some patients present with difficulty with flexion, whereas others may present with classic triggering where the finger gets stuck in the bent position and the patient has to straighten it. Morning stiffness is a common form of presentation.

The patient tells you that while this does not affect her functional activity she finds it to be painful in the mornings. However, she is not interested in having any kind of invasive intervention.

The choice of treatment that you could offer her at this point in time would include which of the following?

A. Periodic observation
B. Splinting
C. Local steroid injection
D. Percutaneous ultrasound guided release of the A1 pulley
E. Open release of A1 pulley

Discussion

The correct answer is either (A) or (B). This patient does not appear to have any functional issues and finds this to be more of a nuisance and uncomfortable first thing in the morning. She is also not interested in having invasive intervention. Therefore, options which include a steroid injection or release of the A1 pulley be it percutaneous or open are incorrect responses to this question. Since the patient has minimal functional issues, periodic observation in this situation is entirely reasonable. On the other hand, if the patient is willing to try a splint, there is some data to show that splinting in patients such as this can be effective up to 50% of the time. In most instances, the patients are asked to wear a splint at night. However, if their occupation allows it, wearing a splint over a few weeks for most of the day is also known to have some degree of success.

The patient returns 3 months later and now has pronounced triggering with the patient being able to demonstrate full composite fist in the office but, when trying to open the fingers, the ring finger remains stuck in the bent position. It requires considerable effort to straighten it and is accompanied by severe pain.

The most appropriate form of treatment at this point in time would be which of the following?

A. Percutaneous release of the A1 pulley
B. Ultrasound guided release of the A1 pulley
C. Open release of the A1 pulley
D. Steroid injection at the level of the A1 pulley

Discussion

The correct answer is (D). In patients who are willing to accept a steroid injection it is certainly reasonable to inject the vicinity of the A1 pulley with steroid. Data suggests that there is no superiority of any one steroid preparation over the other. Numerous methods of steroid instillation have been described. However, none of these methods have been shown to be superior to the other. Simple instillation of the steroid preparation at the level of the A1 pulley is successful in over 75% of the patients. However, the duration of symptom relief is unpredictable. The patient should be cautioned about the possibility of increasing pain for the first day or two after steroid instillation. They should also be informed about the pharmacokinetics of mechanism of action. Most patients notice gradual relief of symptoms over a period of a few weeks. It is now accepted that recurrence of symptoms despite two successful attempts at steroid instillation are best treated by surgical release of the A1 pulley, which has a lasting relief from symptoms of triggering.

Objectives: Did you learn...?

• Describe the clinical presentation of trigger finger?
• Perform Nonoperative management in trigger finger?
• Select invasive treatment options?

CASE 16

A 61-year-old, diabetic male presents with difficulty moving his dominant right index and middle fingers. He has noticed swelling and difficulty bending both fingers over the last 3 months. Occasionally when he wakes up in the morning, he finds that his fingers are stuck in the bent position. Running warm water over his fingers has helped them to open gradually.

The most likely diagnosis is:

A. Trigger fingers of the index and middle fingers
B. Multifocal small joint arthritis
C. Carpal tunnel syndrome
D. None of the above

Discussion

The correct answer is (A). This patient is a diabetic. Presentation of multiple trigger fingers is a well-described phenomenon in diabetics. While multiple trigger fingers can occur in any patient, this presentation appears to favor diabetics. Trigger finger presentation in diabetics, as much as in other populations, can vary from difficulty with generation of a composite fist, to swelling of the affected fingers, to involvement of multiple digits, to the classic form of triggering with clicking and popping with every act of flexion or getting stuck in the bent position.

The pathology in trigger fingers includes which of the following structures?

A. Volar plate of the MP joint
B. A1 pulley
C. Flexor tendon
D. Combination of B and C
E. A, B and C

Discussion

The correct answer is (D). Trigger fingers are a condition characterized by stenosing tenosynovitis at the level of the A1 pulley. Thickening of the A1 pulley, which is very well-documented especially in diabetics, is combined with tenosynovial hypertrophy, which can be most marked at the level of the A1 pulley and just proximal to it. This discrepancy between the size of the A1 pulley, flexor tendons, and the tenosynovium which excurse within it is thought to be responsible for the phenomenon of triggering or catching.

The most appropriate treatment at this time would be which of the following?

A. Splinting at night
B. Splinting for 24 hours for 6 weeks
C. Local instillation of steroid preparations
D. Open release of A1 pulleys
E. Either C or D

Discussion

The correct answer is (E). Instillation of local steroid at the level of the A1 pulley is a treatment option which is successful in most patients including diabetics. However, there is data to show that the responses in diabetics are not as predictable as those in nondiabetics, the duration of relief after steroid injection is less compared to nondiabetics, and the response to steroid preparations as well as the recurrence of the symptoms appears to be related to the control of diabetes. There does not appear to be any convincing evidence to show a difference in response to steroids or the recurrence after steroid instillation in patients who have type 1 versus type 2 diabetes. At all times, when diabetics are injected with steroids at the level of A1 pulley as well as in other locations, they should be cautioned about a transient increase in blood sugar. This is all the more critical in patients who are type 1 diabetics as it may affect the insulin dosage. This transient increase in blood sugar usually lasts for less than 72 hours.

While instilling steroids at the level of the A1 pulley, the location of the A1 pulley is best described by which of the following techniques?

A. At the level of the digito-palmar flexion crease
B. At the level of a line joining the radial edge of the proximal palmar crease to the ulnar edge of a distal palmar crease or just distal to it
C. At the level of the distal palmar crease
D. At the level of the proximal palmar crease
E. None of the above

Discussion

The correct answer is (B). There are numerous methods described to identify the location of the A1 pulley. Among the choices offered in this, the most appropriate answer is B. The line joining the radial edge of the proximal palmar crease to the ulnar edge of the distal palmar crease is a skin representation of the location of the metacarpophalangeal joint. The A1 pulley overlies the volar aspect of the metacarpophalangeal joint. Therefore, it follows that this line would be a good representation of the approximate location of the A1 pulley. However, the A1 pulley is located a few millimeters distal to this line. Therefore, while instilling steroids one must remember that the A1 pulley is located slightly distal to this line, and while the needle may be introduced at the level of this line, it is directed distally at an angle of about 45 degrees so the steroid is placed at the approximate location of the proximal edge of the A1 pulley.

Objectives: Did you learn...?

• Describe the pathophysiology of trigger finger?
• Identify the clinical presentation of trigger finger in diabetics?
• Pinpoint various treatment options?

CASE 17

During the course of examination of finger injuries in the emergency room, it is important to be facile with the placement of local anesthetic. This local anesthetic may be administered in the form of flexor sheath block, a web space block, or a digital nerve block which is administered at the level of the metacarpal neck often referred to as the metacarpal block.

The correct relationship of the digital nerve to the vessels at the level of the proximal phalanx would be which of the following?

A. The proper digital vessel is volar to the digital nerve
B. The digital nerve and the vessel run side by side
C. The digital nerve lies volar to the vessel
D. The exact relationship is undefined and can vary from digit to digit

Discussion

The correct answer is (C). At the level of the base of the palm, the digital vessels, after they come off the superficial arch, lie volar to the digital nerves which are common digital nerves. At the level of the metacarpal necks, the common digital nerve then divides into proper digital nerves which supply contiguous sides of each web space. Shortly thereafter, the digital nerves and vessels change relationships so that by the time the digital nerve is at the level of the proximal phalanx, the nerve comes to lie volar to the vessel.

During the course of placement of local anesthetic for the management of an index finger laceration over the proximal phalanx of the index finger, you place a lidocaine block at the level of the metacarpal neck. The patient's laceration extends on to the dorsal surface of the proximal phalanx of the index finger. The suturing of the volar aspect of the laceration is accomplished uneventfully. As you are suturing the dorsal aspects of the laceration over the index finger proximal phalanx, the patient experiences considerable pain.

The most likely reason for this patient's discomfort is which of the following?

A. The local anesthetic that you placed on the volar side has worn off.
B. The patient has aberrant nerve supply.
C. The patient is simply experiencing nervous anxiety.
D. Sensory supply to the dorsal aspect of the proximal phalanx of the index finger comes from terminal branches of the radial sensory nerve, which need

to be anesthetized separately during the course of performance of the procedure on the dorsal aspect of the proximal phalanx of the index finger.

Discussion

The correct answer is (D). Digital nerves reliably supply the entire volar aspect of all the fingers as well as the thumb. In the fingers, sensory supply to the dorsal aspect of the finger distal to the PIP articulation in most studies appears to be performed by a digital branch, which arises from the radial digital nerve of the finger. However, the dorsal aspect of the proximal phalanx of the index finger and the dorsal aspect of the proximal phalanx of the small finger, respectively, receives cutaneous nerve supply from terminal branches of the radial sensory nerve and the dorsal cutaneous branch of the ulnar nerve, respectively. In performing procedures over the dorsal aspect of these fingers at this level, it is vital to separately anesthetize these nerve branches prior to performing the procedure.

Objectives: Did you learn...?

• Describe the anatomy of the neurovascular structures of the hand?

CASE 18

A 30-year-old radiographer from your institution was helping to set up a backyard barbeque when a plate broke in her hand, and she sustained a laceration at the base of her left small and ring fingers. She was seen in the Emergency Room. Neurovascular examination was intact. However, the patient had no ability to flex her small finger. A clinical appearance is shown in Figure 4–13.

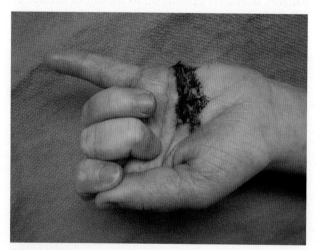

Figure 4–13

The most likely diagnosis is:

A. Lacerated FDP to the small finger
B. Lacerated FDS to the small finger
C. Lacerations of both FDS and FDP to the small finger
D. Pain inhibition of motion of small finger

Discussion

The correct answer is (C). This patient has no ability to flex either her PIP or the DIP joint. This indicates that neither her FDS nor her FDP is functioning. Given the transverse nature of the laceration across the long axis of the flexor tendons, a clinical diagnosis of FDS and FDP lacerations can be made effectively. In a painful situation, the diagnosis can be made by utilizing local anesthetic to provide pain relief and then asking the patient to flex to confirm presence or absence of flexor function. Conversely, to avoid the patient's effort and involvement, the simple act of flexion and extension of the wrist may be utilized to provide tenodesis effect and to see if the fingers flex passively when the wrist is extended. This is a reliable sign of confirming intactness of the flexor mechanism.

The patient wishes to return to her occupation as a radiographer at the earliest. The most suitable form of treatment at this point in an effort to allow her to be a radiographer would be which of the following?

A. Placement in a splint in the intrinsic plus position with early active range of motion
B. Open exploration and repair of flexor digitorum profundus tendon
C. Exploration and repair of both the FDS and FDP
D. Excision of flexor digitorum superficialis and repair of profundus tendons only

Discussion

The correct answer is (C). This patient has a wound, which lies over the distal portion of the palm. At this level, given that she has no flexor function, one has to presume that both tendons are injured. However, the injury has occurred in the act of clasping. Therefore, although the injury may be considered to be a zone 3 injury, one has to presume that in the act of clasping, the fingers were flexing, and therefore the flexor tendon injury itself would be more distal and thereby a zone 2 injury. The readers must familiarize themselves with the zones of flexor tendon injury, with zone 2 injuries being the most challenging. Zone 2 injuries consist of injury that occur between the insertion of superficialis at the base of the middle phalanx to the proximal extent of the A1 pulley. This has been referred to traditionally as "no man's land" and was often thought to be associated with poor outcomes. These outcomes were related to the complexities of flexor digitorum superficialis splitting to allow the profundus to pass through, thereby creating 3 tendons within the flexor sheath at this level. Repair of tendons in this level is often associated with increased bulk and reduced gliding leading to adhesions and poor flexor pull through which then leads to suboptimal outcomes. However, with contemporary techniques, it is possible to perform strong repairs of flexor tendons in zone II and have satisfactory outcomes. In situations where the bulk appears to be inordinately large, it is not uncommon to excise one slip of the FDS to reduce the bulk within the flexor sheath to allow satisfactory function. Repair of both tendons where possible must be performed.

Rehabilitation after such tendon repairs should include which of the following rehabilitation protocols?

A. Unlimited active motion within a few days after surgery
B. Active assisted range of motion within a few days after surgery
C. Passive differential glide motion at DIP and PIP and MP within a few days after surgery
D. No motion for 6 weeks, placement in a short-arm cast

Discussion

The correct answer is (C). Various protocols have been described for flexor tendon rehabilitation after open repair. In the contemporary setting, the most popular and favored means of rehabilitation appears to be that described by Duran and Houser. This protocol relies on passive range of motion of the PIP and the DIP joints as well as the MP joints, which are demonstrated to the patient by a hand therapist. This leads to passive gliding of the repaired flexor tendons within the sheath allowing minimization of adhesions of the flexor tendon to the sheath and also to each other while promoting gliding. This small amount of motion also encourages deposition of collagen fibers along the lines of stress, thereby allowing an early start to an active assisted range of motion program after 3 or 4 weeks of the repair. Other rehabilitation techniques include a dynamic protocol including the use of rubber bands as described by Kleinert as well as early, gently controlled active range of motion.

Objectives: Did you learn...?

- Identify the clinical presentation of lacerations of the FDS?

- Describe various treatment options?
- Pinpoint postoperative treatment options?

CASE 19

A 64-year-old, right-hand-dominant, Caucasian female presents to your office with several months of pain in the right hand. More specifically, she has noticed the pain is worse on doing pinching activities and when trying to do needlepoint and crochet. In gripping these needles, she finds her index finger to be maximally painful as does the rest of the hand. When questioned closely, it appears that the index finger is the most painful. Radiographs are shown in Figure 4–14A and B.

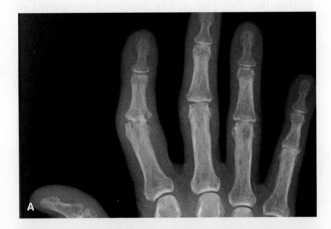

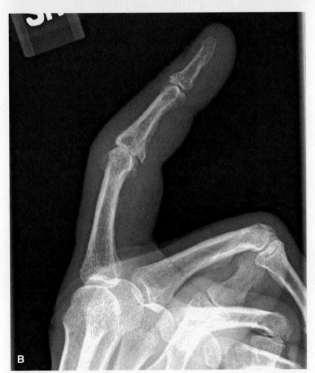

Figure 4–14 **A–B**

The most likely diagnosis is:

A. Posttraumatic osteoarthritis of the index finger PIP
B. Erosive osteoarthritis of the index finger PIP
C. Infectious destruction of the proximal phalangeal condyle
D. Trigger finger

Discussion

The correct answer is (B). This patient has radiographs which show multifocal small joint osteoarthritic change. This is most notable in the PIP joint of the right index finger. The PIP joint of the index finger is unique in that it provides the stability in the act of pinching against the thumb. Therefore, it is not surprising that this patient has developed symptoms of pain as well as a sense of instability on attempting to hold crochet needles.

The patient has tried anti-inflammatories with limited success. She has been seen by other physicians and has undergone a short course of splinting as well as placement of a steroid injection, again with very limited success.

The most appropriate management at this point would be which of the following?

A. Placement of steroid injection using fluoroscopy to confirm appropriate steroid placement
B. A quick cast application to hold the PIP straight and allow it to stiffen in that position
C. Arthrodesis of the index finger PIP
D. Replacement arthroplasty of the index finger PIP
E. Reconstruction of the radial collateral complex of the index finger PIP

Discussion

The correct answer is (C). This patient has radiographs that show that she has angulatory deformity with loss of the height of the ulnar condyle. She has practically no joint space remaining and more importantly has developed a deviation deformity. Therefore, this is an unstable, painful arthritic joint. As mentioned above, the index finger PIP is critical to the act of pinching. Therefore, this patient would be a suitable candidate for PIP arthrodesis. Radial collateral ligament reconstruction is unlikely to be of use since the patient has an extremely arthritic joint. Replacement arthroplasty of the PIP is suitable for the middle or ringer fingers and occasionally for the small finger; however, when the patient requires the ability to pinch strongly, it appears

that replacement arthroplasties do not do as well and tend to wear out and are not as durable. Therefore, replacement arthroplasties are avoided in the index finger PIP.

The most appropriate angle and the choice of implant for fusion would be which of the following?

A. Cannulated screw arthrodesis at 30 degrees
B. Plate and screw fixation at 30 degrees
C. Tension band wire fixation at 30 degrees
D. The choice of implant is not as critical as creation of cancellous bony surfaces which oppose and compress well at an angle between 30 and 50 degrees, customized to the patient's occupational and avocational needs

Discussion

The correct answer is (D). In most circumstances, traditional teaching has involved increasing angles of fusion for the PIP from the index finger to the small finger. However, other schools of thought believe that the appropriate angle for fusion across all digits PIPs would be 40 degrees. Regardless of traditional teaching, in the contemporary setting with patients living longer and having more vocational and avocational needs, it becomes vital to take these into account in planning of patient's PIP arthrodesis. For most circumstances, it appears that fusion at an angle of 40 degrees for the PIP of the index finger is highly desirable.

Objectives: Did you learn...?

• Describe the clinical presentation of erosive arthritis?
• Identify various treatment options of erosive arthritis?

CASE 20

A 69-year-old female presents to office with pain in the right thumb for several years. She has noticed that she has difficulty with holding door knobs, carrying heavy plates, and turning the key in her car. The pain keeps her awake at night, and she has tried various anti-inflammatory medications with limited success. Radiographs are shown in Figure 4–15A and B.

The most likely diagnosis is:

A. Osteoarthritic basal joint of the thumb
B. Trigger thumb
C. Carpal tunnel syndrome
D. Scaphotrapezial trapezoidal arthritis

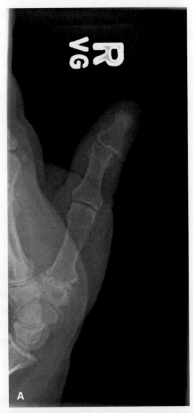

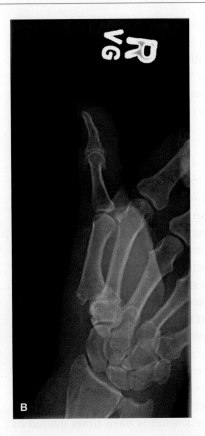

Figure 4–15 **A–B**

Discussion

The correct answer is (A). This is a classic clinical appearance and radiographic presentation in a patient with an arthritic basal joint of the thumb. Basal joints are saddle-shaped biconcave joints, which allow the thumb motion in multiple axes. They tend to degenerate with age and patients oftentimes present with symptomatic degeneration of the basal joint in their 50s and 60s. Women appear to be affected 7 to 10 times more than men. The classic presentation is a prominence at the base of the thumb with difficulty involving actions as those described above.

During the course of clinical examinations, which of the following findings might be expected?

A. Tenderness over the basal joint of the thumb
B. Positive distraction rotation test
C. Positive grind test
D. Difficulty with painful pinch
E. All of the above

Discussion

The correct answer is (E). During the course of the clinical examination, attention should be paid to inspection which usually reveals the presence of fairly large prominence over the basal joint of the thumb as the metacarpal base subluxes from its articulation with the trapezium. This development of the thumb is often referred to as the "shoulder sign." However, this may not be obvious in the early stages of the pathological process. In the early stage of the pathological process, tenderness maybe elicited at the base of the thumb just proximal to the metacarpal base. Grasping the thumb and rotating while putting gentle traction on it can also provoke pain. This is known as the distraction rotation test. Conversely, holding the metacarpal and firmly grinding it against the trapezium (after cautioning the patient that this maneuver could hurt) is known as the grind test. In patients who present with advanced radiographic degenerative changes, it is quite common to have all these signs clinically evident. Patients who present with earlier stages of the radiographic disease process may not present with the grind test.

The patient is keen to avoid surgery and would like to pursue nonoperative means.

Which of the following would be a reasonable choice of treatment for this patient?

A. Splinting with a short opponens splint
B. Splinting with a long opponens splint
C. Neoprene thumb wrap
D. Placement of a steroid injection and any of the splints mentioned above
E. All of the above

Discussion

The correct answer is (E). Patients who present with degenerative basal joint arthritis and who are unwilling to consider surgical intervention even in the age group as this patient is, can be treated with a variety of non-operative interventions. These include: a short course of anti-inflammatory medication after carefully monitoring the renal function in conjunction with the primary care doctor, use of a splint or sleeve as suggested above, or placement of a steroid injection. While comfort and convenience of short splints are often felt to be superior to that of a long splint, the longer splint appears to give the greater degree of support spanning across the CMC joint. However, there is no data to show the superiority of a short opponens splint, long opponens splint, or a Neoprene sleeve over each other. It appears at this time that the decision for a splint is often times guided by patient comfort and choice and personal preferences of the treating physician. The use of a steroid injection can provide patient's long lasting relief; however, they should be cautioned that placement of steroid injections can be painful for the first 24 to 48 hours, and the duration of relief remains unpredictable. They should also be cautioned that any steroid injections can be associated with side effects such as subcutaneous fat atrophy and localized depigmentation.

Objectives: Did you learn...?

- Describe the clinical and radiographic signs of osteoarthritis of the thumb?
- Identify various treatment options?

CASE 21

A 22-year-old patient presents after sustaining an injury to her finger during a softball game. She reports pain and swelling after the trauma, but she was asymptomatic prior to this incident. She went to an urgent care over the weekend and was placed in a splint. She was told that she has a "mass" and presents for further follow up. On physical examination, the digit is swollen and ecchymotic. Range of motion is limited by pain, but no malrotation or scissoring of the digits with flexion

is noted. An x-ray shows a radiolucent intramedullary lesion in the central metaphysis of the proximal phalanx with a transverse nondisplaced fracture through the lesion.

What is the most likely diagnosis of the tumor?

A. Aneurysmal bone cyst
B. Enchondroma
C. Giant cell tumor
D. Fibrous cortical defect
E. Osteoid osteoma

Discussion

The correct answer is (B). Enchondromas are the most common skeletal lesions of the bones of the hand. It is a frequent cause of pathologic fracture. It is asymptomatic prior to fracture, often found in adolescents and young adults, and is located in the central metaphysis.

What is the next step of treatment?

A. Closed reduction and percutaneous pinning of the fracture
B. Curettage and bone grafting of the tumor
C. Splinting the finger
D. Observation with serial radiographs
E. Oncologic ray resection

Discussion

The correct answer is (C). A nondisplaced pathologic fracture through an enchondroma is allowed to heal with closed treatment. At a later time after the fracture has healed, the enchondroma can be treated definitively with curettage and bone grafting.

The patient wants to know what caused this lesion. What do you tell her?

A. The normal ossification of the growth plate was disrupted and the central growth plate became dysplastic
B. Over proliferation of osteoclasts
C. As the bone grew, a defect in the bone filled with fluid
D. Over proliferation of the joint hyaline cartilage eroded into the bone
E. Degeneration of normal bone with immature bone

Discussion

The correct answer is (A). Over proliferation of osteoclasts is associated with giant cell tumor. Unicameral bone cysts are thought to be due to a bone defect filling with fluid. Degeneration of normal bone to immature bone is associated with fibrous dysplasia.

The patient's fracture was treated successfully with immobilization. She presents 6 months later for definitive treatment. During informed consent for curettage and bone grafting, the patient wants to know the risk of malignancy.

What do you tell her?

A. 0%
B. 1% to 2%
C. 10%
D. 25%
E. 100%

Discussion

The correct answer is (B). When associated with multiple enchondromas, also known as enchondromatosis (Ollier disease), the risk is 10% to 25%. When associated with Mafucci syndrome (multiple enchondromas and venous malformations), the risk is near 100%. When the lesion is isolated, the risk is 1% to 2%.

Objectives: Did you learn...?

- Treat an enchondroma with a pathologic fracture?
- Describe the presentation and etiology of enchondroma?
- Identify the risk of malignant degeneration?

CASE 22

A 38-year-old woman is referred to you for "excruciating" pain in the left long fingertip, specifically at the base of the nail. She reports pain throughout the day and exquisite tenderness that has been ongoing for 4 years. There was no antecedent trauma. She reports that it is causing tension in her marriage and that her husband may be considering divorce. The digit and nail appear completely normal on inspection.

What is the most likely diagnosis?

A. Neuroma
B. Neurolemmoma
C. Paronychial infection
D. Glomus tumor
E. Malingering

Discussion

The correct answer is (D). It is a rare, benign neoplasm, which accounts for 1% to 4.5% of hand tumors. The mass is frequently too small to be identified on physical examination. The average length of time to diagnosis is 2 to 7 years from the onset of symptoms. Tragically, many of the patients with glomus tumors suffer for years because they are thought to be malingering or have other psychosocial disorders before a proper diagnosis is made. The masses are typically very painful. The nail bed is a typical location of the mass, although they can be found volarly. Neuromas are less common distal to the trifurcation of the digital nerve and are more typically found after trauma. Neurolemmoma, or schwannoma, is more often painless and is very rare in the fingertip. A paronychial infection would present with swelling and redness on inspection and would not be present for 4 years.

What do you expect on physical examination?

A. Relief of symptoms when the tip of a ballpoint pen presses on the lesion
B. Relief of symptoms when the finger is placed in ice water
C. Relief of symptoms when a blood pressure cuff is raised on an elevated arm
D. Radiating pain when the digital nerve is percussed.

Discussion

The correct answer is (C). Love's pin test (a tip of a pen, head of a pin, or K-wire is pressed on the mass and causes pain) has a reported sensitivity and specificity of 100%. Placing the finger in ice water or cooling it with cold spray increases pain with a sensitivity and specificity of 100%. Cold intolerance is characteristic of glomus tumors. Relief of symptoms with exsanguination and tourniquet elevation (Hildreth's test) is 77% sensitive and 100% specific. A Tinel's test is characteristic of a neuroma, not a glomus tumor.

What is the most appropriate next step in management of this lesion?

A. Fine needle aspiration (FNA)
B. Steroid injection
C. Incisional biopsy
D. Excisional biopsy
E. Amputation

Discussion

The correct answer is (D). Excisional biopsy is both therapeutic and diagnostic. FNA does not have a role in glomus tumor treatment. Steroid injection does not treat glomus tumors. The tumors are typically small (3–5 mm) and well-encapsulated, therefore excisional biopsy is the preferred treatment.

What do you expect to see on pathology?

A. Smooth muscle cells and surrounding vascular tissue
B. Nerve fiber overgrowth
C. Capillary overgrowth with atypical endothelium
D. Fibroblastic proliferation
E. Cystic structure filled with synovial fluid

Discussion

The correct answer is (A). Glomus bodies are a neuromyoarterial apparatus that controls arteriovenous shunting in terminal vessels. The function is to control blood flow in the digits. They are made up of smooth muscle cells and vascular tissue. Nerve fiber overgrowth is associated with a neuroma. Capillary overgrowth with atypical endothelium is found in hemangiomas. Fibroblastic proliferation is typical of fibromas. A cystic structure filled with synovial fluid is consistent with a mucous cyst.

Objectives: Did you learn…?

• Recognize the presentation of glomus tumor?
• Pinpoint the findings on physical examination?
• Understand the treatment and pathology?

CASE 23

A 28-year-old woman presents to your office with complaints of pain with full wrist extension, particularly when she is practicing yoga. She does not report any antecedent trauma. Initial inspection of the wrist at neutral does not reveal any abnormality. The patient is tender over the scapholunate interval. With full flexion, a slight fullness is appreciable at the scapholunate interval. A Watson scaphoid shift test is negative. X-rays are unremarkable.

What is the most likely diagnosis?

A. Kienbock disease (idiopathic avascular necrosis of the lunate)
B. Scapholunate ligament injury
C. Sprain of the extensor carpi radialis longus tendon
D. Occult dorsal wrist ganglion
E. Extensor tenosynovitis

Discussion

The correct answer is (D). Kienbock disease would present with pain over the lunate, not the scapholunate interval. A scapholunate ligament injury would should DISI deformity on x-ray and have a positive Watson scaphoid shift test. A sprain of the ECRL would have pain with resisted wrist extension and would be unlikely to have significant swelling of the dorsal wrist,

nor would there be pain over the scapholunate interval. Extensor tenosynovitis would present with a dorsal wrist swelling that moves with tendon excursion.

The patient refuses MRI evaluation and is lost to follow up. She represents 6 months later with a large mass on the dorsal wrist.

What additional information is not consistent with a presentation of ganglion cyst of the dorsal wrist?

A. A history of the mass increasing and decreasing in size
B. A mobile, firm mass on physical examination
C. Aspiration of clear, thick fluid
D. A mass that does not trans-illuminate with pen light
E. Pain of the dorsal wrist

Discussion

The correct answer is (D). A ganglion cyst will transilluminate. A mass that does not transilluminate is concerning for a solid mass and requires further workup. Ganglion cysts can often change in size secondary to the mass decompressing into the joint and refilling with fluid. The ganglion cyst is expected to be firm and mobile. Aspiration of thick, mucinous fluid is pathognomonic for ganglion cyst. Pain can be associated with ganglion cysts, particularly if it is causing pressure on an adjacent nerve.

Which of the following treatment options has the lowest risk of recurrence?

A. Rupture
B. Injection
C. Aspiration
D. Incision
E. Excision

Discussion

The correct answer is (E). Rupture, aspiration, and incision do not remove the cyst wall or the stalk connecting the cyst to joint fluid. Therefore, excision is the treatment with the lowest recurrence rate.

The patient undergoes dorsal ganglion excision through a transverse approach. She returns to yoga without incident. However, 5 years later she represents with a volar wrist mass.

Which of the following is true regarding volar wrist ganglion cysts?

A. Aspiration to confirm diagnosis is contraindicated
B. The cyst is most likely to arise from the first metacarpotrapezial joint

C. The cyst is confluent with a flexor tendon sheath

D. Volar wrist ganglion cysts rarely cause pain

E. Volar wrist ganglion cysts are not associated with nerve palsy

Discussion

The correct answer is (A). Aspiration of volar ganglia is generally deferred to avoid inadvertent puncture of the radial artery, which often overlies or travels through the cyst on the radial side, or to avoid the ulnar artery and nerve on the ulnar side. The volar cyst is more likely to arise from the radiocarpal joint, followed by the scaphotrapezial joint followed by the metacarpotrapezial joint. The flexor tendon sheath can form a ganglion cyst, or retinacular cyst, but it is not confluent with a volar wrist ganglion. Both volar wrist ganglion and dorsal wrist ganglion cysts are associated with pain. Volar wrist ganglion cysts can cause a compressive neuropathy and associated palsy, particularly of the ulnar nerve within Guyon's canal.

The patient is so pleased with her care that she returns with her 72-year-old grandmother who notes a mass overlying her index distal interphalyngeal joint and nail grooving. The diagnosis is made of mucous cyst.

Which of the following is true regarding mucous cyst management?

A. The nail grooving is completely irreversible

B. Mucous cysts excision is performed without disturbing the underlying bone

C. A ruptured cyst puts the patient at risk of paronychial infection

D. A excision of a large, attenuated cyst often requires a rotational flap for coverage

E. Mucous cysts are often seen overlying normal joints without arthritic changes

Discussion

The correct answer is (D). Nail grooving may be reversible with resolution of the cyst by relieving pressure on the sterile matrix. Excision of the underlying osteophyte is recommended to prevent cyst recurrence. A ruptured cyst puts the patient at risk for septic arthritis. Excision of a large, attenuated cyst often requires excision of overlying poorly perfused skin, and coverage of the underlying joint is achieved with a rotational flap. Mucous cysts are associated with arthritic joints.

Objectives: Did you learn...?

- Recognize the presentation of occult and frank dorsal wrist ganglia?
- Describe the treatment of ganglion cysts with the lowest risk of rupture?
- Understand the difference in management between dorsal and volar wrist ganglia?
- Understand the presentation and management of mucous cysts?

CASE 24

A 34-year-old man presents to the emergency department with pain in his left small finger. He reports that he was cutting meat when his knife slipped and punctured the volar surface of his proximal phalanx. It did not bleed, and he did not seek further medical treatment. He presents with pain in the finger. A diagnosis of flexor tenosynovitis is suspected.

Which of the following is a classic sign of flexor tenosynovitis, as described by Kanavel?

A. A painful finger held in extension

B. Fusiform swelling of the digit

C. Erythema of the digit

D. Pain with axial loading of the digit

E. Tenderness along the lateral aspect of the finger

Discussion

The correct answer is (B). Kanavel's four cardinal signs of flexor tenosynovitis are intense pain with passive extension, a finger held in flexion, fusiform swelling of the entire digit, and percussion tenderness along the course of the tendon sheath. Erythema is not a cardinal sign of flexor tenosynovitis. Pain with axial loading is suggestive of a septic joint.

Which of the following will most likely rule out flexor tenosynovitis?

A. A normal white blood count without a shift

B. A normal ESR

C. A normal CRP

D. A normal x-ray

E. Painless passive extension

Discussion

The correct answer is (E). The earliest sign of flexor tenosynovitis is pain with passive extension. Normal labs and a normal x-ray cannot rule out flexor tenosynovitis, as the negative predictive value of normal inflammatory markers is low for flexor tenosynovitis.

The patient does not improve on antibiotics. His finger is markedly swollen. He needs surgical decompression, irrigation, and debridement.

Which incision should be avoided?

A. An oblique incision over the A1 pulley and a radially based chevron incision over the A5 pulley

B. A Brunner zigzag incision

C. An ulnar posterolateral midaxial longitudinal incision

D. A transverse incision at the proximal edge of the A1 pulley and a transverse incision at the distal interphalyngeal flexion crease

Discussion

The correct answer is (B). The Brunner incision should be avoided because with severe swelling, skin closure may be difficult and the tendons can then desiccate. Incisions accessing the sheath over the A1 and A5 pulleys are used to access the tendon sheath and perform the incision and drainage. Midaxial incisions are preferred if the swelling of the digit is compromising vascularity in order to relieve the pressure and prevent necrosis of the skin.

The patient refuses surgical intervention. As the infection progresses without surgical treatment, which of the following is unlikely?

A. Tendon necrosis

B. Skin necrosis

C. Osteomyelitis

D. Flexor tenosynovitis of the thumb

E. Paronychial infection

Discussion

The correct answer is (E). Increased pressure secondary to infection can lead to skin loss and tendon necrosis, which may require amputation. A direct extension of the infection to the bone causes osteomyelitis. Infection of the small finger may extend to the thumb in what is called a "horseshoe abscess" as the small finger and thumb tendon sheaths communicate. This may involve other digits, as the communications are quite anomalous. A paronychial infection is unlikely as a direct extension of the flexor tenosynovitis because the infection would have to extend through the distal interphalyngeal capsule joint and into the dorsal tissues.

Objectives: Did you learn...?

• Identity the physical examination findings of flexor tenosynovitis?

• Describe the negative predictive value of normal laboratory findings?

• Select which incisions are indicated for drainage?

• Describe the natural course of untreated flexor tenosynovitis?

CASE 25

A 42-year-old man presents to the hospital with pain and swelling of the dorsum of his hand. He reports blunt trauma against a metal shelf, but does not remember a break in the skin. There is a blister of the skin. He reports erythema started approximately 6 hours ago of the hand but it now extends to the wrist. He is febrile to 102 degrees, heart rate is 110, and blood pressure is 92/38. He has significant pain to palpation and induration of the dorsum of the hand.

What is the most appropriate next step in management?

A. Splinting the hand in a position of function, elevation, IV antibiotics, observation for 24 hours

B. Bedside I&D of dorsal hand abscess

C. Echocardiogram to look for valvular vegetation

D. MRI of hand to evaluate underlying abscess

E. Emergent operative debridement

Discussion

The correct answer is (E). The patient is febrile, tachycardic and mildly hypotensive with induration and blistering of the dorsal hand tissues, which is consistent with a diagnosis of necrotizing fasciitis. The rapid spreading of the infection precludes observation. A bedside I&D will be inadequate to debride the affected tissue and control the infection. Echocardiogram will not treat the hand infection, and necrotizing fasciitis is not associated with endocarditis. An MRI will delay the patient's care. Rapid debridement is critical to treat necrotizing soft tissue infections.

The patient is brought to the operating room and dishwater like fluid is drained from the wound. The fascial planes are easily separated with blunt palpation.

Tissue cultures are likely to show what type of bacteria?

A. Group A, Beta hemolytic *Streptococcus*

B. Group B *Streptococcus*

C. Methicillin-resistant *Staphylococcus aureus*

D. *Serratia marcescens*

E. *Clostridium perfringens*

Discussion

The correct answer is (A). Group A Strep and polymicrobial infections are the most common causes of necrotizing fasciitis. Clostridium is also associated with necrotizing soft tissue infections (gas gangrene), but is less common than Group A Strep and polymicrobial infections. Group B strep is largely harmless to adults but is of concern during vaginal deliveries to prevent infections in the newborn. MRSA is associated with hand infections and abscesses. A toxin produced by the bacteria can damage tissue but is not a common pathogen of necrotizing soft tissue infections. *Serratia marcescens* is a gram-negative rod that is not associated with necrotizing soft tissue infections as an isolated pathogen.

Which of the following laboratory values is not associated with a diagnosis of soft tissue necrotizing infection?

A. WBC • 20,000/cc
B. Creatinine • >2.0 mg/dL
C. Sodium • 135 mg/dL
D. Potassium • 3.4 mg/dL
E. Glucose • 180 mg/dL

Discussion

The correct answer is (D). The laboratory risk indicator for necrotizing fasciitis is a scoring system utilized to assist in diagnosis with a score of greater to or equal than 6 raising suspicion for necrotizing fasciitis. Hyperkalemia, not hypokalemia, is consistent with tissue damage and is associated with a poor prognosis and concern for the need for amputation.

C-reactive Protein	Score
<150	0
≥150	4
WBC	
<15	0
15–25	1
>25,000	2
Hemoglobin	
>13.5	0
11–13.5	1
<11	2
Sodium	
≥135	0
<135	2
Creatinine	
<2.0	0
>2.0	2
Glucose	
<180	0
>180	1

4. 24 hours after the initial debridement, the patient has a dorsal hand wound measuring 5 × 4 cm with exposed tendon. His white blood count has decreased from 25,000/cc to 17,000/cc. His temperature is 98 degrees, heart rate is 88 bpm, and blood pressure is 100/64.

What is the most appropriate next step in management?

A. Split thickness skin graft
B. Primary closure
C. Local flap coverage
D. Free flap coverage
E. Second look procedure

Discussion

The correct answer is (E). A second look procedure is indicated in a necrotizing soft tissue infection, particularly without complete resolution of the WBC. Because the infection spreads so quickly, it is prudent to perform repeated debridements to ensure surgical control of the infection. Twenty-four hours after the initial debridement is too early to perform closure, particularly without complete clearance of the infection. In addition, the defect is too large for primary closure. Exposed tendons will not provide a vascularized bed for a split thickness skin graft. Local flaps will not provide adequate coverage of the dorsum of the hand with this large of a defect. Free tissue transfer or regional flap (reverse radial forearm flap) would provide reliable coverage of the described wound after clearance of the infection.

Objectives: Did you learn...?

- Recognize the presentation of necrotizing fasciitis?
- Describe the appropriate treatment?
- Identity the bacteria that cause necrotizing fasciitis?
- Select the expected laboratory values?

CASE 26

A 32-year-old, male patient reports 4 days ago he was fishing in the wilderness when he punctured his long finger with a fishing hook. Over the past 3 days during his trek back, he reports long finger pain with passive extension, fusiform swelling, and pain along the flexor sheath. Flexor tenosynovitis is suspected. He also reports worsening pain in the hand.

Rupture of the flexor sheath and progression of the infection into what space is most concerning?

A. Thenar space
B. Midpalmar space
C. Parona's space

D. Intermetacarpal space
E. Hypothenar space

Discussion

The correct answer is (B). See below for further discussion.

Which of the following is not one of the borders of the midpalmar space?

A. Oblique palmar septum
B. Volar interossei and 3,4,5 metacarpals
C. Hypothenar septum
D. Flexor tendons to the long, ring, and small fingers
E. The adductor pollicis

Discussion

The correct answer is (E). The midpalmar space is a potential space lying between the thenar and hypothenar spaces. It is bordered by the oblique midpalmar septum radially, the flexor tendons to the fingers volarly, the hypothenar septum ulnarly, and the volar interossei and long, ring, and small metacarpals dorsally. The vertical septae of the palmar fascia provides the distal border, and a thin septum at the distal end of the carpal tunnel is the proximal border. This potential space is essentially a bursa to prevent friction between the overlying flexor tendons, the volar interossei, and metacarpals below. The thenar space is bordered by the adductor pollicis (deep), the thenar skin (superficial), and the oblique midpalmar septum (ulnarly). Rupture of the flexor tendon sheath of the ring and long fingers can extend proximally into the midpalmar space.

Parona's space is a potential space of the distal forearm overlying the pronator quadratus and lying deep to the FPL and FDP tendons. The thenar space lies ulnar to the midpalmar fascia and is not usually involved with ring finger flexor tenosynovitis rupture. A collar button abscess extends on both the volar and dorsal side of a web space infection.

Which of the following is consistent with midpalmar space infection?

A. Painless with motion of the ring and long fingers.
B. Maintenance of the palmar concavity
C. Dorsal hand swelling
D. Painless palpation of the mid palm
E. Thumb held in abduction

Discussion

The correct answer is (C). Dorsal hand swelling is often present with deep space hand infections, although it is

usually painless and without erythema. Abduction of the thumb is typical of a thenar space infection. The palm will be tender with a midpalmar space infection, and the palmar concavity is lost. Pain with the ring and long fingers is expected because they pass over the midpalmar space.

What is the appropriate next step in this patient's treatment?

A. Elevation, splinting, antibiotics, and observation
B. Dorsal and volar incisions of the hand for drainage
C. Irrigation and debridement through a midaxial incision on the digit and transverse incision at the midpalmar crease
D. Irrigation and debridement through a longitudinal incision overlying the volar finger extending to the palm
E. Irrigation and debridement through FCR approach to the volar forearm

Discussion

The correct answer is (C). Observation and antibiotics are inadequate to treat this progressive infection. A dorsal incision over the hand is unnecessary to adequately drain the abscess. A midaxial incision and transverse incision will adequately drain the flexor sheath as well as the midpalmar abscess. Longitudinal incisions are avoided across flexion creases of the digits and hand to prevent scar contracture and loss of motion postoperatively. An FCR approach is useful to drain an abscess in Parona's space.

Objectives: Did you learn…?

• Describe the anatomy of the midpalmar space?
• Pinpoint the physical examination findings consistent with midpalmar space infection?
• Describe the correct management of midpalmar abscesses?

CASE 27

A 23-year-old man presents to your office with pain of his fingertip over the past day. He does admit to biting his nails and cuticles, particularly because he is stressed over his upcoming dentistry examinations. He has slight swelling and redness over the ulnar eponychial fold of his index finger. He has tenderness to palpation, but no fluctance is noted.

What is the diagnosis?

A. Paronychial infection
B. Finger felon

C. Distal interphalyngeal septic arthritis
D. Psoriatic arthritis
E. Herpetic Whitlow

Discussion

The correct answer is (A). This is an infection of the tissues around the fingernail. A history of biting of the nails is typical as it results in a break of the skin barrier, a source of bacteria, and a moist environment with tissue maceration. A finger felon is an infection of the fingertip pulp tissue—the pain, swelling, and redness would be volar in that situation. DIP joint septic arthritis would present with generalized swelling of the distal digit. Psoriatic arthritis often presents with pitting of the nails and nails that separate from the underlying nail bed (onycholysis). A herpetic whitlow would present with vesicle formation.

What is the most appropriate next step in management for this patient?

A. Warm soapy water soaks and oral antibiotics
B. Drainage by elevating the paronychial fold away from the nail
C. Drainage by incising over the point of maximal tenderness with the knife directed toward the nail bed and matrix
D. Removal of the ulnar half of the nail
E. Complete removal of the nail

Discussion

The correct answer is (A). Without clear fluctuance and after a short time course, oral antibiotics and soaks in warm soapy water to promote drainage are often adequate. If fluctuance is appreciated, drainage is accomplished by elevating the fold away from the nail after adequate regional block. Alternately, an incision can be made over the point of maximal tenderness but should be directed away from the nail fold to prevent nail deformity. Partial or complete nail removal is utilized with more extensive infections often involving the eponychia and opposite paronychia, respectively.

The patient is treated with antibiotics and has a full recovery. He reports that he passed his examinations and has started his clinical rotations for dental school. However, 3 months later he represents with painful small vesicular lesions with a red base affecting his ulnar paronychia surrounding a confluent, large vesicular lesion extending to the proximal phalanx of his thumb.

What is the most appropriate next step in management?

A. Observation
B. Oral antibiotics and warm soapy soaks
C. Drainage of the infection by elevating the paronychial fold away from the nail.
D. Removal of one half of the nail
E. Removal of the complete nail

Discussion

The correct answer is (A). The vesicular lesions are consistent with a Herpetic Whitlow, or cutaneous Herpes Simplex Virus Infection. Dental workers are at a higher risk because of contact with oral herpetic infections. Young children who suck on their fingers and have an oral infection are also at risk. The condition is usually self-limited, but antivirals are used when the condition is not improving, worsening, or very painful. Surgeons will often receive pressure to drain these infections, but surgical drainage is contraindicated as it does not affect the course of the viral infection and can cause significant wound healing problems, or encephalitis via hematogenous spreading.

Objectives: Did you learn…?

• Describe the presentation of paronychial infection?
• Understand its management?
• Describe the management of herpetic whitlow?

CASE 28

A 19-year-old male mechanic presents with a painless, fleshy mass protruding from the region of his eponychial fold. He reports a metal splinter at that site which he removed 2 weeks ago. He reports that the mass grew quickly and often bleeds.

What is the most likely diagnosis?

A. Inclusion cyst
B. Pyoderma gangrenosum
C. Amelanotic melanoma
D. Pyogenic granuloma
E. Paronychial infection

Discussion

The correct answer is (D). It is an overgrowth of tissue particularly in an area of former trauma or irritation. It is made up of capillary tissue that is not epithelialized; therefore, it is a moist, friable lesion. It is not a truly "pyogenic" or pus producing process, as it is a result of trauma and not infection, and it does not produce purulence. An inclusion cyst is a cyst filled with shed keratinocytes that is caused by trauma that buries epithelialized skin deep to the skin surface. Pyoderma gangrenosum is an ulcerative lesion with a blue-grey or purple irregular border of the surrounding skin, and it is autoimmune in nature. An amelanotic melanoma is a type of skin cancer that does not have pigment. They are quite rare, but the presentation can be similar to pyogenic granuloma with a pinkish red color and rapid growth. Recurrence of amelanotic melanoma is quite high, and it is often fatal despite excision. A paronychial infection is characterized by pain, swelling, and redness of the paronychial tissue.

Which treatment is contraindicated for this mechanic?

A. Curettage
B. Silver nitrate cauterization
C. Electrocauterization
D. Excision and closure
E. Wide local excision and skin grafting

Discussion

The correct answer is (E). The mass is usually friable and treated with simple cautery or excision. A pedunculated stalk is typical of the lesion, so a wide excision is rarely necessary.

The patient undergoes excision of the mass and closure and has an uneventful recovery. On follow-up, he brings his brother to the office who has a history of ulcerative colitis. The brother has a dorsal hand wound that began as a pustule but developed a central area of necrosis and ulceration. The ulcer is enlarging and has been present for several months.

Which of the following is true regarding this condition?

A. Initial treatment is wide local excision
B. The patient should receive systemic steroids and local wound care
C. Treatment of an associated ulcerative colitis flare with immunosuppressants should be avoided with this open wound
D. Skin grafting and closure of the wound halts its progression
E. Topical antifungals are effective

Discussion

The correct answer is (B). The lesion described is of pyoderma gangrenosum. This is an ulcerative lesion associated with autoimmune disorders including ulcerative colitis, Crohn's disease, and rheumatoid arthritis among others. It also occurs in patients without autoimmune disorders. Excision is contraindicated because the

condition can worsen with further tissue damage. Treatment of a flare of ulcerative colitis is recommended as pyoderma gangrenosum is thought to also be a dysfunction of the immune system and often improves with treatment of the associated disease process. Skin grafts do not take well on the ulcerated nonviable tissue. Topical antifungals have no role in the treatment of this immune modulated disease.

Objectives: Did you learn...?

• Recognize the presentation and treatment of pyogenic granuloma?
• Recognize the presentation and treatment of pyoderma gangrenosum?

CASE 29

An 8-month-old patient presents with her parents for evaluation of her right thumb.

The parents report that the left thumb is smaller. At times the patient attempts to use the thumb to pinch, at other times she attempts to pinch objects with her index and long fingers (Fig. 4–16A and B).

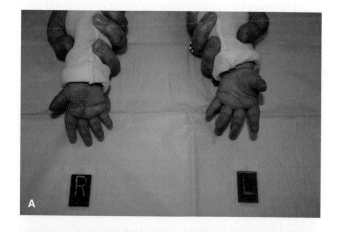

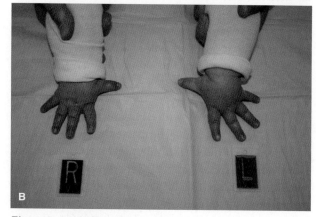

Figure 4–16 **A–B**

Which of the following anomalies is not associated with this condition?

A. Tracheoesophageal fistula
B. Thrombocytopenia present at birth
C. Pancytopenia present at birth
D. Ventricular septal defects
E. Anal atresia

Discussion

The correct answer is (C). This patient has a hypoplastic thumb. Associated syndromes include VACTERRL (vertebral, anal atresia, cardiac defects, trachea-esophageal fistula, renal, and radial limb anomalies), Holt–Oram syndrome, or thumb hypoplasia, and congenital heart defects including atrial or ventricular septal defects. Pancytopenia associated with Fanconi anemia does not often present until later in childhood but can be lethal. Thrombocytopenia with absent radius (TAR) has thrombocytopenia present at birth, and the platelet count typically improves with time.

Which of the following associated conditions is autosomal recessive?

A. VACTERRL
B. VATER
C. Holt–Oram
D. Fanconi Anemia

Discussion

The correct answer is (D). VACTERRL and VATER are often sporadic. Holt–Oram syndrome has an autosomal dominant inheritance pattern. TAR has an autosomal recessive inheritance pattern but can also be sporadic in nature. Fanconi anemia is autosomal recessive.

The patient undergoes genetic testing and is not found to have any associated anomalies. The parents want to know more about possible surgical treatment options.

Which of the following is contraindicated in hypoplastic thumb reconstruction?

A. Abductor digiti quinti opponensplasty
B. Flexor digitorum superficialis tendon transfer opponensplasty
C. Stabilization of the metacarpophalangeal joint with free tendon graft
D. Stabilization of the carpometacarpal joint with free tendon graft
E. Excision of a floating thumb, or pouce flottant

Discussion

The correct answer is (D). Opponensplasty can be performed with either an ADQ (Huber) transfer or an FDS (often from the ring) transfer. The MCP joint is often unstable and can be stabilized as part of reconstruction. The instability of the carpometacarpal joint is most likely due to an underdeveloped proximal metacarpal, so attempts at stabilization with soft tissue will not be successful. A floating thumb has no bony attachment to the hand and no function. Therefore, excising the severely hypoplastic thumb is a common step in thumb reconstruction.

On physical examination, the patient is found to have a thumb in the plane of the hand and absent thenar muscles, a narrow first web space, and instability of the thumb carpometacarpal joint.

What is the most appropriate next step in surgical management?

A. Pollicization
B. Chondrodesis of the carpometacarpal joint
C. First web space deepening with four flap z-plasty
D. Opponensplasty with abductor digiti quinti transfer
E. Progressive splinting to improve the first web space

Discussion

The correct answer is (A). A stable carpometacarpal joint is tantamount to proceeding with thumb reconstruction that preserves the native thumb. Chondrodesis of the CMC joint is contraindicated because it would severely limit opposition. First web space deepening and opponensplasty are utilized in hypoplastic thumbs with stable CMC joints. Progressive splinting will not deepen a congenitally narrow web.

The patient's parents were so inspired by the successful treatment of their son that they adopted a child with radial club hand. They present with this child for treatment. On physical examination, he has an absent thumb, radial deviation of the hand at the wrist, and a foreshortened humerus.

Centralization of the hand is contraindicated in which of the following?

A. A patient without antecedent pollicization
B. Absent scaphoid and trapezium
C. Absent extensor carpi radialis longus and brevis
D. Stiff elbow held in extension
E. Minimal active shoulder abduction

Discussion

The correct answer is (D). The radial longitudinal deficiency often involves multiple radial-sided structures including absence of intrinsic and extrinsic muscles, an absent thumb, and absent radial carpal bones. If the patient is unable to bend the elbow, then the deviated wrist may act as an elbow in order to get the hand to the mouth. By centralizing the hand on the wrist, the patient may therefore lose function if he cannot reach his mouth. Shoulder abduction is not necessary to perform centralization.

Objectives: Did you learn...?

- Recognize the associated syndromes with hypoplastic thumb, their inheritance patterns, and their expected clinical course?
- Identify the indications for opponensplasty versus pollicization?
- Pinpoint the contraindication for wrist centralization in radial hypoplasia?

CASE 30

An 11-month-old patient is brought to you by his parents for "two thumbs on one hand." Examination of the hand is significant for diverging, converging thumb duplication on the right. He has a duplication of the proximal and distal phalanges. On palpation, there is a singular thumb metacarpal.

What is the most appropriate next step in the patient's management?

A. Cardiac ultrasound and renal ultrasound
B. CBC, peripheral blood smear, and chromosome breakage analysis
C. Barium swallow and spine MRI
D. LFTs and chromosome analysis
E. Hand x-ray

Discussion

The correct answer is (E). Thumb duplication is most often sporadic but occasionally autosomal dominant. It is not associated with other conditions, with the exception of triphalyngeal duplicated thumbs (Wassel type VII, see below). The following conditions are associated with thumb hypoplasia, not thumb duplication.

Holt–Oram: cardiac ultrasound

Thrombocytopenia Absent Radius (TAR) CBC, peripheral blood smear

Fanconi anemia: chromosome breakage analysis

VATER/VACTERRL: barium swallow, spine imaging

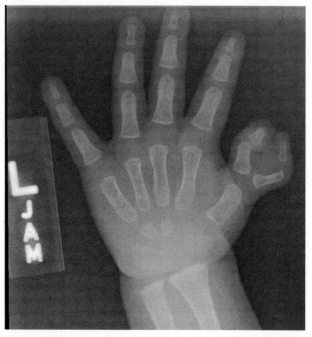

Figure 4–17

A cardiac ultrasound and renal ultrasound are indicated with thumb or radial-sided hypoplasia, not duplication.

The patient undergoes x-ray of the thumb shown in Figure 4–17.

What is the Wassel classification of the thumb?

A. Type II
B. Type III
C. Type IV
D. Type V
E. Type VI

Discussion

The correct answer is (C).

The Wassel classification is as follows:

   I: Bifid distal phalanx
  II: Duplicated distal phalanx
 III: Duplication of the distal phalanx bifid proximal phalanx
 IV: Duplication of the distal phalanx and proximal phalanx
  V: Duplication of the distal phalanx, proximal phalanx, and bifid metacarpal
 VI: Duplication of the distal phalanx, middle phalanx, and metacarpal of the thumb
VII: Thumb duplication with a triphalyngeal thumb.

The classification number corresponds with the number of abnormal bones in the duplication.

Which of the following is likely involved in the etiology of thumb duplication?

A. AER—apical ectodermal ridge
B. ZPA—zone of polarizing activity
C. Vascular insult of the radial artery
D. Separation of chorion from amnion
E. Notochord development

Discussion

The correct answer is (A). The apical ectodermal ridge (AER) is critical in limb development, particularly in the proximal to distal direction. It is thought to be implicated in duplicated thumbs. The zone of polarizing activity on the limb bud has pattern organizing activity for antero/posterior formation (ZPA = AP formation). Vascular insult to the radial artery is one theory in the development of radial club hand. Separation of the chorion from the amnion can result in amniotic band syndrome. Abnormal notochord development can result in spina bifida and other spinal anomalies.

What is the most common and second most common type of thumb duplication?

A. Most common = Type 1; Second most common = Type 2
B. Most common = Type 2; Second most common = Type 1
C. Most common = Type 2; Second most common = Type 4
D. Most common = Type 4; Second most common = Type 2
E. Most common = Type 4; Second most common = Type 6

Discussion

The correct answer is (D). Type 4 is the most common (43%). Type 2 is the second most common (15%).

What is an appropriate step in the initial surgical management of this patient?

A. Removal of the central portion of each thumb and combining the radial half of one thumb with the ulnar half of the other (the Bilhaut–Cloquet procedure)
B. Excision of the divergent/convergent thumbs and pollicization of the index finger
C. Stabilization of the carpometacarpal joint of the thumb

D. Combining the proximal component of the radial thumb with the distal component of the ulnar thumb
E. Excision of the radial thumb and transferring the extrinsic tendons of the radial thumb to the ulnar thumb

Discussion

The correct answer is (E). Combining the two digits into one by removing central tissue is indicated for type 1, 2, and 3 thumbs. This is not performed with type 4 thumbs where four bones would need to be combined to two. The Bilhaut–Cloquet procedure can result in stiffness. Removal of the thumbs and pollicization is indicated in hypoplastic thumbs without a stable CMC joint, not in thumb duplication. The CMC joint is not affected in type four thumbs and does not need to be stabilized. An on-top plasty (combining the proximal component of one thumb with the distal component of the other) is indicated when one digit has a superior proximal component and the other digit has a superior distal component. When the two thumbs are equal in size, such as in this case, the radial thumb is usually excised. Excision of the radial thumb with transfer of the flexor tendons to counteract the Z deforming forces is indicated in this Wassel IV thumb.

Objectives: Did you learn…?

- Classify thumb duplication?
- Describe the appropriate workup of duplicated thumb versus thumb aplasia?
- Identify the embryologic contribution to thumb duplication?
- Pinpoint the most common types of thumb duplication?
- Surgically manage thumb duplication?

CASE 31

A 17-year-old patient presents for evaluation. He reports that after racing his motocross bike for approximately 20 minutes, he reports pain, weakness of grip, forearm swelling and numbness and tingling of all five digits. On physical examination, he has normal sensation, normal strength of all major muscle groups. It resolves with rest.

What is the most likely diagnosis?

A. Carpal tunnel syndrome
B. Chronic exertional compartment syndrome
C. Cervical spinal stenosis
D. Anterior interosseous compressive neuropathy
E. Parsonage–Turner syndrome

Discussion

The correct answer is (B). Chronic exertional compartment syndrome would cause weakness and numbness at times of extreme muscle use. At times of rest, as in the clinic setting, the physical examination is expected to be normal. Treatment is forearm fasciotomy done on a scheduled basis. Carpal tunnel syndrome would involve the radial three and one half digits and would not be expected to cause forearm swelling or grip weakness. Cervical spinal stenosis would not be exertional in nature. Anterior interosseous compressive neuropathy would have weakness without sensation changes. A weakness of thumb, index, and middle pinch and grip is expected. Parsonage–Turner syndrome is an idiopathic brachial plexopathy that presents with usually unilateral shoulder pain followed by numbness and weakness in the upper extremity. It is often posttraumatic, postinfectious, or postvaccination.

Additional Questions

The orthopaedic service is consulted on a 32-year-old patient with severe hand pain. The patient underwent an 8 hour operative procedure in which his hands were tucked during positioning and his hips abducted. After extubation, he began complaining of pain in the left hand. His heart rate is 108 and his blood pressure is 92/54.

Which of the following is most consistent with a diagnosis of compartment syndrome?

A. Compartment pressure of 28
B. Dorsal swelling greater than volar swelling
C. Hand held with MPs flexed and IPs extended
D. Pain with passive flexion greater than extension of the thumb
E. Painless adduction and abduction of the thumb

Discussion

The correct answer is (A). Compartment pressures of 30 to 45 mm Hg or within 30 mm Hg of the diastolic pressure are consistent with a diagnosis of compartment syndrome. The swelling is generally diffuse. The hand is held in intrinsic minus position in compartment syndrome with IPs flexed and MPs extended. Pain with digit extension causes pain as a first sign as well as pain with abduction.

Which of the following is the correct number of compartments in the hand and incisions necessary to release the hand compartments?

A. Eight compartments, four incisions
B. Eight compartments, eight incisions

C. Eight compartments, five incisions
D. 10 compartments, 4 incisions
E. 10 compartments, 10 incisions

Discussion

The correct answer is (D). There are 10 compartments in the hand: thenar, hypothenar, adductor, volar interosseous (3) and dorsal interosseous (4). They can be accessed via two longitudinal incisions centered over the second and fourth metacarpals dorsally to decompress the volar and dorsal interossei as well as the adductor compartment. A longitudinal incision on the radial side of the first metacarpal decompresses the thenar compartment. A longitudinal incision over the ulnar side of the fifth metacarpal decompresses the hypothenar compartment. This is a total of 20 compartments and 4 incisions.

The patient undergoes hand compartment releases and a carpal tunnel release. Herniation of muscle is noted with necrosis of the superficial muscle. The median nerve is exposed within the wound.

Which is indicated?

A. Debridement of muscle and closure of skin to prevent desiccation of tissues
B. Defer excision of necrotic muscle until necrosis is completely demarcated
C. Application of a moist dressing after debridement of necrotic tissue
D. Compressive dressing to prevent hemorrhage and further blood loss
E. Debridement and placement of wound vac sponge within the wounds

Discussion

The correct answer is (D). Wounds should be left open and dressed with a moist dressing in this situation. Early closure of the skin can increase compartment pressures and cause further tissue damage. A second look procedure is indicated and therefore the wounds are left open. Any necrotic tissue should be excised. Delaying excision of necrotic tissue can cause further inflammation and swelling. A compressive dressing can increase compartment pressures and worsen compartment syndrome. A wound vac sponge should not be placed directly on vessels or nerves. This is a contraindication to negative pressure wound therapy. The sponge can erode vessel walls and cause severe bleeding, often occurring at the time of sponge removal.

Objectives: Did you learn...?

- Recognize chronic exertional as well as acute compartment syndrome of the hand including the presentation and diagnosis?
- Describe the anatomy of the hand compartments and how to release each of them?
- Manage compartment syndrome after release?

CASE 32

A 34-year-old, right-hand-dominant man presents with a pinpoint injury to his left index finger. He reports that he was cleaning the nozzle of his paint gun when he accidentally pulled the trigger of the gun. Inspection of the digit reveals a pinpoint skin break at the distal phalanx. He receives tetanus prophylaxis and IV antibiotics in the emergency department.

What is the next appropriate step?

A. Splinting, elevation, and observation
B. Early active motion of the digit
C. Bedside incision and drainage with metacarpal block
D. Formal debridement in the operating room
E. Amputation of the digit

Discussion

The correct answer is (D). High-pressure injection injury requires formal debridement in the operating room. Removal of necrotic tissue and the offending agent is indicated. A bedside I&D will not be adequate in the setting. Without signs of necrosis and without attempting a formal debridement, amputation is not indicated. Splinting and early motion are not adequate treatment of this injury.

Which of the following factors is associated with an improved prognosis?

A. Debridement within 12 to 24 hours
B. Force of injection of 8,000 psi
C. Injection into the palm versus the finger
D. Injection of industrial solvent
E. Injection into the thumb

Discussion

The correct answer is (C). Debridement within 6 to 10 hours shows improved prognosis. Continued contact with caustic materials damages the tissues, and early aggressive debridement on an emergent basis is critical for treatment. Injuries with >7,000 psi have a 100% amputation rate. Injection of the palm has an improved prognosis over the finger as it is not governed by fascial planes. Injection of industrial solvents is associated with a worse prognosis (see below). Injection of the thumb is not associated with improved prognosis. The injected material can extend into the thenar space, and a poorly functioning thumb has a worse prognosis for the overall function of the hand.

Which of the following injection materials is associated with a worse prognosis and increased risk of amputation?

A. Air
B. Latex-based paint
C. Water-based paint
D. Oil-based paint
E. Grease

Discussion

The correct answer is (D). Less tissue damage is associated with grease, latex-based paint, water-based paint, air, and veterinary vaccines.

Objectives: Did you learn...?

- Describe the prognostic factors for paint injection injury?
- Manage paint injection injury?

CASE 33

A 64-year-old man presents with the complaint of inability to place his hand in his pocket and an awkward handshake. On physical examination, he has a flexion contracture involving the ring and small fingers. Dupuytren's contracture is diagnosed.

Which of the following is true regarding this disease process?

A. Ectopic involvement (Ledderhose disease of the feet, Peyronie's disease of the penis) is associated with a less aggressive clinical course
B. The disease is associated with increased Collagen type III production and myofibroblast proliferation
C. Grayson's ligaments are usually spared in the disease process
D. Alcohol intake has a protective effect
E. Bands and cords make up the pathologic anatomy

Discussion

The correct answer is (B). The disease is associated with an increased Collagen type III to type I ratio. Myofibroblast proliferation causes contraction of the collagenous palmar fascia. Platelet-derived growth factor and fibroblast growth factor have also been implicated in the pathogenesis. Ectopic involvement is usually associated with a more aggressive disease course. Cleland's ligaments are usually spared in the disease process; Grayson's ligaments are often involved. Diabetes, antiseizure medications, and alcohol intake are often associated with Dupuytren's contracture. It often has an autosomal dominant pattern with variable penetrance. Cords and nodules make up the pathologic anatomy. Bands represent normal anatomic structures, which then thicken to form cords.

Which of the following is true regarding the pathology of the Dupuytren's disease?

A. Involvement of the natatory ligament causes an abduction contracture
B. A central cord displaced the neurovascular bundles volarly and centrally
C. Involvement of the abductor digiti quinti (ADQ) causes PIP joint contracture in the small finger
D. The neurovascular bundle lies lateral and deep to the spiral cord
E. The DIP joint is not affected by a retrovascular cord

Discussion
The correct answer is (C). The ADQ inserts at the middle phalanx most often, and involvement of the ADQ often leads to PIP joint contracture of the small finger. Involvement of the natatory ligament causes an adduction contracture of the palm. It is also involved in the spiral cord so it may contribute to a PIP joint flexion contracture. The central cord lies between the neurovascular bundles and is an extension of the pretendinous cord. The spiral cord lies deep and lateral to the neurovascular bundle and displaces the bundle central and superficially, putting it at particular risk at the MP flexion crease. It is composed of the natatory band, pretendinous band, spiral band, lateral digital sheath, and Grayson's ligament. The name spiral cord is a misnomer because it does not spiral, rather the bundle spirals around the cord with progressive disease. DIP joint contracture is often from a retrovascular cord.

Which of the following is an indication for surgery?

A. DIP joint contracture of 35 degrees
B. PIP joint contracture of 10 degrees
C. MP joint contracture of 30 degrees
D. Painful palmar nodules
E. Palpable recurrent cord

Discussion
The correct answer is (C). DIP joint contracture is usually not an indication for surgery and rarely occurs in

isolation. A PIP joint contracture of 20 degrees is generally considered an indication for surgery.

Painful nodules are generally not considered an indication for surgery. A recurrent cord without contracture is not an indication for surgery.

Which of the following treatment options is contraindicated?

A. Needle aponeurotomy
B. Collagenase injection followed by manual manipulation
C. Local fasciectomy
D. Subtotal fasciectomy
E. Total fasciectomy

Discussion
The correct answer is (E). Needle aponeurotomy is performed in the office setting or operating room setting. A needle is used to puncture the offending cord multiple times to weaken it before manual traction breaks the cord. It is often done under local anesthesia of the skin that does not block the digital nerves to prevent damaging the digital nerves with the needle. The aponeurotomy is done at the level of the palm to avoid injuring the digital nerves. It is often used for infirmed patients and has a high recurrence rate. Collagenase injection (Xiaflex) has gained popularity. The collagenase is injected into the cord followed by manipulation 24 hours later. Nerve damage and tendon rupture are risks. It is more effective at treating MP joint contractures than PIP joint contractures. A local fasciectomy is an excision of a short segment of diseased tissue. It may be done under local anesthesia, which is of benefit to infirmed patients, but this technique has a high recurrence rate. A subtotal fasciectomy is the most commonly performed procedure for Dupuytren's contracture in which the involved fascia is excised. A total fasciectomy involves removing all fascia of the palm and is associated with an extremely high morbidity. It is of historical interest only.

Which of the following is a contraindicated approach?

A. Longitudinal incision along volar surface of digit followed by z-plasties
B. Transverse palmar incision left open
C. Midaxial digital incision
D. Modified Brunner zig–zag incisions with v-y flap advancement
E. Dermatofasciectomy

Discussion

The correct answer is (C). A midaxial incision is unlikely to provide adequate exposure. Longitudinal incisions followed by z-plasties have the benefit of designing the flaps over the highest quality skin and incorporating inadvertent button hole incisions in the skin. It also converts excess skin in the transverse direction to the longitudinal direction where there is often a deficit in skin after a long-term contracture. Leaving the transverse palmar incision open (McCash technique) is useful in longitudinal skin defects and, unlike skin grafting, allows for immediate active motion protocols. Modified Brunner zigzag incisions are a well accepted technique that allows for wide exposure. Adding a v–y advancement decreases tension on the incisions and allows for further digit extension. A dermatofasciectomy is used often with recurrent disease and is often combined with skin grafting.

Objectives: Did you learn...?

- Describe the fascial anatomy of Dupuytren's disease?
- Pinpoint the indication for surgical intervention?
- Describe the surgical approaches and appropriate techniques?
- Indicate factors associated with the disease process?

CASE 34

A patient sustains a laceration at the level of the middle phalanx of the long finger.

He has an abnormal cascade and undergoes wound exploration. He is noted to have a laceration of the FDP tendon in zone 2. He undergoes repair of both tendons with a four-strand repair and epitendinous suture. He presents 3 days after injury for wound check (Fig. 4–18).

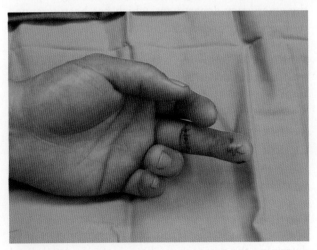

Figure 4–18

What is the most appropriate splint for him postoperatively?

A. A volar splint in the position of function with the wrist extended 30 degrees, MPs flexed 60 degrees, and IPs straight
B. Volar splint with wrist in neutral, MPs flexed 60 degrees, and IPs free
C. Dorsal blocking splint with wrist flexed 30 degrees, MPs flexed 60 degrees, IPs straight
D. Dorsal blocking splint with wrist flexed 30 degrees, MPs extended, IPs flexed 50 degrees
E. Outrigger splint with wrist in neutral and elastic allowing for passive extension and active flexion

Discussion

The correct answer is (C). After flexor tendon repair, a dorsal blocking splint is applied to prevent the digit from extending and placing tension on the repair. The Kleinert splint is also utilized and combines a dorsal blocking splint with a rubber band secured volarly to allow for active extension and passive flexion. The wrist and MPs are placed in flexion, the IPs in extension. A volar splint is avoided because the patient can flex the digit against a volar splint. An outrigger splint is used for radial nerve palsy to allow active flexion and passive extension.

The patient is enrolled in a therapy protocol postoperatively. Which of the following is true regarding therapy?

A. Therapy should begin 10 to 14 days postoperatively at the time of suture removal
B. Passive range of motion protocol is associated with a decreased tendon rupture rate compared to active
C. Passive range of motion protocol is associated with decreased tendon adhesion compared to an active motion protocol
D. The tensile strength of the repaired tendon is adequate for active loading beginning at 8 weeks
E. Gap formation between the repaired tendon ends is associated with a poor prognosis

Discussion

The correct answer is (B). Active motion protocols are associated with less tendon adhesion but a higher rate of tendon rupture. Therapy should begin early after surgery-ideally within 48 hours. The tensile strength of the repaired tendon is adequate for active loading at 4 to 5 weeks postoperatively. Gap formation is not associated with a poor prognosis.

The patient is lost to follow up after a personal issue and presents 3 months later highly motivated to progress with his treatment. He complains of difficulty using the long finger. On physical examination, he has 70 degrees of active flexion of his MP joint and no active flexion of the PIP and DIP joints. He has 80 degrees of passive flexion of his PIP and DIP joints. There is no palpable flexor tendon with attempted flexion of the digit.

What is the appropriate next step?

A. Ultrasonography therapy to treat tendon adhesions
B. Passive motion flexor tendon repair protocol
C. Active motion flexor tendon repair protocol
D. Tenolysis followed by an active motion protocol
E. Excising the flexor tendons and placement of a silicone rod

Discussion

The correct answer is (E). Based on the physical examination, the patient has sustained a tendon rupture. The MPs are likely flexing secondary to lumbrical contraction. The IPs do not have active motion, and the tendon is not palpable on attempted excursion, which would be expected if the tendon were intact but adhesed to the surrounding structures. Flexor tendon repair therapy protocols would not be expected to change this patient's clinical course. Ultrasonography does not have a role after tendon rupture. The only appropriate option is reconstruction.

Objectives: Did you learn...?

- Select the appropriate splint after flexor tendon repair?
- Describe appropriate postoperative therapy?
- Identify tendon rupture and its treatment?

CASE 35

A 28-year-old woman presents after flexor tendon repair in zone 2. Despite an aggressive therapy protocol, she has not achieved sufficient active motion. The tendon is intact on palpation.

Which of the following is true regarding tenolysis?

A. It should be performed 4 to 6 months after primary repair
B. It should be followed by a passive range of motion protocol
C. The A2 pulley should be sacrificed if it is densely adherent to the tendon

D. Tenolysis is indicated to increase passive range of motion as well as active range of motion
E. Postoperative rupture of the tendon is a risk particularly with dense adhesions

Discussion

The correct answer is (E). The tenolysis should be delayed until 6 to 12 months after repair to maximize therapy, minimize risk of tendon rupture, and allow for resolution of inflammation of the digit. Vigorous, active range of motion should be instituted to minimize the risk of postoperative adhesions. Tenolysis will not treat joint contracture, therefore it will not improve passive range of motion of the joints. Postoperative tendon rupture is a known risk of tenolysis. Healing of the tendon to the surrounding structures can indicate weakness of the laceration repair.

Objectives: Did you learn...?

- Identify the appropriate time period to perform tenolysis?

CASE 36

A 26-year-old, right-hand-dominant woman presents to the emergency department 1 hour after sustaining an injury to the tip of her left middle finger (Fig. 4–19A and B). She works as an executive assistant and smokes 1 pack of cigarettes daily but is otherwise healthy. She reports that she sustained the injury when her car door accidentally closed on the tip of the finger, and she sustained a volar oblique amputation of her fingertip. The injury measures 1.8 cm^2 in area, and there is visible exposed bone at the base of the wound. The patient has brought the amputated fingertip into the emergency department, which has been wrapped in moist gauze and placed on ice.

Which of the following is the most appropriate diagnostic test to order/perform at the time of presentation?

A. CBC with differential
B. INR/PT and PTT
C. ESR
D. Plain films of the affected digit
E. CT scan of the hand and wrist

Discussion

The correct answer is (D). Radiographs are important to determine the presence or absence of associated distal

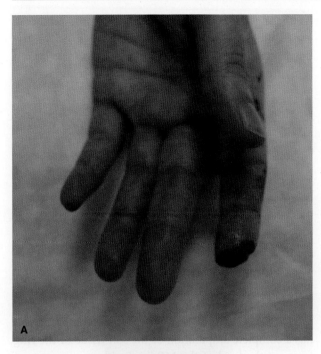

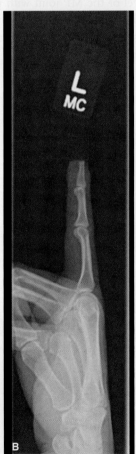

Figure 4–19 **A–B**

phalangeal and other fractures, which can help guide management. The majority of distal phalanx fractures can be treated nonoperatively, but significant displacement often warrants fixation, usually via percutaneous pinning. None of the other diagnostic tests are routinely indicated for this injury in an otherwise healthy young woman.

Which is the most important factor in determining the appropriate treatment for this injury?

A. Presence of exposed bone within the wound
B. Area of the wound >1.5 cm^2
C. Female gender
D. B and C
E. A and B

Discussion
The correct answer is (E). The management of fingertip injuries varies between surgeons and patients, but it is generally accepted that injuries with exposed bone and those with larger defects (generally >1.5 cm^2) require additional intervention to achieve optimal wound closure and soft tissue coverage. The injury geometry is relevant and helps guide treatment options; a variety of surgical procedures exist for volar oblique injuries depending on the digit involved. Female gender by itself does not dictate the optimal treatment.

Which of the following is NOT appropriate initial management of this injury?

A. Irrigation of the wound, closure of available tissue, and application of a moist dressing with prompt clinic follow-up
B. Wound debridement and reverse homodigital neurovascular island flap
C. Immediate shortening of the finger with debridement of the FDP and extensor mechanism proximal to the DIP joint with primary closure
D. Wound debridement and V–Y flap reconstruction
E. Wound debridement and thenar flap reconstruction

Discussion
The correct answer is (C). A variety of surgical options exist for the treatment of fingertip injuries, including homo- and heterodigital island flaps, V–Y flaps, thenar flaps, cross-finger flaps, as well as bony shortening with healing by secondary intention. These can often be performed in semi-elective fashion within the first 1 to 2 weeks post-injury. Immediate shortening of the finger with debridement of the FDP and distal extensor

insertion would not be appropriate in this patient, and would render the finger significantly less functional. Each of the other options constitutes more appropriate treatment of this deformity.

Which deformity may result from proximal retraction of the FDP tendon in management of an injury to the distal part of the finger?

A. Claw finger
B. Lumbrical plus deformity
C. Quadriga
D. Flexion contracture
E. Intrinsic tightness

Discussion

The correct answer is (B). In the lumbrical plus deformity, the finger paradoxically extends at the interphalangeal joints with attempted flexion. This occurs when the proximal end of the FDP tendon retracts proximally, drawing the attached lumbrical. Mechanically, this causes increased tension on the radial lateral band resulting in paradoxical PIP joint extension known as the "lumbrical plus" deformity. Conversely, quadriga occurs when there is tethering of the FDP tendon distally; this results in weak grasp and loss of flexion power in the other digits. Claw finger, flexion contracture, and intrinsic tightness do not result from proximal migration of the FDP tendon.

Objectives: Did you learn...?

• Describe the treatment algorithm for distal phalanx amputations?

CASE 37

A 37-year-old, right-hand-dominant male is referred to the emergency department after sustaining a ring avulsion amputation of his left ring finger (Fig. 4–20A and B). He has mild hypertension, smokes cigarettes occasionally, and works in construction. He sustained the injury while climbing a tree during a hunting expedition, and arrives with the amputated part wrapped in moist gauzed and placed on ice. On examination, the patient has a complete amputation of the soft tissue of the ring finger at the level of the MP joint with preservation of the flexor tendons and extensor mechanism. X-rays demonstrate a subtle fracture of the distal phalanx but no other bony injury (Fig. 4–20C).

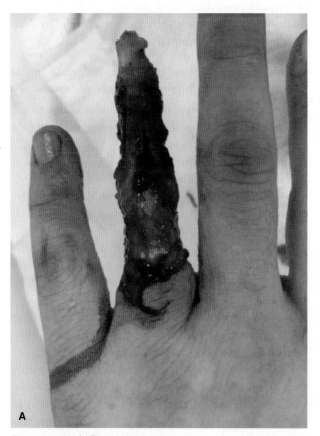

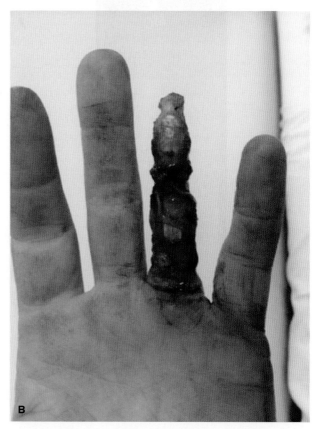

Figure 4–20 **A–B**

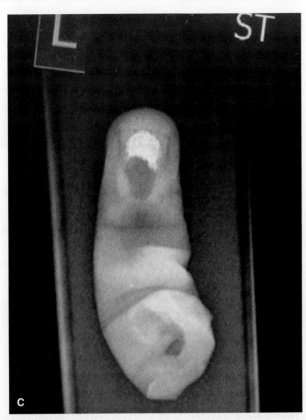

Figure 4–20 **C**

Which of the following is the appropriate Kay classification of this injury?

A. Class I
B. Class 2
C. Class 3
D. Class 4

Discussion

The correct answer is (C). The Kay classification is utilized for the diagnosis and management of ring avulsion injuries. This patient would be classified as Class/Grade 3, which is a complete degloving or complete amputation. Class 1 injuries are avulsion injuries with adequate circulation. Class 2 injuries have arterial compromise only. Class 3 injuries have inadequate circulation with bone, tendon, or nerve injury, and Class 4 injuries represent a complete degloving or complete amputation.

The patient desires all attempts at replantation, even after learning of the lengthy hospital course, requisite postoperative therapy, and possibility of replant failure.

Which of the following factors presents the greatest challenge to performing successful replantation?

A. Absence of significant bony injury
B. Avulsion mechanism of injury
C. Technical challenge of repairing small vessels with operating microscope
D. Age of the patient
E. Amputation level at the MP joint

Discussion

The correct answer is (B). There are many determinants of success during attempted replantation of amputated digits. One important prognostic factor is the mechanism of injury: avulsion amputations have been demonstrated to have a lower success rate than sharp amputations. In general, factors favorable to viable replantation include sharp mechanism of injury, proximal level of amputation, short duration of ischemia, appropriate preservation of the amputated part, and good overall health of the patient with normal platelet count.

Replantation proceeds uneventfully with the use of a vein graft from the volar forearm. On POD 3, the patient's finger becomes increasingly edematous, with violaceous discoloration and capillary refill <1 second.

Which of the following interventions is NOT appropriate at this stage?

A. Immediate return to the operating room for exploration and additional venous anastomosis
B. Removal of the nail plate with application of heparin-soaked gauze to increase efflux of congested blood from the finger
C. Application of medicinal leeches to augment venous outflow
D. Observation only
E. Further discussion with the patient about the option of operative exploration and possible failure of replantation

Discussion

The correct answer is (D). This finger demonstrates signs of venous congestion, which will likely result in failure of replantation unless addressed expeditiously. This can be treated by a variety of different means, including return to the operating room for exploration and provision of additional venous drainage, as well as attempts to augment venous outflow using leeches or topical heparinized saline. In addition, given the single digit nature and mechanism of this injury, it is reasonable to discuss all options with the patient at this stage including the possibility of replant failure.

Leeches are applied with improvement in the color and turgor of the replanted finger.

What is the name of the bacteria present in medicinal leeches and what is the appropriate antibiotic prophylaxis?

A. *Aeromonas hydrophila* and penicillin
B. *Aeromonas hydrophila* and ciprofloxacin
C. *Hirudo medicinalis* and penicillin
D. *Hirudo medicinalis* and ciprofloxacin
E. *Hirudo medicinalis* and tetracycline

Discussion

The correct answer is (B). The primary bacteria found in medicinal leeches are *Aeromonas hydrophila,* and the antibiotic treatment of choice is ciprofloxacin. The name of medicinal leeches is hirudo medicinalis. Other antibiotics which can be used for prophylaxis are trimethoprim/sulfamethoxazole and tetracycline; *Aeromonas hydrophila* is often resistant to penicillin.

Objectives: Did you learn...?

- Describe the Kay classification?
- Pinpoint th challenges that affect outcome in replant failure?
- Identify the signs of venous congestion?
- Treat venous congestion?
- Describe the complications of leeching?

CASE 38

The patient is a 5-year-old boy who is referred into the emergency department with an amputation of his dominant right thumb at the level of the MP joint, sustained during a motor vehicle collision in which a sharp piece of metal lacerated and amputated his thumb. He has no other injuries and is hemodynamically stable. On examination, the patient has a sharp amputation of his thumb through the MP joint, and plain films demonstrate no fractures with preservation of the metacarpal head and proximal phalangeal base.

Which of the following are absolute indications for replantation in this patient?

A. Age of the patient
B. Sharp mechanism of injury
C. Amputation of dominant thumb
D. A and C
E. B and C

Discussion

The correct answer is (D). There are absolute and relative indications for digital replantation. Absolute indications include thumb amputation, multiple digit amputations, amputations in a child, and amputations proximal to the wrist. Relative indications include individual digits distal to the insertion of the FDS (in zone 1). A sharp mechanism of injury is more favorable for success, but by itself is not an absolute indication for replantation.

Which of the following is/are true regarding replantation in this patient?

A. Replantation is more likely to be successful because the patient is a child
B. Replantation is less likely to be successful because the patient's vascular structures are smaller
C. If replantation is successful, the functional outcomes of pediatric patients are superior to that in adults
D. A and C
E. B and C

Discussion

The correct answer is (E). Replantation in children has a lower success rate than in adults. There are many possible reasons for this phenomenon, including more aggressive attempts at replantation in children and the smaller size of vascular structures. If successful, however, the functional results following pediatric replantation are superior to those achieved by adults, possibly due in part to their adaptability and neuroplasticity.

Unfortunately, the replantation is unsuccessful, and the patient is left with absence of the thumb at the level of the MP joint.

Which is the following is the most appropriate reconstruction to offer the patient?

A. No reconstruction
B. Ilizarov thumb lengthening with groin flap reconstruction
C. Toe-to-thumb transfer
D. Pollicization of the index finger
E. Transfer of the contralateral, nondominant thumb

Discussion

The correct answer is (C). The thumb constitutes approximately 50% of hand function, and absence of the thumb at the level of the MP joint is extremely debilitating. The best option for pediatric thumb reconstruction at the MP joint level is a toe-to-thumb transfer. There is some debate about the indications for great toe versus second toe transfer, and each has been performed with success; the choice of donor site is based upon both surgeon experience and patient preference. Thumb lengthening with groin flap reconstruction will provide a longer post for the thumb, but would be inferior to the results of a toe transfer. Pollicization of the index finger is best suited for traumatic absence of the thumb at the CMC joint level.

Objectives: Did you learn...?

- Pinpoint the indications for digital replantation?
- Describe the various treatment options after failed implantation?

CASE 39

The patient is a 68-year-old, right-handed male who presents to the emergency department following a tablesaw injury to his nondominant left index finger (Fig. 4–21A and B). The patient states that he was working at home after having "a few" beers, when his hand slipped and his nondominant index finger was drawn into the blade of the saw. On examination, he has sustained an amputation to the index finger at the mid-shaft of the proximal phalanx, with a stellate, multilevel soft tissue injury to the index finger base. Radiographs demonstrate a comminuted fracture of the proximal phalanx with intra-articular involvement and a fracture of the metacarpal head. The amputated index finger was irretrievable and not brought to the hospital.

What flexor tendon zone is the injury located in, according to Verdan?

A. Zone 1
B. Zone 2
C. Zone 3
D. Zone 4
E. Zone 5

Discussion

The correct answer is (B). There are five flexor tendon zones. Zone 1 is distal to the FDS insertion. Zone 2 is from the A1 pulley to the FDS insertion. Zone 3 is from the carpal tunnel to the A1 pulley. Zone 4 is in the carpal tunnel. Zone 5 is proximal to the carpal tunnel. Injuries in zone 2 are known as "no-man's land," and portend a worse functional prognosis than injuries in other zones.

Which of the following is the most appropriate treatment of this patient?

A. Immediate closure of the laceration in the emergency room
B. Reconnaissance of the amputated part and delayed attempt at replantation
C. Operative exploration with revision amputation of the index finger, without digital neurectomy, leaving the wound open
D. Operative exploration with ray amputation of the index finger and digital neurectomy
E. Application of a dressing and have the patient follow-up in clinic in 3 weeks

Discussion

The correct answer is (D). The functional results of successful single digit replantation in zone 2 have historically been poor. It is often better to perform a revision or a ray amputation with digital neurectomy than to proceed with a single digit replantation at this level,

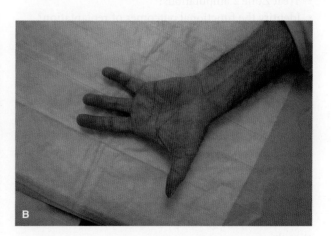

Figure 4–21 **A–B**

particularly in the index finger. A ray amputation for index finger amputations can provide an aesthetic appearance of the hand, while deepening the first web space to allow for pinch grip.

If replantation were to have been attempted, and the finger remained viable postoperatively, what would be the most likely functional result?

A. Significant stiffness of the index finger with bypass of pinch grasp to the middle finger
B. Index finger total active motion of 240 degrees with minimal residual stiffness
C. Index finger total active motion of 140 degrees with two-point discrimination 4 mm at the fingertip
D. Stiffness of the index finger with 170 degrees total active motion, normal sensibility, and normal motion in all other digits
E. Normal range of motion in the index finger but stiffness in all other digits

Discussion

The correct answer is (A). Index finger replantations in zone 2 are notorious for poor functional results, and often lead to significant stiffness with PIP range of motion <40 degrees. If the middle finger is uninjured and the index finger lacks mobility, individuals often bypass the index to the middle finger for pinch grasp. This is the most likely outcome for the patient mentioned in this question. Total active motion in the digits range from 0 to 270 degrees, with 0 to 90 degrees at the MP joint, 0 to 110 degrees at the PIP joint, and 0 to 70 degrees at the DIP joint.

Objectives: Did you learn...?

- Describe the zones of injury according to Verdan?
- Treat Zone 2 amputations?
- Identify the functional outcomes of replantation?

CASE 40

The patient is a 48-year-old, diabetic woman who presents with a 4 months history of numbness and paresthesias of bilateral thumbs, index, and middle fingers. She has had no prior workup for this problem. She reports that her symptoms have been progressive, and that they wake her up from sleep two or three times per week. On physical examination, the patient has grossly normal sensibility in all fingers, and has 5/5 strength to palmar abduction in bilateral thumbs.

What is the most likely diagnosis?

A. Diabetic peripheral neuropathy
B. Cubital tunnel syndrome
C. Pronator syndrome
D. Cervical radiculopathy
E. Carpal tunnel syndrome

Discussion

The correct answer is (E). Carpal tunnel syndrome is the most common compressive neuropathy in the extremity, and can manifest in many ways but often presents with numbness and paresthesias in the volar aspect of the thumb, index finger, middle finger and radial half of the ring finger. It is more common in patients with diabetes, and can result in symptoms that progress over time. This patient's presentation is most consistent with carpal tunnel syndrome.

Which of the following is the most appropriate next step in workup of this patient's symptoms?

A. X-rays of bilateral wrists and hands
B. MRI of bilateral wrists
C. EMG and nerve conduction studies
D. CBC, chemistries, liver function tests
E. TSH and Vitamin B6 levels

Discussion

The correct answer is (C). The most appropriate workup for this patient's symptoms would include electromyography and nerve conduction studies. These tests can provide objective data to determine the presence and severity of the patient's disease. X-rays and MRI are not typically useful in the workup of carpal tunnel syndrome unless other, more rare pathophysiology is suspected.

An EMG is performed which demonstrates mild carpal tunnel syndrome bilaterally, with slight prolongation of distal sensory latencies and no appreciable change in distal motor latencies. The patient is not interested in undergoing surgery.

What is the most appropriate initial management of this patient's condition?

A. Percutaneous carpal tunnel release in the office using an 18 gauge needle
B. Bilateral wrist splints with wrists in 40 degrees of flexion
C. Semi-urgent open bilateral carpal tunnel release
D. Bilateral wrist splints with wrists in neutral position
E. Bilateral corticosteroid injection into the carpal tunnel with 40 cc total of triamcinolone 40 mg/cc mixed with 1% lidocaine with epinephrine

Discussion

The correct answer is (D). This patient has mild carpal tunnel syndrome by EMG. She is not currently interested in undergoing surgical release, and an appropriate first step would be the provision of bilateral wrist splints in neutral position. Studies investigating pressures within the carpal tunnel have demonstrated that the optimal position to splint the wrist are in neutral position or slight extension with slight ulnar deviation. Corticosteroid injections into the carpal tunnel can be effective but at a much lower dose than indicated in answer (E).

Objectives: Did you learn...?

- Poinpoint the clinical presentation of carpal tunnel syndrome?
- Perform workup of carpal tunnel syndrome?
- Initially manage carpal tunnel syndrome?

CASE 41

The patient is a 29-year-old, right-hand-dominant G1 P0 woman, currently 7 months pregnant, who presents with edematous hands and numbness in her thumbs bilaterally. She reports that her symptoms are worst at night and wake her up from sleep. The patient states that she did not have similar symptoms prior to pregnancy. On examination, she has a positive Durkan test but no weakness or thenar atrophy. She is diagnosed with carpal tunnel syndrome of pregnancy.

What is the Durkan test and what is the approximate sensitivity of the test?

A. Wrist flexion test, 25%
B. Wrist flexion test, 50%
C. Wrist flexion test, 90%
D. Direct compression test, 50%
E. Direct compression test, 90%

Discussion

The correct answer is (E). There are many clinical maneuvers which can be used to examine a patient for carpal tunnel syndrome. The Durkan test places direct compression over the median nerve at the carpal tunnel for approximately 30 seconds and is positive with the onset of paresthesias or pain in the median nerve distribution. The approximate sensitivity and specificity are 90%. The wrist flexion, or Phalen test, is performed by asking the patient to flex his/her wrists to 90 degrees—thereby increasing the pressure within the carpal tunnel—and examining for median nerve symptoms.

The sensitivity and specificity are generally thought to be less than that for the Durkan test.

What is the approximate incidence of pregnancy-induced symptoms of carpal tunnel syndrome?

A. 1%
B. 10%
C. 25%
D. 75%
E. 90%

Discussion

The correct answer is (C). Carpal tunnel syndrome during pregnancy is common and is believed to occur in approximately 25% of pregnant women. The etiology appears to be related to whole body edema during the later phases of pregnancy, which in turn causes swelling within the carpal tunnel. In women with prior, asymptomatic compression or a diathesis for compression, symptoms can manifest during pregnancy.

Which of the following is true about carpal tunnel syndrome during pregnancy?

A. Pregnancy is a risk factor for developing carpal tunnel syndrome
B. Surgical intervention for carpal tunnel syndrome during pregnancy is dangerous and should be avoided because it poses significant risks to the mother and fetus
C. Pregnant women frequently experience nocturnal symptoms which can often be treated conservatively
D. A and B
E. A and C

Discussion

The correct answer is (E). It is true that carpal tunnel syndrome is more common within pregnant women, and that most women with this problem can be treated conservatively with the expectation that symptoms will improve and/or resolve following delivery. If surgical intervention is required, it can be safely performed under the direction of an experienced anesthesiologist.

Objectives: Did you learn...?

- Properly perform the Durkan's Test?
- Describe the sensitivity and specificity of Durkan's test?
- Treat pregnancy-induced carpal tunnel syndrome?
- Describe the incidence of pregnancy-induced carpal tunnel syndrome?

CASE 42

The patient is a 65-year-old, diabetic, male carpenter who presents with bilateral carpal tunnel syndrome. His primary symptoms are paresthesias in the median nerve distribution, although he also complains of clumsiness of his hands. On examination, he has weakness to palmar abduction in his thumbs bilaterally with a positive Durkan test. EMG demonstrates moderate bilateral carpal tunnel syndrome. After patient education and counseling, the patient is prepared to undergo carpal tunnel release.

Which of the following is a benefit of endoscopic carpal tunnel release compared to open release?

A.   More complete release of the transverse carpal ligament
B.   Lower complication rate
C.   Faster return of sensation in the median nerve distribution
D.   Faster return to work
E.   Better visualization of critical structures in the palm

Discussion

The correct answer is (D). There are many purported and actual benefits of both open and endoscopic carpal tunnel release, and there are proponents of both techniques. Advantages of the open technique may include better visualization of critical structures in the palm and less required equipment. Some studies have demonstrated a faster return to work with endoscopic release compared with the open technique. In general, both techniques are comparable and can be used successfully in experienced hands.

What structures are at risk during the distal release of the transverse carpal ligament?

A.   The superficial palmar arch vessels
B.   The palmar cutaneous branch of the median nerve
C.   The recurrent motor branch of the median nerve
D.   A and B
E.   A and C

Discussion

The correct answer is (E). There are many structures at risk during the distal release of the transverse carpal ligament, including the superficial palmar arch, the recurrent motor branch of the median nerve, the flexor tendons, and the median nerve, among others. The palmar cutaneous branch of the median nerve arises from the radial side of the median nerve approximately 6cm proximal to the distal volar wrist crease and travels radially onto the thenar eminence. This nerve branch is at risk during proximal, not distal, division of the transverse carpal ligament.

This patient has diabetes. Which of the following is true about diabetic patients and the development of carpal tunnel syndrome?

A.   Patients with diabetes are more likely than nondiabetic patients to develop carpal tunnel syndrome
B.   Patients with diabetes are less likely than nondiabetic patients to develop carpal tunnel syndrome
C.   Patients with diabetes have the same incidence of carpal tunnel syndrome as nondiabetic patients
D.   Patients with diabetes have worse surgical outcomes than those without diabetes
E.   Patients with diabetes have better surgical outcomes than those without diabetes

Discussion

The correct answer is (A). There are many risk factors for the development of carpal tunnel syndrome, including prior wrist fracture, rheumatoid arthritis, hypothyroidism, and diabetes. Patients with diabetes, including those who do not require insulin, are more likely than nondiabetic patients to develop carpal tunnel syndrome. Outcomes following carpal tunnel release, however, appear to be similar in both diabetic and nondiabetic patients.

Objectives: Did you learn...?

• Describe the benefits of endoscopic vs open carpal tunnel release?
• Identify the structures at risk during the release of the transverse carpal ligament?
• Identify the risk factors for carpal tunnel syndrome?

CASE 43

The patient is a 52-year-old, right-hand-dominant male with a history of a nondisplaced right distal radius fracture treated with a short-arm cast for 6 weeks who presents with wrist pain and weakness. His fracture occurred 2 months prior to this presentation, and he initially did well and fully regained range of motion in his wrist and hand. Over the past 3 to 4 weeks, the patient has developed thumb and radial-sided wrist pain. On examination, the patient has crepitation with wrist flexion and wrist extension and has weakness with thumb extension at the MP joint and no appreciable extension at the IP joint.

What is the most specific part of the physical examination to confirm the diagnosis?

A. Thumb flexion with the MP joint held in extension
B. Thumb abduction strength
C. Thumb retropulsion by extending thumb from a palm-down position
D. Thumb extension at the MP joint
E. Finkelstein test

Discussion

The correct answer is (C). The most specific test to isolate and evaluate the extensor pollicis longus tendon is to examine for thumb retropulsion by having the patient place his palm flat down on a table and asking him/her to extend the thumb. The EPL is the only muscle able to perform this function. Thumb flexion and adduction are performed by different muscles; thumb extension at the MP joint is performed primarily by the EPB.

What is the incidence of this complication following treatment for nondisplaced distal radius fractures?

A. 0%
B. 2% to 5%
C. 7% to 10%
D. 10% to 15%
E. 15% to 20%

Discussion

The correct answer is (B). EPL rupture is an uncommon, but recognized complication of distal radius fractures, even those that are nondisplaced and treated without surgery. The incidence of this complication varies in different studies but probably occurs in 2% to 5% of patients. EPL rupture following ORIF of a distal radius fracture with a volar plate may be due to improper screw length, tendon ischemia, or attrition.

What is the most appropriate treatment for this problem?

A. Observation only
B. Urgent direct repair of the ruptured EPL tendon
C. Urgent repair of the EPL tendon with palmaris longus tendon graft
D. Nonurgent repair of the EPL tendon within 2 weeks
E. Extensor indicis proprius tendon transfer

Discussion

The correct answer is (E). Rupture of the EPL tendon following distal radius fracture is rarely amenable to direct repair. The most commonly utilized and best option for this patient would be transfer of the EIP tendon to the EPL. The EIP is an extensor of the index finger, and is identified ulnar to the EDC tendon. This tendon transfer often provides satisfactory extension of the thumb IP joint without sacrificing additional function.

What is the location of the EPL tendon in the distal forearm?

A. First dorsal extensor compartment
B. Second dorsal extensor compartment
C. Third dorsal extensor compartment
D. Forth dorsal extensor compartment
E. Fifth dorsal extensor compartment

Discussion

The correct answer is (C). The extensor pollicis longus is located in the third dorsal extensor compartment. The first compartment contains the APL and EPB, the second contains the ECRL and ECRB, the third the EPL, the fourth the EDC and EIP, the fifth the EDM, and the sixth the ECU.

Objectives: Did you learn...?

- Evaluate maneuvers for the EPL?
- Describe the incidence of EPL rupture after nondisplaced distal radius fracture?
- Describe the anatomy of the dorsal extensor compartments?
- Treat EPL rupture?

CASE 44

The patient is a 31-year-old woman who sustained a laceration to the radial side of her index finger while cutting vegetables at home. She presented to an outside emergency room where her laceration was repaired. Four days later, she presents to the office complaining of numbness along the radial side of her index finger. On examination, the patient has a 1.5 cm oblique laceration along the volar radial aspect of her index finger distal to the MP joint overlying the proximal phalanx, but is able to flex at the PIP and DIP joints without discomfort. You diagnose her with a radial digital nerve laceration and plan for operative repair.

What is a normal two-point discrimination in the tip of the index finger?

A. 0 to 1 mm
B. 2 to 6 mm
C. 6 to 10 mm
D. 10 to 15 mm
E. 15 to 20 mm

Discussion

The correct answer is (B). Two-point discrimination in the fingertips can be measured either with a static or moving examination. Normal values vary between individual patients and between the individual digits, but in general 2 to 6 mm is considered a normal two-point discrimination in the fingertips. Following trauma or reconstructive surgery, two-point discrimination is often decreased.

During surgical exploration, the radial digital nerve to the index finger is completely lacerated. What is the relationship of the digital artery and digital nerve at the level of the proximal phalanx?

A. The relationship of the digital nerve and artery is variable
B. The digital artery is volar to the digital nerve
C. The digital nerve is volar to the digital artery
D. The digital nerve is dorsal to the digital vein
E. None of the above is true

Discussion

The correct answer is (C). Within the digits and distal to the MP joint, the digital nerves lie volar to the digital artery, a relationship which is both predictable and practical. This relationship is reversed proximal to the MP joint, where the common digital vessels lie volar to the common digital nerves.

What is the most common neural structure repaired during digital nerve coaptation?

A. Mesoneurium
B. Epineurium
C. Perineurium
D. Nerve fascicles
E. Endoneurium

Discussion

The correct answer is (B). In addition to the neural components, peripheral nerves are comprised of different layers of connective tissue surrounding the axons and fascicles. The endoneurium is the innermost layer of connective tissue, and surrounds the myelin sheath of individual nerve fibers. The perineurium is connective tissue surrounding fascicles within the nerve, and the epineurium is the outermost layer of dense connective tissue surrounding a peripheral nerve. The most common method of digital nerve repair utilizes an epineural suture technique, which does not require intraneural neurolysis or intrafasicular dissection.

Objectives: Did you learn...?

- Describe the relationship of the digital nerve and artery at the level of the proximal phalanx?
- Identify the structure that is repaired during digital nerve coaptation?

CASE 45

The patient is a 48-year-old, diabetic, male smoker who presents to the emergency room after sustaining a laceration to the volar aspect of his palm with a tablesaw (Fig. 4–22). In addition to injuring multiple tendons, the patient has injuries to multiple digital nerves and digital arteries. He is brought to the operating room urgently for exploration and repair; his fingers are revascularized and his digital nerves and tendons are repaired. Postoperatively, the patient inquires about his expected neural recovery.

What is the typical rate of nerve regeneration following repair?

A. 0.1 to 0.2 mm/day
B. 0.2 to 0.5 mm/day
C. 1 to 2 mm/day
D. 5 to 10 mm/day
E. 1 to 2 cm/day

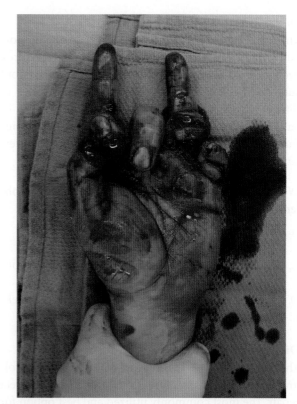

Figure 4–22

Discussion

The correct answer is (C). There are many factors that contribute to the rate of regeneration of peripheral nerves, including mechanism of injury, time until repair, and individual host factors, among others. Most evidence suggests that the average rate of nerve regeneration in peripheral nerves is approximately 1 to 2 mm/day after a brief latency period.

Postoperatively, the patient has incomplete neural recovery of the radial side of his long finger and develops sharp, neuropathic pain at the site of his initial injury with a positive Tinel sign.

What is the likely cause of his neuropathic pain?

A. Tinel lesion
B. Tendon adhesions
C. Joint stiffness
D. Neuroma
E. Wallerian degeneration

Discussion

The correct answer is (D). This patient has developed a neuroma, which is manifest clinically by increased sensitivity and pain following traumatic injury to a nerve. Neuromas can be caused by scarring and incomplete nerve recovery. There are many possible interventions to ameliorate this problem, including embedding the nerve stumps in bone or muscle, injection of substances such as alcohol or phenol, and further resection or cauterization.

What are possible cause(s) of this complication?

A. Failure to resect damaged ends of the digital nerve prior to coaptation
B. Undue tension on the nerve repair
C. Too early wrist and finger extension following repair
D. Unrecognized extent of the zone of injury
E. All of the above

Discussion

The correct answer is (E). There are many possible causes of neuroma following digital nerve repair, including failure to recognize the extent of the injury and resect injured segments of the nerve, undue tension on the nerve repair, and inappropriate mobilization of the nerve coaptation site. Any of these factors, individually or in conjunction, can lead to a painful neuroma.

Objectives: Did you learn...?

- Identify the rate of nerve degeneration?
- Explain the causes of nerve pain in a damaged nerve?
- Describe the causes of neuroma?

CASE 46

The patient is an 18-year-old woman who sustained a laceration to the radial side of her index finger at the level of the PIP joint two and a half weeks prior to her office visit. The injury was sustained when a kitchen knife slipped and accidentally caused a 2 cm laceration to this area. On examination, the patient has anesthesia of the radial side of her index finger distal to the injury, but is able to flex at the PIP and DIP joints without difficulty. Surgery is planned for digital nerve exploration and repair.

Which of the following reasons might predict the existence of a nerve gap and worse prognosis following repair?

A. Female gender
B. Time elapsed between injury and surgical intervention
C. Sharp laceration
D. Patient's age
E. Anatomic location of the laceration

Discussion

The correct answer is (B). Of the factors listed, a time delay to nerve repair is most likely to result in a nerve gap and poor recovery. Female gender is not predictive of a poor outcome. The sharp laceration and the patient's young age make her a good candidate to experience more complete nerve recovery.

What is the accepted limit of nerve gap for which a nerve conduit can be used?

A. 5 mm
B. 1 cm
C. 2 cm
D. 3 cm
E. 4 cm

Discussion

The correct answer is (D). In a seminal paper, Mackinnon and Dellon demonstrated that clinical results of nerve reconstruction using a nerve conduit were comparable to standard nerve graft techniques up to 3.0 cm. Although newer conduits and synthetic nerve grafts are available and are becoming more widely used in various clinical settings, the largest gap for which conduits are recommended is 3.0 cm.

If autologous nerve is desired for use in a digital nerve graft, which nerve is commonly utilized and expendable in the upper extremity?

A. Radial sensory nerve at the wrist
B. Lateral antebrachial cutaneous nerve proximal to the elbow
C. Anterior interosseous nerve 5 cm distal to the elbow
D. Dorsal ulnar sensory nerve at the wrist
E. Posterior interosseous nerve at the wrist

Discussion

The correct answer is (E). Of the options presented, the posterior interosseous nerve at the wrist provides the best caliber and fascicle match for the digital nerve in zone 1. The radial sensory and dorsal sensory nerves at the wrist should not be harvested for digital nerve reconstruction because of donor site morbidity. The anterior interosseous nerve, although suitable for nerve reconstruction when harvested distally, should not be utilized immediately distal to the elbow because of motor innervation to the FPL and FDP to the index finger. The lateral antebrachial cutaneous nerve can be harvested distally for a good size match to the digital nerve but should not be harvested proximal to the elbow for this purpose.

Objectives: Did you learn...?

- Identify factors that contribute to poor recovery in nerve repair?
- Indicate uses for nerve conduit?
- Identify nerves used for autologous nerve grafting?

CASE 47

The patient is a 74-year-old man involved in a motor vehicle collision who sustained a soft tissue injury to the dorsum of his left hand when it was caught out the window (Fig. 4–23). He has no other injuries and is

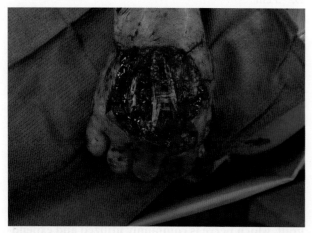

Figure 4–23

otherwise healthy. He underwent initial debridement followed by extensor tendon repair (extensor digitorum communis to the index and middle fingers as well as the extensor indicis proprius) and is left with an 8 × 8 cm wound over the dorsum of the hand, with exposed extensor tendons.

Which of the following will have the greatest impact on the likely take of skin graft reconstruction of this wound?

A. The presence of underlying fractures
B. The smoking status of the patient
C Whether or not the skin graft is meshed
D. The presence of intact paratenon coverage of the tendons
F. None of these factors will have an impact

Discussion

The correct answer is (D). Skin grafting is often a viable option for reconstruction in the extremity. In order to obtain predictable success with skin grafting along tendon surfaces, the most important component is the presence of intact paratenon, which will allow take of the skin graft because of its vascularity. The other factors will also contribute to the overall success rate, but the graft will not survive if it is placed over a traumatized, avascular bed.

Given the patient's exposed critical structures, more robust soft tissue coverage is warranted, and a reverse radial forearm flap is chosen.

Which of the following is NOT TRUE about this flap?

A. Perfusion through the ulnar artery into the hand must be intact to use this flap for reconstruction
B. This flap is distally based, with arterial inflow through the distal aspect of the radial artery
C. There is no need for venous drainage for this flap, since venous flow would be against the direction of the valvular system
D. This flap can be included as a "fascia-only" flap or a fasciocutaneous flap (with a skin paddle)
E. This flap is capable of resurfacing the entire dorsum of the hand and allows for adequate tendon gliding

Discussion

The correct answer is (C). The reverse radial forearm flap is a conventional reconstructive option for dorsal hand wounds, and is capable of resurfacing the entire dorsum of the hand. It can be used as a "fascia-only" or a "fasciocutaneous" flap. In order to use this flap, perfusion through the ulnar artery must be intact. Importantly, this flap has a reliable arterial supply with a robust venous drainage system; despite the presence of unidirectional valves it appears that denervation, vascular engorgement, and elevated venous pressure contribute to the ability to drain the flap in retrograde fashion.

In patients who cannot undergo a reverse fore-arm flap, what other options for soft tissue coverage are available?

A. Posterior interosseous artery flap
B. Integra® placement followed by skin graft coverage in 2 to 4 weeks
C. Free flap coverage using an anterolateral thigh flap
D. A and C
E. All of the above

Discussion

The correct answer is (E). There are many options for soft tissue coverage of the dorsum of the hand. In addition to the reverse radial forearm flap, coverage with a posterior interosseous artery flap or a free flap, such as the anterolateral thigh flap, is commonly utilized. In addition to autologous options, Integra® and other skin substitutes can be used as a bridge to skin grafting such difficult wounds; Integra has been shown to have >90% success over exposed tendons, although the resultant gliding of these structures has not been well studied.

Objectives: Did you learn...?

• Access the risk factors for poor outcomes of skin grafting?
• Describe the characteristics of a reverse radial forearm flap?

CASE 48

The patient is a 47-year-old male who sustained a table-saw injury to the volar aspect of his nondominant left thumb (Fig. 4–24). He has no other injuries and the remainder of his hand and fingers is uninjured. On examination, there is a 3 × 2 cm soft tissue defect on the volar aspect of his thumb distal to the IP joint, with preservation of the dorsal skin and nailbed of his thumb. The FPL tendon is intact but exposed at the base of the wound with a 30% laceration. The distal dorsal aspect of the thumb is perfused.

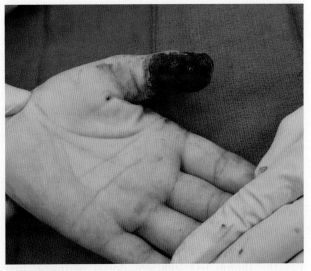

Figure 4–24

Which of the following is the best reconstructive option for this patient?

A. Full thickness skin graft from the hypothenar eminence
B. Allow to heal by secondary intention with dressing changes alone
C. Thenar flap
D. First dorsal metacarpal artery flap ("Kite" flap)
E. Moberg advancement flap

Discussion

The correct answer is (D). This patient has a volar thumb soft tissue defect which measures 3 × 2 cm in area. Given the exposed FPL tendon at the base of the wound, soft tissue coverage with a flap is the most appropriate reconstructive option. Allowing the thumb to heal by secondary intention would likely result in a paucity of coverage and/or a flexion contracture. A thenar flap is not possible for the thumb and is a better option for middle finger volar pulp defects. The Moberg advancement flap is a good option for volar thumb defects but is generally limited to defects 1.5 cm² in area.

If the defects of the distal volar thumb were smaller, 1 cm², but had exposed FPL tendon at the base, what would be another acceptable option for reconstruction unique to the thumb?

A. Full thickness skin graft from the hypothenar eminence
B. Healing by secondary intention with dressing changes
C. Thenar flap
D. Cross-finger flap
E. Moberg advancement flap

Discussion

The correct answer is (E). As mentioned above, the Moberg flap is a good reconstructive option for volar thumb defects less than 1.5 cm². This reconstruction is unique to the thumb because of the robust dorsal circulation, allowing perfusion to be maintained when the volar advancement flap is raised. A cross-finger flap is another acceptable reconstruction in this situation but is not unique to the thumb.

Why is the Moberg flap possible for thumb reconstruction but is not typically possible for similar reconstruction in other digits?

A. The thumb is shorter in length than other digits

B. The thumb has a greater width than other fingers

C. The thumb has sufficient dorsal perfusion that allows for this reconstruction

D. The thumb has less sensory requirement than other digits

E. The thumb is more expendable than other digits

Discussion

The correct answer is (C). The blood supply to the thumb predominantly arises from the princeps pollicis artery, which emerges from the radial artery. The princeps pollicis artery runs between the first dorsal interosseous artery and the adductor pollicis, and branches into the radial and ulnar digital arteries to the thumb. There are axial dorsal arterial branches that supply the dorsum of the thumb, which are reliable and can provide sufficient inflow to maintain perfusion to the thumb tip.

Objectives: Did you learn...?

- Describe the indications of a Kite Flap?
- Describe the indications for a Moberg advancement flap?
- Identify the anatomy of the thumb?

CASE 49

The patient is a 36-year-old otherwise healthy male who presents with a volar soft tissue defect overlying the distal phalanx of the index finger (Fig. 4–25). The patient reports that this is the result of a locally aggressive infection which required surgical debridement. The infection has been clinically eradicated with local wound care and a course of antibiotics. On examination, the patient has a 2 × 2 cm soft tissue defect of the volar distal phalanx of the index finger extending proximal to the DIP joint, with exposed flexor tendon sheath. The finger is stiff but is sensate and perfused.

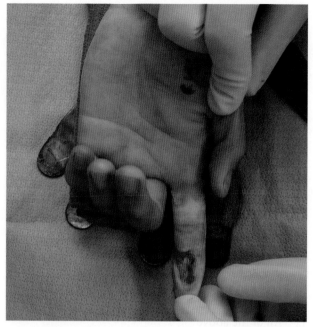

Figure 4–25

Which of the following is NOT a reconstructive option for the patient?

A. Reverse radial forearm fascial flap with full thickness skin graft

B. Cross-finger flap from the dorsum of the ring finger

C. Free arterialized venous "flow through" flap from the volar forearm

D. Split thickness skin graft

E. Heterodigital island flap

Discussion

The correct answer is (D). There are many possible reconstructive solutions for this problem, including a cross-finger flap, arterialized venous flow through flap, heterodigital island flap, and reverse radial forearm flap with full thickness skin graft. A split thickness skin graft is not a good option for this patient given the exposed tendon and open wound that crosses the PIP joint. A split thickness skin graft undergoes significant secondary contracture and would likely result in progressive deformity with functional limitation at the PIP joint.

A cross-finger flap is performed from the dorsal aspect of the middle finger middle phalanx, with skin graft placement over the donor site. Seven days later, there is no appreciable take of the skin graft at the flap donor site and an open wound has resulted.

Which of the following reasons may have resulted in failure of skin graft take at the donor site?

A. Infection
B. Hematoma or seroma deep to the skin graft
C. Failure of adequate immobilization of the skin graft
D. Shear forces preventing continual adherence of the graft to the underlying tissue
E. All of the above

Discussion

The correct answer is (E). There are many reasons for failure of skin graft take, including infection, hematoma/seroma, shear forces on the graft, failure of adequate immobilization, and poor vascularity of the underlying tissue bed. These are best preempted prior to the operation to ensure the best chance for optimal graft take.

How long should one wait before confidently performing division of the cross-finger flap between the two fingers?

A. 2 to 3 days
B. 4 to 6 days
C. 7 to 9 days
D. 2 to 3 weeks
E. 5 to 6 weeks

Discussion

The correct answer is (D). Traditionally, pedicled flaps are divided approximately 3 weeks after creation to allow for development of sufficient neovascularization from the recipient bed. There is evidence that flap division can be performed earlier than 3 weeks but this depends on the anatomic area, the patient's overall medical condition, and the defect size, among other factors. Pedicled flaps are often challenged with a tourniquet in the office prior to formal division to ensure that adequate vascularity has developed prior to division.

Objectives: Did you learn...?

• Identfiy indications for split thickness skin graft?
• Describe reasons for failure of skin graft take?
• Access timing of division for cross finger flaps?

CASE 50

The patient is a 51-year-old male construction worker who presents with pain in his proximal left palm and a superficial 1 × 1 cm ulcer along the radial aspect of his small finger tip. He reports that he has had pain in his hand for approximately 4 months, but has had the ulcer for only 3 weeks. He operates heavy machinery at work and often uses a jackhammer. On examination, the patient has a normal appearing, sensate hand with an ulcer of his small fingertip. There is no muscular wasting. He has normal range of motion in all fingers and his grip and pinch strength are normal.

Which of the following additional components of the physical examination is likely to be abnormal for this patient?

A. Two-point discrimination in the median nerve distribution
B. Scaphoid shift test
C. Allen test
D. Bunnell intrinsic tightness test
E. Elbow compression test

Discussion

The correct answer is (C). The most appropriate test to evaluate the perfusion to the hand is the Allen test, first described in 1929 to evaluate the differential vascular inflow into the hand from the radial and the ulnar arteries. In this patient, this test would be the most appropriate to evaluate the perfusion to the hand. The other tests mentioned, while important components of a thorough upper extremity evaluation, would not likely reveal pathology in this case.

The patient undergoes additional imaging and is found to have thrombosis of the ulnar artery as it passes through Guyon's canal. What is this condition called?

A. Carpal tunnel syndrome
B. Buerger's disease
C. Scleroderma
D. Hypothenar hammer syndrome
E. Raynaud disease

Discussion

The correct answer is (D). Hypothenar hammer syndrome is characterized by finger ischemia, caused by occlusion of palmar ulnar artery in a person repetitively striking objects with the hypothenar surface of the hand. This patient's presentation is classic for hypothenar hammer syndrome. The other diagnoses, although part of the differential diagnosis, are less likely in this case.

Which of the following objective measures can determine the degree to which arterial inflow into the digits is affected and help guide the decision for treatment?

A. Capillary refill in the digits
B. Color of the digits
C. Digital brachial index
D. Systolic blood pressure
E. Two-point discrimination in the digits

Discussion

The correct answer is (C). The digital brachial index is an objective measure of arterial inflow into each of the digits, and can guide the various treatment options. One study concluded that patients with digital brachial indices of less than 0.7 required reconstruction with a vein graft or primary arterial anastomosis, whereas those above this level warranted only vessel ligation. The remaining options, although important components of the hand examination, are less objective than the digital brachial index in this patient.

Which of the following are treatment options for this patient?

A. Aspirin, calcium channel blockers, and/or systemic anticoagulation
B. Resection and ligation of the affected ulnar artery segment
C. Smoking cessation
D. Reconstruction of the affected ulnar artery with vein graft
E. All of the above

Discussion

The correct answer is (E). All of the listed treatment options may be helpful for this patient. Smoking cessation, independent of surgical intervention, may be helpful for this patient to prevent disease progression. The choice of ulnar artery ligation vs. reconstruction with a vein graft is surgeon- and patient-dependent; either option might be indicated in this scenario as described above. Adjunctive medications such as anti-platelet therapy (Aspirin), anticoagulation, and vasodilators such as calcium channel blockers may be helpful in cases of distal finger ischemia.

Objectives: Did you learn...?

• Identify the indications for the use of the Allen's test?
• Identify the indications for Digital Brachial Index?
• Describe the pathoanatomy of Hypothenar Hammer Syndrome?
• Treat Hypothenar Hammer Syndrome?

BIBLIOGRAPHY

Case 1

Souer JS, Mudgal CS. Plating for multiple closed metacarpal fractures. *J Hand Surg.* 2008;33(6):740–744.

Case 2

Watanabe H, Hamada Y, Toshima T. Conservative management of infantile trigger thumb: indications and limitations. *Tech Hand Up Extrem Surg.* 2003;7(1):37–42.

Case 3

Ritting AW, Baldwin PC, Rodner CM. Ulnar collateral ligament injury of the thumb metacarpophalangeal joint. *Clin J Sport Med.* 2010;20(2):106–112.

Case 4

Ruchelsman DE, Christoforou D, Wasserman B, Lee SK, Rettig ME. Avulsion injuries of the flexor digitorum profundus tendon. *J Am Acad Orthop Surg.* 2011;19(3):152–162.

Case 5

Huang JI, Fernandez DL. Fractures of the base of the thumb metacarpal. *Instr Course Lect.* 2010;59:343–356.

Case 6

Bloom JM, Hammert WC. Evidence-based medicine: Metacarpal fractures. *Plast Reconstr Surg.* 2014;133(5): 1252–1260.

Case 7

Mudgal CS. Staged management of tophaceous gout with DIP arthritis in the elderly: A preliminary technique report. *J Hand Surg.* 2006;31B(1):101–103.
Ruchelsman DE, Hazel A, Mudgal CS: Percutaneous arthrodesis of the DIP joint. *Hand.*2010;5(4):434–439.

Case 8

Neuhaus V, Thomas MA, Mudgal CS. Type IIb bony mallet finger: is anatomical reduction of the fracture necessary? *Am J Orthop (Belle Mead NJ).* 2013;42(5):223–226.
Tuttle HG, Olvey SP, Stern PJ. Tendon avulsion injuries of the distal phalanx. *Clin Orthop Relat Res.* 2006;445:157–168.

Case 9

Neuhaus V, Wong G, Russo KE, Mudgal CS. Dynamic splinting with early motion following zone IV/V and TI to TIII extensor tendon repairs.*J Hand Surg Am May.*2012;37(5):933–937.

Case 10

Mangelson JJ, Stern PJ, Abzug JM, Chang J, Osterman AL. Complications following dislocations of the proximal interphalangeal joint. *Instr Course Lect.* 2014;63:123–130.

Case 11

Lee DH, Mignemi ME, Crosby SN. Fingertip injuries: an update on management. *J Am Acad Orthop Surg*. 2013; 21(12):756–766.

Case 12

Mangelson JJ, Stern PJ, Abzug JM, Chang J, Osterman AL. Complications following dislocations of the proximal interphalangeal joint. *Instr Course Lect*. 2014;63:123–130.

Case 13

Eberlin KR, Babushkina A, Neira JR, Mudgal CS. Outcomes of closed reduction and periarticular pinning of base and shaft fractures of the proximal phalanx. *J Hand Surg Am*. 2014;39(8):1524–1528.

Case 14

Meurer WJ, Kronick SL, Lowell MJ, Desmond JS, Mudgal CS. Complex metacarpophalangeal dislocation. *Int J Emerg Med*. 2008;1(3):227–228.

Mudgal CS, Mudgal S. Volar open reduction of complex metacarpophalangeal dislocation of the index finger: a pictorial essay. *Tech Hand Up Extrem Surg*. 2006;10(1):31–36.

Case 15

Mol MF, Neuhaus V, Becker SJ, Jupiter JB, Mudgal C, Ring D. Resolution and recurrence rates of idiopathic trigger finger after corticosteroid injection. *Hand (NY)*. 2013;8(2):183–190.

Ring D, Lozano-Calderón S, Shin R, Bastian P, Mudgal C, Jupiter J. A prospective randomized controlled trial of injection of dexamethasone versus triamcinolone for idiopathic trigger finger. *J Hand Surg Am*. 2008;33(4):516–522.

Case 16

Mol MF, Neuhaus V, Becker SJ, Jupiter JB, Mudgal C, Ring D. Resolution and recurrence rates of idiopathic trigger finger after corticosteroid injection. *Hand (NY)*. 2013;8(2):183–190.

Ring D, Lozano-Calderón S, Shin R, Bastian P, Mudgal C, Jupiter J. A prospective randomized controlled trial of injection of dexamethasone versus triamcinolone for idiopathic trigger finger. *J Hand Surg Am*. 2008;33(4):516–522.

Case 17

Zenn MR, Hoffman L, Latrenta G, Hotchkiss R. Variations in digital nerve anatomy. *J Hand Surg Am*. 1992;17(6):1033–1036.

Case 18

Neumeister MW, Amalfi A, Neumeister E. Evidence-based medicine: Flexor tendon repair. *Plast Reconstr Surg*. 2014; 133(5):1222–1233.

Case 19

Belhorn LR, Evelyn VH. Erosive osteoarthritis. *Seminars in Arthritis and Rheumatism*. Vol. 22. No. 5. WB Saunders; 1993.

Ehrlich GE. Erosive osteoarthritis: presentation, clinical pearls, and therapy. *Curr Rheumatol Rep*. 2001;3(6):484–488.

Case 20

Hartigan BJ, Stern PJ, Kiefhaber TR. Thumb carpometacarpal osteoarthritis: arthrodesis compared with ligament reconstruction and tendon interposition. *J Bone Joint Surg Am*. 2001;83-A(10):1470–1478.

Slutsky DJ. Osteoarthritis of the thumb. *Disorders of the Hand*. London: Springer; 2015: 71–91.

Case 21

Sassoon AA, Fitz-Gibbon PD, Harmsen WS, Moran SL. Enchondromas of the hand: factors affecting recurrence, healing, motion, and malignant transformation. *J Hand Surg Am*. 2012;37(6):1229–1234.

Case 22

Hamdi MF. Glomus tumour of fingertip: report of eight cases and literature review. *Musculoskelet Surg*. 2011;95(3):237–240.

Case 23

Gude W, Morelli V. Ganglion cysts of the wrist: pathophysiology, clinical picture, and management. *Curr Rev Musculoskelet Med*. 2008;1(3–4):205–211.

Case 24

Bishop GB, Born T, Kakar S, Jawa A. The diagnostic accuracy of inflammatory blood markers for purulent flexor tenosynovitis. *J Hand Surg Am*. 2013;38(11):2208–2211.

Case 25

Espandar R, Sibdari SY, Rafiee E, Yazdanian S. Necrotizing fasciitis of the extremities: a prospective study. *Strategies Trauma Limb Reconstr*. 2011;6(3):121–125.

Wong CH, Khin LW, Heng KS, Tan KC, Low CO. The LRINEC (Laboratory risk indicator for necrotizing fasciitis) score: a tool for distinguishing necrotizing fasciitis from other soft tissue infections. *Crit Care Med*. 2004;32(7): 1535–1541.

Case 26

Jebson PJ. Deep subfascial space infections. *Hand Clin*. 1998; 14(4):557–566, viii.

Case 27

Franko OI, Abrams RA. Hand infections. *Orthop Clin North Am*. 2013;44(4):625–634.

Case 28

Badri T, Ishak F. Images in clinical medicine. Pyogenic granuloma of the finger. *N Engl J Med*. 2012;366(6):e10.

Wall LB, Stern PJ. Pyoderma gangrenosum. *J Hand Surg Am*. 2012;37(5):1083–1085.

Case 29

Bednar MS, James MA, Light TR. Congenital longitudinal deficiency. *J Hand Surg Am*. 2009;34(9):1739–1747.

Light TR, Gaffey JL. Reconstruction of the hypoplastic thumb. *J Hand Surg Am*. 2010;35(3):474–479

Case 30

Xu YL, Shen KY, Chen J, Wang ZG. Flexor pollicis longus rebalancing: a modified technique for Wassel IV-D thumb duplication. *J Hand Surg Am*. 2014;39(1):75–82.

Case 31

Jans C, Peersman G, Peersman B, Van Den Langenbergh T, Valk J, Richart T. Endoscopic decompression for chronic compartment syndrome of the forearm in motocross racers. *Knee Surg Sports Traumatol Arthrosc*. 2014.

Kanj WW, Gunderson MA, Carrigan RB, Sankar WN. Acute compartment syndrome of the upper extremity in children: diagnosis, management, and outcomes. *J Child Orthop*. 2013;7(3):225–233.

Case 32

Amsdell SL, Hammert WC. High-pressure injection injuries in the hand: current treatment concepts. *Plast Reconstr Surg*. 2013;132(4):586e–591e.

Lozano-Calderón SA, Mudgal CS, Mudgal S, Ring D. Latex paint-gun injuries of the hand: are the outcomes better? *Hand (NY)*. 2008;3(4):340–345.

Case 33

Eaton C. Evidence-based medicine: Dupuytren contracture. *Plast Reconstr Surg*. 2014;133(5):1241–1251.

Meathrel KE, Thoma A. Abductor digiti minimi involvement in Dupuytren's contracture of the small finger. *J Hand Surg Am*. 2004;29(3):510–513.

Case 34

Chow JA, Thomes LJ, Dovelle S, Monsivais J, Milnor WH, Jackson JP. Controlled motion rehabilitation after flexor tendon repair and grafting. A multi-centre study. *J Bone Joint Surg Br*. 1988;70(4):591–595.

Klein L. Early active motion flexor tendon protocol using one splint. *J Hand Ther*. 2003;16(3):199–206.

Sokol SC, Robert MS. Flexor Tendon Surgery. *Evid Based Orthop*. 2012:1057–1071.

Case 35

Strickland JW. Flexor tenolysis. *Hand Clin*. 1985;1(1):121–132.

Silfverskiöld KL, May EJ, Törnvall AH. Gap formation during controlled motion after flexor tendon repair in zone II: a prospective clinical study. *J Hand Surg Am*. 1992;17(3):539–546.

May EJ, Silfverskiöld KL. Rate of recovery after flexor tendon repair in zone II. A prospective longitudinal study of 145 digits. *Scand J Plast Reconstr Surg Hand Surg*. 1993;27(2):89–94.

Case 36

Dean BJ, Little C. Fractures of the metacarpals and phalanges. *Orthop Trauma*. 2011;25:43–56.

Dolich BH, Schultz RJ, Kaplan EB. The post traumatic "lumbrical plus" finger: etiology and treatment. *Bull Hosp Joint Dis*. 1973;34:107–116.

Lemmon JA, Janis JE, Rohrich RJ. Soft-tissue injuries of the fingertip: methods of evaluation and treatment. An algorithmic approach. *Plast Reconstr Surg*. 2008;122:105e–117e.

Momeni A, Zajonc H, Kalash Z, Stark GB, Bannasch H. Reconstruction of distal phalangeal injuries with the reverse homodigital island flap. *Injury*. 2008;39:1460–1463.

Verdan C. Syndrome of the quadriga. *Surg Clin North Am*. 1960;40:425–426.

Case 37

Kay S, Werntz J, Wolff TW. Ring avulsion injuries: classification and prognosis. *J Hand Surg Am*. 1989;14:204–213.

Lineaweaver WC, Hill MK, Buncke GM, et al. Aeromonas hydrophila infections following use of medicinal leeches in replantation and flap surgery. *Ann Plast Surg*. 1992;29:238–244.

Smoot EC 3rd, Debs N, Banducci D, Poole M, Roth A. Leech therapy and bleeding wound techniques to relieve venous congestion. *J Reconstr Microsurg*. 1990;6:245–250.

Waikakul S, Sakkarnkosol S, Vanadurongwan V, Un-nanuntana A. Results of 1018 digital replantations in 552 patients. *Injury*. 2000;31:33–40.

Case 38

Boulas HJ. Amputations of the fingers and hand: indications for replantation. *J Am Acad Orthop Surg*. 1998;6:100–105.

Saies AD, Urbaniak JR, Nunley JA, Taras JS, Goldner RD, Fitch RD. Results after replantation and revascularization in the upper extremity in children. *J Bone Joint Surg Am*. 1994;76:1766–1776.

Wei FC, Chen HC, Chuang CC, Chen SH. Microsurgical thumb reconstruction with toe transfer: selection of various techniques. *Plast Reconstr Surg*. 1994;93:345–351; discussion 352–347.

Case 39

Urbaniak JR, Roth JH, Nunley JA, Goldner RD, Koman LA. The results of replantation after amputation of a single finger. *J Bone Joint Surg Am*. 1985;67:611–619.

Urbaniak JR, Roth JH, Nunley JA, Goldner RD, Koman LA. The results of replantation after amputation of a single finger. *J Bone Joint Surg Am*. 1985;67:611–619.

Verdan CE. Primary repair of flexor tendons. *J Bone Joint Surg Am*. 1960;42-A: 647–657.

White WL. Why I hate the index finger. *Orthopaed Rev*. 1980; 9:23–29.

Case 40

Katz JN, Stirrat CR. A self-administered hand diagram for the diagnosis of carpal tunnel syndrome. *J Hand Surg Am*. 1990;15:360–363.

Levine DW, Simmons BP, Koris MJ, et al. A self-administered questionnaire for the assessment of severity of symptoms and functional status in carpal tunnel syndrome. *J Bone Joint Surg Am.* 1993;75:1585–1592.

Thomas JE, Lambert EH, Cseuz KA. Electrodiagnostic aspects of the carpal tunnel syndrome. *Arch Neurol.* 1967;16: 635–641.

Weiss ND, Gordon L, Bloom T, So Y, Rempel DM. Position of the wrist associated with the lowest carpal-tunnel pressure: implications for splint design. *J Bone Joint Surg Am.* 1995;77:1695–1699.

Case 41

Osterman M, Ilyas AM, Matzon JL. Carpal tunnel syndrome in pregnancy. *Orthop Clin North Am.* 2012;43:515–520.

Szabo RM, Slater RR Jr., Farver TB, et al. The value of diagnostic testing in carpal tunnel syndrome. *J Hand Surg Am.* 1999;24:704–714.

Voitk AJ, Mueller JC, Farlinger DE, et al. Carpal tunnel syndrome in pregnancy. *Can Med Assoc J.* 1983;128:277–281.

Case 42

Agee JM, McCarroll HR Jr, Tortosa RD, Berry DA, Szabo RM, Peimer CA. Endoscopic release of the carpal tunnel: a randomized prospective multicenter study. *J Hand Surg Am.* 1992;17:987–995.

Geoghegan JM, Clark DI, Bainbridge LC, Smith C, Hubbard R. Risk factors in carpal tunnel syndrome. *J Hand Surg Br.* 2004;29:315–320.

Samarakoon LB, Guruge MH, Jayasekara M, Malalasekera AP, Anthony DJ, Jayasekara RW. Anatomical landmarks for safer carpal tunnel decompression: an experimental cadaveric study. *Patient Saf Surg.* 2014;8:8.

Vella JC, Hartigan BJ, Stern PJ. Kaplan's cardinal line. *J Hand Surg Am.* 2006;31:912–918.

Zyluk A, Puchalski P. A comparison of outcomes of carpal tunnel release in diabetic and non-diabetic patients. *J Hand Surg Eur Vol.* 2013;38:485–488.

Case 43

Benson EC, DeCarvalho A, Mikola EA, Veitch JM, Moneim MS. Two potential causes of EPL rupture after distal radius volar plate fixation. *Clin Orthop Relat Res.* 2006;451:218–222.

Magnussen PA, Harvey FJ, Tonkin MA. Extensor indicis proprius transfer for rupture of the extensor pollicis longus tendon. *J Bone Joint Surg Br.* 1990;72:881–883.

Rockwell WB, Butler PN, Byrne BA. Extensor tendon: anatomy, injury, and reconstruction. *Plast Reconstr Surg.* 2000;106:1592–1603; quiz 1604, 1673

Roth KM, Blazar PE, Earp BE, Han R, Leung A. Incidence of extensor pollicis longus tendon rupture after nondisplaced distal radius fractures. *J Hand Surg Am.* 2012; 37:942–947.

Case 44

Eaton RG. The digital neurovascular bundle. A microanatomic study of its contents. *Clin Orthop Relat Res.* 1968;61:176–185.

Louis DS, Greene TL, Jacobson KE, Rasmussen C, Kolowich P, Goldstein SA. Evaluation of normal values for stationary and moving two-point discrimination in the hand. *J Hand Surg Am.* 1984;9:552–555.

Siemionow M, Brzezicki G. Chapter 8: Current techniques and concepts in peripheral nerve repair. *Int Rev Neurobiol.* 2009;87:141–172.

Case 45

Dellon AL, Mackinnon SE. Treatment of the painful neuroma by neuroma resection and muscle implantation. *Plast Reconstr Surg.* 1986;77:427–438.

Gutmann E, Gutmann L, Medawar PB, et al. The rate of regeneration of nerve. *J Exp Biol.* 1942;19:41–44.

Herndon JH, Eaton RG, Littler JW. Management of painful neuromas in the hand. *J Bone Joint Surg Am.* 1976;58:369–373.

Case 46

Higgins JP, Fisher S, Serletti JM, Orlando GS. Assessment of nerve graft donor sites used for reconstruction of traumatic digital nerve defects. *J Hand Surg Am.* 2002;27:286–292.

Mackinnon SE, Dellon AL. Clinical nerve reconstruction with a bioabsorbable polyglycolic acid tube. *Plast Reconstr Surg.* 1990;85:419–424.

Reissis N, Stirrat A, Manek S, Dunkerton M. The terminal branch of posterior interosseous nerve: a useful donor for digital nerve grafting. *J Hand Surg Br.* 1992;17:638–640.

Ruijs AC, Jaquet JB, Kalmijn S, Giele H, Hovius SE.. Median and ulnar nerve injuries: a meta-analysis of predictors of motor and sensory recovery after modern microsurgical nerve repair. *Plast Reconstr Surg.* 2005;116:484–494; discussion 495–486.

Case 47

Eberlin KR, Chang J, Curtin CM, et al. Soft-tissue coverage of the hand: a case-based approach. *Plast Reconstr Surg.* 2014;133:91–101.

Eberlin KR, Chang J, Curtin CM, et al. Soft-tissue coverage of the hand: a case-based approach. *Plast Reconstr Surg.* 2014; 133:91–101.

Robson MC, Krizek TJ. Predicting skin graft survival. *J Trauma.* 1973;13:213–217.

Shores JT, Hiersche M, Gabriel A, Gupta S. Tendon coverage using an artificial skin substitute. *J Plast Reconstr Aesthet Surg.* 2012;65:1544–1550.

Timmons MJ. The vascular basis of the radial forearm flap. *Plast Reconstr Surg.* 1986;77:80–92.

Case 48

Chang SC, Chen SL, Chen TM, Chuang CJ, Cheng TY, Wang HJ. Sensate first dorsal metacarpal artery flap for resurfacing extensive pulp defects of the thumb. *Ann Plast Surg.* 2004;53:449–454.

Earley MJ. The arterial supply of the thumb, first web and index finger and its surgical application. *J Hand Surg Br.* 1986;11:163–174.

Macht SD, Watson HK. The Moberg volar advancement flap for digital reconstruction. *J Hand Surg Am*. 1980;5:372–376.

Yang JY. The first dorsal metacarpal flap in first web space and thumb reconstruction. *Ann Plast Surg*. 1991;27:258–264.

Case 49

George P, DeJesus RA. Venous flow-through flap reconstruction following severe finger wound infection: case report. *J Reconstr Microsurg*. 2009;25:267–269.

Hallock GG. Preliminary assessment of laser Doppler flowmetry for determining timing of division of the cross-finger flap. *J Hand Surg Am*. 1990;15:898–901.

Kappel D, Burech J. The cross-finger flap. An established reconstructive procedure. *Hand Clin*. 1985;1:677.

Teh BT. Why do skin grafts fail? *Plast Reconstr Surg*. 1979;63:323–332.

Case 50

Carpentier PH, Biro C, Jiguet M, Maricq HR. Prevalence, risk factors, and clinical correlates of ulnar artery occlusion in the general population. *J Vasc Surg*. 2009;50:1333–1339.

Ferris BL, Taylor LM Jr., Oyama K, et al. Hypothenar hammer syndrome: proposed etiology. *J Vasc Surg*. 2000;31:104–113.

Lifchez SD, Higgins JP. Long-term results of surgical treatment for hypothenar hammer syndrome. *Plast Reconstr Surg*. 2009;124:210–216.

Zimmerman NB, Zimmerman SI, McClinton MA, Wilgis EF, Koontz CL, Buehner JW. Long-term recovery following surgical treatment for ulnar artery occlusion. *J Hand Surg Am*. 1994;19:17–21.

5

Foot and Ankle

Jeremy T. Smith

CASE 1

Dr. Tom Douglas

A 40-year-old male, recreational basketball player presents 1 week after feeling like he was kicked in the back of the leg while coming down from a rebound. He was initially seen at an outside facility where he was diagnosed with an ankle sprain. One week prior to the injury he reports that he was given antibiotics for a sore throat.

Which of the following antibiotics would increase the chance of an Achilles tendon rupture?

A. Keflex
B. Clindamycin
C. Ciprofloxacin
D. Azithromycin

Discussion

The correct answer is (C). Fluoroquinolones have been implicated in tendon rupture secondary to two theories. One theory is a decrease in blood flow, which causes an increase rate of rupture. The second theory is that there is a decrease in transcription of decorin, which modifies the biomechanics of the tendon itself, resulting in increased fragility. The mechanism of action of fluoroquinolones is inhibition of DNA topoisomerase II, which results in an inability for the cell to replicate. Keflex, clindamycin, and azithromycin have not been implicated in tendon pathology. The mechanism of action of keflex is disruption of cell wall synthesis. The mechanism of action of clindamycin is inhibition of protein synthesis through binding to the 50S ribosome. The mechanism of action of azithromycin is binding to the 50S ribosome and inhibiting protein synthesis.

Other risk factors for Achilles rupture include steroid use, steroid injections into the tendon, inflammatory arthropathy, and prodromal Achilles tendinosis.

Fortunately you learn that the patient had been started on azithromycin. On examination it is noted that he has no plantar flexion with calf squeeze, a palpable gap, and tenderness around his Achilles.

Based upon ischemic regions of the tendon, what is the most likely location of rupture?

A. Musculotendinous junction
B. 12 cm proximal to the insertion
C. 5 cm proximal to the insertion
D. Avulsion off the calcaneus

Discussion

The correct answer is (C). The blood supply for the Achilles tendon is predominantly from the muscular region and from the bony insertion, resulting in a relative watershed area located at the midportion of the tendon approximately 2 to 6 cm proximal to the insertion of the tendon. The average location of rupture is 4.7 cm proximal to the insertion site.

The diagnosis of Achilles tendon rupture is made with clinical examination including a palpable gap, lack of dorsiflexion with calf squeeze, and increased passive dorsiflexion of the ankle. Additional tests include placement of a needle percutaneously into the proximal Achilles and dorsiflexing the ankle looking for movement of the needle. Another test involves placing a sphygmomanometer around the calf with the cuff inflated to 100 mm Hg while the foot is plantar flexed.

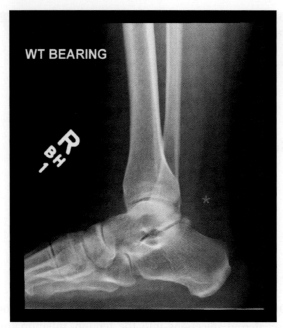

Figure 5–1 The normal outline of Kager's triangle on the lateral x-ray is the radiolucent region bordered by the Achilles posteriorly, flexor hallucis longus muscle belly anteriorly, and superior border of the calcaneus inferiorly.

Dorsiflexion of the foot should result in an increase in pressure to 140 mm Hg.

Radiographic findings of an Achilles rupture may include disruption of Kager's triangle on the lateral x-ray. This is the fat-filled region located superior to the calcaneus, anterior to the Achilles, and posterior to the flexor hallucis longus (Fig. 5–1). Ultrasound and MRI will demonstrate a gap in the Achilles at the location of rupture.

The patient is interested in treatment options for his rupture. Based upon the latest data available, which of the following is unable to be recommended as a treatment option?

A. Cast in plantar flexion for 10 weeks followed by mobilization in a cam boot
B. Splint placement followed by early rehabilitation with physical therapy
C. Acute repair through a percutaneous approach
D. Acute repair through an open approach followed by weight bearing in a boot at 4 weeks

Discussion

The correct answer is (A). The AAOS clinical practice guidelines give a moderate recommendation to employ a protective device that allows mobilization by 2 to 4 weeks postoperatively. Classically there has been reported an increased re-rupture rate with nonoperative management of acute Achilles tendon ruptures when compared to surgical treatment. Re-rupture rates after nonoperative treatment of the Achilles have been quoted at 12% or higher, with re-rupture rates of surgical treatment quoted at 4%. The higher rates of re-rupture have occurred in groups with prolonged immobilization of their nonoperatively treated rupture.

Recently there has been a push for earlier motion following either operative or nonoperative treatment. Level 1 evidence from Willits et al. (*J Bone Joint Surgery Am,* 2010) demonstrated similar outcomes of surgical and nonsurgical treatment utilizing an early motion protocol. There was a statistically significant difference in strength favoring operative treatment, however there were more soft tissue complications in the surgical treatment group. Percutaneous repair of Achilles tendon rupture is an option and has been demonstrated to yield similar benefits as standard open repair based on level 2 evidence with potentially fewer soft tissue complications.

The patient elects for surgical treatment. He undergoes repair via a standard open repair. What is the most common complication associated with this surgery?

A. Superficial wound complications
B. Saphenous nerve injury
C. Sural nerve transection
D. Deep wound infection

Discussion

The correct answer is (A). This has been reported as high as 17% (Bhattacharyya, 2009) with open operative treatment, although the true incidence is likely significantly lower. The sural nerve lies superficial to the tendinous portion of the Achilles at approximately 10 cm proximal to the insertion of the Achilles tendon and may be encountered during the approach, especially with more proximal ruptures. The saphenous, deep peroneal, and superficial peroneal nerves should not be at risk during an Achilles repair. Although deep wound infection is a major complication associated with Achilles tendon repair, it is most commonly reported at approximately 1%.

Objectives: Did you learn...?

• Identify association between fluoroquinolone antibiotics and Achilles tendon rupture?
• Pinpoint watershed region of the Achilles tendon?
• Treat for acute Achilles tendon ruptures?

CASE 2

Dr. Thomas Dowd

A 55-year-old woman complains of great toe pain and arrives in your office wearing narrow, high-heeled shoes. She notes that the pain is worse with shoewear and activity. She states that she doesn't want her feet to end up like her mother's. Physical examination demonstrates a prominent, tender medial eminence without pain on passive range of motion of the first metatarsophalangeal joint (MTPJ). She demonstrates no instability or pain at the first tarsometatarsal joint (TMTJ). An AP foot radiograph is obtained (Fig. 5–2).

The most appropriate initial treatment recommendation is:

A. Correction with distal soft tissue release and first TMTJ corrective arthrodesis

B. An orthotic with a Morton's extension

C. Toe spacer, shoe wear modification, and a ball-ring shoe stretcher

D. First MTPJ medial capsule imbrication, lateral soft tissue release, and corrective osteotomy

E. First MTPJ arthrodesis

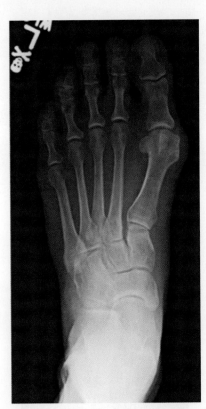

Figure 5–2 AP radiograph of the foot showing a hallux valgus deformity.

Discussion

The correct answer is (C). The initial treatment for hallux valgus is nonsurgical and is focused on eliminating the use of constrictive shoes and passively correcting the deformity. Morton's extensions are primarily used for hallux rigidus. Surgical options are employed after nonoperative measures have failed. Among the surgical options, first TMTJ arthrodesis is typically reserved for patients who demonstrate first TMTJ instability or excessive metatarsus primus varus. First MTPJ arthrodesis is reserved for bunions that are associated with arthritic change and pain with first MTPJ range of motion.

The patient returns 6 months later, having changed to flat shoes with a wide toe box. She notes that NSAIDs have had a diminishing effect in helping her pain. She asks you to explain her radiographs to her.

The AP radiograph (Fig. 5–2) demonstrates all but which of the following?

A. Increased hallux valgus angle (HVA)

B. Increased intermetatarsal angle (IMA)

C. Uncovered fibular sesamoid

D. Prominent medial eminence

E. Congruent joint

Discussion

The correct answer is (E). This radiograph reflects a moderate deformity (Table 5–1) with evidence of an increased HVA, IMA, uncovered fibular sesamoid, and a prominent medial eminence. This radiograph demonstrates an incongruent joint at the first MTPJ with lateral subluxation of the proximal phalanx base relative to the metatarsal head.

Satisfied that you know what you are talking about, she asks you to discuss the complications associated with the various treatment options.

Table 5–1   HALLUX VALGUS DEFORMITY SEVERITY IS DEFINED BY HALLUX VALGUS ANGLE (HVA) AND INTERMETATARSAL ANGLE (IMA)

	HVA (degrees)	IMA (degrees)
Mild	<20	<11
Moderate	20–40	11–16
Severe	>40	>16

Which is the incorrectly paired procedure and complication?

A. Proximal opening wedge osteotomy—hallux stiffness
B. Fibular sesamoid excision—hallux varus
C. First TMTJ arthrodesis—capital necrosis
D. Ludloff osteotomy—transfer metatarsalgia

Discussion

The correct answer is (C). First TMTJ arthrodesis is not typically associated with capital segment necrosis. Capital necrosis is more classically associated with the combination of a distal osteotomy with an aggressive soft tissue release about the first MTPJ. A Ludloff osteotomy is a first metatarsal osteotomy that has the potential to shorten the first MT relative to the lateral metatarsals, which may result in transfer metatarsalgia. A proximal opening wedge osteotomy relatively lengthens the first ray and, when combined with distal soft tissue correction of hallux valgus, can result in stiffness of the tendons that cross the first MTPJ. Fibular sesamoid excision, lateral FHB tenotomy, excessive imbrication of the medial capsule, and excessive metatarsal head resection (lateral to the sagittal sulcus) can all result in hallux varus.

Objectives: Did you learn...?

- Describe radiographic findings associated with hallux valgus?
- Identify initial treatment options for hallux valgus?
- Describe the spectrum of severity for hallux valgus?

CASE 3

Dr. Daniel Guss

A 16-year-old male presents noting frequent sprains to his right ankle. He notes that he rolls his right ankle several times a day, and also describes pain along the lateral border of his foot. His left ankle is similarly symptomatic, but not quite as severe. Radiographs are obtained (Figs. 5–3 and 5–4).

Based on the radiographs (Figs. 5–3 and 5–4), which of the following do you expect to observe on clinical examination?

A. Pes cavus
B. Pes planus
C. Hindfoot valgus
D. Forefoot varus

Discussion

The correct answer is (A). Radiographic characteristics of a pes cavus deformity include an elevated dorsiflexion

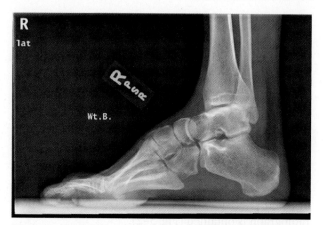

Figure 5–3 Lateral weight-bearing radiograph of the foot.

pitch of the calcaneus, so that the angle between the calcaneus and the floor often exceeds 30 degrees on weight-bearing radiographs (Fig. 5–5A). A plantar-flexed first ray may also be characteristic, in which case the straight line normally formed by the talus and the first metatarsal on lateral radiograph is abnormal. This is known as Meary's angle (Fig. 5–5B).

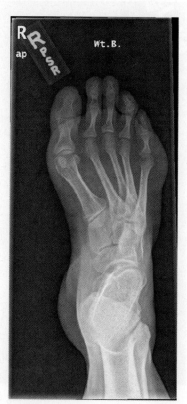

Figure 5–4 AP weight-bearing radiograph of the foot.

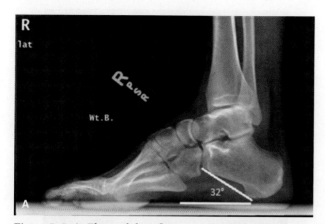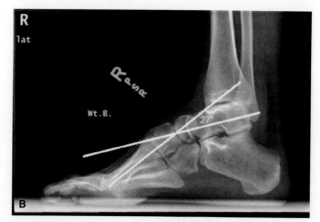

Figure 5–5 **A:** Elevated dorsiflexion pitch of the calcaneus with pes cavus. **B:** Abnormal Meary's angle with pes cavus.

Pes planus is further characterized by hindfoot varus and forefoot valgus. Adult-acquired flatfoot deformity would be characterized by hindfoot valgus and forefoot varus.

What additional information are you likely to elicit on patient history?

A. A history of clubfoot as an infant
B. A history of multidirectional instability of the shoulder
C. A family member with similar symptoms
D. Frequent fractures as a young child

Discussion

The correct answer is (C). While pes cavus may have diverse etiology, one study found that neurologic findings were apparent in approximately two-thirds of patients. Of patients with neurologic findings, half were diagnosed with Charcot–Marie–Tooth disease (CMT). A more recent pediatric study found that 78% of children with bilateral pes cavus are ultimately diagnosed with CMT. CMT refers to a heterogenous array of genetic disorders that collectively affect either nerve axons or their surrounding myelin sheaths, ultimately resulting in nerve dysfunction. This underscores the importance of a thorough neurological examination in patients presenting with pes cavus.

Patients presenting early with CMT often have flexible joint deformities. Assuming this patient has flexible deformities, what would you expect to find with Coleman block testing?

A. Elevation of the first ray
B. Correction of forefoot adduction

C. Normalization of the talar-first metatarsal angle (Meary's angle)
D. Correction of hindfoot varus

Discussion

The correct answer is (D). Coleman block testing refers to having the patient stand with the lateral border of the foot on flat blocks. This allows the plantar-flexed first ray to contact the ground at a lower level. With a forefoot-driven hindfoot varus deformity and a flexible hindfoot, standing on the Coleman blocks will correct the hindfoot varus into a more neutral alignment. If, alternatively, the varus hindfoot is not driven by the cavus deformity, the Coleman block test will not permit correction of the varus hindfoot.

Assuming the hindfoot varus corrects with Coleman block testing, and the patient has failed conservative management, the bony components of operative intervention would include which of the following?

A. Shortening osteotomy of the first ray
B. Dorsiflexion osteotomy of the first ray
C. Calcaneal osteotomy with medial heel slide
D. None of the above

Discussion

The correct answer is (B). Correction of the hindfoot varus with Coleman block testing confirms that the subtalar joint remains flexible and that the cavus deformity is driving the hindfoot varus. A dorsiflexion osteotomy of the first ray will raise the first metatarsal from its pathologic plantar-flexed position. With subsequent weight bearing, the head of the first metatarsal must still contact the ground. When doing so postoperatively,

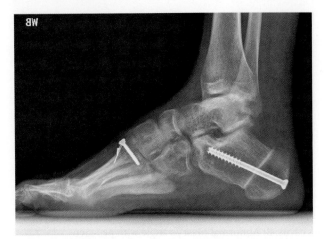

Figure 5–6 Dorsiflexion osteotomy of the first ray and calcaneal osteotomy with lateral heel slide for pes cavus.

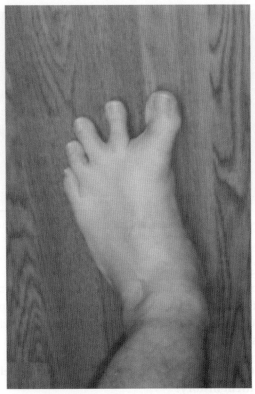

Figure 5–7 Photograph of the left foot with patient standing.

however, it forces the hindfoot out of pathologic varus into a more neutral position. This can be supplemented with a calcaneal osteotomy with lateral heel slide if necessary (Fig. 5–6); a medial slide would accentuate the hindfoot varus deformity.

Objectives: Did you learn...?

- Describe radiographic findings of pes cavus?
- Assess familial aspect of CMT?
- Describe the role of Coleman block testing?
- Describe the role of osteotomies in treating CMT-related deformity?

CASE 4

Dr. Jeremy T. Smith

A 53-year-old man presents to your office 2 months after a motor vehicle accident. He reports that he had to slam on the break prior to a collision and noted the immediate onset of pain in his left foot. He was taken by ambulance to an emergency room, where he underwent a reduction of a dislocated great toe. He reports that he has been wearing a walking boot since the time of the injury. A photograph and x-ray of his foot are shown (Figs. 5–7 and 5–8). On examination, you are able to passively push his toes into proper alignment.

What is your diagnosis?

A. Ligamentous Lisfranc injury
B. Hallux varus
C. Hallux valgus
D. Turf toe

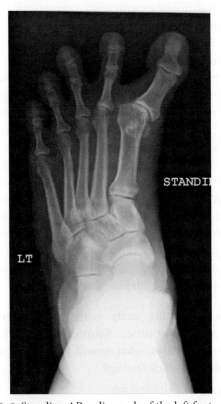

Figure 5–8 Standing AP radiograph of the left foot.

Discussion

The correct answer is (B). The patient likely sustained a varus-directed dislocation at the first metatarsophalangeal (MTP) joint. This was presumably closed-reduced, but a hallux varus deformity has persisted. There is no widening between the medial cuneiform and second metatarsal base to suggest Lisfranc injury. The photograph and x-ray show hallux varus, not hallux valgus. And while a turf toe that differentially ruptured the lateral aspect of the plantar plate of the hallux could result in hallux varus, the better answer to this question is hallux varus.

Which of the following structures around the first MTP joint are restraints preventing hallux varus?

A. Lateral capsule, lateral ligaments, adductor hallucis, lateral aspect of the flexor hallucis brevis, fibular sesamoid
B. Lateral capsule, lateral ligaments, abductor hallucis, lateral aspect of the flexor hallucis brevis, fibular sesamoid
C. Lateral capsule, lateral ligaments, adductor hallucis, lateral aspect of the flexor hallucis brevis, tibial sesamoid
D. Lateral capsule, lateral ligaments, abductor hallucis, lateral aspect of the flexor hallucis brevis, tibial sesamoid

Discussion

The correct answer is (A). The first MTP joint is balanced by both bony and soft tissue stabilizers. The soft tissue stabilizers on the lateral aspect of the joint prevent the toe from drifting into a hallux varus position.

The most common cause of hallux varus is:

A. Congenital
B. Traumatic
C. Shoe-wear related
D. Over-correction during hallux valgus surgery

Discussion

The correct answer is (D). Hallux varus has been reported to occur between 2% and 15% of the time after hallux valgus surgery. This can result from a number of technical causes, including over-correction with a metatarsal osteotomy or fusion, excessive resection of the medial first metatarsal head, excessive tightening of the medial capsule, and excessive lateral soft tissue release. Postoperative hallux varus has been described with the

true McBride procedure, in which the fibular sesamoid is excised.

After you meet this patient, your initial management should include all of the following except:

A. Closed reduction and percutaneous pinning of the hallux
B. Shoe modifications with the use of wider shoes and/or shoe stretching
C. Strapping or taping of the hallux into a neutral position
D. Counseling on the importance of avoiding narrow toe-box shoes

Discussion

The correct answer is (A). This patient presents to you 2 months after his injury. For hallux varus, the initial treatment is most often nonsurgical and should involve patient counseling and shoe modifications to avoid shoes that rub against the hallux. Sometimes taping or strapping of the hallux into a neutral position can manage symptoms.

This patient undergoes a period of attempted taping and shoe modifications, yet finds that he has persistent pain at his hallux MTP joint and also from his toe rubbing against his shoes. You decide to proceed with operative reconstruction.

What is the most appropriate procedure for this patient?

A. First MTP joint arthrodesis
B. Proximal metatarsal osteotomy
C. Extensor tendon transfer
D. Reverse distal Chevron osteotomy

Discussion

The correct answer is (C). Extensor tendon transfer, either with extensor hallucis longus (EHL) or extensor hallucis brevis (EHB), has been shown to effectively correct a nonarthritic flexible hallux varus deformity. If using the EHL—either the entire EHL or a split portion of the EHL—the tendon is released distally and then passed deep to the transverse metatarsal ligament and attached to the hallux proximal phalanx to correct the deformity. If using EHB, the attachment distally is maintained and the proximal portion of the tendon is passed deep to the transverse metatarsal ligament and then attached to the first metatarsal head to hold the deformity corrected. These procedures are often coupled with a medial soft tissue release.

Objectives: Did you learn...?

• Identify structures that contribute to maintenance of alignment of the hallux MTP joint?
• Pinpoint causes of hallux varus?
• Describe various treatment options for hallux varus?

CASE 5

Dr. John Paul Elton

A 50-year-old otherwise healthy and active gentleman fell from a height of approximately 8 ft while rock climbing. He had immediate pain in his left ankle and was unable to bear weight on that extremity. He presented to the emergency department with pain isolated to the left ankle and foot. Initial radiographs of the left ankle are obtained and the lateral view is shown (Fig. 5–9).

What is the most appropriate next step?

A. CT scan of the left ankle
B. Short-leg splint with crutches and referral to orthopaedic clinic
C. Physical examination
D. Open reduction and internal fixation

Discussion

The correct answer is (C). Severe pain from the calcaneus fracture may present as a distracting injury and the patient may not recognize additional inju-

ries. Patients presenting with calcaneus fractures have been shown to have a 25% chance of having an associated injury to the lower extremities or lumbar spine. Focused physical examination and appropriate radiographs, if there is any spine or extremity tenderness to palpation, should be the first step in evaluation of this patient. While the other management options in this question may be appropriate, the initial step should be physical examination.

What other diagnostic study should be obtained?

A. Compartment pressures
B. Stress radiographs
C. MRI of the ankle
D. CT of the ankle

Discussion

The correct answer is (D). The bony anatomy, in particular displacement and comminution of the posterior facet, are best seen with CT and should be considered mandatory for evaluation of displaced, joint depression calcaneus fractures. The Sanders classification is widely accepted in describing the articular comminution and displacement of the posterior facet and is based on the coronal view of the CT at the widest portion of the posterior facet of the talus (Fig. 5–10). This view allows the

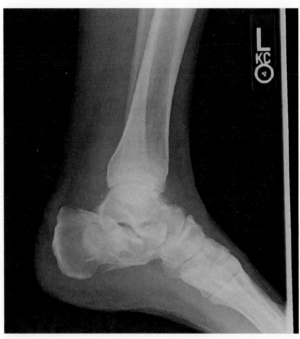

Figure 5–9 Lateral radiograph of the ankle.

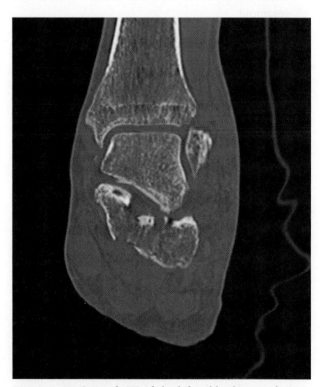

Figure 5–10 Coronal CT of the left ankle showing fracture lines in the posterior facet used in the Sanders classification.

posterior facet of the calcaneus to be divided into thirds by two vertical lines, thereby designating the lateral, central, and medial columns of the facet. The sustentaculum tali may also be fractured, resulting in four possible fragments. Lateral radiographs also allow for measurement of the angle of Gissane, measured by the intersection of two lines drawn from a point at the most anterior-inferior point of the posterior facet, one line drawn to the superior surface of the posterior facet and the second line to the most superior point of the anterior process. Bohler's angle is also measured on the lateral radiograph, formed by a line from the most superior point of the posterior tuberosity directed to the most superior point of the posterior facet, and a line directed from the most superior aspect of the anterior process back to the same superior point of the posterior facet.

The patient's ankle is splinted and he is referred to orthopaedics for further evaluation. The patient now presents to clinic with improved pain, moderate edema to the left hindfoot, and questions about treatment options. He reminds you that he still enjoys a very active lifestyle, is busy on his feet as a site engineer for an energy company, and has never smoked.

What is the most important predictor that he may benefit from surgical fixation of his fracture?

A. He is a male
B. He has a heavy workload
C. Severity of his joint depression-type fracture
D. His age

Discussion

The correct answer is (C). A prospective randomized controlled study of calcaneus fractures by Buckley et al. (*J Bone Joint Surg*, 2002) found that patients who had severe joint depression-type fractures, as described by Essex–Lopresti, fared better with operative than with nonoperative treatment. They also found that patients with female sex, a light workload, and age 20 to 29 also had improved outcomes with operative treatment if they were not receiving worker's compensation.

Objectives: Did you learn...?
• Describe the associated risk of additional musculoskeletal injury in patient with a joint depression type calcaneus fracture?
• Describe Sanders' classification of intra-articular joint depression calcaneus fractures?
• Identify factors affecting the decision to treat these fractures operatively or nonoperatively?

CASE 6

Dr. Daniel Guss

A 60-year-old male presents noting left foot pain of over a year's duration. He was originally diagnosed with plantar fasciitis, but a progressive feeling of fullness was subsequently confirmed to be a mass on magnetic resonance imaging. A plain x-ray and MRI are shown (Figs. 5–11 to 5–13).

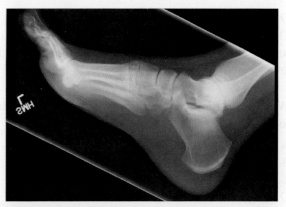

Figure 5–11 Lateral radiograph of the foot.

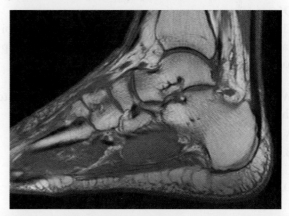

Figure 5–12 MRI sagittal T1 image.

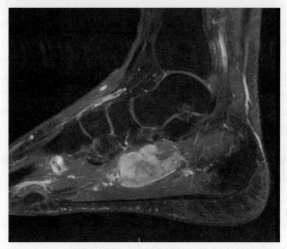

Figure 5–13 MRI sagittal T1 fat-suppressed image with IV contrast.

From a purely statistical point of view and ignoring the presented images, what is the most likely diagnosis?

A. Benign tumor
B. Primary malignant tumor
C. Metastatic malignant tumor
D. Both A and C are equally likely

Discussion

The correct answer is (A). Approximately 75% of tumors or tumor-like conditions in the foot and ankle are benign in origin.

What is the most common soft tissue sarcoma in the foot?

A. Synovial sarcoma
B. Clear cell sarcoma
C. Epithelioid sarcoma
D. Angiosarcoma

Discussion

The correct answer is (A). Synovial sarcomas are typically slow growing with a prolonged duration of symptoms prior to diagnosis.

Which tumors are most likely to metastasize to the foot?

A. Breast
B. Thyroid
C. Lung
D. Renal

Discussion

The correct answer is (C). The skeletal system is the most frequent region of metastasis by tumors of the breast, lung, thyroid, kidney, and prostate. Metastases distal to the knee or elbow are rare, however, and acrometastasis (metastasis to the hand and foot) account for less than 0.5% of metastases. In such cases, primary tumor in the lung or prostate should be investigated.

What is the next recommended step in treating the above patient?

A. CT scan of the lungs
B. Needle biopsy
C. Open biopsy
D. Referral to an orthopaedic oncologist

Discussion

The correct answer is (D). Biopsy should be the final step of tumor identification. Given the concern for malignancy in the described patient, the decision to biopsy should be handled by the treating oncologic surgeon who will decide the location of any potential surgical incision. Given that biopsy tracts potentially seed tumor, they are frequently excised.

Objectives: Did you learn...?

• Discuss the likelihood of benign versus malignant tumors in the foot?
• Describe the most common soft tissue sarcoma in the foot?
• Describe the concept and most likely source of acrometastasis?
• Assess the role of referral to orthopaedic oncologists?

CASE 7

Dr. Thomas Dowd

A 54-year-old woman presents to clinic reporting discomfort on the dorsum of her foot with shoewear and pain in the middle of her foot with activity, especially when she goes upstairs.

All but which of the following comprise the midfoot?

A. Second and third tarsometatarsal joints (TMTJs)
B. Subtalar joint
C. First TMTJ
D. Articulation between the navicular and cuneiforms
E. Fourth and fifth TMTJs

Discussion

The correct answer is (B). The subtalar joint is not part of the midfoot; it is part of the hindfoot. The remaining answers comprise portions of the midfoot.

She is interested in avoiding surgery for her midfoot arthritis and asks you what options she has for a type of shoe or orthotic that might alleviate her pain.

Your first suggestion would be:

A. Arizona brace
B. UCBL orthotic
C. Stiff-soled shoe with or without rocker bottom modification
D. Half-length carbon fiber insert
E. Budin splint

Discussion

The correct answer is (C). Stiff-soled shoes with rocker bottom modification have long been the initial non-operative therapy for midfoot arthritis. Recently, in an effort to address the cumbersome nature of these shoes, exchangeable full-length carbon fiber inserts have been employed. Both are acceptable first-line treatments. Half-length inserts are unlikely to span the affected joints and will not help in minimizing pain in the midfoot. The Arizona brace is typically used to address ankle or hindfoot arthritis. The UCBL is a stiff, custom orthotic that is used to address adult-acquired flatfoot disorder. It employs a deep heel cup to stabilize the hindfoot and a built-up lateral wall to address an abducted foot. The UCBL's rigid medial arch may offer some midfoot pain relief but the UCBL is not a first-line treatment of midfoot arthritis. Budin splints are used to address hammertoes.

The patient returns the following year and reports that her pain has gradually worsened with nonsurgical management. Radiographic findings demonstrate arthritic changes, primarily at the second TMTJ (Fig. 5–14).

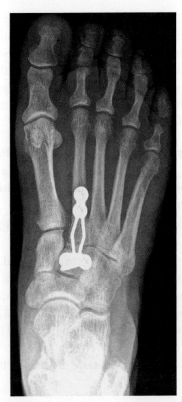

Figure 5–15 Postoperative WB AP foot radiograph demonstrating second TMTJ arthrodesis, associated with 95% relief of pain.

Prior image-guided injection at the second TMTJ relieved the vast majority of her pain. She states that her pain is not limited to the "bumps at the top of her foot," and is a deeper achy discomfort. You recommend a second TMTJ arthrodesis (Fig. 5–15).

When dealing with midfoot arthritis, which of the following pairings of location and surgical intervention is least appropriate?

A. Dorsal bossing with dorsal pain associated with shoewear only: exostectomy
B. 1–3 TMTJ arthritis: arthrodesis
C. 4–5 TMTJ arthritis: arthrodesis
D. 4–5 TMTJ arthritis: interpositional arthroplasty

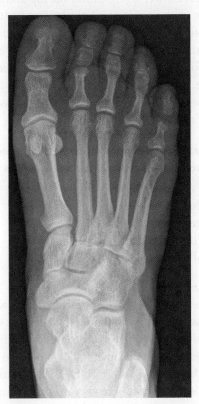

Figure 5–14 Weight-bearing AP radiograph of the foot demonstrating joint space narrowing at the second TMTJ with relative sparing of the first TMTJ.

Discussion

The correct answer is (C). Pain that is dorsally based and associated with pressure on prominences from shoewear may be addressed with exostectomy. Medial and midfoot arthritis that has failed nonoperative treatment is best addressed with arthrodesis. Range of motion in the sagittal plane at this location is around

7 degrees. However, lateral midfoot range of motion is approximately 20 degrees and lateral midfoot flexibility plans an important role in accommodating the ground. Accordingly, lateral midfoot arthrodesis is rarely recommended. If intervention is pursued for lateral midfoot arthritis, interpositional arthroplasty is often considered.

You are planning the surgical procedure at the beginning of the case and reviewing standard measurements and anatomical relationships. Which of the following is incorrect?

A. The second TMTJ is approximately 1 to 2 cm proximal to the first TMTJ

B. The first TMTJ is often between 2.5 and 3 cm deep

C. The distance from the tip of the hallux to the first metatarsophalangeal joint is nearly equivalent to that from the first MTPJ to the first TMTJ

D. On cross section, the midfoot is shaped like an arch with a dorsal apex

E. The second TMTJ is distal to the first and third TMTJs

Discussion

The correct answer is (E). The second TMTJ is proximal to the adjacent joints by approximately 1 to 2 cm. The remaining options are correct and can be valuable in planning surgical incisions. Of particular note is the depth of the first TMTJ (Fig. 5–16). Failure to fully prepare the plantar aspect of the TMTJs can lead to nonunion, partial union, or malunion.

Objectives: Did you learn...?

• Assess anatomic considerations about the midfoot (range of motion, osseous relationships, depth of first TMTJ)?

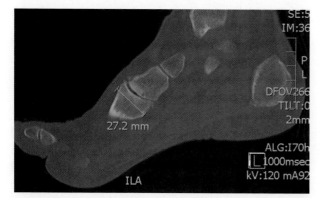

Figure 5–16 Sagittal CT section of first TMTJ demonstrating joint space narrowing, cuneiform subchondral cyst and dorsal osteophytes with a measured depth of ~2.7 cm.

• Describe nonsurgical treatment options for midfoot arthritis?

• Describe surgical options for midfoot arthritis?

CASE 8

Dr. Joshua Lamb

A 48-year-old female presents to your office with worsening right ankle pain. Twenty years ago she sustained an ankle fracture, which was treated by open reduction and internal fixation. She subsequently underwent removal of hardware. She now is experiencing pain and swelling throughout the ankle, which is exacerbated by weight-bearing activities. Weight-bearing radiographs are obtained (Fig. 5–17A and B).

What is the most common cause of ankle arthritis?

A. Inflammatory disease

B. Chronic ligamentous instability

C. Previous trauma

D. Primary degenerative disease (osteoarthritis)

Discussion

The correct answer is (C). Unlike the hip and knee, osteoarthritis of the ankle is relatively rare (<10%). Most patients who develop ankle arthritis have sustained previous trauma. Nonanatomic fracture healing alters joint contact forces and changes load bearing mechanics of the ankle, potentially leading to arthritis in the future. Inflammatory disease and instability are less common causes of ankle arthritis.

What forms of bracing and shoe wear modification may be helpful to control symptoms in this patient?

A. Lace up ankle support

B. Ankle foot orthosis (AFO)

C. Rocker bottom shoe

D. Patellar tendon weight-bearing orthosis

E. All of the above

Discussion

The correct answer is (E). Many patients with ankle arthritis will discover on their own that their symptoms can be mitigated using a high-top boot or shoe. A lace up ankle support is well tolerated and helps to minimize motion through the ankle. An AFO or Arizona brace (lace up leather brace) are more rigid bracing options that often require the use of larger shoes. A patellar tendon weight-bearing orthosis offers the advantage of decreasing load across the ankle, although it is not typically well tolerated as a long-term solution. A rocker

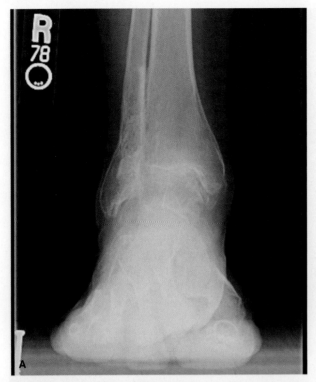 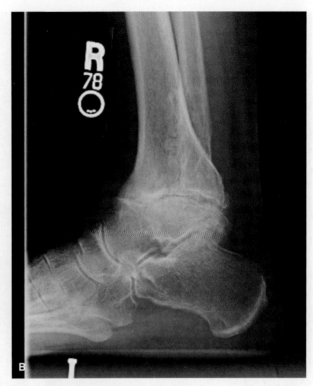

Figure 5–17 **A, B:** AP and lateral weight-bearing ankle radiographs.

bottom shoe can be beneficial by transferring sagittal plane motion to the bottom of the shoe. A rocker bottom shoe can be combined with a cushioned heel to help absorb impact at heel strike.

Despite extensive nonoperative management, the patient has persistent pain and elects to proceed with ankle arthrodesis. Postoperative radiographs were obtained at 6 weeks (Fig. 5–18A and B).

What is the recommended positioning of the ankle for arthrodesis?

A. Neutral plantar flexion, hindfoot valgus of 5 degrees, rotation equal to contralateral limb
B. 10 degrees of plantar flexion, neutral hindfoot varus/valgus, rotation equal to contralateral limb
C. 10 degrees of plantar flexion, hindfoot varus of 5 degrees, 10 degrees of external rotation
D. Neutral plantar flexion, hindfoot varus of 5 degrees, 10 degrees of external rotation

Discussion

The correct answer is (A), neutral plantar flexion, hindfoot valgus of 5 degrees, and rotation equal to contralateral limb (typically 5–10 degrees external rotation).

Excessive hindfoot valgus will reduce the locking phenomenon of the transverse tarsal joints during the stance and push off phase of gait. This will in turn result in an excessively flexible midfoot and forefoot. Conversely, placing the hindfoot in varus will lock the transverse tarsal joints and result in excessive midfoot and forefoot rigidity.

Following ankle arthrodesis, what is this patient most likely to experience?

A. Painful hardware
B. Ipsilateral hip and knee arthritis
C. Nonunion
D. Ipsilateral adjacent hindfoot arthritis

Discussion

The correct answer is (D). Adjacent hindfoot and midfoot arthritis eventually develops in most patients after an ankle arthrodesis. Adjacent joint arthritis is often seen on radiographs but may remain asymptomatic. Pain associated with the hardware may occur but is not a common complaint. Hip and knee arthritis have not been associated with ankle arthrodesis. Reported nonunion rates vary but on average are about 10%.

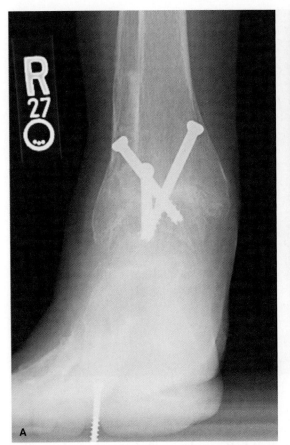
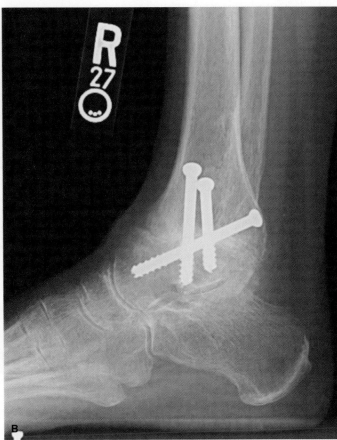

Figure 5–18 **A, B:** AP and lateral ankle radiographs 6 weeks following ankle arthrodesis.

Objectives: Did you learn...?

- Identify the most common cause of ankle arthritis?
- Describe nonoperative bracing and orthotic options to treat ankle arthritis?
- Optimally position an ankle arthrodesis?

CASE 9

Dr. Jeffrey R. Jockel

A 59-year-old female with a longstanding history of bilateral foot pain presents with a recurrent painful callus on her feet and difficulty with ambulation. She describes a history of multiple orthopaedic surgeries in the past addressing her hands, hip, knee, and spine. Weight-bearing radiographs of the foot are obtained (Fig. 5–19A and B).

What is the most likely underlying diagnosis?

A. Charcot arthropathy
B. Osteomyelitis
C. Posttraumatic arthropathy
D. Inflammatory arthropathy
E. Osteoporosis

Discussion

The correct answer is (D), inflammatory arthropathy (specifically rheumatoid arthritis). Figure 5–19 demonstrates the classic radiographic findings of rheumatoid arthritis (RA), as the forefoot is the most commonly affected region of the foot. RA presents as a symmetric polyarthropathy, with increased deformity with a longer duration of active rheumatoid disease. Patients often develop difficulties with shoeware and metatarsalgia pain from a combination of MTP joint instability, joint synovitis, and hammer toes, followed by ambulation difficulty due to progressive deformity. Charcot arthropathy most commonly affects the midfoot joints, and can also present with joint instability and dislocation.

What is the underlying pathophysiology for this patient's forefoot deformity?

A. Inflammatory synovial proliferation
B. Factor VIII deficiency with repetitive hemorrhage
C. Synovial crystalline deposition

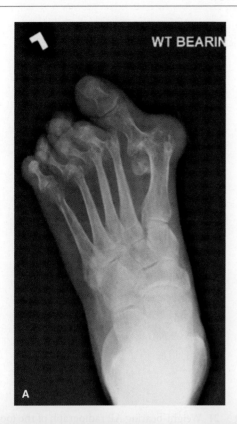

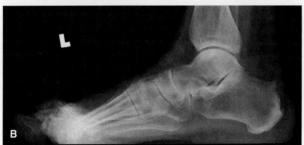

Figure 5-19 **A, B:** AP and lateral radiographs of the foot.

D. Intra-articular immune complex deposition and antibody formation
E. Neurotraumatic and autosympathetic destruction

Discussion

The correct answer is (A). The common forefoot deformity of rheumatoid arthritis includes MTP joint instability due to chronic capsular distention from inflammatory synovium, leading to attenuation of capsuloligamentous attachments. Metatarsophalangeal joint instability progresses to subluxation/dislocation, and is accompanied by tendon contractures of the lesser toes resulting in PIP/DIP deformities including hammer toes. In addition, the plantar fat pad migrates

distally with dorsal MTP subluxation and toe contracture, further increasing metatarsalgia symptoms. The incidence of hallux valgus increases with rheumatoid chronicity. Factor VIII deficiency is associated with hemophilic arthropathy, and gout/pseudogout is caused by crystalline deposition of monosodium urate or calcium pyrophydrate dehydrate, respectively.

The patient has had prior treatment by her primary care physician with medical management, callus trimming, and custom orthotics with extra-depth shoes. She continues to report persistent metatarsalgia pain, plantar callus formation, and skin breakdown over her "bunion."

Surgical treatment for this patient should consist of:

A. Lapidus procedure (first tarsometatarsal arthrodesis), lesser toe hammer toe correction with PIP resection arthroplasty
B. First MTP arthrodesis, lesser toe metatarsal head resections, lesser toe hammer toe corrections
C. First metatarsal double osteotomy and distal soft tissue reconstruction, lesser toe plantar plate repair with hammer toe corrections
D. Transmetatarsal amputation
E. Keller procedure (first MTP resection arthroplasty), lesser toe metatarsal head plantar condylectomy and hammer toe corrections

Discussion

The correct answer is (B), first MTP arthrodesis, lesser toe metatarsal head resections, and lesser hammertoe corrections (Fig. 5–20). Multiple descriptions of this procedure have been reported (*Hoffman procedure, Clayton procedure, Fowler procedure*) including modifications. With chronic lesser MTP joint subluxation/dislocation, soft tissue reconstruction of the MTP joints traditionally is not performed, and therefore resection arthroplasty of the lesser metatarsal heads is performed to address metatarsalgia symptoms. An appropriate resection cascade of lesser metatarsal lengths is created to allow approximately 1 cm of space for lesser MTP joint decompression. The first metatarsal length is then adjusted to fit the lesser MT cascade, prior to first MTP arthrodesis. Hammer toe correction may be performed with an open procedure addressing the PIP joint for a fixed deformity, or a closed toe osteoclasis for mild/flexible hammer toe deformity. Surgical complications from rheumatoid forefoot reconstruction include recurrent toe deformities, floppy toes, recurrent intractable plantar keratosis, and wound healing problems. Discontinuation of biologic and disease-modifying antirheumatic

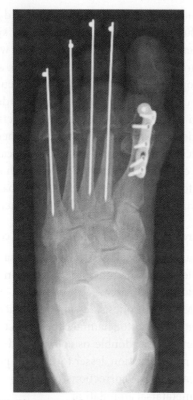

Figure 5–20 Rheumatoid forefoot reconstruction.

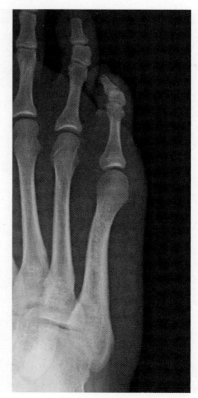

Figure 5–21 Weight-bearing AP radiograph of the foot.

medications perioperatively in this patient population is currently controversial.

Objectives: Did you learn...?
• Describe the pathophysiology of rheumatoid arthritis?
• Describe rheumatoid forefoot deformity?
• Conservatively treat forefoot deformity?
• Surgically treat rheumatoid forefoot?

CASE 10

Dr. Richard J. De Asla

An otherwise healthy 19-year-old female presents with a 6-week history of progressive pain over the lateral aspect of the right fifth metatarsal head. She denies a history of foot trauma. She prefers to wear high-heeled shoes at her part time job. Physical examination reveals mild swelling and a small callus over the lateral fifth metatarsal head. Passive range of motion of the fifth metatarsophalangeal (MTP) joint is painless. A weight-bearing AP x-ray of the right foot was obtained (Fig. 5–21).

What is the most appropriate treatment at this time?

A. Conservative management including a discussion about avoiding constrictive shoe wear

B. Refer the patient to a rheumatologist for serum hematologic and immunologic testing
C. Aspirate the fifth MTP joint and evaluate for crystals and elevated white blood cell count
D. Rotational osteotomy of the fifth metatarsal
E. Lateral condylectomy of the fifth metatarsal head

Discussion
The correct answer is (A). The patient has a bunionette deformity. Irritation over the lateral aspect of the fifth metatarsal head results from mechanical rubbing of ill-fitting footwear against the bony prominence. Callus formation and an inflamed bursa may be noted on physical examination. Initial treatment is conservative and may include paring of the callus, orthotics, and well-fitting shoes. Rheumatology referral is not necessary as nothing in the patient history suggests a systemic inflammatory condition. Joint aspiration is not indicated in the face of painless joint range of motion and focal tenderness. Surgical measures are not indicated unless nonsurgical measures fail and symptoms are deemed unacceptable by the patient.

Despite regular callus debridement and shoe wear modification the same patient returns 1 year later with similar complaints. She is contemplating surgical intervention for symptomatic relief.

Which is the most appropriate surgical option?

A. Excision of the fifth metatarsal head
B. Lateral condylectomy of the fifth metatarsal head
C. Rotational osteotomy of the fifth metatarsal
D. Arthrodesis of the fifth MTP joint

Discussion

The correct answer is (C). The patient has a type 2 bunionette, characterized by a lateral curvature in the diaphysis. A type 2 bunionette is best corrected with a rotational osteotomy of the distal or midshaft region of the fifth metatarsal. Type 1 bunionette deformities are characterized by an enlarged lateral head prominence. In these cases, a simple lateral condylectomy can be performed. Type 3 bunionettes result from an increased 4–5 intermetatarsal angle. Both type 2 and 3 deformities can be treated with rotational osteotomy. There is typically not a role for excision of the fifth metatarsal head or fifth MTP joint arthrodesis for bunionette correction.

Objectives: Did you learn...?

• Initially manage a bunionette deformity?
• Classify bunionettes?
• Identify surgical management options for a bunionette?

CASE 11

Dr. Jeremy T. Smith

A 45-year-old woman presents to your office and notes that she has had a several years history of pain at the plantar medial hindfoot. She reports that the pain is present throughout the day and seems to be worse when she is active. She denies any trauma or recent change in shoewear. A lateral foot radiograph is reviewed (Fig. 5–22).

Your differential diagnosis includes all of the following except:

A. Plantar fasciitis
B. Entrapment first branch lateral plantar nerve (Baxter's nerve)
C. Noninsertional Achilles tendinosis
D. Calcaneal stress fracture

Discussion

The correct answer is (C). The patient presents with heel pain. While plantar fasciitis is far and away the most common cause of heel pain, one must also consider less

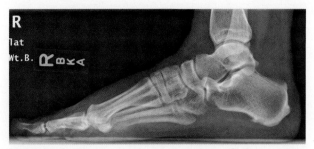

Figure 5–22 Lateral weight-bearing radiograph of the foot.

common diagnoses including calcaneal stress fracture, entrapment of the first branch of the lateral plantar nerve, and central heel pain (fat pad atrophy). Noninsertional Achilles tendinosis would not cause pain in this location.

Upon examination she is focally tender at the site marked with the dot and black arrow (Fig. 5–23). Based upon this site of tenderness, you suspect which of the diagnoses?

A. Plantar fasciitis
B. Entrapment first branch lateral plantar nerve (Baxter's nerve)
C. Central heel pain
D. Calcaneal stress fracture

Discussion

The correct answer is (B). The first branch of the lateral plantar nerve can be entrapped by the deep fascia of the abductor hallucis muscle at the site where this patient is tender. It is important to distinguish between this site of pain and other sites of heel pain. Plantar fasciitis typically causes pain at the origin of the plantar fascia (*white*

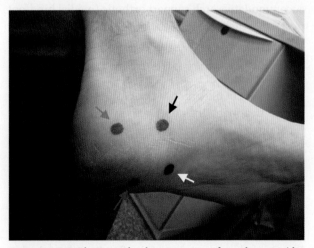

Figure 5–23 Photograph showing site of tenderness (dot with *black arrow*).

arrow). Central heel pain typically causes pain at the plantar aspect of the heel (*red arrow*), and a calcaneal stress fracture at the medial and lateral hindfoot (*blue arrow*).

Terminal branches of the tibial nerve distal to the tarsal tunnel include which of the following?

A. Lateral plantar nerve, deep peroneal nerve, medial calcaneal nerve
B. Lateral plantar nerve, sural nerve, medial calcaneal nerve
C. Lateral plantar nerve, medial plantar nerve, superficial peroneal nerve
D. Lateral plantar nerve, medial plantar nerve, medial calcaneal nerve

Discussion

The correct answer is (D). The superficial and deep peroneal nerves are branches of the common peroneal nerve. The sural nerve originates typically at the level of the knee or proximal calf.

Your initial treatment for Baxter's nerve entrapment should involve which of the following?

A. Medial posting accommodative hindfoot orthotic, anti-inflammatory medications, activity modification
B. Surgical release of the nerve
C. Nerve transection and burial
D. Lateral posting accommodative hindfoot orthotic, anti-inflammatory medications, activity modification

Discussion

The correct answer is (A). The initial goal of treatment is to reduce local inflammation and also to attempt to remove pressure from the site of nerve entrapment. An accommodative arch support orthotic (medial hindfoot post), may help to push the hindfoot into varus a bit, taking pressure off structures stretched at the medial hindfoot. This type of orthotic would be of particular use if the hindfoot were in valgus.

Your patient undergoes an extensive course of nonoperative treatment, including activity modification, anti-inflammatory medications, icing, and physical therapy yet has persistent pain that she finds to be very limiting.

You discuss operative treatment, specifically planning for which of the following procedures?

A. Transection and burial of the first branch of the lateral plantar nerve
B. Open decompression of the first branch of the lateral plantar nerve

C. Endoscopic plantar fascia release
D. Excision of the first branch of the lateral plantar nerve and intercalary sural nerve grafting

Discussion

The correct answer is (B). The goal of this operation is to decompress the entrapped area of nerve. This often involves transecting the deep fascia of the abductor hallucis muscle. Transection of the nerve is not recommended as maintenance of plantar sensation is critical.

Objectives: Did you learn...?

• Describe the anatomy of the plantar-medial hindfoot and common sources of pain?
• Discuss nonoperative and operative treatment for Baxter's nerve entrapment?

CASE 12

Dr. Tom Douglas

A 22-year-old, police officer presents to your office with bilateral leg pain and foot numbness while partaking in group physical training. He states that as he has been increasing his activities, there is a progressive tight feeling in the front of his lower legs. He also reports that if

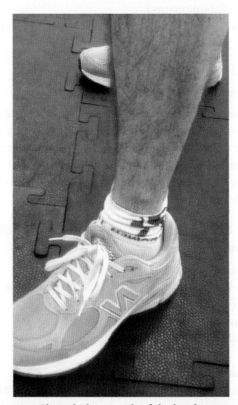

Figure 5–24 Clinical Photograph of the leg demonstrating a fascial herniation.

he runs long enough his feet sound like they are slapping the ground. The only thing abnormal in the appearance of his leg is a bump which appears on the distal/lateral lower leg with exercise. He has been through a course of physical therapy without any improvements.

On physical examination this is a fit male in no distress. He walks with a normal gait and has a neutral alignment of his hindfoot. He is nontender across his anterior tibia. He demonstrates 5/5 strength throughout his bilateral lower extremities. There is a visible and palpable fascial herniation at the distal leg approximately 2×2 cm in size (Fig. 5–24). Radiographic evaluation demonstrates no stress fracture of the tibia, no masses, and no arthrosis at either the ankle or the knee.

Your next step in evaluation of this patient is:

A. Triple phase bone scan

B. Noncontrast MRI of bilateral tibia

C. Compartment pressure measurements

D. Vascular ultrasound

Discussion

The correct answer is (C). This patient presents with a history consistent with exertional compartment syndrome. A bone scan would be valuable for the evaluation of a stress fracture. An MRI would assist in the evaluation of either a stress fracture or tumor. Vascular ultrasound is valuable for the evaluation of DVT or popliteal artery entrapment syndrome.

The patient obtains pressure measurements of his bilateral legs, which are as follows (mm Hg).

	Resting	Post Exercise (5 minutes)
Right anterior compartment	6	43
Right lateral compartment	10	35
Right superficial posterior compartment	11	17
Right deep posterior compartment	11	18
Left anterior compartment	7	47
Left lateral compartment	10	33
Left superficial posterior compartment	11	19
Left deep posterior compartment	12	15

The patient reports that during the compartment testing there was a burning, electric-like pain that shot down to the space between his great and second toes, and he has since had numbness in this region which is gradually improving.

What compartment was most likely being tested when the nerve injury occurred?

A. Anterior compartment

B. Lateral compartment

C. Superficial posterior compartment

D. Deep posterior compartment

Discussion

The correct answer is (A). The deep peroneal nerve innervates the first web space and is localized in the anterior compartment. The superficial peroneal nerve is located within the lateral compartment. The deep posterior compartment contains the tibial nerve, which provides sensory innervation to the plantar surface of the foot.

The patient's dysesthesias resolve after approximately a week, and he is continuing to have symptoms and an inability to continue with his physical training program. He is now potentially going to be "booted out of the force" due to his inability to stay within physical fitness standards.

Your recommendation at this point is:

A. Continued observation and continued physical therapy

B. Night splints

C. Bilateral anterior and lateral compartment fasciotomy

D. Bilateral four compartment fasciotomy

Discussion

The correct answer is (C). This patient had elevated post exercise compartment pressures in the anterior and lateral compartments only. The diagnostic numbers for chronic exertional compartment syndrome are the same for both the upper and lower extremities. Pre exercise compartment pressures should be below 15 mm Hg, 1 minute post exercise they should be no higher than 30 mm Hg, and at 5 minutes post exercise they should be no higher than 20 mm Hg. There is no indication for deep and superficial posterior compartment releases in this patient. Night splints have been shown to be effective for many problems in the foot and ankle including plantar fasciitis and Achilles tendinosis but not for exertional compartment syndrome.

The patient undergoes an uneventful anterior and lateral compartment release on the left side and is extremely happy with the results. Approximately 6 weeks postoperatively he undergoes surgery on the right side. On the right side, at his first postoperative visit he reports an area of numbness on his foot.

Which nerve was most likely injured during this surgery?

A. Sural
B. Deep peroneal nerve
C. Tibial
D. Superficial peroneal nerve

Discussion

The correct answer is (D). During approach to the anterior and lateral compartments, the superficial peroneal nerve is often encountered. It exits the fascia of the lateral compartment approximately 12.5 cm proximal to the tip of the fibula, placing it at risk during distal release. The sural nerve lies posterior and heads laterally placing it at risk during Achilles repairs and lengthening of the tendo-Achilles complex. The deep peroneal nerve is at risk during anterior to posterior screw placement as well as during the anterior approach to the ankle. The tibial nerve lies in the deep posterior compartment.

Objectives: Did you learn...?

- Describe clinical findings of chronic exertional compartment syndrome?
- Describe intracompartmental pressure measurements consistent with an exertional compartment syndrome?
- Pinpoint the location of the superficial peroneal nerve in relation to the fibula?

CASE 13

Dr. Joshua Lamb

A 45-year-old man presents to your office with pain and stiffness in his big toe. He denies any history of trauma. He has noticed increased pain with exercise. His pain is primarily over the dorsal aspect of first metatarsophalangeal (MTP) joint. On physical examination, there is a negative MTP joint grind test and dorsiflexion is limited to 30 degrees. He complains of pain when jogging. Weight-bearing AP and lateral radiographs were obtained (Fig. 5–25A and B).

Which of the following orthoses may be effective in reducing symptoms?

A. Orthotic with Morton's extension
B. Hinged AFO

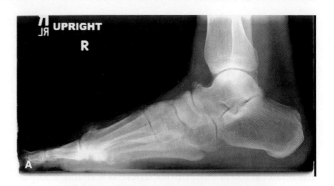

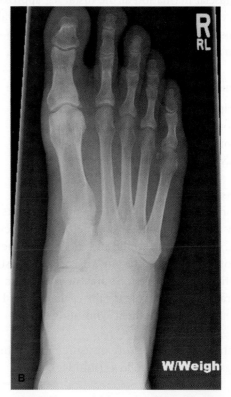

Figure 5–25 **A, B:** AP and lateral radiographs demonstrating degenerative changes in the first MTP joint with a dorsal osteophyte and <50% loss of joint space.

C. UCBL
D. Arizona brace

Discussion

The correct answer is (A). A Morton's extension provides added stiffness under the first MTP joint to limit dorsiflexion through the first MTP joint. Alternative forms of shoe modification include a carbon fiber insert, stiff soled shoe, and toe box stretching. A hinged AFO and Arizona brace would stabilize the ankle and would not address the pain at the hallux. A UCBL (University California Biomechanics Laboratory) orthosis is used to stabilize flexible deformities such as flexible pes planus or flexible metatarsus adductus/abductus.

After failing treatment with a Morton's extension orthosis and shoe wear modification, the patient has elected to proceed with surgery.

What would be the most appropriate surgical treatment option at this point?

A. Cheilectomy
B. Lapidus procedure
C. Clayton–Hoffman procedure
D. Keller procedure
E. First MTP arthrodesis

Discussion

The correct answer is (A). A cheilectomy is a good treatment option for younger patients wanting to preserve motion of first MTP joint. It is best for patients with "bump" pain and no pain in the mid arch of motion (grind test). It has been shown to be effective in grade I–II first MTP joint arthritis and can be combined with a Moberg (proximal phalanx) osteotomy to treat grade III disease. A Lapidus procedure is an arthrodesis of the first tarsometatarsal joint. A Clayton–Hoffman procedure combines a first MTP fusion with resection of the lesser metatarsal heads and is typically used to treat severe forefoot deformities associated with inflammatory arthritis. A Keller procedure is a resection arthroplasty of the first MTP joint and is best used in very low-demand patients with severe hallux rigidus. The Keller procedure often leads to a "cock-up" toe deformity and poor push off strength. Arthrodesis can be used to treat more severe or global forms of first MTP arthritis, such as grade III and IV diseases.

After performing a cheilectomy, range of motion is limited to 20 degrees of dorsiflexion. What is the best option for increasing dorsiflexion in this setting?

A. Keller procedure
B. Akin osteotomy
C. Release of the flexor hallucis brevis
D. Moberg osteotomy

Discussion

The correct answer is (D). The Moberg, or dorsiflexion osteotomy of the proximal phalanx, can be combined with a cheilectomy procedure to increase effective dorsiflexion through the first MTP joint. It can be used if the cheilectomy does not achieve 30 to 40 degrees of dorsiflexion or if the patient is a runner. Runners require >60

degrees of dorsiflexion. A Keller procedure is poorly tolerated in young, active patients hoping to preserve push off strength. An Akin osteotomy is a varus producing proximal phalanx osteotomy used to treat hallux valgus interphalangeus. Release of the flexor hallucis brevis will result in unopposed pull from the extensor hallucis brevis and flexor hallucis longus, resulting in a claw toe deformity.

Branches from which sensory nerve are at risk from the dorsomedial approach to the great toe?

A. Medial plantar
B. Superficial peroneal
C. Tibial
D. Saphenous
E. Deep peroneal

Discussion

The correct answer is (B). The superficial peroneal nerve branches into the medial dorsal cutaneous and the intermediate dorsal cutaneous nerves, providing sensation to the dorsal foot. The first web space is innervated by the deep peroneal nerve. The medial plantar nerve is a branch off of the tibial nerve and provides sensation to the plantar medial foot. The saphenous nerve is the largest cutaneous nerve from the femoral nerve and provides sensation to the medial foot up to the level of the first MTP joint.

Objectives: Did you learn...?

• Describe approach to nonoperative management of hallux rigidus?
• Identify the indications for cheilectomy?
• Identify when it is appropriate to consider the addition of a Moberg osteotomy?

CASE 14

Dr. Tom Douglas

A 52-year-old female with a past medical history significant for long-term type 2 diabetes presents with a right foot ulcer. She is now 3 years post gastric bypass surgery which in effect cured her diabetes, however she has residual foot deformity and neuropathy with decreased sensation to the level of the mid tibia. She is afebrile, has a normal white blood cell count, and a mildly elevated erythrocyte sedimentation rate and C-reactive protein. On examination of her right foot she has an ulcer present over the plantar aspect of her first metatarsal head which extends to bone. There is no purulence or foul odor present. She has palpable dorsalis pedis and posterior tibial pulses, but her skin is dry and cracked in regions. Her last hemoglobin A1c was 5.9. An MRI was performed which demonstrates osteomyelitis of the metatarsal head. In addition to recommending an irrigation and debridement you recommend a Strayer procedure (lengthening of the gastrocnemius tendon).

Your indications for performing this are:

A. Isolated soleus contracture
B. Isolated Achilles contracture
C. Isolated gastrocnemius contracture
D. Negative Silfverskiold test

Discussion

The correct answer is (C). A lengthening of the Achilles tendon has been shown to decrease forefoot pressure and reduce the recurrence of forefoot ulcers. Because the gastrocnemius crosses the knee as well as the ankle, a positive Silfverskiold test (equinus contracture with knee extended which resolves when the knee is flexed) will be seen with an isolated gastrocnemius contracture. This contracture can be addressed by a lengthening of the gastrocnemius at the musculotendinous junction (Fig. 5–26). In a patient with an equinus contracture with the knee both flexed and extended, a formal Achilles lengthening procedure, such as a triple hemisection or z-lengthening, should be performed. An additional posterior capsulotomy may be required.

Following debridement of the ulcer, Strayer procedure, and 6 weeks of culture specific antibiotics, the ulcer is healed on her right foot. At 12-week follow-up she reports a superficial ulcer on the contralateral foot at the plantar aspect of her second toe. Treatment

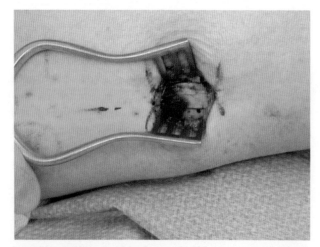

Figure 5–26 Clinical photograph of the musculotendinous junction of the gastrocnemius muscle.

options are discussed with her, and she is started with local wound care and diabetic shoes to unload this area. Prior to her next follow-up appointment, the following week she arrives in the emergency department with fevers, chills, an elevated white blood cell count and increased inflammatory markers. An MRI obtained by the emergency department demonstrates osteomyelitis of the distal phalanx of the second toe (Fig. 5–27).

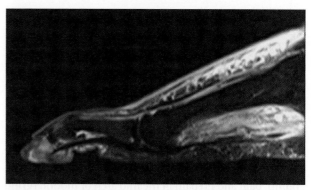

Figure 5–27 Sagittal T2 MRI demonstrating edema in the distal phalanx of the second toe.

Debridement of the second toe at this point should also include potential:

A. Amputation
B. Evaluation of adequate vascular inflow to the foot
C. Heel cord lengthening
D. All of the above

Discussion

The correct answer is (D). Debridement of diffuse osteomyelitis at a distal phalanx often results in a complete or partial amputation of the toe. When a patient has osteomyelitis, it is important to assess the blood flow, potential pressure overload from a contracture, neuropathy, and a potential abscess. Reversible causes of an ulcer should be addressed such as debridement of the osteomyelitis, drainage of any abscess, and addressing any potential contractures. Addressing inadequate blood flow via a vascular intervention is recommended prior to any definitive amputations.

The patient heals a toe amputation uneventfully and asks what the likelihood of her having an additional amputation on her foot is. Your best reply is:

A. You are at very high risk of an amputation
B. It is very unlikely that you will require an amputation
C. There is not enough information present in the literature

Discussion

The correct answer is (A). In a patient who has had a previous diabetic ulcer, there is a very high risk for a recurrent ulcer (greater than 50% 5-year recurrence) and amputation (greater than 10% at 5 years). For patients with a prior amputation, the risk of ipsilateral repeat amputation is great than 20%.

Objectives: Did you learn...?

- Discuss the value of addressing equinus contracture in a patient with forefoot ulcer?
- Describe how to differentiate between an isolated gastrocnemius contracture and an Achilles contracture?
- Pinpoint the importance of having adequate sensation in prevention of ulcer formation?

CASE 15

Dr. Jeffrey R. Jockel

A 52-year-old female presents to you reporting left foot pain that has been present for the past 3 months. She describes discomfort over the medial hindfoot region, which began without a traumatic inciting event. Her pain is minimal in the morning, however becomes progressively worse after extended walking and standing. She has worn inserts in her shoes for many years due to "low arches." Physical examination reveals a flexible valgus hindfoot, with midfoot abduction, and forefoot supination. The patient has tenderness and swelling along the posterior tibial tendon, and difficulty with single-limb rise. Radiographs of the foot and ankle are obtained (Fig. 5–28A–C).

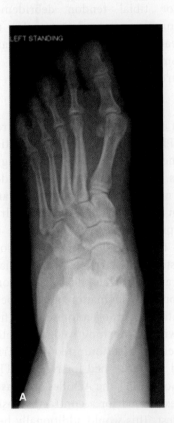
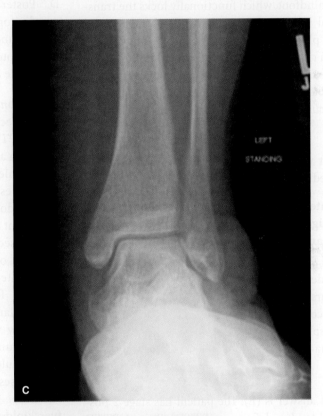
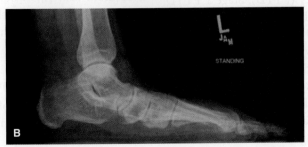

Figure 5–28 **A–C:** Initial foot and ankle radiographs.

Which muscle is the functional antagonist to the posterior tibial tendon?

A. Achilles
B. Gastrocnemius
C. Peroneus brevis
D. Peroneus longus
E. Peroneus tertius

Discussion

The correct answer is (C). The posterior tibialis muscle is a component of the deep posterior compartment of the leg. The posterior tibial tendon (PTT) courses along the posterior border of the medial malleolus, along with the flexor digitorum longus, posterior tibial neurovascular bundle, and flexor hallucis longus tendon. The PTT broadly attaches to the navicular, and functions to invert the hindfoot, which functionally locks the transverse tarsal joints (talonavicular and calcaneocuboid joints) and plantarflexes the ankle. This locking motion allows for a rigid lever during the push off phase of gait. The peroneus brevis is the functional antagonist to the PTT and acts to evert the hindfoot. The tibialis anterior and peroneus longus are functional antagonists to one another.

The patient was previously seen by another physician who ordered an MRI of the ankle (Fig. 5–29A–C).

Appropriate initial conservative treatment for this patient might include activity modification, nonsteroidal anti-inflammatories, and which of the following?

A. Extra-depth shoes
B. Metatarsal bar
C. Ankle compression sleeve
D. Night splint
E. Arizona brace

Discussion

The correct answer is (E). The patient has stage 2 posterior tibial tendon deficiency (PTTD). Stage 1 PTTD includes tenosynovitis of the PTT without degeneration or deformity. Stage 2 PTTD is a flexible planovalgus deformity, which is passively correctable. MRI images show longitudinal split tearing and tendinopathy of the PTT, consistent with this finding. Stage 3 PTTD is a rigid flatfoot deformity, while stage 4 includes involvement of the tibiotalar joint as well as the foot. Initial conservative treatment for stage 2 PTTD can be with the use of an Arizona brace. A night splint would be more appropriate for the treatment of plantar fasciitis, and an ankle compression sleeve might be for lower extremity edema.

The patient returns to clinic after 6 months of conservative treatment, and continues to report pain in the medial hindfoot. She would like to discuss surgical treatment options.

The recommended surgical treatment would include:

A. Posterior tibial tendon debridement
B. Posterior tibial tendon debridement, flexor digitorum longus tendon transfer
C. Posterior tibial tendon debridement, flexor digitorum longus tendon transfer, and lateralizing calcaneal osteotomy
D. Posterior tibial tendon debridement, flexor digitorum longus tendon transfer, medializing calcaneal osteotomy, and first ray plantar flexion osteotomy
E. Triple arthrodesis

Discussion

The correct answer is (D). The surgical treatment for stage 2 PTTD should include both soft tissue reconstruction and joint-preserving bone realignment with osteotomies. Posterior tibial tendon debridement alone does not correct deformity, and transfer of the FDL tendon to the navicular without addressing malalignment predisposes to failure of the reconstruction. Based upon the degree of correction required, calcaneal osteotomies may include a medial slide osteotomy, lateral column lengthening osteotomy, or both. Residual forefoot supination should be addressed with a plantar flexion osteotomy of the first ray, traditionally with an opening wedge osteotomy of the medial cuneiform (Cotton osteotomy). Triple arthrodesis would be performed for rigid PTTD (stage 3). In all cases of PTTD, the Achilles and gastrocnemius should be examined for a contracture using the Silfverskiold test. This would additionally be addressed at the time of surgery with a tendo-Achilles lengthening or Strayer/gastrocnemius lengthening in the same surgical setting.

Objectives: Did you learn...?

- Describe the anatomy of the medial ankle/hindfoot?
- Identify the function and mechanics of the posterior tibial tendon?
- Assess nonsurgical and surgical treatment of PTTD?

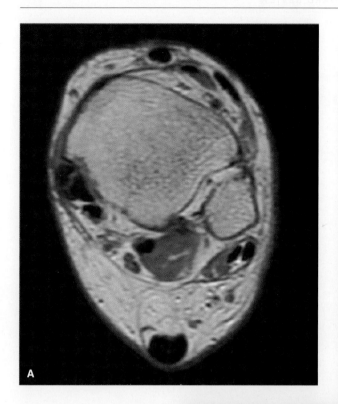
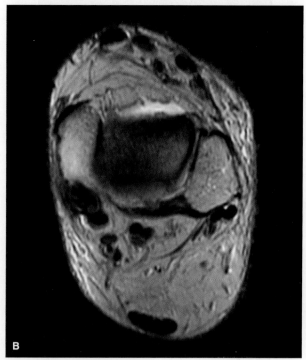
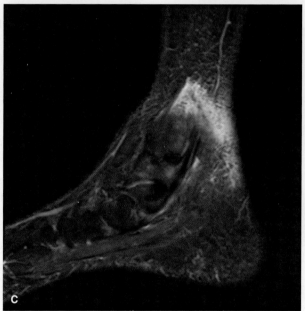

Figure 5–29 **A–C:** MRI images of the ankle.

CASE 16

Dr. Christopher P. Chiodo

A 47-year old woman presents with 2 years of atraumatic hindfoot pain. She has noticed the gradual onset of pain that is worse in the morning and when first standing after sitting for long periods. Her review of systems is remarkable for episodic hip pain and diffuse morning stiffness. On examination, she is tender just anterior to the ankle joint, which has full motion. There is no heel tenderness. Radiographs of the foot were obtained (Fig. 5–30A and B).

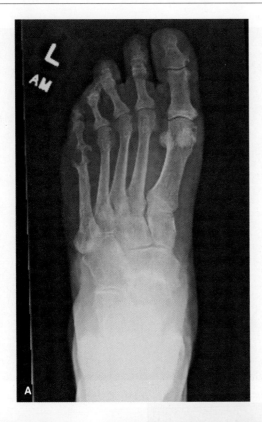

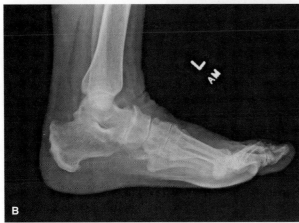

Figure 5–30 **A, B:** AP and lateral radiographs of the foot.

What is the most likely diagnosis?

A. Plantar fasciitis
B. Posterior tibial tendon dysfunction
C. Talonavicular osteoarthritis
D. Talonavicular rheumatoid arthritis

Discussion

The correct answer is (D). It is not uncommon for RA to occur in the joints of the hindfoot and, in some patients, this is the initial presentation of the disease. The radio-

graphs show isolated narrowing of the talonavicular joint. The lack of previous injury, combined with history of morning stiffness and other associated joint pain, support an inflammatory process as the diagnosis. Posterior tibial tendon dysfunction would not necessarily be associated with joint space narrowing. While "start-up" pain is characteristic of plantar fasciitis, the heel is not tender and symptoms have been present for 2 years.

Your patient returns 1 year later having been treated with medical management provided by a rheumatologist, who confirmed the diagnosis or RA. Further, there has been no relief with custom orthotics and a radiology-guided corticosteroid injection. Unfortunately, there is daily pain that significantly interferes with activities of daily living.

The most appropriate procedure would be:

A. Joint synovectomy and debridement
B. Isolated talonavicular arthrodesis
C. Triple arthrodesis
D. Interpositional arthroplasty

Discussion

The correct answer is (B). The diagnosis has been confirmed, nonoperative measures have been tried, and the patient remains substantially symptomatic. As such, surgery is reasonable. Isolated talonavicular fusion is the most appropriate option. The joint damage is too advanced for joint debridement. The other hindfoot joints are not significantly involved and therefore triple arthrodesis is not necessary. In the foot, interpositional arthroplasty is sometimes considered for the first metatarsal–phalangeal joint, but not for the talonavicular joint.

The patient has a nephew who is entering his first year of orthopaedic residency. She is concerned about loss of motion with isolated hindfoot fusion and decides to call him to inquire about this.

Loss of motion in which joint has the greatest effect on overall hindfoot motion?

A. Talonavicular
B. Calcaneocuboid
C. Talocalcaneal (subtalar)
D. Navicular–cuneiform

Discussion

The correct answer is (A). The three joints of the hindfoot are the talonavicular, talocalcaneal (subtalar), and calcaneocuboid. Together, these joints allow inversion and eversion of the foot, which in turn allows the foot to adapt to uneven ground. Another important concept to consider is that when the hindfoot is in valgus, as with heel strike, it is flexible and can better absorb ground reaction forces. When it is in neutral or varus, as with push off, it is more rigid and is a more effective lever.

A biomechanical study has demonstrated that eliminating motion at the talonavicular joint essentially eliminated motion at the other joints and that the talonavicular joint was the "key joint" of the triple joint complex.

Objectives: Did you learn...?

- Discuss that it is not uncommon for inflammatory arthritis to affect the hindfoot?
- Describe the anatomy of the hindfoot as well as the associated biomechanics?
- Describe the initial treatment of hindfoot inflammatory disease?
- Assess the appropriate surgical treatment for recalcitrant disease?

CASE 17

Dr. Richard J. De Asla

A 60-year-old female presents with a chief complaint of an intermittently painful mass on the medial border of the plantar medial arch in the left foot. It has been present for approximately 5 years but has not grown in size over the past 2 years. When pain occurs, it is only in shoes with an arch support. She is pain-free walking barefoot. Physical examination reveals a subcutaneous firm nodule along the medial cord of the plantar fascia. There are no overlying skin lesions. Tinel's sign is negative. Plain x-rays (Figs. 5–31 and 5–32) and an MRI of the foot were obtained. Figures 5–33 and 5–34 are pregadolinium and Figure 5–35 is postgadolinium.

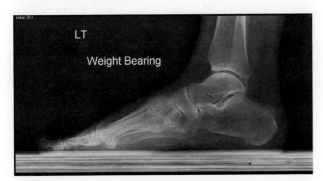

Figure 5–31 Lateral radiograph of the foot.

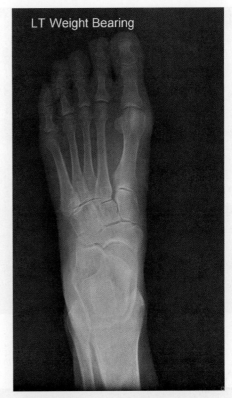

Figure 5–32 AP radiograph of the foot.

The most appropriate treatment is:

A. Referral to an orthopaedic oncologist for definitive management
B. An excisional biopsy of the lesion

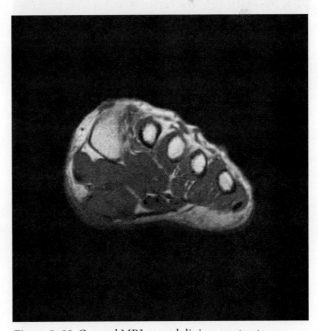

Figure 5–33 Coronal MRI pregadolinium contrast.

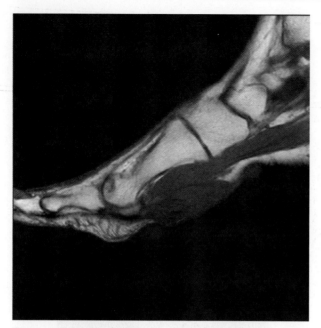

Figure 5–34 Sagittal MRI pregadolinium contrast.

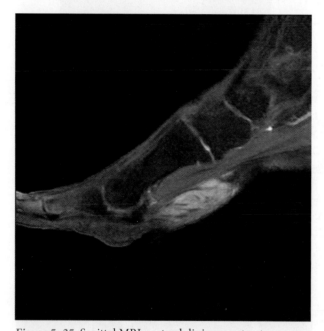

Figure 5–35 Sagittal MRI postgadolinium contrast.

C. To obtain a plain chest x-ray and plan for a wide margin resection of the lesion

D. To obtain a needle biopsy of the lesion and await pathology findings for definitive management

E. To consider a custom-molded orthotic to accommodate the lesion and provide reassurance

Discussion

The correct answer is (E). The patient has a plantar fibroma. Fibromas are typically solitary tumors located along the medial cord of the plantar fascia that contain dense, mature fibrocytes. In older patients, plantar fibromas may be associated with Dupuytren's or Peyronie's disease. Most often they are painless and require no treatment at all. When pain does occur, it is usually the result of the incongruous border rubbing against the insole of a shoe. Surgical excision is ill-advised in the vast majority of cases. Post surgery recurrence is very high because extensions of the lesion infiltrate the dermis and fascia making obtaining clean margins exceedingly difficult. Malignant degeneration of these lesions is essentially unheard of. An MRI can be obtained if the diagnosis is uncertain. Gadolinium will increase the specificity of the examination. A T1 image demonstrates low signal comparable to muscle. The lesion will demonstrate variable enhancement with gadolinium. Soft tissue sarcomas of the foot and ankle do exist but are quite rare. The most common soft tissue sarcoma in the foot is a synovial cell sarcoma. These malignant tumors generally occur in patients younger than 30 years of age. There is a propensity for these tumors to metastasize to the lungs and wide margin surgical excision is required for treatment.

Objectives: Did you learn...?

• Identify typical clinical presentation for a plantar fibroma?

• Treat a plantar fibroma?

CASE 18

Dr. Thomas Dowd

You are asked to evaluate a 40-year-old man with medial forefoot pain. The patient's primary care provider (PCP) tells you the patient has had the insidious onset of a chronic ache that is worsened with barefoot walking, particularly when pushing off, and made better by stiff shoe wear. No imaging studies are available, but the PCP would like to know what to do before sending the patient to your clinic.

You ask the primary care provider to:

A. Obtain an MRI of the foot

B. Obtain a bone scan

C. Obtain weight-bearing x-rays of the foot

D. Provide a Morton's extension (rigid orthosis to protect the first metatarsophalangeal joint [MTPJ])

Discussion

The correct answer is (C). Weight-bearing views of the foot are requisite for the initial evaluation of medial forefoot pain. Additional views may include contralateral comparison radiographs, an axial sesamoid view, and lateral/medial oblique radiographs. MRI can be a very specific study in differentiating the various structures about the first MTPJ but is not an effective screening tool. Bone scan is a useful study but is not specific and is not the first-line of study for these patients. With a bone scan, uptake should be compared with the contralateral side given the occasional increased uptake in asymptomatic patients. A Morton's extension may eventually be employed, especially if hallux rigidus is identified, but a diagnosis should be established first.

Weight-bearing foot radiographs are obtained (Fig. 5–36). You do not notice a bipartite sesamoid.

Regarding the findings of bipartite sesamoid(s), which is least accurate?

A. The medial sesamoid is bipartite in 50% of the population
B. The lateral sesamoid is rarely bipartite

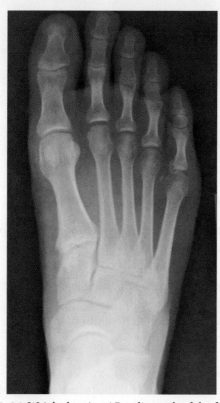

Figure 5–36 Weight-bearing AP radiograph of the foot.

C. The medial sesamoid is bipartite in 10% of the population
D. In patients with a bipartite sesamoid, the finding is bilateral in 25% of the population

Discussion

The correct answer is (A). The prevalence of a bipartite medial sesamoid is 10%, not 50%. A bipartite lateral sesamoid is rarely encountered and is less frequently noted than a bipartite medial sesamoid. One-quarter of patients found to have a bipartite sesamoid have a similar finding on the contralateral foot.

You evaluate the patient and note maximal tenderness at the lateral sesamoid with reproduction of plantar pain with passive dorsiflexion and resisted plantar flexion at the first MTPJ. Passive and active motion at the interphalangeal joint is not painful, and the medial eminence is not tender. There is no dorsal tenderness. Your initial treatment involves activity modification and orthotic wear with a recess under the first MTPJ. During this lengthy nonoperative course, an MRI is obtained (Fig. 5–37).

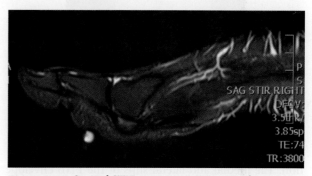

Figure 5–37 Sagittal STIR sequence MRI image demonstrating the lateral sesamoid.

Having failed nonoperative treatment, the patient requests surgical intervention. What is the most appropriate surgical intervention?

A. Microfracture of the lateral sesamoid
B. Excision of medial and lateral sesamoids
C. Plantar flexion osteotomy of the first metatarsal
D. Excision of the lateral sesamoid with flexor hallucis brevis (FHB) repair

Discussion

The correct answer is (D), excision of the lateral sesamoid with FHB repair (Fig. 5–38). The physical examination and MRI findings suggest lateral sesamoiditis. The sesamoids act as pulleys for the FHB, thus placing the FHB on stretch or resisting its active function can reproduce

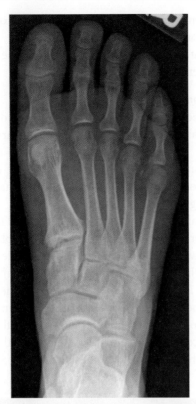

Figure 5–38 AP radiograph demonstrating excision of the lateral sesamoid.

the patient's pain. The increased signal on MRI provides objective evidence to support the diagnosis.

The mainstay of surgical intervention for lateral sesamoiditis is excision. A plantar approach is employed. Care is taken to protect the flexor hallucis brevis tendon. The medial and lateral slips of the FHB envelope the plantar aspect of their respective sesamoids. After the lateral sesamoid is excised from the flexor hallucis brevis and surrounding plantar plate complex, it is of utmost importance to perform a meticulous soft tissue repair. If not performed, iatrogenic hallux varus may result. Alternatively, failure to perform this repair during a medial sesamoidectomy may result in the development of hallux valgus. Excision of both sesamoids may result in claw toe deformity, and is therefore not recommended. A plantar flexion osteotomy of the first ray would likely exacerbate the problem and load the sesamoids further. Those patients with a plantar-flexed first ray may benefit from a dorsiflexion osteotomy.

Objectives: Did you learn...?

- Describe the prevalence of bipartite sesamoids?
- Describe considerations for imaging studies used to assess the sesamoids?

- Identify the anatomic location of the medial and lateral sesamoids within the medial and lateral slips of the flexor hallucis brevis?
- Assess the considerations for surgical treatment of sesamoiditis?

CASE 19

Dr. Jeffrey R. Jockel

A 65-year-old female with a history of osteopenia presents complaining of hindfoot pain for the past 2 years. She denies any traumatic inciting event, but notices the pain primarily while ambulating. She has had to wear orthotics for many years but recently developed new ankle pain during the past 6 months. She reports particular difficulty when on uneven surfaces and that her ankle brace and orthotics do not seem to be working. Radiographs are obtained (Figs. 5–39 and 5–40).

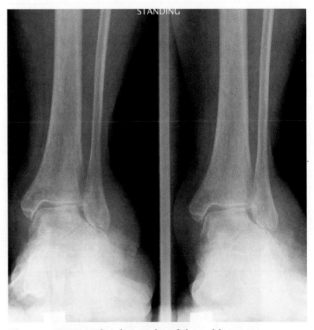

Figure 5–39 Initial radiographs of the ankle.

The most likely underlying etiology of the patient's deformity is:

A. Talonavicular arthritis
B. Posterior tibial tendon deficiency
C. Charcot arthropathy
D. Spastic peroneal flatfoot disorder
E. Subtalar arthritis

Discussion

The correct answer is (B). The patient has stage 4 PTTD, which is characterized by tibiotalar joint involvement

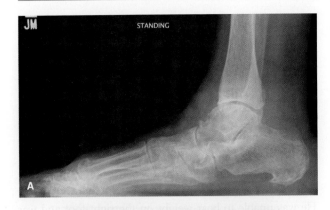

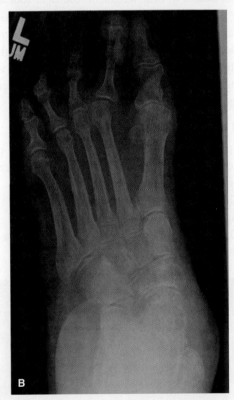

Figure 5–40 **A, B:** Initial radiographs of the foot.

in addition to an adult-acquired planovalgus hindfoot deformity. The patient does have a dorsal talonavicular joint osteophyte indicating that there is some talonavicular arthritis, although this does not underlie the patient's deformity. Spastic peroneal flatfoot disorder is primarily seen in children. Charcot arthropathy often present with deformity and reactive bone changes, which are not present.

Physical examination of the patient reveals a prominent callus underlying the talar head, with swelling and tenderness to palpation along the course of the posterior

tibial tendon, as well as tibiotalar joint line. Hindfoot motion is rigid, while ankle motion is full with correctable alignment.

In addition to the patient's foot deformity, the ligamentous deficiency most responsible for her ankle pain is:

A. The anterior talofibular ligament
B. The calcaneofibular ligament
C. The anterior-inferior tibiofibular ligament
D. The deltoid ligament
E. The transverse tibiofibular ligament

Discussion

The correct answer is (D). Longstanding planovalgus deformity due to PTTD may progress to medial ligamentous involvement of the ankle. The specific anatomy of the deltoid ligament is complex and controversial. The ligament is composed of a superficial and deep component. The superficial ligament attaches to the anterior colliculus, while the deep portion attaches to the posterior colliculus and intercollicular groove. The anterior talofibular ligament (ATFL) and calcaneofibular ligament (CFL) are components of the lateral ligamentous complex, while the anterior-inferior tibiofibular ligament and transverse tibiofibular ligaments are components of the syndesmosis complex.

The patient elects to proceed with conservative management for her foot and ankle pain utilizing a customized ankle-foot orthosis. She returns to the office 10 months later reporting new lateral ankle pain and swelling which began approximately 8 weeks ago. New radiographs are obtained (Fig. 5–41). Her ankle motion remains full with a completely flexible deformity through the ankle. Hindfoot motion remains rigid. The patient would like to consider surgical intervention at this time.

Recommended surgery would include which of the following?

A. Ankle arthrodesis with distal fibulectomy
B. Triple arthrodesis
C. Triple arthrodesis with deltoid ligament reconstruction
D. Posterior tibial tendon debridement, flexor digitorum longus transfer, calcaneal osteotomy
E. Open reduction internal fixation of the fibula
F. Medial closing wedge osteotomy of the distal tibia

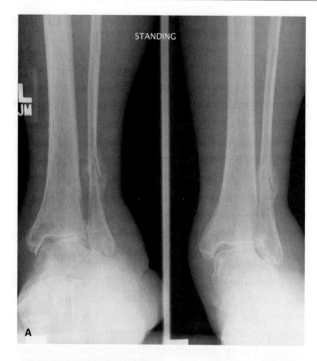

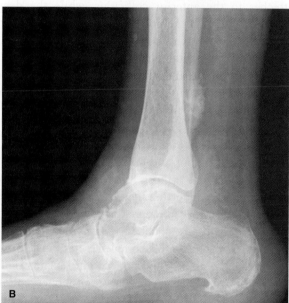

Figure 5–41 **A, B:** Follow-up radiographs of the ankle.

Discussion

The correct answer is (C). As the patient has a rigid planovalgus foot deformity, triple arthrodesis would be required to correct this deformity. The valgus ankle malalignment, which contributed to the fibular stress fracture seen in Figure 5–41A and B, should also be addressed with deltoid reconstruction. Both ankle arthrodesis and tibial osteotomies would not address the underlying foot deformity.

Objectives: Did you learn...?

- Describe the stages of PTTD?
- Describe the anatomy and pathophysiology of the deltoid ligament failure?
- Treat PTTD?

CASE 20

Dr. John Paul Elton

A 26-year-old man sustained an injury to his right ankle when he was caught in an avalanche while snowboarding. He was unable to bear weight on the right foot and was taken to the emergency department for evaluation. His right ankle is noted to have mild to moderate edema with soft foot compartments, intact pulses, and intact light touch sensation. There are no fracture blisters or open wounds. Radiographs and CT of the right ankle are obtained in the emergency room (Figs. 5–42 and 5–43A and B).

What is the best course of treatment?

A. Splinting the ankle in neutral position to prevent equinus contracture and plan for nonsurgical management
B. Urgent external fixation placement
C. Application of short-leg cast
D. Open treatment of the talus fracture in a timely manner

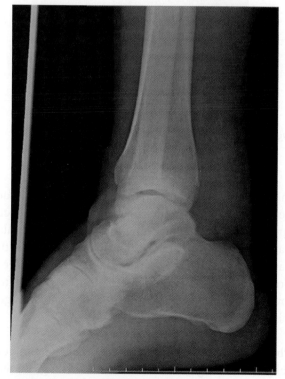

Figure 5–42 Lateral radiograph of the ankle.

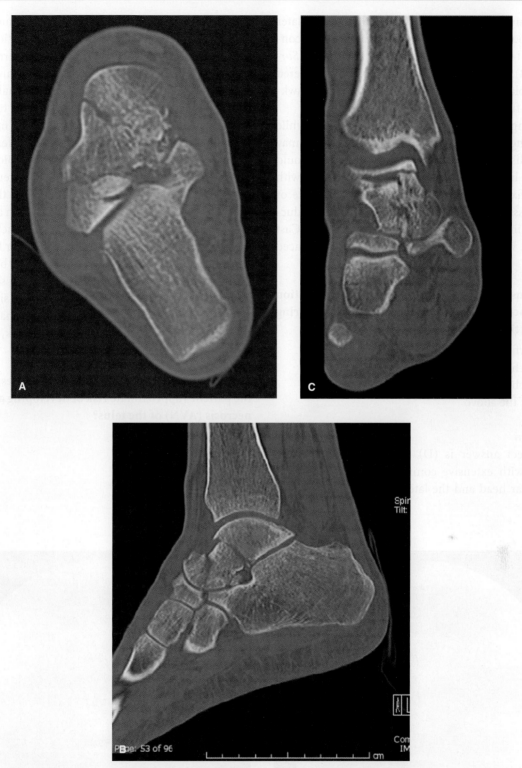

Figure 5–43 **A:** Axial CT. **B:** Sagittal CT. **C:** Coronal CT.

Discussion

The correct answer is (D). The imaging studies show a comminuted and displaced talar neck fracture. Hawkins described a classification system for talar neck fractures. Type I fractures are nondisplaced, type II fractures are displaced with subluxation or dislocation of the subtalar joint, and type III fractures are displaced with subluxation or dislocation of both the subtalar and tibiotalar joints. Canale and Kelly later added a fourth type that is a type III fracture with concomitant talonavicular dislocation (*J Bone Joint Surgery*, 1978). Operative treatment should be considered in all displaced talar neck fractures, including Hawkins type I fractures.

Splinting the ankle in neutral dorsiflexion, while minimizing the chance of equinus contracture, may further displace the fracture. This fracture would likely not have significantly improved alignment with external fixation placement, and the current state of his soft tissue envelope does not preclude open reduction with internal fixation at the index procedure. Cast treatment would not be appropriate for this displaced fracture.

When considering the surgical approach for fixation of this fracture, what structures may be at risk during the dissection?

A. Superficial peroneal nerve
B. Branches of the dorsalis pedis artery
C. Branches of the posterior tibialis artery
D. All of the above

Discussion

The correct answer is (D). A displaced talar neck fracture with extensive comminution and extension to the talar head and the lateral process/body is best approached through a dual incision technique. The dual incision approach allows for mobilization of the fracture and verification of an adequate reduction. Often, the medial talus has extensive comminution. A dual incision technique allows for internal fixation along the medial and lateral aspects of the talus (Fig. 5–44), which often helps to prevent varus malunion. Medial dissection, particularly along the inferior talar neck should be done very carefully to avoid further injury to the deltoid branches and the artery of the tarsal canal, which supply the majority of the blood supply to the talar body. Extensive dissection along the dorsal talar neck may disrupt vascular branches from the dorsalis pedis artery that supply the talar head and neck. The superficial peroneal nerve may be at risk during the lateral approach to the talus and should be identified and protected. The artery of the sinus tarsi from the peroneal artery, which forms an anastomotic sling on the inferior surface of the talar neck, is also at risk with the lateral approach.

Based on the preoperative imaging studies, what is the patient's approximate risk of developing avascular necrosis (AVN) of the talus?

A. Less than 15%
B. 15% to 50%
C. 50% to 75%
D. Greater than 75%

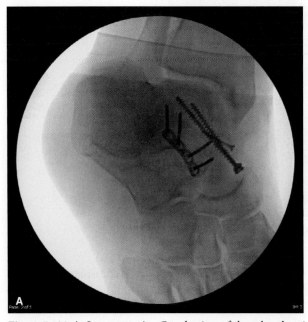 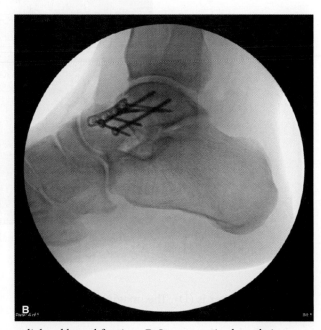

Figure 5–44 **A:** Intraoperative Canale view of the talus showing medial and lateral fixation. **B:** Intraoperative lateral view.

Discussion

The correct answer is (B). The Hawkins classification system is predictive of the risk of development of avascular necrosis of the talus. Based on the imaging studies, this fracture is classified as a Hawkins II fracture because of the mild subluxation of the subtalar joint seen best on the sagittal CT image. In Hawkins' study on talar neck fractures, a 42% rate of AVN was seen in type II fractures. Subsequent studies, including Vallier et al. (*J Bone Joint Surg*, 2004) found that Hawkins type II fractures had an AVN rate of 39%.

Objectives: Did you learn...?

- Describe the Hawkins classification for talar neck fractures?
- Describe the importance of using a dual incision technique to obtain an anatomic reduction and avoid varus malunion?
- Identify relevant vascular supply of the talus?

CASE 21

Dr. Tom Douglas

A 29-year-old male presents with the chief complaint of weakness in his right leg. He reports that 6 months ago he was playing basketball and when jumping felt that he was kicked in the back of the leg. He never sought medical care, and since that point he has been unable to recover strength in his leg. He takes no steroids, never had an injection into his Achilles, was not on antibiotics, and there was no family history of inflammatory arthropathy.

On physical examination, he is a fit male in no distress. He is unable to perform a single leg heel rise on the right and there is marked atrophy of his gastrocnemius on this side. In the prone position with his knees flexed there is no plantar flexion with calf squeeze, and the resting position of his right foot is in 5 degrees of plantar flexion compared with 25 degrees of plantar flexion of his left foot.

His radiographs are unremarkable. An MRI is reviewed (Fig. 5–45), which shows a gap of 4 cm between the proximal and distal ends of the Achilles tendon. Treatment options were discussed with him and you recommend surgery.

Which of the following is unlikely to be utilized in the upcoming surgery?

A. Gore tex graft
B. Flexor hallucis longus (FHL) tendon transfer
C. V to Y advancement of the Achilles
D. Gastrocnemius turndown flap

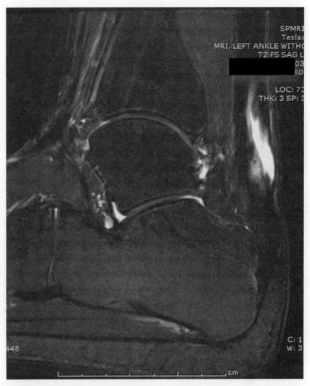

Figure 5–45 Sagittal T2 MRI of Achilles tendon demonstrating rupture with a gap of 4 cm.

Discussion

The correct answer is (A). Synthetic graft has not been proven to be successful nor should it be utilized as a first-line of treatment for chronic Achilles tendon ruptures. There is some degree of evidence to support the use of allograft in a patient who has undergone multiple revisions or has a very large gap between the proximal and distal segments (>6 cm). The flexor hallucis longus can be easily harvested through the same incision and placed into the calcaneus. Another option is to harvest the FHL more distally and double it on itself to provide more collagen to the repair. Utilizing a Strayer, V to Y advancement, or gastrocnemius turndown can also address a gap in the Achilles. Usually a gap of up to 6 cm can be addressed with some form of a lengthening procedure of the Achilles. Beyond this distance, utilization of allograft may be considered.

The patient undergoes an FHL transfer in addition to a V to Y advancement secondary to a residual gap following mobilization of the proximal tendon (Fig. 5–46). The FHL tendon was harvested through the posterior approach, placed into the calcaneus, and secured with an interference screw. You considered the need for increased length of the FHL tendon and thought of harvesting the tendon at the hallux interphalangeal (IP) joint of the great toe.

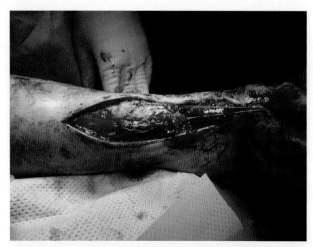

Figure 5–46 Clinical photograph demonstrating residual gap present after initial mobilization of the proximal gastrocsoleus complex.

When the FHL is harvested at the IP joint, one must perform a release of the FHL tendon where?

A. Release of the FHL from adhesions of the plantar fascia

B. Nothing more needs to be released

C. The FHL must be freed from the fibroosseus tunnel below the sustentaculum

D. Release at the master knot of Henry

Discussion

The correct answer is (D). The FHL and FDL are connected at the knot of Henry. This is located dorsal and lateral to the abductor hallucis musculature. Significant adhesions at the sustentaculum are rarely encountered. There is no connection between the FHL and the plantar fascia.

The patient asks when he will be able to return to playing basketball. You inform him that it will likely be no earlier than:

A. 4 weeks

B. 8 weeks

C. 12 weeks

D. 6 months

Discussion

The correct answer is (D). Even among the most aggressive rehabilitation protocols for a primary repair of an Achilles tendon, it would be extremely aggressive to return a player to basketball in less than 3 months. Willits et al. demonstrated good success with an early rehabilitation program,

however even in this protocol the patient was weaning from the boot in the 8- to 12-week period. A few studies have demonstrated return to jogging at 3 months, but the earliest successful return to sports reported has been 4 months. Many studies have demonstrated a return to sports between 6 to 12 months postoperatively.

Objectives: Did you learn…?

• Identify physical examination findings of a chronic Achilles rupture?

• Describe various treatment options of chronic Achilles tendon ruptures?

• Describe the anatomy flexor hallucis longus in relation to the master knot of Henry?

CASE 22

Dr. Daniel Guss

A 22-year-old female presents complaining of pain along the lateral border of her left foot. She has a known history of Charcot–Marie–Tooth disease (CMT) and a clinically evident pes cavus. Radiographs are obtained (Figs. 5–47 and 5–48).

Physical examination is notable for hindfoot varus. Which of the following muscle imbalances contribute to this alignment?

A. Strong anterior tibialis and weak posterior tibialis

B. Strong peroneus longus and weak anterior tibialis

C. Strong anterior tibialis and weak peroneus brevis

D. Strong peroneus brevis and weak peroneus longus

Discussion

The correct answer is (B). For reasons that are not entirely understood, muscles of the anterior compartment of the

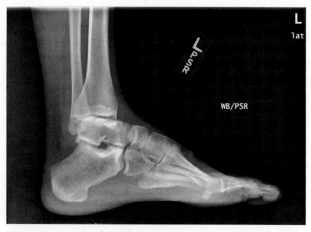

Figure 5–47 Lateral weight-bearing radiograph of the foot.

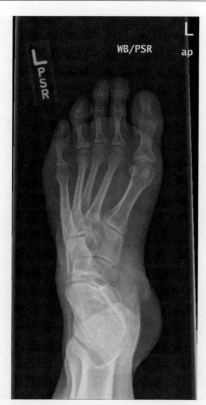

Figure 5–48 AP weight-bearing radiograph of the foot.

leg are selectively predisposed to weakness in CMT. The lateral compartment is also predisposed to weakness, but this specifically affects the peroneus brevis while sparing the peroneus longus. Thus, the anterior tibialis and peroneus brevis are weak while the posterior tibialis and peroneus longus remain strong, causing a force imbalance. This imbalance precipitates hindfoot varus through two mechanisms. First, the intact peroneus longus plantarflexes the first ray without the opposing dorsiflexion force normally provided by the anterior tibialis. The plantar-flexed first ray in turn drives hindfoot varus. Second, the intact posterior tibialis exerts an inversion force on the subtalar joint without the counterbalancing eversion force normally provided by the peroneus brevis. These two phenomena combine to create subtalar inversion and clinically apparent hindfoot varus.

Why is a dorsiflexion osteotomy of the first ray unlikely to correct hindfoot varus in the setting of significant subtalar arthritis?

A. The peroneus brevis remains weak
B. One must first correct the drop-foot caused by a weakened tibialis anterior

C. The strong peroneus longus will still provide an inversion force
D. None of the above

Discussion
The correct answer is (D). Before any deformity-correcting surgery for pes cavus, one must first assess whether the hindfoot position is flexible or rigid. A hindfoot varus is deemed flexible when hindfoot alignment can be moved into more neutral position, either with passive testing of subtalar range of motion or with Coleman block testing. Flexible deformities progressively become rigid over time through degenerative changes in the affected joints. Once the subtalar joint is arthritic, the hindfoot varus can no longer be corrected through subtalar range of motion. In such cases, a corrective arthrodesis of the subtalar joint is necessary to correct hindfoot alignment.

Why do patients with CMT often develop claw toes?

A. Intrinsic muscle weakness
B. Extensor digitorum longus weakness (EDL)
C. Flexor digitorum longus weakness (FDL)
D. All of the above

Discussion
The correct answer is (A). CMT is characterized by wasting of the intrinsic musculature of the foot. Similar to the intrinsics of the hand, the intrinsics of the foot plantar flex the metatarsophalangeal (MTP) joints and extend the interphalangeal (IP) joints. Weakness allows overpull by the intact extrinsic muscles, including the EDL and FDL. This causes claw toes, which are characterized by hyperextension at the MTP joints and flexion at the IP joints.

Which of the following soft tissue procedures frequently accompany bony procedures in reconstruction of foot deformities caused by CMT?

A. Release of the plantar fascia
B. Transfer of the peroneus longus (PL) to the peroneus brevis (PB)
C. Transfer of the extensor hallucis longus (EHL) to the neck of the first metatarsal
D. All of the above

Discussion
The correct answer is (D). Soft tissue procedures may prevent deformity if performed early enough in the course of CMT. In pes cavus, the raised arch tightens

the windlass mechanism provided by the plantar fascia, potentially necessitating a plantar fascia release. By transferring the strong PL to the weak PB, one converts the PL's function from one of first ray plantar flexion (which exacerbates the cavus and hindfoot varus) to one of hindfoot eversion (which helps correct the hindfoot varus). The EHL is often intact in CMT, and patients frequently use it to compensate for a weak anterior tibialis. Unfortunately, this can also lead to a claw toe deformity in the large toe. By transferring the EHL to the neck of the first metatarsal, one allows it to dorsiflex the foot without precipitating a claw deformity. When this EHL transfer is accompanied by a fusion of the first toe interphalangeal joint, this procedure is titled a "Jones procedure."

Objectives: Did you learn...?

- Describe muscle imbalance characteristics of CMT?
- Identify the role of flexible versus rigid deformities in operative planning?
- Describe interplay between intrinsic and extrinsic foot musculature that contributes to CMT deformities?
- Assess the role of tendon transfers in CMT?

CASE 23

Dr. Tom Douglas

A 29-year-old woman presents to you with pain on the medial aspect of the ankle and numbness and tingling on the plantar aspect of the foot. She reports no trauma and describes an insidious onset of symptoms over the past month. On physical examination she has neutral hindfoot alignment and no palpable masses. She has a positive Tinnel's sign just posterior to her medial malleolus which worsens the paresthesias on her plantar foot. Plain radiographs of the ankle demonstrate no masses, no fractures, and no significant arthritis.

You are concerned that the patient has tarsal tunnel syndrome, your next step is:

A.   Corticosteroid injection into the tarsal tunnel
B.   Tibial nerve decompression
C.   Lateral posting orthotics
D.   MRI

Discussion

The correct answer is (D). A subset of patients with tarsal tunnel syndrome will have a space occupying mass located in or adjacent to the tarsal tunnel causing tibial nerve compression. This space-occupying lesion may be tenosynovitis, a ganglion cyst, varicosities, lipoma, or tumor.

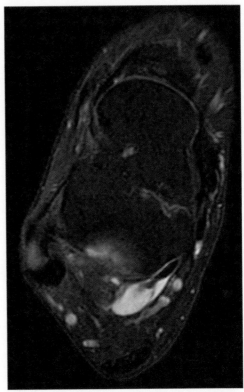

Figure 5–49 Axial MRI demonstrating tenosynovitis along the course of the flexor digitorum longus and flexor hallucis longus.

Although at some point a single corticosteroid injection may be considered, there is concern about injecting steroid into weight-bearing tendons of the foot. A lateral posting orthotic would likely increase tension on the medial structures and provide no benefit to a patient with a neutral hindfoot alignment. An MRI is performed (Fig. 5–49).

Based on the imaging you now recommend which of the following?

A.   Soft tissue rest and anti-inflammatory medications
B.   Tarsal tunnel release
C.   Tenosynovectomy
D.   Flatfoot reconstruction

Discussion

The correct answer is (A). The MRI demonstrates tenosynovitis of the flexor hallucis longus. The initial treatment of this will include soft tissue rest, anti-inflammatories, and activity modifications. For the majority of patients, tarsal tunnel syndrome resolves with nonoperative treatment. A period of nonoperative management should be attempted prior to surgical treatment of tarsal tunnel syndrome. A flatfoot reconstruction would

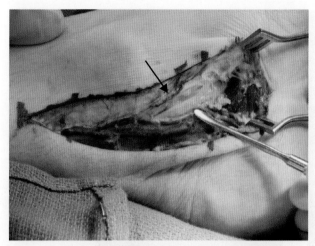

Figure 5–50 Clinical photograph of the completed tarsal tunnel release demonstrating complete release of the fascia overlying the tarsal tunnel.

typically address pathology associated with the posterior tibial tendon.

Following the MRI and approximately 12 weeks of conservative treatment, it is noted that the patient is still having symptoms. A repeat MRI demonstrates resolution of the tenosynovitis along the FHL and FDL. An EMG/nerve conduction study is ordered which demonstrates nerve compression within the tarsal tunnel. At this point you discuss the risks and benefits of a tarsal tunnel release and the patient requests to proceed with the surgery. During the release, a thickened region of fascia is identified before entering the tarsal tunnel. This is labeled with an arrow in Figure 5–50.

What is the name of the tissue marked with the black arrow?

A. Extensor retinaculum
B. Laciniate ligament
C. Epineurium
D. Retrocalcaneal bursa

Discussion

The correct answer is (B). The laciniate ligament is also known as the flexor retinaculum and is a thickening of the fascia overlying the posterior medial ankle. Additional structures located in this region are anteriorly the posterior tibial tendon and flexor digitorum longus. Posterior and lateral to the neurovascular bundle is the flexor hallucis longus. The extensor retinaculum lies on the anterior aspect of the ankle joint. The epineurium directly overlies nerves. The retrocalcaneal bursa is located behind the calcaneus and anterior to the Achilles.

While exploring the tibial nerve, a branch of the posterior tibial nerve that passes deep to the abductor hallucis is noted. This nerve is released and the fascia of the abductor hallucis is incised and the muscle belly of the abductor hallucis mobilized.

Which nerve was just released?

A. Medial plantar nerve
B. Calcaneal branch of the tibial nerve
C. First branch of the lateral plantar nerve
D. Second branch of the lateral plantar nerve

Discussion

The correct answer is (C). This nerve, also known as Baxter's nerve, can be a source of medial heel pain. The course of the nerve is from the tibial nerve distally where it crosses deep to the abductor hallucis muscle belly, a common location of compression. Following this, it courses between the flexor digitorum brevis and quadratus plantae before innervating the abductor digiti quinti. The medial plantar nerve runs toward the knot of Henry and innervates the medial three toes. The calcaneal branch of the tibial nerve comes directly off the tibial nerve and is directed posteriorly to the calcaneus.

Objectives: Did you learn...?

• Initially treat tarsal tunnel syndrome?
• Describe the role of an MRI in the diagnosis of a mass causing tarsal tunnel syndrome?
• Anatomy of the posteromedial ankle?

CASE 24

Adrienne Bonvini; Dr. Christopher P. Chiodo

A 50-year-old male presents with 6 months of atraumatic forefoot pain. He has noticed the gradual onset of pain that is worse with running and prolonged weight bearing. There has been no trauma, and he has not recently changed his exercise regimen. He denies numbness, tingling, or burning. On physical examination, there is mild hammering of the second toe. He is focally tender at the second metatarsophalangeal joint, which can be translated dorsally (positive "drawer" test). There is no web space tenderness. Weight-bearing radiographs of the foot were obtained (Fig. 5–51).

What is the most likely diagnosis?

A. Morton's neuroma
B. Metatarsal stress fracture

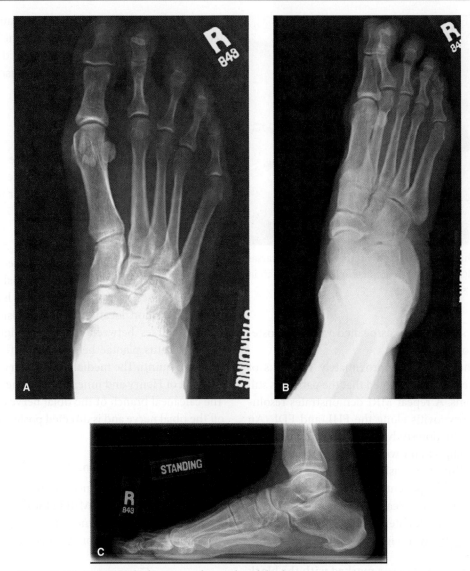

Figure 5-51 **A–C:** Weight-bearing radiographs of the foot.

C. Second metatarsophalangeal synovitis and instability
D. Freiberg's infraction

Discussion

The correct answer is (C). The history, physical examination, and radiographs are most consistent with second metatarsophalangeal synovitis and instability. The second metatarsophalangeal joint can become inflamed, injured, and unstable, which can lead to pain and sometimes deformity. Most often pain in this joint is the result of thinning or a tear of the *plantar plate*, which essentially is a thickening of the plantar joint capsule. Due to the instability, the joint does not track properly and becomes inflamed and painful. This con-

dition is often associated with a long second metatarsal, which is visible on the radiographs. He is nontender in the web space and denies any burning sensation, making Morton's neuroma less likely. While a gradual onset may be seen in metatarsal stress fractures, they typically occur with a change in exercise frequency, duration, or intensity. The second metatarsal head is characteristically the site of Freiberg's infraction, but there is no evidence of an irregular bony surface, sclerosis, or flattening of the metatarsal head.

Initial treatment might include all of the following treatment EXCEPT:

A. Metatarsal pads or a custom orthotic
B. Taping or a "Budin" splint

C. A short walking boot

D. A corticosteroid injection

Discussion

The correct answer is (D). All of the above are appropriate initial treatments except for injection. This is the most invasive choice and is also associated with joint dislocation due to further attenuation and weakening of the plantar plate from the corticosteroid.

Despite these treatments, the patient remains symptomatic 6 months later and reports unchanged pain that interferes with activities of daily living. He requests surgery.

Of the following, which is the most appropriate surgical intervention?

A. Shortening metatarsal osteotomy

B. Extensor tendon transfer

C. Syndactylization of the second and third toes

D. Partial second metatarsal head resection

Discussion

The correct answer is (A). The long second metatarsal is felt to contribute to the attenuation of the plantar plate. As such, most surgeons use a shortening osteotomy, with or without a plantar plate repair, if surgery is indicated.

Objectives: Did you learn...?

- Differentially diagnose second metatarsophalangeal joint pain?
- Identify initial treatment options for second metatarsophalangeal joint synovitis?
- Describe the relationship between a long second metatarsal and second metatarsophalangeal joint synovitis and instability?

CASE 25

Dr. Richard J. De Asla

A healthy 43-year-old female developed insidious onset of plantar right heel pain 2 months ago. She describes an exacerbation of symptoms when initiating weight bearing after getting out of bed in the morning and when transitioning from a seated to standing position during the day. There is no swelling or discoloration around the heel and no complaints of right lower extremity radiculopathy. Pain resolves quickly when the heel is off-loaded. Physical examination demonstrates significant and focal tenderness to directed pressure over the medial tubercle of the calcaneus.

What is the most likely diagnosis?

A. Calcaneal stress fracture

B. Plantar fasciitis

C. Tarsal tunnel syndrome

D. Compression of the first branch of the lateral plantar nerve

E. Symptomatic plantar calcaneal spur

Discussion

The correct answer is (B). The patient presents with a typical history of plantar fasciitis. The onset of pain is often insidious without any prior traumatic or overuse event. Pain is often exacerbated when the heel is loaded after a period of offloading or rest. Pain is most pronounced to direct palpation at the origin of the plantar fascia on the medial tubercle of the calcaneus. Symptoms are relieved quickly when the foot is off-loaded. Calcaneal stress fractures typically present with heel swelling and pain to compression of the calcaneal tuber. Tarsal tunnel syndrome is an uncommon condition caused by compression of the posterior tibial nerve within the tarsal tunnel located immediately posterior to the medial malleolus. Symptoms include radiating pain into the plantar aspect of the foot and, less commonly, up the medial aspect of the leg. Compression of the first branch of the lateral plantar nerve (Baxter's nerve) between the deep fascia of the abductor hallucis muscle and the medial edge of the quadratus plantae muscle can be associated with plantar fasciitis. Pain is aggravated by weight-bearing activity, may radiate to the lateral foot, and often lingers after rest (so-called after burn). Symptoms are reproduced by direct pressure over the nerve deep to the abductor hallucis muscle belly. Approximately 15% of the population has a plantar calcaneal spur with only 5% of this subgroup reporting a history of heel pain. About 50% of patients with plantar fasciitis have a heel spur. Although heel spurs may be present in patients with plantar heel pain, they are not considered the cause.

An appropriate diagnostic workup would include which of the following?

A. HLA-B27 testing

B. MRI

C. Technetium bone scan

D. No further workup is required

Discussion

The correct answer is (D). In the vast majority of cases, obtaining a complete history and performing an appropriate physical examination is all that is necessary in making the diagnosis of plantar fasciitis. MRI or bone scan can be helpful when the history and physical examination are not straightforward and obtaining an accurate diagnosis is challenging. Typical MRI findings in cases of plantar fasciitis include increased T2 signal intensity and thickening at the origin of the plantar fascia. Technetium bone scan demonstrates marked increased uptake at the origin of the plantar fascia. The clinician can consider HLA-B27 testing in patients with protracted symptoms, other joint complaints, and bilateral symptoms as part of a greater rheumatological workup.

Objectives: Did you learn...?

• Identify typical symptoms of plantar fasciitis?
• Describe differential diagnosis of heel pain?
• Perform a workup for plantar fasciitis?

CASE 26

Dr. Tom Douglas

You are called by the emergency department to see a 50-year-old male who reported a wound on his leg yesterday. He initially did not have any problems, however in the past 4 hours he has noted increased erythema, pain requiring IV narcotics, and tachycardia. The emergency department asks what laboratory information may be helpful in determining if this is necrotizing fasciitis or just cellulitis.

Based upon the Laboratory Risk Indicator for Necrotizing Fasciitis (LRINEC) criteria, which of the following is not of value?

A. CRP
B. WBC
C. Sodium
D. ESR

Discussion

The correct answer is (D). Although valuable for nearly every other infectious process in orthopaedics, the erythrocyte sedimentation rate (ESR) is not a component of the LRINEC criteria. The LRINEC criteria have been described as a means of differentiating necrotizing fasciitis from cellulitis. A score is given based upon CRP level (greater or less than 150 mg/L), WBC (less than 15,000, between 15,000 and 25,000, and greater than 25,000), hemoglobin (greater than 13.5, between 11 and 13.5, or less than 11), sodium (greater or less than 135), creatinine (greater or less than 1.6), and glu-

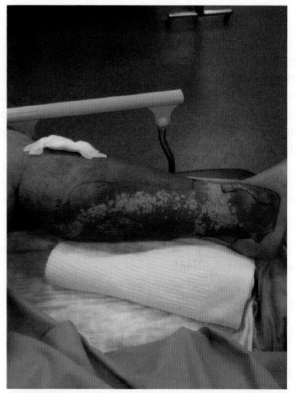

Figure 5–52 Clinical image of the left leg demonstrating bullae with surrounding erythema.

cose (greater or less than 180). With a score less than or equal to 5, there is less than 50% chance of necrotizing fasciitis, however with a score greater than or equal to 8, there is a 75% chance of necrotizing fasciitis.

Upon evaluation of the patient in the emergency department there is a noted waxy appearance of the skin with bullae formation and erythema spreading beyond the borders drawn by the emergency department physician 20 minutes ago (Fig. 5–52). You decide at that point to bring the patient to the operating room for an emergent irrigation and debridement. In the operating room there is murky dishwater fluid at the level of the fascia. You take cultures at this point and perform an irrigation and debridement using your gloved finger to undermine skin in regions which are affected.

Which of the following is the most likely causative organism?

A. *Staphylococcus aureus*
B. *Escherichia coli*
C. *Vibrio vulnificus*
D. Polymicrobial
E. Group A beta hemolytic Streptococcus

Discussion

The correct answer is (D). Necrotizing fasciitis can be classified into three groups based upon causative organism. The most common type is type 1, which is caused by a polymicrobial infection with multiple organisms growing on culture. Type 2 necrotizing fasciitis is caused by Group A beta hemolytic strep-tococci or methicillin-resistant *Staphylococcus aureus*. This is the typical "flesh eating bacterial" presenta-tion. This is more typical in healthy individuals. Type 3 necrotizing fasciitis is caused by marine organisms such as vibrio vulnificus and often occurs in patients with liver disease. This is the least common form of necrotizing fasciitis.

Following surgery, he is admitted to the ICU. Initial Gram stain from intraoperative cultures comes back with gram-positive cocci in clusters. In addition to vancomycin, which other antibiotic should be added to the treatment protocol?

A. Zosyn
B. Penicillin
C. Cefazolin
D. Clindamycin

Discussion

The correct answer is (D). Based upon coverage of varying forms of necrotizing fasciitis, the addition of clindamycin seems to provide the best coverage for all variations of gram-positive Gram stains. Clindamycin inhibits exotoxin production of staph aureus. In addi-tion, it has been shown to blunt the systemic affects of the disease. Finally, it has been demonstrated to clini-cally decrease the in-house mortality of necrotizing fasciitis.

Postoperatively, he is relatively stable in the ICU. Based upon the degree of necrosis present and how sick the patient was at initial surgery, you decide to take him back to the operating room at 24 hours for a repeat irri-gation and debridement. In the operating room again you notice that there is skin which can be undermined with a gloved finger along the posterior medial calf. This skin does not bleed when cut.

Based upon these findings you decide to:

A. Perform an amputation
B. Debride all necrotic skin edges back to viable tissue
C. Utilize this tissue as a biologic dressing
D. Remove all skin from the extremity and place a wound vac

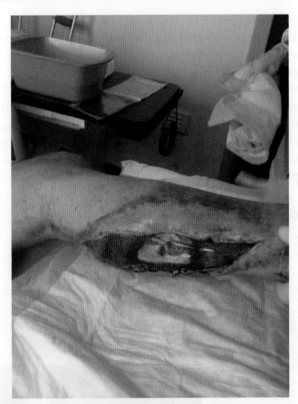

Figure 5–53 Clinical photograph of the limb after multiple irrigations and debridements.

Discussion

The correct answer is (B). Amputation, although fre-quently encountered in patients with necrotizing soft tissue infections, is not indicated at this point as he is clini-cally stable. As in dealing with debridement of all wounds, it is important to remove all nonviable tissue even if it will require skin graft or flap coverage in the future.

Following the second trip to the operating room, the patient remains stable and you have placed a wound vac. At the second wound vac change the wound is healthy appear-ing and surrounding erythema is resolving (Fig. 5–53). In addition to replacing the wound vac and discussing cov-erage options with the plastic surgeon, you also request assistance from the intensivist service to provide adequate nutrition, glucose control, and antibiotic coverage.

The patient asks whether he should have received hyperbaric oxygen instead of surgery. You explain that:

A. There is no role for hyperbaric oxygen in patients with necrotizing soft tissue infections
B. There is a role but it is secondary to surgical debridement and antibiotic therapy
C. Hyperbaric oxygen is an alternative to surgical debridement for early onset necrotizing fasciitis

Discussion

The correct answer is (B). The mainstay of treatment for necrotizing soft tissue infections is aggressive irrigation and debridement, however there are adjunctive therapies including hyperbaric oxygen, IVIG, and recombinant protein C which may be beneficial in patients with necrotizing soft tissue infections. The evidence for utilizing these are limited to retrospective studies at this point, however there have been some promising results.

Objectives: Did you learn...?

- Classify necrotizing fasciitis by organism?
- Describe initial antibiotic regimen for treating necrotizing soft tissue infections?
- Use the LRINEC criteria in differentiating between cellulitis and necrotizing fasciitis?

CASE 27

Dr. Jeffrey R. Jockel

A 52-year-old male presents to your office reporting increased medial and lateral hindfoot pain for the past 8 months. He describes having "problems" with his left foot for many years and previously has worn orthotics and a custom brace to relieve symptoms. Physical examination reveals no ankle tenderness or pain with full ankle range of motion. The patient has tenderness to palpation at the lateral hindfoot and talonavicular region and limited hindfoot motion that is not correctable to a plantigrade position. Radiographs are obtained (Fig. 5–54A–C).

What is the most likely cause of the patient's pain?

A. Sinus tarsi and subfibular impingement
B. Talonavicular arthritis
C. Achilles tendinopathy

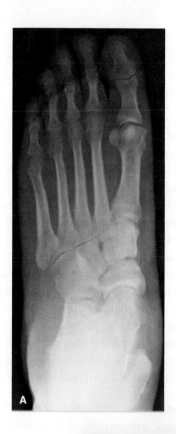
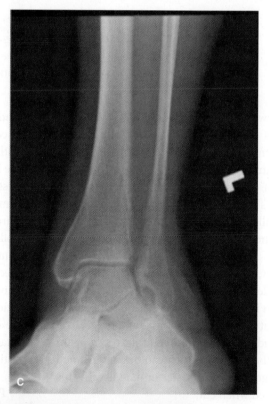
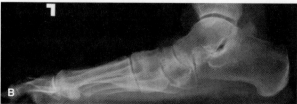

Figure 5–54 **A–C:** Weight-bearing radiographs of the foot and ankle.

D. Extensor digitorum brevis contracture

E. Tarsal tunnel syndrome

Discussion

The correct answer is (A). The patient has stage 3 posterior tibial tendinopathy, which is characterized by a rigid non-correctable deformity during attempted passive hindfoot joint manipulation. This deformity consists of a planovalgus subtalar joint and abduction deformity across Chopart's joints with talonavicular uncoverage. Radiographs show loss of talo-first metatarsal alignment (Meary's angle) on both the lateral and AP images. Hindfoot valgus leads to subfibular impingement as the calcaneus abuts the fibula. Sinus tarsi impingement occurs when the anterior process of the calcaneus abuts the lateral process of the talus due to abduction deformity with talotarsal subluxation. Medial-sided hindfoot pain, when present, is most commonly due to posterior tibial tendinopathy. There are no radiographic signs of talonavicular joint space narrowing or degeneration, which would suggest arthritis.

The patient works as an independent truck driver and is frustrated with persistent pain despite bracing and analgesics. He is currently in the off-season for his job and would like to consider surgical options.

Surgical treatment should consist of:

A. Posterior tibial tendon debridement, flexor hallucis longus tendon transfer, calcaneal osteotomy

B. Posterior tibial tendon debridement, flexor digitorum longus tendon transfer, calcaneal slide osteotomy

C. Posterior tibial tendon debridement, flexor digitorum longus tendon transfer, calcaneal slide osteotomy, and calcaneal lateral column lengthening

D. Posterior tibial tendon debridement, flexor digitorum longus tendon transfer, subtalar arthroereisis

E. Triple arthrodesis

Discussion

The correct answer is (E). Stage 3 posterior tibial tendon dysfunction is a rigid deformity and often will have some degree of arthritic change in the hindfoot joints. Therefore, joint sparing procedures including tendon transfers and osteotomies are not the treatment of choice. Triple arthrodesis of the talonavicular, subtalar, and calcaneocuboid joints (Fig. 5–55A and B) relieves hindfoot pain and allows for deformity correction. Patients with flexible posterior tibial tendon dysfunction (PTTD) should be treated with soft tissue and joint sparing procedures, traditionally including PTT debridement, FDL tendon transfer, and calcaneal osteotomy. All PTTD patients also should be examined for an associated Achilles or gastrocnemius contracture, which should be addressed if needed at the time of surgery.

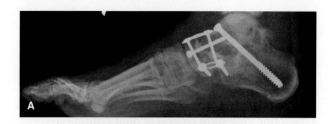

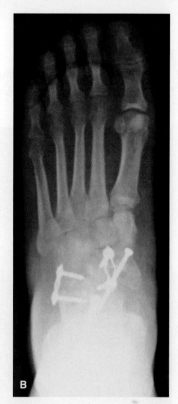

Figure 5–55 **A, B:** Postoperative radiographs following triple arthrodesis.

Prior to surgery, the patient should be counseled about which associated risk in the future following triple arthrodesis?

A. Achilles tendinopathy

B. Ankle arthritis

C. Peroneal tendinopathy

D. Deep peroneal neuralgia

E. Fibular stress fracture

Discussion

The correct answer is (B). Following surgical reconstruction with triple arthrodesis, signs and symptoms of associated joint arthritis may be seen within 5 years. The most common location for arthritis following triple arthrodesis is at the ankle joint. Tarsometatarsal arthritis has not been clinically correlated with hindfoot arthrodesis. Fibular stress fracture may be seen in PTTD, although a planovalgus foot deformity due to subfibular impingement would not be expected following a triple arthrodesis in a plantigrade position.

Objectives: Did you learn…?

• Describe mechanisms for pain with PTTD?
• Treat rigid posterior tibial tendinopathy?
• Describe long-term sequela of joint arthrodesis?

CASE 28

Dr. John Paul Elton

A 20-year-old otherwise healthy woman injured her right foot in a fall while skateboarding 1 week ago. She was seen at the emergency room where x-rays of the foot were obtained (Fig. 5–56A–C). She was splinted and referred to your orthopaedic clinic. She has moderate edema of the right foot and tenderness through the midfoot and slight forefoot abduction compared to the contralateral foot.

Which of the following is the LEAST likely sequela of this injury?

A.   Development of a pes cavus deformity
B.   Avascular necrosis
C.   Posttraumatic arthrosis
D.   Loss of subtalar motion

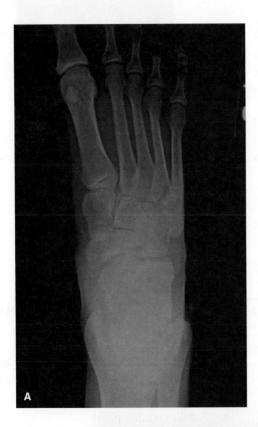
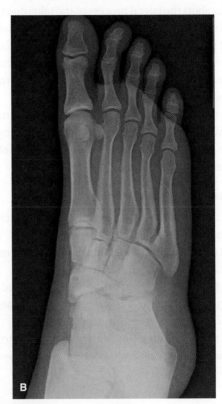
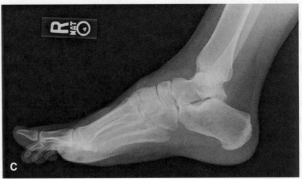

Figure 5–56   **A:** AP radiograph of the foot. **B:** Oblique radiograph of the foot. **C:** Lateral radiograph of the foot.

Discussion

The correct answer is (A). This patient has sustained what Sangeorzan described as a type 3 navicular body fracture resulting in comminution of the lateral pole of the tarsal navicular. The loss of support of the lateral pole of the navicular has allowed the forefoot to abduct, making a cavus deformity unlikely. The amount of articular surface of the navicular limits its blood supply to dorsal branches fed by the dorsalis pedis artery and plantar branches supplied by the medial plantar branch of the posterior tibial artery. This anatomy makes avascular necrosis a concern when treating navicular fractures. The comminution at the talonavicular joint predisposes these fractures to development of posttraumatic arthrosis and subsequent loss of subtalar motion because of the intimate coupling of the talonavicular joint with subtalar motion.

A CT scan is obtained of the foot (Fig. 5–57A–C).

What is the recommended treatment for this fracture?

A. Short-leg cast and protected weight bearing
B. Open reduction with internal fixation of the navicular fracture

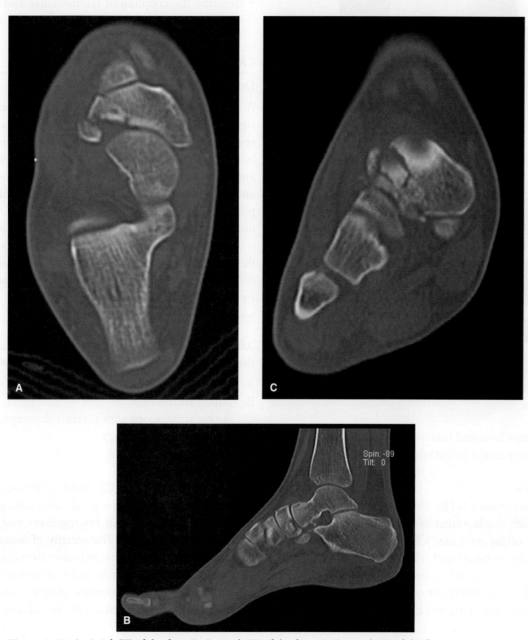

Figure 5–57 **A:** Axial CT of the foot. **B:** Sagittal CT of the foot. **C:** Coronal CT of the foot.

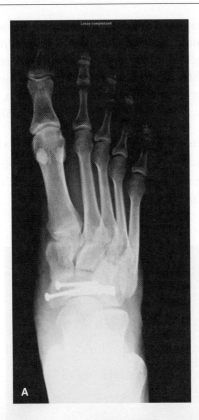

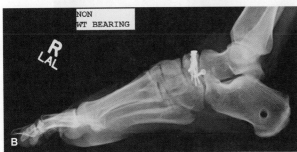

Figure 5–58 **A:** Postoperative AP radiograph showing plate and screw fixation. **B:** Lateral postoperative radiograph showing internal fixation and autograft harvest site from calcaneal tuberosity.

C. Fracture boot and functional rehabilitation
D. Primary fusion of the talonavicular joint

Discussion

The correct answer is (B). The CT scan shows comminution with displacement of the fragments of the lateral pole of the navicular. Closed treatment would be reserved for nondisplaced fractures, typically Sangeorzan type 1 or some stress fractures of the navicular. A removable boot would not offer adequate support for this fracture, and if treated closed, motion should not

be instituted until radiographic union is seen. Primary talonavicular arthrodesis may be the salvage procedure needed in severe fractures when a sufficient reconstruction of the articular surface or restoration of length cannot be obtained. However, in a young and active individual, every attempt to reconstruct the joint surface, support length (which may require bone grafting), and maintain function should be made (Fig. 5–58A and B).

Objectives: Did you learn...?

- Use Sangeorzan classification of navicular fractures?
- Describe the vascular supply to the tarsal navicular?
- Describe the coupling of talonavicular and subtalar motion?

CASE 29

Dr. Joshua Lamb

A 32-year-old, professional ballet dancer presents with right ankle pain. She reports that she has had several severe ankle sprains in the past but denies ankle instability. She localizes the pain to the anterior aspect of the ankle and reports that it is worse with deep knee bends and activities requiring ankle dorsiflexion. She complains of intermittent locking of her ankle as well. On physical examination there is tenderness to palpation over the anterior aspect of the ankle with ankle dorsiflexion of only 5 degrees compared to 15 degrees on the contralateral ankle. There is anterior ankle pain with passive ankle dorsiflexion. Radiographs and a CT scan were obtained (Figs. 5–59 and 5–60).

After failure of nonoperative management, what is the best surgical treatment option for this patient?

A. Distraction arthroplasty
B. Ankle arthrodesis
C. Ankle arthroscopy with anterior decompression
D. Total ankle arthroplasty

Discussion

The correct answer is (C). Ankle arthroscopy with anterior decompression is a good treatment option for patients with symptoms of impingement and without global tibiotalar arthritis. The severity of osteoarthritic change is a better prognostic indicator for outcome after arthroscopic surgical treatment for anterior impingement than the size and location of spurs. Distraction arthroplasty is more appropriate for advanced ankle

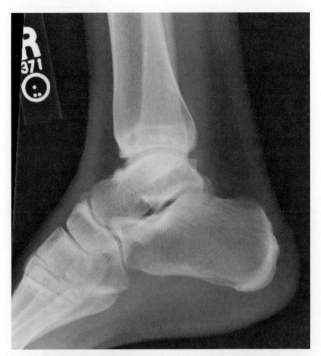

Figure 5–59 Lateral ankle radiograph depicting mild degenerative changes in the ankle with anterior tibial and talar osteophyte formation and a loose body posteriorly.

arthritis. Ankle arthrodesis is not a good option for this young ballet dancer with only mild degenerative changes. Total ankle arthroplasty is an alternative to arthrodesis in some patients with end-stage arthritis, but would not be a good choice in this individual.

What is the most common complication associated with ankle arthroscopy?

A. Deep peroneal nerve injury
B. Superficial peroneal nerve injury
C. Saphenous nerve injury
D. Tibialis anterior tendon injury

Discussion

The correct answer is (B). An injury to the dorsal intermediate cutaneous branch of the superficial peroneal nerve is the most common complication following ankle arthroscopy. Injury to this nerve occurs at the anterolateral portal. The superficial peroneal nerve and the course of its branches can typically be visualized by flexing the fourth toe. Visualizing the course of the nerve prior to portal placement may help to protect the nerve from injury. The deep peroneal nerve is at risk

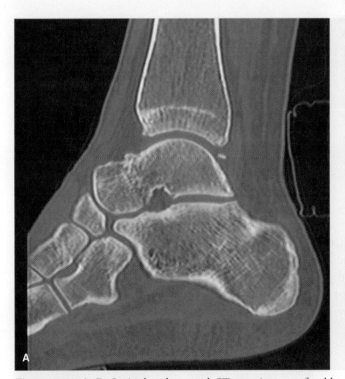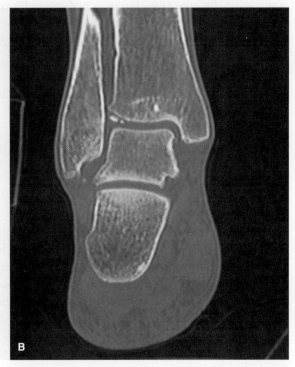

Figure 5–60 **A, B:** Sagittal and coronal CT scan images of ankle showing anterior tibial and talar osteophyte formation and multiple loose bodies.

from an anterocentral portal. The saphenous nerve and vein are at risk from an anteromedial portal. The tibialis anterior tendon is not commonly injured during ankle arthroscopy. Ferkel reports an overall complication rate during ankle arthroscopy of 9.0%, with neurologic complications in 4.4%. Most nerve complications are transient and resolve within 6 months.

Which one of the following is a contraindication to total ankle arthroplasty (TAA)?

A. Patient weight of 200 lb
B. Preoperative hindfoot valgus of 10 degrees
C. Massive talar avascular necrosis
D. Posttraumatic arthritis

Discussion

The correct answer is (C). Massive or unresectable osteonecrosis is a contraindication to TAA because there is not a stable platform on which to seat the talar component. In addition, peripheral vascular disease, severe osteoporosis, neuropathy, neuropathic joint disease, and history of infection are considered contraindications to TAA. The ideal candidate for TAA would have end-stage ankle arthritis, weigh less than 250 lb, be greater than 50 years old, have a moderate activity level, have no significant comorbidities, and have less than 20 degrees of varus or valgus hindfoot deformity with excellent bone stock. Posttraumatic arthritis is not a contraindication to TAA.

Objectives: Did you learn...?

• Identify the risk of nerve injury with ankle arthroscopy?
• Describe some of the indications and contraindications for total ankle arthroplasty?

CASE 30

Dr. Daniel Guss

A 54-year-old male presents with right forefoot pain, swelling, and a sense of pressure. He reports that he was previously evaluated by a podiatrist who aspirated fluid from a lump in his foot, but that the lump subsequently recurred. The patient arrives with a foot x-ray (Fig. 5–61) and MRI (Figs. 5–62 and 5–63).

What is the most likely diagnosis?

A. Angiosarcoma
B. Ganglion cyst
C. Clear cell sarcoma
D. Lipoma

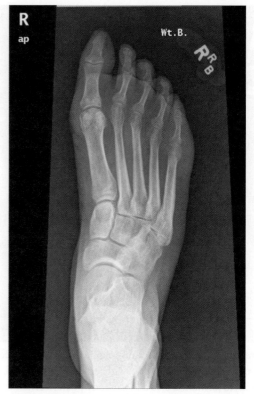

Figure 5–61 AP radiograph of the foot.

Discussion

The correct answer is (B). Unlike other areas of the body that may have higher concentrations of somatic tissue, the foot has a high concentration of tendons, fascia, and synovium. Ganglion cysts consist of mucinous fluid intimately connected with a joint or, more frequently in the foot, a tendon sheath. The foot is the third most common place for ganglion cysts after the hand and

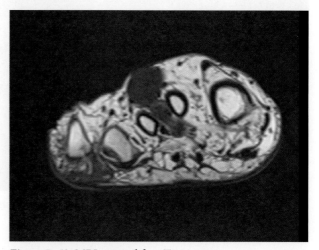

Figure 5–62 MRI coronal foot T1 image.

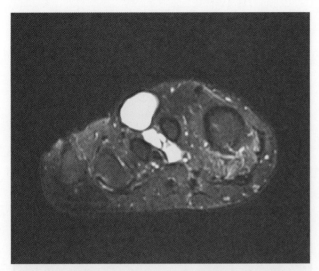

Figure 5–63 MRI coronal foot T2 fat-suppressed image.

wrist. On MRI ganglions can be round, lobulated, or septated, but generally have a sharp outline with clear T2 signal.

Had the above lesion been similar in shape on MRI, but bright on T1 and dark on T2, what would be the most likely diagnosis?

A. Angiosarcoma

B. Ganglion cyst

C. Clear cell sarcoma

D. Lipoma

Discussion

The correct answer is (D). Lipomas generally show a signal intensity similar to normal fat, which is bright on T1 and dark on T2. Areas of inflammation or fibrosis, however, can make some lipomas more difficult to distinguish from liposarcomas.

Giant cell tumor (GCT) of tendon sheath is an extra-articular tumor that can be found in the foot. What is its intra-articular equivalent?

A. Pigmented villonodular synovitis

B. Synovial sarcoma

C. Clear cell sarcoma

D. Ganglion cyst

Discussion

The correct answer is (A). GCTs of tendon sheath are of synovial origin and may arise from tendon sheaths as well as ligaments bursa, and joint capsules. This tumor is commonly found in the hand, where it has a low recurrence rate after resection. In the lower extremity

it is the most commonly found tumor in the digits, but can also occur elsewhere in the foot. A nonfocal, diffuse and infiltrative variety (florid proliferative synovitis) is thought to be an extra-articular version of pigmented villonodular synovitis. Characteristic appearance on MRI includes inhomogenous T1 and T2 signals with solid areas as well as areas of tumor necrosis. Its pathologic appearance is highly vascular with interspersed giant cells, macrophages, fibroblasts, and deposits of hemosiderin.

Objectives: Did you learn...?

• Identify MRI appearance of common benign lesions in the foot?

• Describe the pathologic origin of some foot and ankle tumors?

CASE 31

Dr. Joshua Lamb

A 57-year-old female presents with an 8-month history of pain at the Achilles tendon insertion. She reports a burning pain that is worse with activity. She is only able to wear backless shoes. On physical examination, she has point tenderness at the insertion of the Achilles tendon. She has a positive Silfverskiold sign, with ankle dorsiflexion to 0 degrees with the knee extended that increases to 10 degrees with the knee flexed to 90 degrees. A radiograph is shown in Figure 5–64.

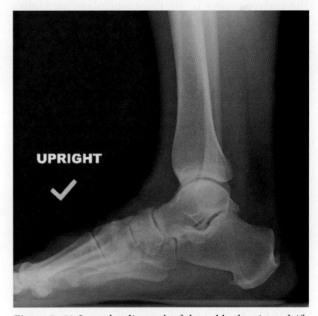

Figure 5–64 Lateral radiograph of the ankle showing calcification at the insertion of the Achilles tendon.

The most appropriate initial management of Achilles tendinopathy includes:

A. Cortisone injection
B. A nonweight-bearing cast for 4 weeks
C. Surgical debridement
D. Eccentric calf stretching and physical therapy

Discussion

The correct answer is (D). Eccentric calf stretching (application of load during muscle lengthening) has been shown to decrease pain and shorten the time to return to sport. Insertional Achilles tendinopathy does not respond as well to eccentric calf stretching as noninsertional tendinopathy but should still be considered as a first-line treatment. A nonweight-bearing cast may help improve symptoms but will result in calf atrophy and poor organization of the collagen repair. Cortisone should be avoided around the Achilles tendon; case reports of Achilles tendon rupture following corticosteroid injections exist. Surgical debridement should be used to treat refractory cases of tendinosis.

Acute tendinitis has been associated with which class of medication?

A. Aminoglycosides
B. Fluoroquinolones
C. β-Lactam antibiotics
D. Lincosamides
E. Macrolides

Discussion

The correct answer is (B). Fluoroquinolone antibiotics have been linked to Achilles tendinitis and Achilles tendon rupture. Ciprofloxacin is the most commonly implicated fluoroquinolone and has been associated with a 4.1-fold increase in risk of Achilles rupture. Median onset of tendinitis is 6 days (85% of cases within first month) after starting the ciprofloxacin and symptoms typically precede tendon rupture by up to 2 weeks. While other tendons can be involved, the Achilles is most commonly affected (90% of cases). Aminoglycosides, such as gentamycin, have been associated with renal toxicity and hearing loss. β-Lactam antibiotics, such as penicillin, may be associated with GI symptoms or a rash. Lincosamides, such as clindamycin, may be associated with pseudomembranous colitis. Macrolides, such as erythromycin, may be associated with GI symptoms.

This patient has persistent pain despite extensive conservative treatment and wishes to consider surgery. An MRI is obtained to determine the extent of involvement of the Achilles tendon (Fig. 5–65).

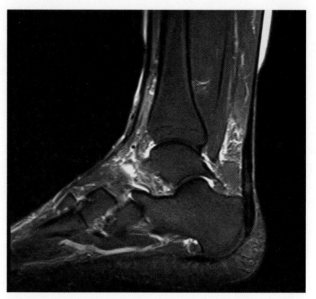

Figure 5–65 A T2 sagittal MRI showing insertional thickening of the Achilles tendon and >50% involvement of the tendon.

What is the best surgical treatment option for this patient?

A. Multiple percutaneous longitudinal tenotomies
B. Excision of Haglund deformity
C. Achilles tendon debridement, excision of the Haglund deformity, and flexor hallucis longus (FHL) tendon transfer
D. Calcaneal osteotomy

Discussion

The correct answer is (C). Excision of the Haglund deformity alone will not address the tendinopathy; the degenerative portion of the tendon should be debrided. Tendon transfer to supplement Achilles debridement should be considered when >50% of the tendon is involved and in older patients (>55 years). A recent study evaluating FHL tendon transfer showed more improvement in functional outcomes in patients older than 50 years compared with patients younger than 50 years. Multiple percutaneous longitudinal tenotomies can be used as a minimally invasive treatment option for noninsertional Achilles tendinopathy. A calcaneal osteotomy may be used to address hindfoot malalignment but does not address tendon pathology.

Objectives: Did you learn...?

• Importance of eccentric stretching and strengthening for Achilles tendinopathy?
• Describe the relationship between fluoroquinolone antibiotics and Achilles tendon pathology?

CASE 32

Dr. John Paul Elton

A 33-year-old man jumped off a 6-ft ledge, injuring his right ankle. He presented to the emergency department shortly thereafter, unable to bear weight on the right foot. The ER physician confirmed that he was in no acute distress, had no open wounds, and had palpable pedal pulses with soft foot compartments. He had moderate edema and ecchymosis around his foot and no other lower extremity or back injuries. Lateral radiograph of the right ankle is shown (Fig. 5–66).

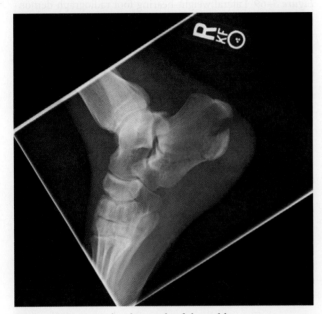

Figure 5–66 Lateral radiograph of the ankle.

What is the appropriate next step in management?

A. X-rays of the contralateral ankle
B. Padded splint and crutches with referral to clinic
C. Urgent orthopaedic evaluation and surgical treatment
D. Delayed surgical intervention once soft tissue edema has resolved

Discussion

The correct answer is (C). Fractures of the posterior tuberosity may be intra-articular or extra-articular. Figure 5–66 shows a beak fracture of the calcaneus with intra-articular extension. This fracture has a significant risk of damaging the thin layer of skin and soft tissue over the posterior calcaneus by pressure necrosis. Urgent evaluation of the soft tissues will frequently show puckering of the soft tissues in the fracture gap, and blanching of the skin overlying the prominent fracture fragment posteriorly. This injury should be

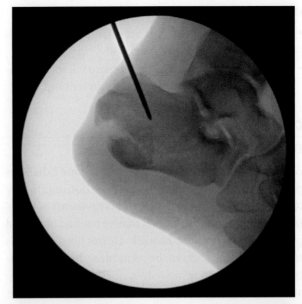

Figure 5–67 A percutaneous guide pin is placed into the posterior calcaneal tuberosity to control the main fragment and lever it into an anatomically reduced position.

evaluated urgently and treated with reduction before the pressure on the skin causes necrosis. Despite swelling and ecchymosis, this fracture is not appropriate to be referred to clinic for delayed fixation. The procedure can often be performed with a limited open approach and screw fixation to minimize further injury to the soft tissues (Figs. 5–67 and 5–68).

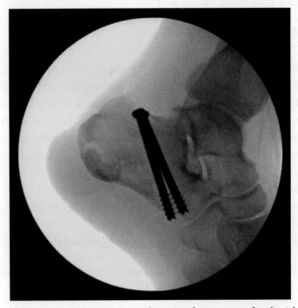

Figure 5–68 The posterior tuberosity fragment is fixed with two large fragment screws after anatomic reduction, thereby preserving the posterior soft tissue envelope.

Objectives: Did you learn...?

- Identify the importance of soft tissue injury associated with calcaneal beak fractures?
- Discuss the standard treatment approach for a calcaneal beak fracture with posterior skin tenting?

CASE 33

Dr. Tom Douglas

A 55-year-old man with a long history of type 2 diabetes presents with a swollen, erythematous, hot, and mildly tender right foot. The majority of his erythema is localized in his midfoot. He reports that he has had increased pain in his foot for the past week. He has been doing his regular foot care without any skin breakdown. In addition, he has had no fevers, chills, or elevated blood sugars. On physical examination his vital signs are stable. He has swelling in his right foot, but no visible ulcer. His pulse is strongly palpable, but he has decreased sensation bilaterally in a stocking distribution to the level of the mid tibia. In addition to concern for infection you wish to evaluate the patient for Charcot foot.

Which of the following is a more consistent physical examination finding in a Charcot foot than in an infected diabetic foot?

A. Erythema which does not resolve with elevation
B. Warmth
C. Swelling
D. Intact skin on the foot

Discussion

The correct answer is (D). Charcot foot is often confused with infection as both often present as red, hot, swollen, and occasionally painful feet. Classically, elevation of the Charcot foot will result in resolution of erythema, whereas in an infection erythema will remain with elevation. Osteomyelitis in a diabetic foot most often results from an adjacent ulcer as opposed to hematogenous spread. The definitive diagnosis however would be made from a pathologic specimen that demonstrates no organisms and bone fragments within the synovium.

A lateral x-ray of the patient's foot is obtained (Fig. 5–69).

The patient asks if this location for neuropathic joint changes in the foot is common. You respond:

A. No this is very uncommon and almost case reportable
B. This is the most common location for Charcot arthropathy

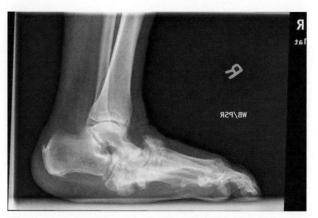

Figure 5–69 Lateral weight-bearing foot radiograph demonstrating fragmentation and collapse through the midfoot.

C. Yes, this is a common location in the lower extremity, however there are other places which are more common locations

Discussion

The correct answer is (B). Charcot neuropathy is classified based both upon the location of the pathology in the foot (Brodsky) and stage of the disease (Eichenholtz). In the Brodsky classification, type 1 disease is in the midfoot, type 2 is in the hindfoot, type 3a is tibiotalar joint involvement, and type 3b is calcaneal tuberosity involvement. The most commonly affected region is the midfoot (type 1), often resulting in the classic rocker bottom deformity of the foot. Types 2 and 3 are less common. Type 3a however tends to be very difficult to control and can result in varus or valgus collapse and subsequent ulcer formation and osteomyelitis.

The Eichenholtz classification describes the stages based upon the pathologic progression of the disease from fragmentation through coalition. The pathologic changes of a Charcot joint begin with the fragmentation stage. This typically presents with osteopenia and joint subluxation, fracture, or dislocation. This is followed by the coalescence phase during which the progression of radiographic deformity halts as demonstrated on serial radiographs. The final stage is reconstruction, during which there is resolution of the inflammation and union of the fragmented regions. The end result often includes residual deformity, which may or may not be problematic.

The patient wants to know if he needs surgery at this point in time. You explain that there is no clear indication for surgery at this point given that there is no ulcer formation, or skin at risk.

You recommend initially treating him with a total contact cast, and nonweight bearing for this stage of his disease. The reason for this is:

A. To prevent progression of collapse

B. To increase rate of union

C. For pain control

Discussion

The correct answer is (A). The goal of casting in the inflammatory stage is to prevent the progression of deformity which would result in ulcers. At the early fragmentation stage, there is a great degree of instability across the midfoot which may result in collapse and deformity. This can lead to worsened arch collapse and progression of the rocker bottom. The progression through the stages of Charcot neuropathy has not been tied to immobilization and often takes months to resolve. Many of these patients are non-painful due to neuropathy. This results in the need for frequent skin evaluation to prevent skin breakdown in the cast.

After 8 months of follow-up the patient is found to have no further progression of his deformity and no erythema or warmth present. He still is having difficulty in shoewear, even with accommodative orthotics. He now presents with an ulcer on the plantar aspect of his foot (Fig. 5–70). Radiographs demonstrate no progression of deformity.

The best treatment option at this point is:

A. Below knee amputation

B. Plantar exostectomy

C. Triple arthrodesis

D. Ankle arthrodesis

Discussion

The correct answer is (B). Since the patient has passed through the coalescence phase and failed accommodative orthotics, it is reasonable to proceed with a surgical intervention to relieve the pressure on the skin from the bony prominence. In this instance, the foot has a classic rocker bottom deformity. A plantar exostectomy can relieve the pressure on the skin at this location. A below knee amputation is necessary in the setting of uncontrolled infection resulting in risk of life to the patient. A triple arthrodesis will correct deformity present in the talocalcaneal, talonavicular, and calcaneocuboid joints, however in this case the deformity is distal to the transverse tarsal joint, so would be of no benefit. The same is true for

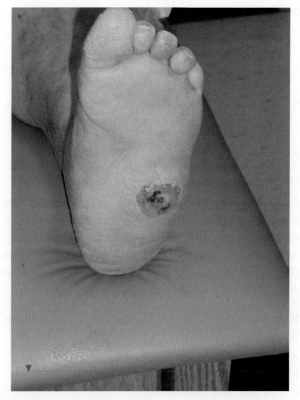

Figure 5–70 Clinical photograph of the plantar foot.

ankle arthrodesis. Additional procedures for correcting residual deformity of a Charcot foot include open reduction with internal fixation either with plates and screws or with intramedullary fixation (Fig. 5–71).

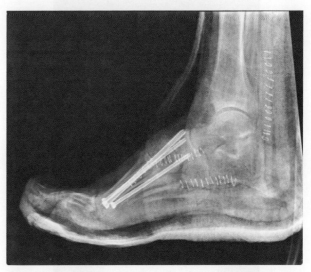

Figure 5–71 Postoperative lateral radiograph demonstrating intramedullary fixation of midfoot Charcot arthropathy.

Objectives: Did you learn...?

- Describe physical examination maneuvers to differentiate between osteomyelitis and Charcot joint?
- Identify classification and staging systems of Charcot arthropathy?
- Discuss procedures available for the treatment of residual deformity from neuroarthropathy in the midfoot?

CASE 34

Dr. Thomas Dowd

A 58-year-old woman comes to clinic reporting that her previous surgeon has performed two procedures on her foot and that she is quite unhappy. She brings with her radiographs taken after her first operation (Fig. 5–72). You note a prior medial eminence resection and a recurrent hallux valgus deformity.

Which of the following is not associated with recurrent hallux valgus?

A. Incomplete sesamoid reduction
B. Inadequate correction of the IMA
C. Fibular sesamoid excision
D. Premature weight bearing
E. Juvenile/adolescent patient

Discussion

The correct answer is (C). Fibular sesamoid excision, as described by McBride, is associated with the development of hallux varus and should be avoided. The remaining options are associated with recurrence. Optimally, the sesamoids will be positioned plantar to the crista as the valgus and pronation is corrected. The intermetatarsal angle (IMA) should be corrected to minimize the return of deforming forces across the first metatarsophalangeal joint (MTPJ). Premature weight bearing has been shown to increase the risk of recurrence. Hallux valgus correction in the young patient is notorious for its association with recurrence, with a rate of over 50% in some series.

You obtain new radiographs that show an opening wedge proximal first metatarsal osteotomy with now a hallux varus deformity (Fig. 5–73).

What technical error is not associated with postoperative hallux varus?

A. Excessive dorsiflexion at the osteotomy site
B. Excessive plication of the medial capsule
C. Fibular sesamoid excision
D. Excessive medial eminence resection
E. Lateral flexor hallucis brevis transection

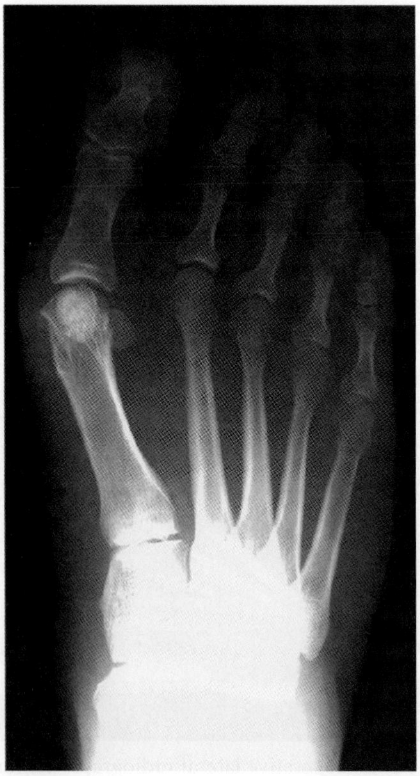

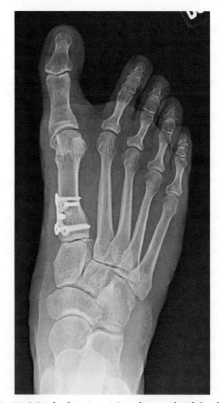

Figure 5–72 AP weight-bearing radiograph of the foot.

Figure 5–73 Weight-bearing AP radiograph of the foot.

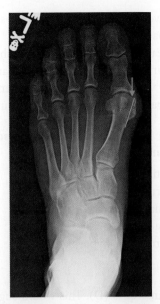

Figure 5-74 AP weight-bearing radiograph of the foot with appropriate path of saw blade for medial eminence resection (*line*) with relationship to the sagittal sulcus (*arrow*).

Discussion

The correct answer is (A). Excessive dorsiflexion at the osteotomy site is associated with transfer metatarsalgia, not postoperative hallux varus. As the first ray is dorsiflexed, the distal lesser toes are exposed to increased postoperative pressure. The medial capsule should be provisionally imbricated with assessment prior to completion of the case. Excessive tightening of the medial capsule will result in varus. Fibular sesamoid excision has largely been abandoned due to its association with hallux varus. Medial eminence resection should be performed with a distal starting point medial to the sagittal sulcus. The cut should be completed in line with the medial cortex of the first metatarsal, taking care to avoid notching (Fig. 5–74).

Objectives: Did you learn...?

• Assess the causes for postoperative recurrence and hallux varus after hallux valgus procedures?

CASE 35

Dr. Thomas Dowd

A 40-year-old woman reports pain in her forefoot, especially when wearing dress shoes. She notes a shooting, electrical quality to the pain. Her pain improves with rest and unshod feet. You suspect that she has a Morton's neuroma.

What physical examination finding best supports your suspicion?

A. Positive drawer test at the second metatarsophalangeal joint (MTPJ)

B. Pain with passive dorsiflexion at the first MTPJ

C. Decreased sensation at the lateral second toe and medial third toe

D. Pain and click with a plantarly applied, dorsally directed force at the third web space with simultaneous forefoot compression

Discussion

The correct answer is (D), which describes the Mulder's click test (Fig. 5–75). Classically, a Morton's neuroma occurs in the third web space, as branches from the medial and lateral plantar nerves join to form the interdigital nerve and are compressed between the surrounding metatarsals and the transverse metatarsal ligament (Fig. 5–76). A Morton's neuroma may arise in the second web space or both the second and third web spaces. Reproduction of pain with Mulder's click suggests a diagnosis of Morton's neuroma. Drawer testing of the second MTPJ is important for assessing instability that is more commonly associated with plantar plate injury and MTPJ synovitis.

Your patient states that she cannot tolerate this condition any longer and desires surgical intervention. She has not tried changing her footwear or trying any inserts. She is concerned with the location of her scar.

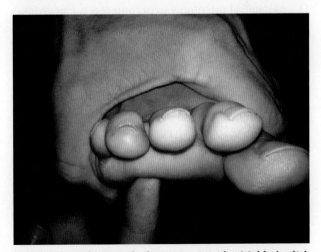

Figure 5-75 Photograph demonstrating the Mulder's click test. This test involves compression of the metatarsals with a dorsally directed force between the third and fourth metatarsals.

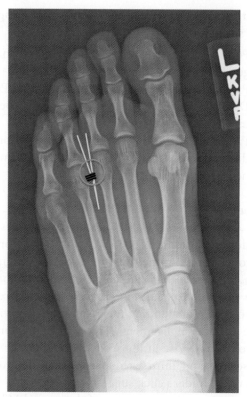

Figure 5–76 Note the area of concern (*gray circle*) depicting compression of nerve (*white lines*) between the metatarsal heads just distal to the transverse metatarsal ligament (*black lines*).

What initial treatment do you recommend?

A. Neurolysis via a dorsal approach
B. Neurectomy via a dorsal approach
C. Shoewear modification and the use of a metatarsal pad
D. Metatarsal osteotomy to decompress the neuroma
E. Neurectomy via a plantar approach

Discussion

The correct answer is (C). Treatment of a Morton's neuroma is initially nonoperative. Conservative treatment consists of shoewear modification, metatarsal pad placement, and NSAID use. Diagnostic and therapeutic injections may also be performed in the region of the affected nerve. If the aforementioned measures fail, primary surgical treatment of this disorder typically consists of release of the transverse metatarsal ligament with neurectomy via a dorsal approach. Some reports have demonstrated promising results with neurolysis. Plantar approaches are typically reserved for recurrent or refractory cases that have failed intervention employing a dorsal incision. The nerve is subcutaneous relative to the plantar skin and is more readily accessed through a plantar approach. In cases with involvement of adjacent nerves, a transverse plantar approach may be advantageous.

Despite the use of a metatarsal pad and shoewear modifications, your patient has persistent pain and undergoes a neurectomy via a dorsal approach. You send the excised tissue to the pathologist for histologic evaluation.

What is the characteristic finding associated with Morton's neuroma?

A. Proliferative synovitis
B. Reed Sternberg cells
C. Demyelinated nerve
D. Perineural fibrosis
E. Angiofibroblastic hyperplasia

Discussion

The correct answer is (D). This would suggest that the term "neuroma" is a misnomer. Nevertheless, use of the term continues for ease of communication. Proliferative synovitis is associated with several diagnoses, including rheumatoid arthritis, pigmented villonodular synovitis, and giant cell tumor of tendon sheath. Demyelinated nerve is seen peripherally with conditions such as Charcot–Marie–Tooth and Guillain–Barré syndrome. Angiofibroblastic hyperplasia was coined by Nirschl to describe pathologic changes associated with lateral epicondylitis (tennis elbow).

Objectives: Did you learn…?

• Describe anatomic considerations that contribute to location of pathology?
• Identify histologic finding classically seen with Morton's neuroma?
• Describe nonsurgical treatment options and recommendations?
• Discuss options for surgical intervention and when to consider plantar and dorsal approaches?

CASE 36

Dr. Jeremy T. Smith

While on call, you receive a consult to see a 75-year-old male who had been admitted to the medical service with fevers, swelling, redness, and drainage from a forefoot ulcer. He has a history of diabetes for which he takes insulin, coronary artery disease status-post bypass grafting, and atrial fibrillation for which he takes coumadin. Upon examination, you observe the following (Fig. 5–77). You attempt to palpate pulses and are unable to palpate a dorsalis pedis or posterior tibial pulse. Ankle range of motion

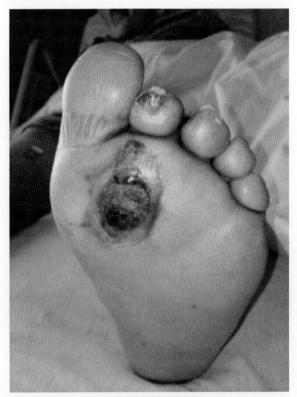

Figure 5–77 Photograph of plantar aspect of the foot.

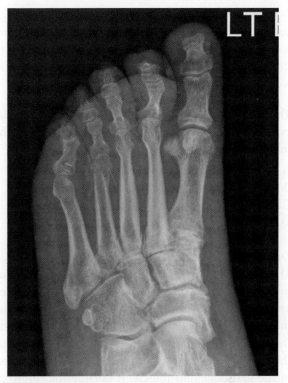

Figure 5–78 Plain radiograph showing multiple insulin syringe needles in the soft tissues.

is tested and is noted to be from zero degrees dorsiflexion to 40 degrees of plantar flexion, with dorsiflexion increasing to 10 degrees when you flex his knee.

You obtain an x-ray of the foot, which shows multiple insulin syringe needles in the soft tissues (Fig. 5–78).

In addition to the physical examination, the most appropriate additional studies include which of the following?

A. Erythrocyte sedimentation rate, C-reactive protein, white blood cell count, vascular studies
B. Erythrocyte sedimentation rate, C-reactive protein, white blood cell count, MRI
C. Erythrocyte sedimentation rate, C-reactive protein, white blood cell count, vascular studies, MRI
D. Erythrocyte sedimentation rate, C-reactive protein, white blood cell count

Discussion

The correct answer is (A). Given the patient's presentation, you should be concerned about a foot infection. Because of this, basic laboratory work that includes inflammatory markers and a WBC count is appropriate. While an MRI is a reasonable study to obtain

in most situations, you may be concerned about an MRI in the setting of multiple metallic foreign bodies (insulin syringes) in his foot. For this reason, an MRI should probably be deferred. Vascular studies should be obtained because of the lack of palpable pulses.

Noninvasive vascular studies are obtained and reveal infrapopliteal stenosis in the extremity with the ulceration.

Based upon the vascular studies, you recommend the following?

A. Below knee amputation
B. Consultation with a vascular surgeon
C. Transmetatarsal amputation
D. No further vascular intervention as his blood flow seems to be adequate

Discussion

The correct answer is (B). With absent pulses and abnormal vascular studies, it is appropriate to involve a vascular surgeon to determine the need for a revascularization procedure to accompany further treatment of the foot ulcer. While this patient may at some point come to require an amputation, obtaining further vascular input is appropriate before an amputation.

Based upon your clinical evaluation, you have a high concern that this patient has osteomyelitis of the fore-foot associated with the plantar ulcer. You take him to the operating room for irrigation and debridement as well as a gastrocnemius recession.

The Silfverskiold test, performed during your initial evaluation of the patient, tests for which of the following?

A. Isolated soleus contracture
B. Foot drop
C. Achilles contracture
D. Isolated gastrocnemius contracture

Discussion

The correct answer is (D). The Silfverskiold test is done by measuring ankle dorsiflexion with the knee extended and then again with the knee flexed. The gastrocnemius muscle spans both the ankle and knee joints, and therefore examining ankle dorsiflexion while altering the flexion of the knee specifically measures the effect of the gastrocnemius muscle. If dorsiflexion improves with knee flexion, then a gastrocnemius contracture is present. Alternatively, if ankle dorsiflexion does not improve, then a contracture of the tendo-Achilles is present.

Objectives: Did you learn…?

• Discuss basic laboratories to be sent upon initial evaluation of a patient with a foot ulcer?
• Describe the importance of evaluating and treating the vascular status, pressure overload, and infection in the setting of a foot ulcer?

CASE 37

Dr. John Paul Elton

A 24-year-old professional tennis player presents to clinic 2 days after twisting her ankle while playing tennis. She reports swelling and pain with walking at the lateral aspect of her foot. She is otherwise healthy, without previous fracture or antecedent pain. Oblique and lateral radiographs are shown in Figure 5–79A and B.

What is the most appropriate treatment for this individual?

A. Surgical fixation
B. Hard-soled shoe
C. Short-leg weight-bearing cast
D. Bone scan

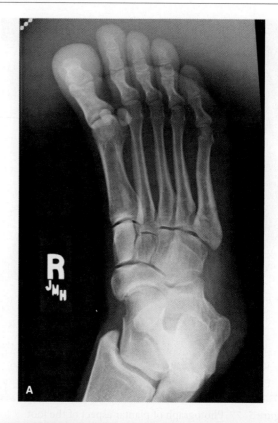

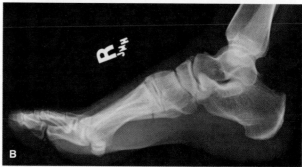

Figure 5–79 **A:** Oblique radiograph of the right foot. **B:** Lateral radiograph of the right foot.

Discussion

The correct answer is (A). This patient has a fracture of the fifth metatarsal base at the junction of zones II and III. Fifth metatarsal base fractures are divided into fracture of three zones. Zone I represents an avulsion fracture of the tuberosity, which occurs from pull of the peroneus brevis and plantar fascia. Zone II fractures occur in the metaphysis approximately 1.5 cm distal to the base and adjacent to the 4–5 metatarsal articulation. Zone II injuries occur with an adduction moment placed on the foot, such as with inversion injuries with weight bearing on the lateral border of the foot. Zone III fractures frequently represent stress fractures of the proximal shaft of the fifth metatarsal.

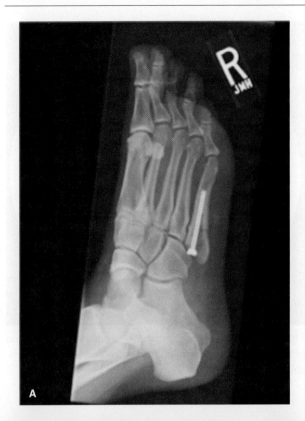

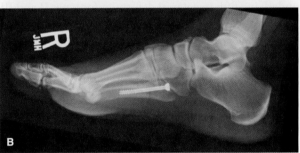

Figure 5–80 **A, B:** Postoperative radiographs showing intramedullary screw placement across fracture.

Fractures of Zone II are significant in that they occur in a watershed area of blood supply to the fifth metatarsal between the metaphyseal vessels and the nutrient artery of the diaphysis. Because of the relatively poor blood supply in Zone II, these fractures are susceptible to nonunion and are treated more aggressively than a tuberosity fracture, which can be treated with a hard-soled shoe. If closed treatment of a Zone II fracture is undertaken, a short-leg cast with nonweight bearing for 6 to 8 weeks is recommended. Closed treatment is appropriate in the majority of patients, but for high level athletes such as the professional tennis player presented in this case, surgical treatment may be preferred (Fig.

5–80). A bone scan or MRI would be useful to evaluate for stress fracture in a patient with persistent pain with activity and no evidence of fracture with plain radiographs.

Objectives: Did you learn...?

- Describe the mechanism of injury for different types of fifth metatarsal fractures?
- Assess the risk of delayed- or nonunion with Zone II fifth metatarsal fractures?
- Discuss treatment approaches for different types of fifth metatarsal fractures?

CASE 38

Dr. Joshua Lamb

A 39-year-old female presents with increasing pain over the lateral aspect of her foot. She complains of difficulty with shoe wear. She reports pain specifically at the lateral aspect of her fifth metatarsophalangeal joint. A weight-bearing AP radiograph was obtained (Fig. 5–81).

What is the best initial treatment for a bunionette (tailor's bunion) deformity?

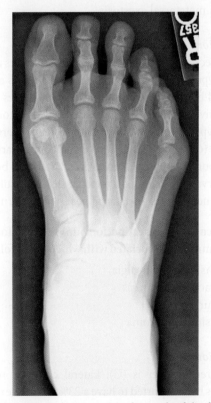

Figure 5–81 Weight-bearing AP radiograph of the foot.

A. Arizona brace

B. Fifth metatarsal head excision

C. Fifth metatarsal lateral condylar resection

D. Shoe wear modification, keratosis padding, and shaving

Discussion

The correct answer is (D). Nonoperative management has a 75% to 90% success rate. An Arizona brace is used to manage hindfoot or ankle pathology. Metatarsal head excision should be used as a salvage procedure as it will destabilize the fifth MTP joint. Lateral condylar resection is appropriate for some patients after failure of conservative management.

After failure of nonsurgical management, a diaphyseal fifth metatarsal osteotomy is the best treatment for which of the following?

A. A 45-year-old female with a normal 4–5 intermetatarsal angle and an enlarged lateral prominence of the fifth metatarsal head with an intractable lateral keratotic lesion

B. A 45-year-old female with a widened 4–5 intermetatarsal angle (>8 degrees) and a painful prominence over the fifth metatarsal head

C. A 60-year-old diabetic with an ulceration over a fifth metatarsal exostosis

Discussion

The correct answer is (B). This scenario describes a patient with a type III bunionette. Type III bunionettes are characterized by an increase in the IMA >8 degrees and can be effectively treated with a diaphyseal osteotomy (Fig. 5–82). Type I bunionettes have a normal 4–5 intermetatarsal angle (6.5–8 degrees) and an enlarged metatarsal head. Type II bunionettes are characterized by a lateral bow (outward curvature) in the fifth metatarsal shaft, resulting in a prominence over the metatarsal head, with a normal IMA.

Lateral condylar resection for bunionette deformity is most commonly associated with which of the following?

A. Transfer metatarsalgia

B. Intractable keratosis

C. Recurrence

D. Incisional neuroma

Discussion

The correct answer is (C). Lateral condylar resection alone has been reported to have a 23% incidence of recurrence or persistent lateral forefoot pain. Failure to address

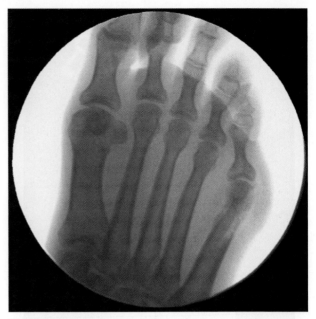

Figure 5–82 Intraoperative image demonstrating correction of the 4–5 IMA using a diaphyseal osteotomy and bioabsorbable fixation.

underlying fifth metatarsal deformity, for types II and III bunionettes, may result in persistent pain. Transfer metatarsalgia may occur following resection of the metatarsal head or if the fifth metatarsal is excessively shortened. Intractable keratosis may occur if a lateral condylar resection is performed for a type II or III deformity, although this is less common than recurrence. Incisional neuroma is a possible complication, although not the most commonly associated complication with this procedure.

Objectives: Did you learn...?

• Discuss the importance of nonoperative management for bunionette deformity?

• Assess the three types of bunionette deformities?

• Describe the surgical approach to addressing different bunionette deformities?

CASE 39

Dr. John Paul Elton

A 27-year-old, competitive triathlete sustained an injury to her left foot while trail running when she had a misstep impacting her foot and twisting it. She was seen at a local emergency department, had supine x-rays performed, and was diagnosed with a foot sprain. She presents to clinic now 3 weeks post injury with persistent pain upon weight bearing and an inability to run. There is mild edema, faint plantar ecchymosis, and tenderness to palpation in the midfoot without obvious deformity.

What is the most appropriate next step in treatment?

A. CT scan of the foot
B. MRI of the foot
C. Physical therapy
D. Weight-bearing radiographs

Discussion

The correct answer is (D). This patient has signs and symptoms consistent with a Lisfranc complex injury. Her plantar ecchymosis, in particular, is concerning for a more involved injury than a simple sprain. The Lisfranc complex is composed of the distal intertarsal, tarsometatarsal, and proximal intermetatarsal joints and their supportive bony and ligamentous structures. Together, these structures form a strong bony and capsuloligamentous structure likened to a Roman arch, which maintains the longitudinal and transverse support of the foot. The apex of the arch, or the so-called keystone, is at the second tarsometatarsal joint. The base of the second metatarsal sits in a recessed mortise between the medial and lateral cuneiforms and is supported by the stout Lisfranc ligament. There is no proximal intermetatarsal ligament between the first and second metatarsals, rather, the Lisfranc ligament connects the plantar base of the second metatarsal to the medial cuneiform. This ligament may be torn, or may contribute to a small avulsion fracture at the base of the second metatarsal, referred to as the fleck sign (Fig. 5–83). Static, nonweight-bearing radiographs may show concentric reduction of more subtle injuries, and so weight-bearing x-rays or stress x-rays of the foot should be obtained if clinical suspicion is high. CT scan may aid in preoperative planning, and MRI may be useful in patients unable to tolerate weight-bearing or stress radiographs. Physical therapy may be useful if instability is ruled out.

What is the most appropriate treatment recommendation for this patient?

A. Short-leg cast with weight bearing as tolerated
B. Short-leg cast with nonweight bearing
C. Closed reduction with percutaneous fixation
D. Open reduction and internal fixation (ORIF) or primary arthrodesis

Discussion

The correct answer is (D). In a healthy young athletic patient with diagnosed instability on radiographs, cast treatment is not recommended. Closed reduction may

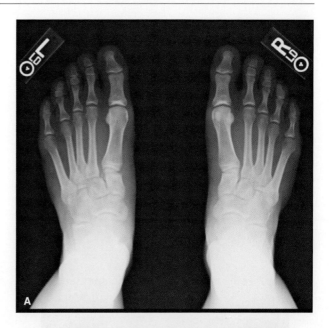

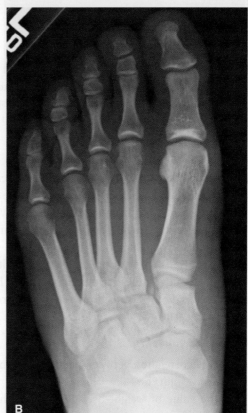

Figure 5–83 **A:** AP weight-bearing radiographs of the bilateral feet for comparison, showing diastasis of the first intermetatarsal space and a positive fleck sign. **B:** Magnified view of AP weight-bearing radiograph showing the small avulsion from the medial base of the second metatarsal and lateral translation of the second base on the middle cuneiform—the medial borders of these bones should be in line on the AP view.

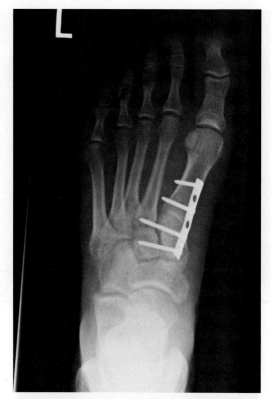

Figure 5–84 Postoperative AP radiograph showing anatomic reduction of the Lisfranc complex with extra-articular stabilization of the medial column with plate and screw construct.

not allow for anatomic reduction of the injury. There is some controversy as to whether open repair of the Lisfranc injury (Fig. 5–84) or primary arthrodesis provides the best long-term treatment for these injuries, and a discussion with the patient should be undertaken presenting these options. The intermediate-term results of these treatments suggest these two treatments may have similar outcomes, with less need for secondary procedures if primary arthrodesis is performed.

Objectives: Did you learn...?

• Describe the correlation between plantar ecchymosis and a Lisfranc injury?
• Discuss the value of weight-bearing radiographs in diagnosing a Lisfranc injury?
• Discuss the treatment options for a Lisfranc injury?

CASE 40

Dr. Thomas Dowd

A 21-year-old, collegiate football player noted acute medial forefoot pain when he axially loaded a dorsiflexed great toe and plantar-flexed ankle while blocking

during a game. He noted gradual swelling and ecchymosis about his first metatarsophalangeal joint (MTPJ). He was unable to return to the game. He denies pain near his midfoot. An AP foot radiograph is shown (Fig. 5–85).

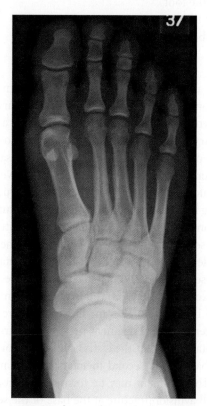

Figure 5–85 AP foot radiograph. Image courtesy of Tom Douglas, MD.

What is the most likely diagnosis?

A. First MTPJ dislocation
B. First MTPJ plantar plate rupture
C. Hallux valgus
D. Flexor hallucis longus (FHL) rupture

Discussion

The correct answer is (B). Plantar plate rupture, or "turf toe," is associated with this mechanism of injury, radiographic findings, and associated disability. MTPJ dislocation and FHL rupture may occur with this mechanism, however, axial loading of a dorsiflexed or hyper-dorsiflexed first MTPJ is more frequently associated with turf toe. Hallux valgus may be encountered with a partial medial plantar plate rupture and/or displaced tibial sesamoid fracture but this would more commonly be seen radiographically with angular deformity.

When compared to a contralateral AP foot radiograph, what radiographic finding best supports the diagnosis of complete plantar plate rupture?

A. Proximal migration of the sesamoids
B. MTPJ dislocation
C. Proximal phalanx fracture
D. Increased hallux valgus angle

Discussion

The correct answer is (A). With avulsion of the plantar plate insertion from the proximal phalanx or tear through the mid-substance of the plantar plate, the sesamoids may retract proximally. This can be identified on films of the injured extremity (Fig. 5–85) and may be confirmed by obtaining comparison views of the contralateral, uninjured extremity. Alternatively, the injury may be associated with fracture of one or both sesamoids. If the diagnosis is not clear by plain radiograph (limited proximal migration, concern for bipartite sesamoid), an MRI may be obtained to evaluate disruption of the plantar plate. MTPJ dislocation would be more easily identified on lateral radiographs of the foot and would not likely require a contralateral AP view. Proximal phalanx fracture is less commonly associated with plantar plate rupture, although a small avulsion fleck(s) may be appreciated. Increased hallux valgus angle may be noted with injuries that are limited to the medial aspect of the plantar plate complex.

Your patient desires to return to football next year for his final college season.

What intervention might you recommend?

A. First MTPJ arthrodesis
B. First MTPJ cheilectomy
C. Plantar plate repair
D. Extensor hallucis transfer

Discussion

The correct answer is (C). With complete plantar plate rupture, especially in the high-level athlete, direct surgical repair is often recommended. This is typically performed with suture repair of the medial and lateral aspects of the plantar capsuloligamentous cuff (Figs. 5–86 and 5–87). If plantar plate rupture is associated with significant displacement of one or both fractured sesamoids, open reduction and internal fixation (ORIF) may be incorporated into the treatment plan. Alternatively, a sesamoid may be excised with repair of the surrounding soft tissue if ORIF is not feasible.

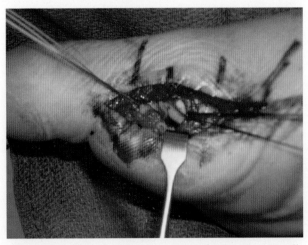

Figure 5–86 Medial approach with sutures placed proximally and distally in plantar plate prior to approximation.

First MTPJ cheilectomy or arthrodesis is performed for hallux rigidus, which may be a delayed consequence of plantar plate rupture. However, this would not be appropriate for initial treatment. Extensor hallucis transfer is not the initial treatment for this injury. With loss of the plantar plate and flexor hallucis brevis complex, unopposed pull of the extensors, and flexor hallucis longus may result in the development of intrinsic minus of the hallux (cock-up toe).

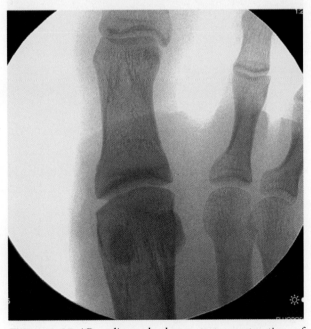

Figure 5–87 AP radiograph demonstrates restoration of proper sesamoid position relative to the metatarsal head.

Objectives: Did you learn...?

- Describe the mechanism of injury for turf toe?
- Describe the relevance of sesamoid retraction?
- Identify indications for surgical repair?
- Discuss reasons for development of intrinsic minus hallux with failed treatment?

CASE 41

Dr. Joshua Lamb

A 31-year-old female presents to your office with increasing pain over the posterior medial ankle and stiffness in the great toe. She works as a professional ballet dancer and complains of increasing pain in the "demi pointe" position. On physical examination, the patient is noted to have decreased motion through the first MTP joint and triggering of the first MTP joint with passive dorsiflexion. Dorsiflexion of the first MTP joint is measured both with the ankle in maximal plantar flexion and in moderate dorsiflexion. A decrease in first MTP motion of 30 degrees is noted when the ankle is brought into dorsiflexion. An MRI of the ankle is obtained (Fig. 5–88).

FHL tenosynovitis can occur at which anatomic location?

A. Posterior ankle
B. Sustentaculum tali

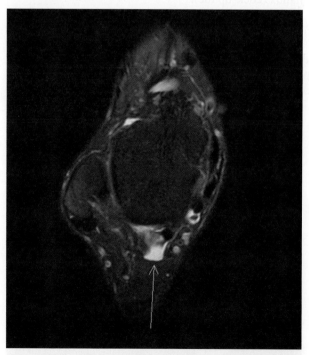

Figure 5–88 Axial T2-weighted MRI showing increased fluid surrounding the FHL tendon (*arrow*), consistent with FHL tenosynovitis.

C. Plantar midfoot
D. Level of the sesamoids
E. All of the above

Discussion

The correct answer is (E). FHL tenosynovitis can occur in four different regions of the foot and ankle. On physical examination, it is important to examine each region to localize the pathology. The muscle belly and musculotendinous region can be palpated at the level of the ankle posterior and lateral to the posterior tibial tendon. FHL tenosynovitis can occur in the setting of posterior ankle impingement associated with a symptomatic os trigonum. Most commonly, FHL tenosynovitis occurs as the tendon enters the fibroosseous canal, which can be palpated inferior to the sustentaculum tali. At the plantar midfoot, at the level of the navicular medial cuneiform articulation, the FHL can be palpated as it traverses the knot of Henry. Distally, FHL tenosynovitis can occur at the level of the sesamoids and the FHL can be palpated plantar to the first metatarsal head.

The patient is diagnosed with FHL tenosynovitis. You initiate conservative treatment with immobilization in a walking boot and physical therapy to focus on FHL stretching. The patient wants to know the success rates of conservative treatment.

True/False: Nonoperative treatment of FHL tenosynovitis is successful 80% of the time?

A. True
B. False

Discussion

The correct answer is (B). The success of nonoperative treatment is low. Failure rates of nonoperative treatment have been reported at 40% to 100%. However, most authors recommend a 6-month trial of nonoperative treatment including rest, immobilization, NSAIDs, and stretching.

The patient fails nonoperative treatment and requires excision of a symptomatic os trigonum and release of the FHL through a posteromedial approach.

What is the intramuscular interval typically used for this approach?

A. Flexor digitorum longus and flexor hallucis longus
B. Flexor hallucis longus and peroneus brevis
C. Tibialis posterior and flexor hallucis longus
D. Peroneus longus and peroneus brevis

Discussion

The correct answer is (A). The posterior medial approach to the ankle is centered over the neurovascular bundle posterior to the medial malleolus. After incising the skin, the fascia and laciniate ligament are split to expose the neurovascular bundle. The bundle is most often retracted posteriorly, protecting the medial calcaneal branch of the tibial nerve. Next the deep aspect of the sheath is released to expose the FHL tendon. At this point, a tenosynovectomy can be performed. The FHL can be retracted posteriorly to gain access to the Os trigonum. This exposure can be extended as needed plantar to the sustentaculum tali to release the fibroosseous tunnel.

Objectives: Did you learn...?

- Describe the physical examination findings for FHL tenosynovitis?
- Identify nonoperative approach to management of FHL tenosynovitis?
- Describe the posterior medial approach to the ankle?

CASE 42

Dr. John Paul Elton

A 28-year-old man falls from a ladder at work from approximately 12 feet, injuring his right ankle. He is taken by ambulance to the emergency room where radiographs of the right ankle are obtained (Fig. 5–89). A closed reduction is attempted in the emergency room.

What is the most likely structure to block a successful closed reduction of the joint?

A. Extensor digitorum brevis muscle
B. Posterior tibial tendon
C. Peroneal tendons
D. Flexor hallucis longus tendon

Discussion

The correct answer is (B). This patient has sustained a closed lateral subtalar dislocation. The vast majority of subtalar dislocations (85%) occur when the calcaneus and remaining foot displace medially, and the talar head is left prominent dorsolaterally. The talar head may even buttonhole through the extensor digitorum brevis muscle/tendon unit leaving that structure and the capsule of the talonavicular joint to interpose between the talus and navicular blocking a successful attempt at closed reduction. The lateral subtalar dislocation is more likely to have the reduction attempt blocked by an interposed posterior tibial tendon or flexor digitorum longus tendon.

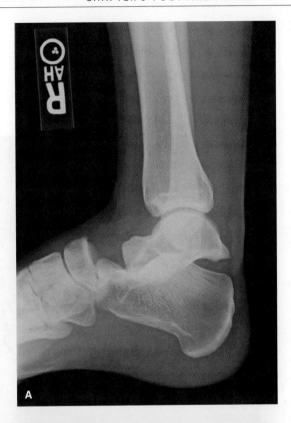

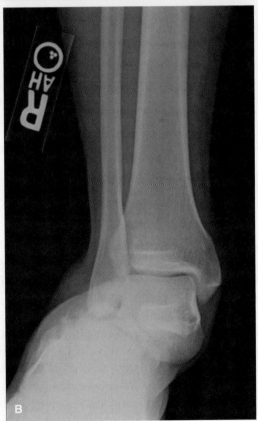

Figure 5–89 **A:** Lateral ankle radiograph. **B:** AP ankle radiograph.

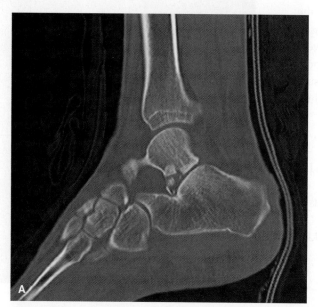
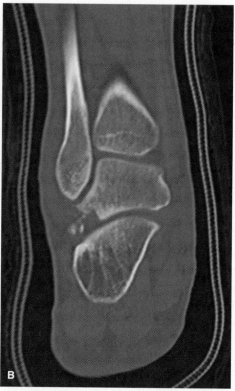

Figure 5–90 A: Sagittal CT reconstruction of the ankle after reduction showing fracture of the lateral process of the talus with fragmentation. **B:** Coronal CT reconstruction of the ankle after reduction.

The joint is successfully reduced and splinted in the ER and the patient is now comfortable, without any signs of compartment syndrome or open wounds.

What is the most appropriate next step in treatment?

A. Measurement of ankle brachial index (ABI)
B. Referral for ligament reconstruction
C. Referral to physical therapy
D. CT scan of the ankle

Discussion

The correct answer is (D). A postreduction CT scan (Fig. 5–90) is recommended to evaluate for congruency of the joints, incarcerated bone fragments in the subtalar and talonavicular joints, and associated fractures. Vascular compromise is not a frequent complication in subtalar dislocation, and the ABI is measured above the most significant zone of injury. The ligaments about the subtalar joint are significantly injured in a subtalar dislocation, but stiffness, rather than instability, is a more common sequela of the injury. The patient will likely benefit from therapy to combat stiffness, but the postreduction CT scan is more appropriate in the acute setting.

Objectives: Did you learn...?

• Describe which structures often block reduction of a subtalar dislocation?
• Discuss the importance of a CT scan after reduction?

BIBLIOGRAPHY

Case 1

Ahmed IM, Lagopoulos M, McConnell P, Soames RW, Sefton GK. Blood supply of the Achilles tendon. *J Orthop Res.* 1998;16(5):591–596.

Bhattacharyya M, Gerber B. Mini-invasive surgical repair of the Achilles tendon—does it reduce post-operative morbidity? *Int Orthop.* 2009;33(1):151–156.

Huston KA. Achilles tendinitis and tendon rupture due to fluoroquinolone antibiotics. *N Engl J Med.* 1994;331(11):748.

Willits K, Amendola A, Bryant D. Operative versus nonoperative treatment of acute Achilles tendon ruptures: a multicenter randomized trial using accelerated functional rehabilitation. *J Bone Joint Surg Am.* 2010;92(17):2767–2775.

Case 2

Robinson AH, Limbers JP. Modern concepts in the treatment of hallux valgus. *J Bone Joint Surg Br.* 2005;87(8):1038–1045.

Case 3

Aktas S, Sussman MD. The radiological analysis of pes cavus deformity in Charcot Marie Tooth disease. *J Pediatr Orthop B*. 2000;9(2):137–140.

Boyer MI. *AAOS Comprehensive Orthopaedic Review 2*. Rosemont, IL: American Academy of Orthopaedic Surgeons, Copyright; 2014:687–689.

Franco AH. Pes Cavus and Pes Planus Analyses and Treatment. *Phys Ther*. 1987;67(5):688–694.

Case 4

Boyer MI. *AAOS Comprehensive Orthopaedic Review 2*. Rosemont, IL: American Academy of Orthopaedic Surgeons, Copyright; 2014:1469–1470.

Goldman FD, Siegel J, Barton E. Extensor hallucis longus tendon transfer for correction of hallux varus. *J Foot Ankle Surg*. 1993;32(2):126–131.

Skalley TC, Myerson MS. The operative treatment of acquired hallux varus. *Clin Orthop Relat Res*. 1994;(306):183–191.

Turner RS. Dynamic post-surgical hallux varus after lateral sesamoidectomy: treatment and prevention. *Orthopedics*. 1986;9(7):963–969.

Case 5

Boyer MI. *AAOS Comprehensive Orthopaedic Review 2*. Rosemont, IL: American Academy of Orthopaedic Surgeons, Copyright; 2014:464–466.

Buckley R, Tough S, McCormack R, et al. Operative compared with nonoperative treatment of displaced intra-articular calcaneal fractures a prospective, randomized, controlled multicenter trial. *J Bone Joint Surg Am*. 2002;84-A(10):1733–1744.

Rammelt S, Zwipp H. Calcaneus fractures: facts, controversies and recent developments. *Injury*. 2004;35(5):443–461.

Case 6

Cockshott S, Hayward K, Grimer R. Synovial sarcoma of the foot. *J Bone Joint Sur, Br Vol*. 2011;93(Supp III):315–316.

Ozdemir HM, Yildiz Y, Yilmaz C, Saglik Y. Tumors of the foot and ankle: analysis 196 cases. *J Foot Ankle Surg*. 1997;36(6):403–408.

Zindrick MR, Young MP, Daley RJ, Light TR. Metastatic tumors of the foot: case report and literature review. *Clin Orthop Relat Res*. 1982;(170):219–225.

Case 7

Boyer MI. *AAOS Comprehensive Orthopaedic Review 2*. Rosemont, IL: American Academy of Orthopaedic Surgeons, Copyright; 2014:1451–1452.

Boyer MI. *AAOS Comprehensive Orthopaedic Review 2*. Rosemont, IL: American Academy of Orthopaedic Surgeons, Copyright; 2014:1504–1505.

Myerson MS. The diagnosis and treatment of injury to the tarsometatarsal joint complex. *J Bone Joint Surg Br*. 1999;81(5):756–763.

Rao S, Baumhauer JF, Becica L, Nawoczenski DA. Shoe inserts alter plantar loading and function in patients with midfoot arthritis. *J Orthop Sports Phys Ther*. 2009;39(7):522–531.

Case 8

Boyer MI. *AAOS Comprehensive Orthopaedic Review 2*. Rosemont, IL: American Academy of Orthopaedic Surgeons, Copyright; 2014:1499–1501.

Kitaoka HB, Crevoisier XM, Harbst K, Hansen D, Kotajarvi B, Kaufman K. The effect of custom-made braces for the ankle and hindfoot on ankle and foot kinematics and ground reaction forces. *Arch Phys Med Rehabil*. 2006;87(1):130–135.

Martin RL, Stewart GW, Conti SF. Posttraumatic ankle arthritis: an update on conservative and surgical management. *J Orthop Sports Phys Ther*. 2007;37(5):253–259.

Scranton PE Jr. An overview of ankle arthrodesis. *Clin Orthop Relat Res*. 1991;(268):96–101.

Thomas RH, Daniels TR. Current concepts review: ankle arthritis. *J Bone Joint Surg Am*. 2003;85-A(5):923–936.

Case 9

Abdo RV, Iorio LJ. Rheumatoid arthritis of the foot and ankle. *J Am Acad Orthop Surg*. 1994;2:326–332.

Cannada LK. *Orthopaedic Knowledge Update 11*. Rosemont, IL: American Academy of Orthopaedic Surgeons, Copyright; 2014:645–646.

Karbowski A, Schwitalle M, Eckhardt A. Arthroplasty of the forefoot in rheumatoid arthritis: long-term results after Clayton procedure. *Acta Orthop Belg*. 1998;64(4):401–405.

Case 10

Coughlin MJ. Common causes of pain in the forefoot in adults. *J Bone Joint Surg Br*. 2000;82(6):781–790.

Coughlin MJ. Treatment of bunionette deformity with longitudinal diaphyseal osteotomy with distal soft tissue repair. *Foot Ankle*. 1991;11(4):195–203.

Case 11

Alshami AM, Souvlis T, Coppieters MW. A review of plantar heel pain of neural origin: differential diagnosis and management. *Man Ther*. 2008;13(2):103–111.

Baxter DE, Pfeffer GB. Treatment of chronic heel pain by surgical release of the first branch of the lateral plantar nerve. *Clin Orthop Relat Res*. 1992;(279):229–236.

Cannada LK. *Orthopaedic Knowledge Update 11*. Rosemont, IL: American Academy of Orthopaedic Surgeons, Copyright; 2014:52–65.

Case 12

Fronek J, Mubarak SJ, Hargens AR, et al. Management of chronic exertional anterior compartment syndrome of the lower extremity. *Clin Orthop Relat Res*. 1987;(220):217–227.

Rorabeck CH, Fowler PJ, Nott L. The results of fasciotomy in the management of chronic exertional compartment syndrome. *Am J Sports Med*. 1988;16(3):224–227.

Wilder RP, Magrum E. Exertional compartment syndrome. *Clin Sports Med*. 2010;29(3):429–435.

Case 13

Mann RA, Clanton TO. Hallux rigidus: treatment by cheilectomy. *J Bone Joint Surg Am*. 1988;70(3):400–406.

Yee G, Lau J. Current concepts review: hallux rigidus. *Foot Ankle Int.* 2008;29(6):637–646.

Case 14

Armstrong DG, Lavery LA, Harkless LB. Validation of a diabetic wound classification system: the contribution of depth, infection, and ischemia to risk of amputation. *Diabetes Care.* 1998;21(5):855–859.

Lipsky BA, Berendt AR, Deery HG, et al. Diagnosis and treatment of diabetic foot infections. *Clin Infect Dis.* 2004; 39(7):885–910.

Pinney SJ, Sangeorzan BJ, Hansen ST Jr. Surgical anatomy of the gastrocnemius recession (Strayer procedure). *Foot Ankle Int.* 2004;25(4):247–250.

Case 15

Cannada LK. *Orthopaedic Knowledge Update 11.* Rosemont, IL: American Academy of Orthopaedic Surgeons, Copyright; 2014:650–651.

DiPaola M, Raikin SM. Tendon transfers and realignment osteotomies for treatment of stage II posterior tibial tendon dysfunction. *Foot Ankle Clin.* 2007;12(2):273–285.

Mizel MS, Temple HT, Scranton PE Jr. Role of the peroneal tendons in the production of the deformed foot with posterior tibial tendon deficiency. *Foot Ankle Int.* 1999; 20(5):285–289.

Case 16

Cracchiolo A 3rd. Rheumatoid arthritis: hindfoot disease. *Clin Orthop Relat Res.* 1997;(340):58–68.

Kindsfater K, Wilson MG, Thomas WH. Management of the rheumatoid hindfoot with special reference to talonavicular arthrodesis. *Clin Orthop Relat Res.* 1997;(340):69–74.

Wülker N, Stukenborg C, Savory KM, Alfke D. Hindfoot motion after isolated and combined arthrodeses: measurements in anatomic specimens. *Foot Ankle Int.* 2000; 21(11):921–927.

Case 17

Aluisio FV, Mair SD, Hall RL. Plantar fibromatosis: treatment of primary and recurrent lesions and factors associated with recurrence. *Foot Ankle Int.* 1996;17(11):672–678.

Sammarco GJ, Mangone PG. Classification and treatment of plantar fibromatosis. *Foot Ankle Int.* 2000;21(7):563–569.

Case 18

Chisin R, Peyser A, Milgrom C. Bone scintigraphy in the assessment of the hallucal sesamoids. *Foot Ankle Int.* 1995; 16(5):291–294.

Cohen BE. Hallux sesamoid disorders. *Foot Ankle Clin.* 2009; 14(1):91–104.

Richardson EG. Hallucal sesamoid pain: causes and surgical treatment. *J Am Acad Orthop Surg.* 1999;7:270–278.

Case 19

Bluman EM, Myerson MS. Stage IV posterior tibial tendon rupture. *Foot Ankle Clin.* 2007;12(2):341–362.

Deland JT, de Asla RJ, Sung IH, Ernberg LA, Potter HG. Posterior tibial tendon insufficiency: which ligaments are involved? *Foot Ankle Int.* 2005;26(6):427–435.

Myerson MS. Instructional Course Lectures, The American Academy of Orthopaedic Surgeons-Adult Acquired Flatfoot Deformity. Treatment of Dysfunction of the Posterior Tibial Tendon. *J Bone Joint Sur.* 1996;78(5):780–792.

Case 20

Fortin PT, Balazsy JE. Talus fractures: evaluation and treatment. 2001;9:114–127.

Hawkins LG. Fractures of the neck of the talus. *J Bone Joint Surg Am.* 1970;52:991–1002.

Vallier HA, Nork SE, Barei DP, Benirschke SK, Sangeorgzan BJ. Talar neck fractures: results and outcomes. *J Bone Joint Surg Am.* 2004;86-A(8):1616–1624.

Case 21

Maffulli N. Current Concepts Review-Rupture of the Achilles Tendon. *J Bone Joint Surg Am.* 1999;81(7):1019–1036.

Tashjian RZ, Hur J, Sullivan RJ, Campbell JT, DiGiovanni CW. Flexor hallucis longus transfer for repair of chronic Achilles tendinopathy. *Foot Ankle Int.* 2003;24(9):673–676.

Willets K, Amendola A, Bryant D, et al. Operative versus nonoperative treatment of acute achilles rupture. *J Bone Joint Surg Am.* 2010;92:2767–2775.

Case 22

Alexander IJ, Johnson KA. Assessment and management of pes cavus in Charcot-Marie-Tooth disease. *Clin Orthop Relat Res.* 1989;(246):273–281.

Guyton GP. Current concepts review: orthopaedic aspects of Charcot-Marie-Tooth disease. *Foot Ankle Int.* 2006; 27(11): 1003–1010.

Reilly MM, Murphy SM, Laurá M. Charcot-Marie-Tooth disease. *J Peripher Nerv Syst.* 2011;16(1):1–14.

Case 23

Baxter DE, Pfeffer GB. Treatment of chronic heel pain by surgical release of the first branch of the lateral plantar nerve. *Clin Orthop Relat Res.* 1992;(279):229–236.

Frey C, Kerr R. Magnetic resonance imaging and the evaluation of tarsal tunnel syndrome. *Foot Ankle.* 1993;14(3):159–164.

Sammarco GJ, Cooper PS. Flexor hallucis longus tendon injury in dancers and nondancers. *Foot Ankle Int.* 1998;19(6):356–362.

Case 24

Bhutta MA, Chauhan D, Zubairy AI, Barrie J. Second metatarsophalangeal joint instability and second metatarsal length association depends on the method of measurement. *Foot Ankle Int.* 2010;31(6):486–491.

Shirzad K, Kiesau CD, DeOrio JK, Parekh SG. Lesser toe deformities. *J Am Acad Orthop Surg.* 2011;19(8):505–514.

Case 25

Neufeld SK, Cerrate R. Plantar fasciitis: evaluation and treatment. *J Am Acad Orthop Surg.* 2018;16:338–346.

Case 26

Bilton BD, Zibari GB, McMillan RW, Aultman DF, Dunn G, McDonald JC. Aggressive surgical management of necrotizing fasciitis serves to decrease mortality: a retrospective study. *Am Surg*. 1998;64(5):397–400.

Brook I, Frazier EH. Clinical and microbiological features of necrotizing fasciitis. *J Clin Microbiol*. 1995;33(9):2382–2387.

Courvalin P. Vancomycin resistance in gram-positive cocci. *Clin Infect Dis*. 2006;42(Suppl 1):S25–S34.

Escobar SJ, Slade JB Jr, Hunt TK, Cianci P. Adjuvant hyperbaric oxygen therapy (HBO2) for treatment of necrotizing fasciitis reduces mortality and amputation rate. *Undersea Hyperb Med*. 2005;32(6):437–443.

Stevens DL, Wallace RJ, Hamilton SM, Bryant AE. Successful treatment of staphylococcal toxic shock syndrome with linezolid: a case report and in vitro evaluation of the production of toxic shock syndrome toxin type 1 in the presence of antibiotics. *Clin Infect Dis*. 2006;42(5):729–730.

Wong CH, Khin LW, Heng KS, Tan KC, Low CO. The LRINEC (Laboratory Risk Indicator for Necrotizing Fasciitis) score: A tool for distinguishing necrotizing fasciitis from other soft tissue infections. *Crit Care Med*. 2004;32(7):1535–1541.

Case 27

Beals TC, Pomeroy GC, Manoli A 2nd. Posterior tendon insufficiency: diagnosis and treatment. *J Am Acad Orthop Surg*. 1999;7(2):112–118.

Cannada LK. *Orthopaedic Knowledge Update 11*. Rosemont, IL: American Academy of Orthopaedic Surgeons, Copyright; 2014:651.

Deland JT, Page A, Sung IH, O'Malley MJ, Inda D, Choung S. Posterior tibial tendon insufficiency results at different stages. *HSS J*. 2006;2(2):157–160.

Malicky ES, Crary JL, Houghton MJ, Agel J, Hansen ST Jr, Sangeorzan BJ. Talocalcaneal and subfibular impingement in symptomatic flatfoot in adults. *J Bone Joint Surg Am*. 2002;84-A(11):2005–2009.

Case 28

Cannada LK. *Orthopaedic Knowledge Update 11*. Rosemont, IL: American Academy of Orthopaedic Surgeons, Copyright; 2014:635–636.

Sangeorzan BJ, Benirschke SK, Mosca V, Mayo KA, Hansen ST Jr. Displaced intra-articular fractures of the tarsal navicular. *J Bone Joint Surg Am*. 1989;71(10):1504–1510.

Case 29

Drez D Jr, Guhl JF, Gollehon DL. Ankle arthroscopy: technique and indications. *Foot Ankle*. 1981;2(3):138–143.

Ferkel RD, Heath DD, Guhl JF. Neurological complications of ankle arthroscopy. *Arthroscopy*. 1996;12(2):200–208.

van Dijk CN, Scholte D. Arthroscopy of the ankle joint. *Arthroscopy*. 1997;13(1):90–96.

Case 30

Llauger J, Palmer J, Monill JM, Franquet T, Bagué S, Rosón N. MR imaging of benign soft-tissue masses of the foot and ankle. *Radiographics*. 1998;18(6):1481–1498.

Lucas DR. Tenosynovial giant cell tumor: case report and review. *Arch Pathol Lab Med*. 2012;136(8):901–906.

Rozbruch SR, Chang V, Bohne WH, Deland JT. Ganglion cysts of the lower extremity: an analysis of 54 cases and review of the literature. *Orthopedics*. 1998;21(2):141–148.

Case 31

Alfredson H. Conservative management of Achilles tendinopathy: new ideas. *Foot Ankle Clin*. 2005;10(2):321–329.

Richardson DR, Willers J, Cohen BE, Davis WH, Jones CP, Anderson RB. Evaluation of the hallux morbidity of single-incision flexor hallucis longus tendon transfer. *Foot Ankle Int*. 2009;30(7):627–630.

van der Linden PD, Sturkenboom MC, Herings RM, Leufkens HG, Stricker BH. Fluoroquinolones and risk of Achilles tendon disorders: case-control study. *BMJ*. 2002;324(7349):1306–1307.

Case 32

Cannada LK. *Orthopaedic Knowledge Update 11*. Rosemont, IL: American Academy of Orthopaedic Surgeons, Copyright; 2014:633–635.

Sanders R. Current concepts review – displaced intra-articular fractures of the calcaneus. *J Bone Joint Surg Am*. 2000;82:225–250.

Case 33

Boyer MI. *AAOS Comprehensive Orthopaedic Review 2*. Rosemont, IL: American Academy of Orthopaedic Surgeons, Copyright; 2014:1549–1552.

Cannada LK. *Orthopaedic Knowledge Update 11*. Rosemont, IL: American Academy of Orthopaedic Surgeons, Copyright; 2014:219.

Laurinaviciene R, Kirketerp-Moeller K, Holstein PE. Exostectomy for chronic midfoot plantar ulcer in Charcot deformity. *J Wound Care*. 2008;17(2):53–55, 57–58.

van der Ven A, Chapman CB, Bowker JH. Charcot neuroarthropathy of the foot and ankle. *J Am Acad Orthop Surg*. 2009;17:562–571.

Case 34

Chou L. *AAOS Orthopaedic Knowledge Update 5: Foot and Ankle*. Rosemont, IL: American Academy of Orthopaedic Surgeons, Copyright; 2014:183–189.

Donley BG. Acquired hallux varus. *Foot Ankle Int*. 1997;18(9):586–592.

Case 35

Bennett GL, Graham CE, Mauldin DM. Morton's interdigital neuroma: a comprehensive treatment protocol. *Foot Ankle Int*. 1995;16(12):760–763.

Graham CE, Graham DM. Morton's neuroma: a microscopic evaluation. *Foot Ankle*. 1984;5(3):150–153.

Case 36

Boyer MI. *AAOS Comprehensive Orthopaedic Review 2*. Rosemont, IL: American Academy of Orthopaedic Surgeons, Copyright; 2014:1546–1548.

Cannada LK. *Orthopaedic Knowledge Update 11*. Rosemont, IL: American Academy of Orthopaedic Surgeons, Copyright; 2014:640.

Malhotra R, Chan CS, Nather A. Osteomyelitis in the diabetic foot. *Diabet Foot Ankle*. 2014;5.

Case 37

Den Hartog BD. Fracture of the proximal fifth metatarsal. *J Am Acad Orthop Surg*. 2009;17:458–464.

Lawrence SJ, Botte MJ. Jones' fractures and related fractures of the proximal fifth metatarsal. *Foot Ankle*. 1993;14(6):358–365.

Porter DA, Duncan M, Meyer SJ. Fifth Metatarsal Jones Fracture Fixation With a 4.5-mm Cannulated Stainless Steel Screw in the Competitive and Recreational Athlete A Clinical and Radiographic Evaluation. *Am J Sports Med*. 2005;33(5):726–733.

Case 38

Boyer MI. *AAOS Comprehensive Orthopaedic Review 2*. Rosemont, IL: American Academy of Orthopaedic Surgeons, Copyright; 2014:468.

Cohen BE, Nicholson CW. Bunionette deformity. *J Am Acad Orthop Surg*. 2007;15:300–307.

Case 39

Ly TV, Coetzee JC. Treatment of primary ligamentous lisfranc joint injuries: primary arthrodesis compared with open reduction and internal fixation. *J Bone Joint Surg Am*. 2006;88-A(3):514–520.

Thompson MC, Mormino MA. Injury to the tarsometatarsal joint complex. *J Am Acad Ortho Surg*. 2003;11:260–267.

Case 40

Anderson RB. Turf toe injuries of the hallux metatarsophalangeal joint. *Tech Foot Ankle Surg*. 2002;1(2):102–111.

McCormick JJ, Anderson RB. The great toe: failed turf toe, chronic turf toe, and complicated sesamoid injuries. *Foot Ankle Clin*. 2009;14(2):135–150.

McCormick JJ, Anderson RB. Turf Toe Anatomy, Diagnosis, and Treatment. *Sports Health*. 2010;2(6):487–494.

Rodeo SA, O'Brien S, Warren RF, Barnes R, Wickiewicz TL, Dillingham MF. Turf-toe: an analysis of metatarsophalangeal joint sprains in professional football players. *Am J Sports Med*. 1990;18(3):280–285.

Case 41

Michelson J, Dunn L. Tenosynovitis of the flexor hallucis longus: a clinical study of the spectrum of presentation and treatment. *Foot Ankle Int*. 2005;26(4):291–303.

Case 42

Mulroy RD. The tibialis posterior tendon as an obstacle to reduction of a lateral anterior subtalar dislocation. *J Bone Joint Surg Am*. 1955;37-A(4):859–863.

Perugia D, Basile A, Massoni C, Gumina S, Rossi F, Ferretti A. Conservative treatment of subtalar dislocations. *Int Orthop*. 2002;26(1):56–60.

6

Trauma

Daniel J. Stinner

CASE 1

Dr. Christina M. Hylden

You are the sole provider in a small rural hospital when a 56-year-old female is brought in after a MVC rollover. The patient is brought on a backboard in a cervical collar by EMS who reports a prolonged extrication. She has an obviously deformed left thigh and is bleeding from a scalp wound.

What is the first step in assessing the patient upon arrival?

A. Put direct pressure on the scalp wound.

B. Have someone apply direct in-line traction to the left lower extremity to stabilize the fracture.

C. Call the closest trauma center to prepare for transport of the patient.

D. Ask the patient to state her name.

Discussion

The correct answer is (D). ATLS principles should be followed in surgical management such as this. Although all of the answers are actions that are likely to be taken, the first priority is to assess the patient's airway. This can quickly be done by asking her to state her name. As she answers, you know that her airway is patent, and she is alert enough to follow directions.

On the same patient, you get a set of vitals which shows her blood pressure at 90/40, heart rate 120, and pulse-ox of 99%. She has a GCS of 14, and you note that she appears drowsy and confused, leading you to be concerned for hemorrhagic shock.

What amount of blood loss has she most likely sustained?

A. 10%

B. 25%

C. 40%

D. 55%

Discussion

The correct answer is (C). Class I hemorrhage is when there is a loss of <15% blood volume. This is equivalent to donating a unit of blood and usually shows no systemic cardiovascular changes. Class II hemorrhage is a loss of between 15% and 30% blood volume. At that point, tachycardia is seen, but most people are able to sustain a normal blood pressure. Class III hemorrhage, 30% to 40%, is when systolic blood pressure drops, which is where our patient is in this example. More blood loss than this is Class IV hemorrhage, and the patient is considered on the verge of dying unless drastic measures are taken immediately.

What is the most appropriate fluid resuscitation to initiate at this time?

A. Give 1 L of crystalloid at 200 cc/hr.

B. Administer 2 L of crystalloid as a fluid bolus. Alert the blood bank for possible transfusion needs.

C. Give 1 unit PRBCs now, alert the blood bank to start bringing platelets and plasma.

D. Monitor her urine output and administer fluid to keep UOP at 1 to 2 cc/kg/hr.

Discussion

The correct answer is (B). The standard ATLS protocol includes giving 2 L of warmed crystalloid fluid prior to initiating blood transfusions. However, when transfusions are expected, the blood bank should be alerted soon in the process with an initiation of a massive transfusion protocol as allowed by your facility. Using urine output is appropriate for maintaining fluids but not during an initial trauma resuscitation.

Objectives: Did you learn...?

- Principles of ATLS?
- Classes of hemorrhagic shock?

CASE 2

Dr. Christina M. Hylden

A 19-year-old male ranch-hand was accidently shot in the left leg while pursuing a coyote. His coworker fired, and the bullet ricocheted before striking him in the thigh.

If the patient sustained a fracture that did not require surgical stabilization, a gunshot wound from which of the following weapons likely does NOT need to be treated surgically as an open fracture, i.e., does not need to undergo operative debridement?

A.   8-mm round shot from a pistol
B.   277 hunting rifle
C.   "Buckshot" from a shotgun at 12 ft
D.   22 caliber bullet from an M16

Discussion

The correct answer is (A). Gunshot fractures caused by low-velocity weapons do not need to be treated surgically unless the fracture itself requires operative fixation. Low-velocity weapons include most handguns (except magnums) and any weapon with a muzzle velocity <350 m/s. Hunting rifles and military rifles (such as the M16) have muzzle velocities >600 m/s and are high-velocity weapons. A shotgun, regardless of the type of shot used, is an intermediate velocity, and the level of energy imparted to the patient depends on the range from which it was shot. Close range for a shotgun is anything less than 21 ft.

Upon examination of the patient, it is noted that he has an entrance wound proximal and lateral to the superior pole of the patella and no exit wound. His radiographs show a stable fracture of the lateral femoral condyle and a retained bullet fragment within the soft tissues adjacent to the distal femur. From the history, the patient believes he was shot with a handgun.

What is the next step in management?

A.   Local wound care, IV antibiotics, knee immobilizer
B.   Load the knee with up to 155 cc of sterile saline
C.   Surgical debridement of the wound with removal of retained bullet
D.   Immediate surgical debridement with open reduction and internal fixation of the bone fragment

Discussion

The correct answer is (B). In this case, you need more information before deciding on the definitive plan of care. Since the wound was caused by a low-velocity weapon, it may not need to go to the operating room. Local wound care may be appropriate, but due to the proximity of the wound to the knee, you need to determine if there is an open joint first. If the saline load test is positive, then irrigation of the knee is the next appropriate step. The question stem states that the fracture is stable, and therefore does not need immediate open reduction and internal fixation. Also, if the bullet is retained in the muscle and not in the joint, it does not necessarily need to be removed.

Which of the following statements regarding retained bullets is true?

A.   A bullet fragment in the superior patella does not need to be removed.
B.   A bullet that passed through the abdomen and is located in the vertebral body of L1 should be surgically removed.
C.   A bullet with a posterior entrance wound and located in the spinal canal at L3 with weak knee extension should be excised.
D.   A bullet with viscous penetration before lodging in the ilium should be excised with copious irrigation.

Discussion

The correct answer is (C). Any intra-articular retained metallic fragment should be removed due to risk of plumbism. Bullets that pass through abdominal organs before going into bone, such as the spine and ilium, do not require removal if the associated fractures are stable. A 7- to 14-day course of IV antibiotics to cover intestinal bacteria is the preferred treatment unless the fractures require fixation. However, if there is a retained bullet in the spinal cord and a corresponding incomplete motor deficit, surgical excision of the fragment is indicated.

Objectives: Did you learn...?

- The difference in management of high-velocity and low-velocity gunshot wounds?

- The treatment of various gunshot injuries depending on the course of the missile or the location of the retained fragment?

CASE 3

Dr. Christina M. Hylden

A 19-year-old male is brought in after an ATV accident when he was off-roading on his grandparent's farm. He has an obvious deformity to the right tibia with exposed bone visualized through a 12-cm open wound and gross organic contamination.

According to the Gustillo–Anderson classification of open fractures, which of the following is INCORRECT?

A. The difference between Types I, II, and III is related to wound size.
B. The difference between Types IIIA, IIIB, and IIIC is related to contamination.
C. Both Type II and IIIA injuries can be covered with local muscle and skin.
D. Type II injuries include comminution of the bone.

Discussion

The correct answer is (B). The different categories within Type III are delineated by soft tissue coverage needs as well as vascular status of the extremity as shown in Table 6–1.

What is the most appropriate antibiotic prophylaxis for the patient upon presentation?

A. First-generation cephalosporin
B. Cephalosporin and an aminoglycoside
C. Cefezolin, gentamicin, and penicillin
D. Clindamycin, gentamicin

Table 6–1   GUSTILO FRACTURES

Type	Subtype	Definition
I		Low energy with <1 cm wound
II		Low to moderate energy with >1 cm wound size
III	A	High energy with severe bony comminution or segmental fracture
	B	Wound with exposed bone that requires soft tissue coverage
	C	Any open fracture with arterial damage that requires repair

Discussion

The correct answer is (C). Because this patient has a large wound which is most likely to be a Type III and was injured on a farm, antibiotic prophylaxis should include coverage of gram-positive, gram-negative, and anaerobic bacteria. In addition, the patient should be given tetanus prophylaxis. However, there is a growing body of evidence that a second-generation cephalosporin only is adequate antibiotic prophylaxis for the majority of open fractures.

For the initial irrigation and debridement, which of the following options is most appropriate for this patient?

A. At least 12 L of fluid on high-pressure
B. 3 L of fluid and placement of an antibiotic pouch
C. 6 L of fluid that includes a soapy material
D. Low-pressure saline, 9 L

Discussion

The correct answer is (D). At least 3 L should be used for irrigation for each Gustillo–Anderson type, meaning that a Type III should be irrigated with a minimum of 9 L of fluid, and a Type I and Type II open fracture, 3 L and 6 L, respectively. The most effective lavage to reduce bacterial count is low-pressure, and it does not matter if there is soap or antibiotics in the fluid as long as there is enough volume, and the irrigation is accompanied by a thorough debridement of foreign material and dead tissue.

Objectives: Did you learn...?

- The Gusillo–Anderson classification system of open fractures?
- Optimal method of irrigation when performing a debridement and irrigation of open fractures?

CASE 4

Dr. Christina M. Hylden

A 20-year-old, male, college football player tackled a fellow teammate in practice and had subsequent pain and decreased range of motion to the left shoulder. He was brought to the ED to be assessed the same day and notices that he is having trouble breathing when asked to lie supine on the gurney. His shoulder radiographs are negative for fracture or glenohumeral dislocation, and based on physical examination, you suspect a sternoclavicular dislocation.

What imaging study is preferred to make this diagnosis?

A. Bilateral clavicle AP
B. Plain film of clavicle with beam aimed at a 40-degree cephalic tilt
C. CT scan
D. MRI

Discussion

The correct answer is (C). Sternoclavicular dislocations, both anterior and posterior, are difficult to visualize on plain films. The serendipity view (beam at 40 degrees cephalic tilt) can help, but CT scan is still the preferred modality. The benefits of a CT scan include determining direction of dislocation, differentiation from a physeal fracture in patients less than 25 years of age, and can visualize mediastinal structures and associated injuries or compromise that should be addressed. MRI in an acute setting does not contribute any additional information for immediate treatment and takes longer to obtain.

You are concerned for a posterior sternoclavicular dislocation in this patient. All of the following is a physical finding related to a posterior dislocation but not an anterior dislocation EXCEPT:

A. Tachypnea
B. Decreased range of motion (ROM) of upper extremity
C. Stridor
D. Venous congestion in upper extremity

Discussion

The correct answer is (B). Decreased ROM due to pain can happen with a sternoclavicular dislocation in either direction. The main physical finding with an anterior dislocation is a palpable prominence at the joint which increases with abduction and elevation. A posterior dislocation happens when the clavicle moves posterior to the sternum. This can result in compression of mediastinal structures to include the bronchus (stridor and shortness of breath, especially when supine), the recurrent laryngeal nerve (dysphagia), the brachiocephalic vein (venous congestion), brachiocephalic artery (diminished pulses compared to contralateral side), and the brachial plexus (paresthesias). All of these physical examination findings should be looked for as they are included in the indications for surgical intervention.

What is the most important structure for sternoclavicular anterior–posterior stability?

A. Posterior capsular ligament
B. Anterior sternoclavicular ligament
C. Rhomboid ligament
D. Intra-articular disk ligament

Discussion

The correct answer is (A). This ligament is the primary restraint to AP displacement. The anterior sternoclavicular ligament is the primary restraint to superior displacement of the clavicle. The rhomboid ligament is also called the costoclavicular ligament and prevents rotational and medial/lateral displacement with two fascicles. The intra-articular disk ligament prevents medial and superior displacement of the clavicle.

After imaging and physical examination are complete, it is determined that our patient has a posterior sternoclavicular displacement. Physical examination findings are notable only for decreased ROM of the left shoulder and dyspnea when lying supine.

What is the optimal treatment for this patient?

A. Medial clavicle excision
B. Sling for comfort, referral to physical therapy for range of motion, and instructions to sleep in a recliner until dyspnea improves
C. Closed reduction under general anesthesia with or without thoracic surgery
D. Open reduction and soft tissue reconstruction with thoracic surgery backup

Discussion

The correct answer is (D). Since this patient is experiencing shortness of breath, he should have surgery to relieve the pressure. This will need to be done open with a plan for reconstruction or other internal fixation to maintain a stable joint. Because of the mediastinal compromise, this should not be attempted without thoracic surgery backup available. Another indication for immediate open reduction is decreased peripheral pulses in the affected upper extremity. A medial clavicle excision is a treatment for chronic or recurrent sternoclavicular dislocations. Sling and physical therapy are treatment options for atraumatic subluxations or chronic dislocations (>3 weeks). Acute (<3 weeks) anterior and posterior sternoclavicular dislocations that are not associated with neurovascular or mediastinal compromise can have an attempted closed reduction.

Objectives: Did you learn...?

- Diagnosis of sternoclavicular joint dislocations?
- Treatment of sternoclavicular joint dislocations?

CASE 5

Dr. Christina M. Hylden

A 32-year-old, right-hand-dominant male who works as a rancher fell off his horse onto an outstretched left upper extremity with immediate pain and deformity to his left clavicle. He presents later the same day. His injury radiograph is shown in Figure 6–1.

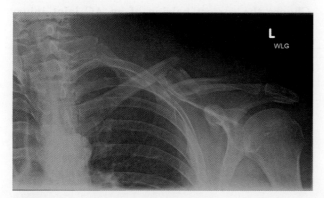

Figure 6–1

How would this fracture be classified?

A. Neer classification Type IIB
B. Group I, complete displacement
C. Group II, Type IIB
D. Group III, anterior displacement

Discussion

The correct answer is (B). Clavicle fractures are first placed into a group by location of the fracture. Group I fractures occur in the middle third of the clavicle. These are the most commonly encountered (80–85%) and are further classified as completely displaced with >100% displacement versus minimally or incompletely displaced when there is still some bone overlap between the main medial and lateral fragments. Group II clavicle fractures occur in the lateral third and are further classified using the Neer classification for Types I through V. Medial third fractures are Group III and are further defined by either anterior or posterior displacement.

Indications to perform open reduction with internal fixation for a middle-third clavicle fracture include all of the following EXCEPT:

A. Skin compromise over the fracture site
B. Displaced fracture with 2.5 cm of shortening
C. Ipsilateral scapular neck fracture
D. Asymptomatic nonunion

Discussion

The correct answer is (D). Nonunions are not uncommon with nonoperative treatment (4.5% of completely displaced middle-third fractures), but unless symptomatic, are not an indication for surgical intervention. Taut skin over a bony prominence which decreases blood blow to the skin can lead to a closed fracture becoming an open fracture and should be addressed in a timely fashion. Midshaft clavicle fractures with severe shortening (>2 cm) are likely to lead to a nonunion and may change shoulder kinematics if the fracture is untreated and left in this shortened position. A scapular neck fracture on the same side as a clavicle fracture is a floating shoulder, and stability of the suspensory shoulder complex should be restored for best chance of return to function. Other relative indications for operative treatment include inability to self-protect (closed head injury, seizure disorder), brachial plexus injury, and a polytrauma patient.

After discussion of management options, the patient chooses to proceed with operative treatment. The postoperative radiograph is shown in Figure 6–2.

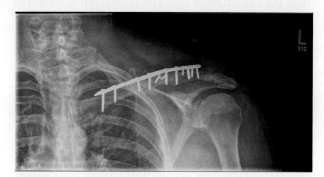

Figure 6–2

Which of the following statements is true in regard to operative options?

A. Intramedullary screw fixation has a lower complication rate than plate and screw fixation.
B. Superior plating has a higher rate of soft tissue irritation than anterior plating.
C. Anterior plating is biomechanically stronger than superior plating.
D. Anterior plating has a higher risk of neurovascular injury during placement than superior plating.

Discussion

The correct answer is (B). Studies demonstrate that approximately 30% of patients with plate and screw fixation request hardware removal due to soft tissue irritation, and this rate is higher for superior plates. Intramedullary screw or nail fixation is an alternative for length-stable fractures, but there is a higher overall complication rate due to hardware migration. Superior plating can sustain a higher load before failure and bending strength, and it is generally preferred for inferior bony comminution. However, there is an increased risk of penetrating the subclavian artery or vein during drilling intraoperatively for superior plates.

Objectives: Did you learn...?

• Surgical indications for middle-third clavicle fractures?
• Advantages and disadvantages of various operative techniques for fixation of clavicle fractures?

CASE 6

Dr. Christina M. Hylden

A 25-year-old, right-hand-dominant male presents to clinic complaining of right shoulder pain which started 1 week ago when he tried to open a jammed door with the point of his shoulder. He is tender over the acromioclavicular joint and has a bony prominence greater than the contralateral side. His radiograph is shown in Figure 6–3.

What is true of the anatomy of the AC joint?

A. There is no synovial fluid associated with this joint.
B. The posterior component of the acromioclavicular ligament is most important for this joint's vertical stability.
C. The trapezoid ligament inserts on the clavicle 3 cm proximal to the lateral border.
D. The motion at the joint includes gliding and rotation.

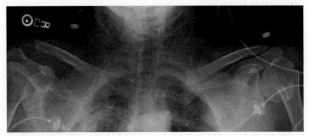

Figure 6–3

Discussion

The correct answer is (C). The trapezoid ligament is the more lateral coracoclavicular ligament at 3 cm from the distal clavicle while the conoid ligament is 4.5 cm proximal to the lateral border of the clavicle. These two ligaments together provide the vertical stability of the joint. The AC joint is diarthrodial and does produce synovial fluid. The acromioclavicular ligament provides horizontal stability, and the strongest component is the superior ligament. Most of the motion is from the bones, and their ability to rotate, not the joint itself; the only movement at the AC joint is gliding.

Choose the correct pairing of an AC joint injury classification with its description.

A. Type I: sprained AC and CC ligaments with slight vertical separation noted on radiographs
B. Type II: torn AC and CC ligaments with a CC distance of 25% to 100% of the contralateral side
C. Type IV: torn AC and CC ligaments with lateral clavicle displaced posteriorly
D. Type V: torn AC and CC ligaments with distal clavicle under the conjoined tendon

Discussion

The correct answer is (C). Type I is a sprained acromioclavicular ligament only and shows no change on plain radiographs. Type II is sprained AC and CC ligaments with slight vertical separation noted on radiographs. A Type III sprain is torn AC and CC ligaments with a CC distance of 25% to 100% of the contralateral side. Type IV is torn AC and CC ligaments with lateral clavicle displaced posteriorly. A Type V sprain has torn acromioclavicular and coracoclavicular ligaments and a coracoclavicular distance >100% as compared to the contralateral side. A Type VI sprain is described in choice D; these are rare injuries, and the clavicle can either be subacromial or subcoracoid.

When considering operative intervention for an AC joint separation, which of the following statements is true?

A. ORIF with CC suture fixation has an associated risk of hardware migration.
B. Modified Weaver–Dunn uses a technique that only returns 20% strength of vertical stability compared to a free tendon graft.
C. Primary AC joint fixation generally has a low incidence of complications.
D. A hook plate is preferred for its low profile and low rate of soft tissue irritation.

Discussion

The correct answer is (B). The Modified Weaver–Dunn is a CC ligament reconstruction that uses a transfer of the coracoacromial ligament to the distal clavicle. This recreates the CC ligament but has only 20% strength as the normal CC ligament. A CC ligament reconstruction, which uses a free tendon graft, can more closely recreate the strength of the CC ligament. An ORIF with suture fixation does not have a risk of hardware failure or migration, but it can be associated with suture erosion, which can cause a clavicle fracture. Primary AC joint fixation is not routinely done due to pin migration and a high complication rate. Hook plate fixation requires a second surgery for hardware removal due to soft tissue irritations.

Objectives: Did you learn...?

- The anatomy of the CC ligaments?
- Then classification of AC joint injuries?
- Advantages and disadvantages of various treatment options for AC joint injuries?

CASE 7

Dr. Christina M. Hylden

A 38-year-old, left-hand-dominant male was brought to the ED after a high-speed MVC. He sustained a closed injury but is alert and able to participate fully in his physical examination. He has a couple of broken ribs and is being monitored, and complains of left shoulder pain. His radiographs and CT scan is shown in Figure 6–4A–E.

Which statement is true regarding scapula fractures?

A. They are common and are a result of low-energy trauma.
B. There is an 80% rate of associated injuries.
C. The most common associated injury is to the head.
D. Associated brachial plexus injuries leave permanent disability 50% of the time.

Discussion

The correct answer is (B). Scapula fractures are uncommon (<1% all fractures) and are typically a result of a high-energy mechanism. There is a 2% to 5% mortality rate. The most common associated injury is rib fractures, with over 50% incidence. Head injuries occur 34% of the time. Other associated injuries include clavicle fracture, spine fractures, pneumothorax, pulmonary contusions, and vascular injury. Brachial plexus inju-

ries occur in 5% of scapula fractures, and 75% of them resolve over time.

Which of the following would NOT be an indication for surgery?

A. Coracoid fracture with 4 mm displacement.
B. Scapula neck fracture with 12 mm of translation.
C. Ipsilateral middle-third clavicle fracture with <100% displacement.
D. Glenoid medialization.

Discussion

The correct answer is (A). Surgical Indications for scapula fractures includes: open fractures, loss of rotator cuff function, a coracoid fracture with more than 10 mm displacement, a neck fracture with either 40 degrees angulation or 10 mm displacement, or glenohumeral instability. The joint is generally considered to be unstable if one of the following is true: more than 25% glenoid involvement and humeral subluxation, more than 5 mm of articular surface step-off, or excessive medialization of the glenoid. Another indication for surgery is a floating shoulder, and thus ipsilateral clavicle fractures as well as AC joint separation must be considered.

The patient underwent operative fixation and his postoperative radiographs are shown in Figure 6–5.

Upon initial presentation, if the patient was found to have global decreased sensation to his left upper extremity as well as decreased pulses compared to the contralateral side, another condition would have been considered.

Which of the following statements regarding this condition is true?

A. The axillary artery is the most common associated vascular injury.
B. Vascular injury is more common than neurological injury.
C. The mortality rate is 25%.
D. If neurological function does not return, early amputation is recommended.

Discussion

The correct answer is (D). The condition that should be considered in this situation is scapulothoracic dissociation. This is typically caused by a lateral traction injury to the shoulder girdle resulting in disruption of the scapulothoracic articulation. A flail extremity, complete loss of motor and sensory function, is seen in over 50% of cases. Neurological injury is more common than vascular. The subclavian artery is the most

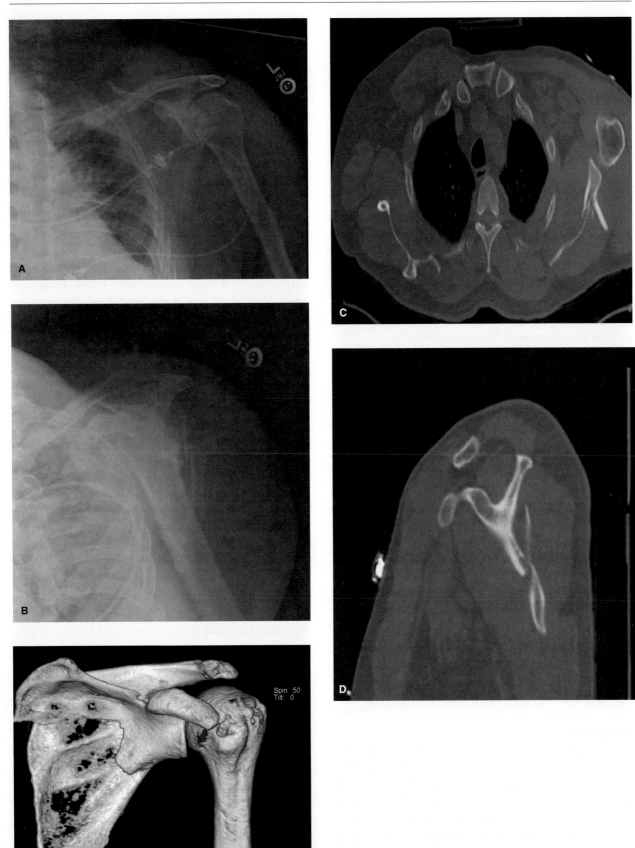

Figure 6–4 **A–E**

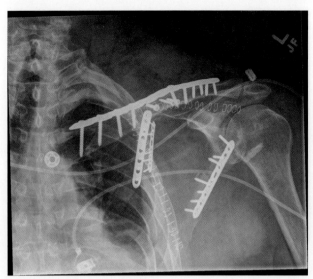

Figure 6–5

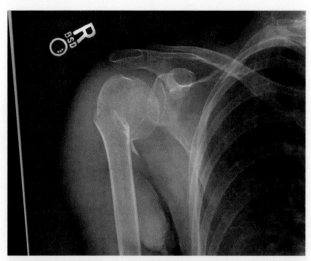

Figure 6–6

common vascular structure injured. The mortality rate is 10%, and it is recommended that early amputation be performed if the return of neurological function is unlikely. On plain chest x-ray, a diagnosis of scapulothoracic dissociation is suggested by a scapula laterally displaced more than 1 cm from the spinous processes (in comparison to the contralateral scapula), a widely displaced clavicle fracture, acromioclavicular separation, or sternoclavicular dislocation. Advanced imaging includes angiogram which looks for an injury to either the subclavian or axillary arteries.

Objectives: Did you learn...?

• Surgical indications for scapular fractures?
• Diagnosis of scapulothoracic dissociation?

CASE 8

Dr. Christina M. Hylden

A 57-year-old, right-hand-dominant female fell in her house while walking up the stairs with a laundry basket. She complains of immediate right shoulder pain and decreased range of motion. Her injury radiograph is seen in Figure 6–6.

Which of the following statements regarding this type of fracture is true?

A. The primary vascularity to the articular surface travels parallel to the long head of the biceps tendon.
B. The epiphyseal plate is the weakest portion of the humeral head and therefore most common fracture location.

C. There is a rare incidence of associated nerve injury.
D. The most commonly used classification is based on the anatomic relationship of four segments of bone.

Discussion

The correct answer is (D). The primary blood supply to the humeral head is from the posterior humeral circumflex artery; the vascularity to the articular component is most likely to be maintained if at least 8 mm of the medial calcar is attached to the segment. The anterior humeral circumflex artery runs parallel to the lateral tendon in the bicipital groove, as described in A. The epiphyseal plate is the anatomic neck. It is the surgical neck that is the weakened area of bone and the most common fracture site. Studies have shown as high as a 45% incidence of axillary nerve injury with proximal humerus fractures. These fracture are frequently classified by the Neer classification which uses four parts of the proximal humeral anatomy. These four parts are as follows: The articular surface, greater tuberosity, lesser tuberosity and the humeral shaft.

In choosing a surgical approach, what is true of the anatomy in the deltopectoral surgical approach?

A. The musculocutaneous nerve enters the biceps 5 cm distal to the coracoid.
B. The axillary nerve is at risk during the release of the subscapularis tendon.
C. The deltopectoral approach uses the internervous plane between the axillary nerve and the musculocutaneous nerve.

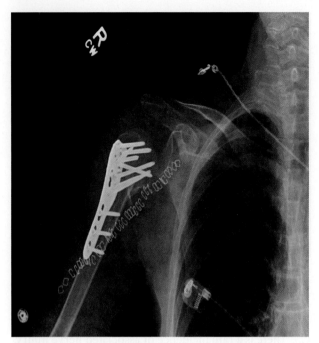

Figure 6–7

D. The anterior circumflex humeral artery runs just distal to the pectoralis major tendon.

Discussion

The correct answer is (B). The muscolocutaneous nerve enters the biceps only 5 to 8 cm from the coracoid, meaning that retraction should be done with care. It uses the internervous plane between the deltoid (axillary nerve) and the pectoralis major (medial and lateral pectoral nerves). The axillary nerve runs distal to the subscapularis tendon and proximal to the teres major and latissimus dorsi tendons. The anterior humeral circumflex artery runs anteriorly around the proximal humerus and is proximal to the pectoralis major tendon.

The patient underwent operative fixation through a deltopectoral approach. The postoperative radiographs are shown in Figure 6–7.

Objectives: Did you learn...?

• The Neer classification for proximal humerus fractures?
• The anatomy of the deltopectoral surgical approach?

CASE 9

Dr. Christina M. Hylden

A 68-year-old, right-hand-dominant female fell onto her left arm while walking her dog. An injury radiograph is shown in Figure 6–8.

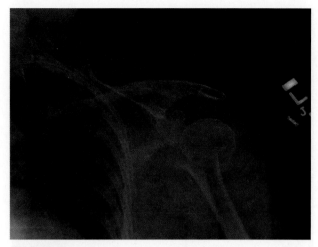

Figure 6–8

What is her best treatment option?

A. Closed reduction followed by 4 weeks of immobilization
B. Sling for comfort followed by early range of motion
C. Closed reduction with percutaneous pinning of the humeral head
D. Early total shoulder arthroplasty

Discussion

The correct answer is (B). This is a two-part fracture in an elderly patient, and clinical outcomes with nonoperative treatment are overall good. Long-term immobilization is not ideal because of the significant decrease in functional range of motion. Instead, early passive ROM should be initiated with early physical therapy follow-up (within 2 weeks from injury). A closed reduction with percutaneous pinning carries risks of axillary nerve injury and pin migration, especially in osteoporotic bone, without significant benefit over nonoperative treatment. This patient will most likely have a rotator cuff injury and possible deltoid atony after her injury and would not be a good surgical candidate for a total shoulder arthroplasty in the acute setting.

The patient heals her fracture as shown in Figure 6–9.

In another 6 months, she returns with radiographic signs of avascular necrosis of the humeral head, Cruess stage III, although she does not have any clinical complaints at this time.

How does this affect your treatment plan?

A. Discuss diagnosis and reassure the patient as she is currently asymptomatic.

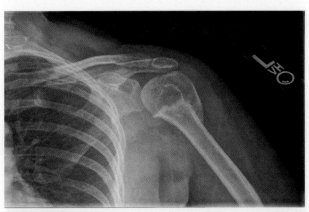

Figure 6–9

B. Recommend a core decompression of the humeral head now with physical therapy and weight-bearing restrictions.

C. Order an MRI to assess whether patient is a better candidate for a hemiarthroplasty or reverse shoulder arthroplasty.

D. Recommend she proceed with a total shoulder arthroplasty.

Discussion

The correct answer is (A). Although avascular necrosis of the humeral head is more common in four-part fractures, it can occur in any proximal humerus fracture. It is unclear in the shoulder that radiographic signs correlate with clinical deficits. In the case of this patient, since her pain is gone, and she has no complaints, the osteonecrosis can be treated conservatively with reassurance and an explanation of possible future symptoms. If symptoms arise and lead to lifestyle changes, surgical options can be discussed at that time.

Objectives: Did you learn...?

• Nonoperative management of proximal humerus fractures?
• Management of osteonecrosis of the humeral head?

CASE 10

Dr. Christina M. Hylden

A 42-year-old, right-hand-dominant, male, government contractor sustains blunt trauma to his right arm while using a jackhammer. He has immediate pain and deformity to his right upper extremity and presents immediately to the emergency department with this isolated injury. Physical examination shows skin to be intact, and patient has wrist extensor weakness. Plain radiographs reveal a spiral fracture of the right humerus mid-diaphysis with 30 degrees of anterior and 30 degrees of varus angulation.

Which of the following is NOT a contraindication to nonoperative treatment with a coaptation splint?

A. 20 degrees of varus angulation
B. Vascular injury
C. Radial nerve injury
D. Brachial plexus injury

Discussion

The correct answer is (C). Acceptable alignment for nonoperative management of a humeral shaft fracture is less than 20 degrees in the sagittal plane, less than 30 degrees in the coronal plane, or less than 3 cm of shortening. Radial nerve palsy in a closed fracture is most likely a neuropraxia, and it is not a contraindication to closed treatment. Vascular injuries that require repair and a brachial plexus injury are both considered absolute indications for surgery and repair or exploration. Another absolute indication is an open fracture.

Which of the following about the radial nerve is true?

A. It courses across the posterior humerus from lateral to medial.
B. It can be found 5 cm proximal to the lateral epicondyle of the humerus.
C. It can be found 10 cm proximal to the medial epicondyle.
D. It has an increased incidence of injury with a distal one-third humeral shaft fracture.

Discussion

The correct answer is (D). A spiral fracture of the distal one-third of the humeral shaft (eponym Holstein–Lewis fracture) has a 22% incidence of radial nerve neuropraxia. The radial nerve travels from the medial humerus proximally, crossing posteriorly to the lateral side. On average it is 14 cm proximal to the lateral epicondyle and 20 cm proximal to the medial epicondyle.

The above patient is treated with an intramedullary nail and is later lost to follow-up. He presents to clinic 9 months later with a complaint of persistent right arm pain. Radiographs and advanced imaging reveal that he has a hypertrophic nonunion.

What is the most appropriate definitive treatment?

A.   Nail removal and open reduction with internal fixation with autologous bone grafting
B.   Revision intramedullary nailing
C.   Nail removal and functional bracing
D.   Continued observation

Discussion

The correct answer is (A). In this case, the patient is more than 6 months out from his procedure but does not show cortical healing. The question defines that his nonunion is hypertrophic, which means that he has poor stability of the fracture fragments from the intramedullary nail. The best option is to create a more stable fixation with open reduction and plating. Adding a bone graft will augment this fixation and give him the best chance of healing with one procedure. Exchanging the nail, functional bracing, and observation will not obtain the stability that he needs.

Objectives: Did you learn...?

• Indications for nonoperative management of a humeral shaft fracture?
• Anatomic location of the radial nerve?
• Treatment of humeral shaft nonunion?

CASE 11

Dr. James N. Foster

A 54-year-old, right-hand-dominant, high school principal presents to the emergency department with severe left elbow pain after a fall onto the extremity which she sustained earlier that morning while walking her dog. She notes pain with any movement of the elbow, and her clinical examination finds this to be a closed injury with an intact median, radial, and ulnar nerve examination. Injury radiographs are shown in Figure 6–10A and B.

How would you classify this distal humerus fracture?

A.   Extra-articular (AO/OTA 13A)
B.   Partial articular (AO/OTA 13 B)
C.   Complete articular (AO/OTA 13C)
D.   Further imaging is required in order to make determination

Discussion

The correct answer is (C). These images show an intra-articular fracture involving both the medial and lateral

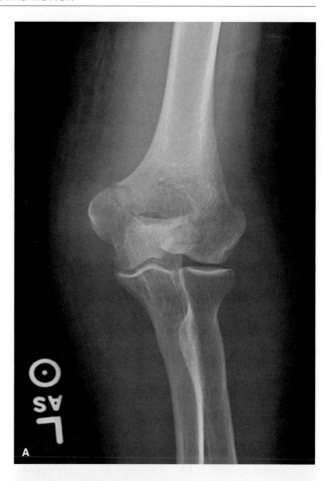

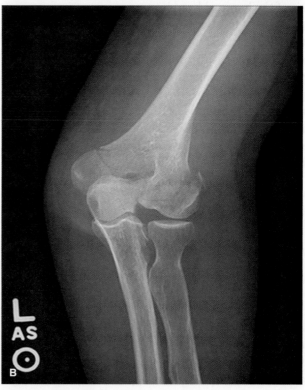

Figure 6–10 **A–B**

columns of the distal humerus with no articular portion remaining in continuity with the diaphysis. Multiple radiographic views may be necessary in order to make this determination, especially when there is minimal displacement. A CT scan can be useful for both classification and operative planning purposes. Multiple classification systems are used to describe these fractures, and below are figures showing two of the more commonly cited: the AO/OTA classification in Figure 6–11A and the scheme described by Jupiter and Mehne in Figure 6–11B.

Further imaging reveals a coronal shear fracture of the capitellum. In considering your surgical approach

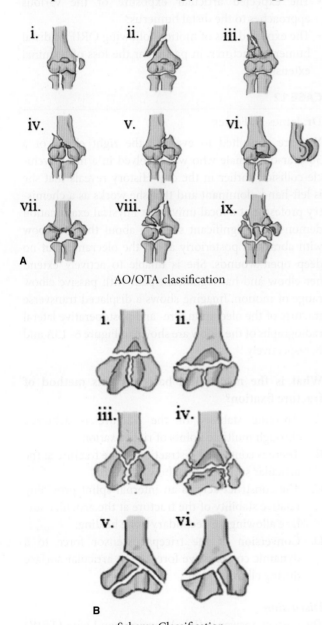

AO/OTA classification

Scheme Classification

Figure 6–11 **A–B** (Illustrated by David Beavers.)

for open reduction internal fixation (ORIF), which will provide you with the most extensive exposure of the distal humerus articular surface?

A. Triceps splitting approach
B. Lateral (Kocher) approach
C. Volar Henry approach
D. Olecranon osteotomy approach
E. Triceps reflecting (Bryan–Morrey) approach

Discussion

The correct answer is (D). In an anatomic study by Wilkinson et al., the triceps splitting, triceps reflecting, and transolecranon osteotomy approaches were found to allow direct visualization of 35%, 46%, and 57%, respectively, of the distal humerus articular surface. This study found all three of these approaches provided adequate access to both the radial and ulnar columns of the distal humerus for plating purposes. In the presence of a coronal shear component or a capitellum fracture, an olecranon osteotomy should be considered as a means to obtain improved joint visualization in order to achieve a congruent articular reduction. The Kocher approach is a lateral approach to the elbow used commonly for radial head fractures or LUCL reconstruction, and the volar Henry approach is used to address forearm fractures, not fractures of the humerus.

The surgeon elects to use an olecranon osteotomy and performs ORIF using orthogonal plating in combination with several headless compression screws to address the capitellum fracture. The post-op radiographs are shown in Figure 6–12A and B.

What complication is the patient most likely to experience?

A. Nonunion of the distal humerus fracture
B. Iatrogenic ulnar nerve injury
C. Wound-healing complications
D. Loss of elbow motion
E. Symptomatic hardware requiring removal

Discussion

The correct answer is (D). It is extremely common to lose some elbow range of motion after elbow fractures, particularly with distal humerus fractures. This loss of motion may be due to a number of variables including articular incongruity, capsular contractures, loose bodies, heterotopic ossification, and/or prominent hardware. The average flexion contracture following ORIF of distal humerus fractures is 20 to 25 degrees, and an expected total arc of motion is 100 to 110 degrees.

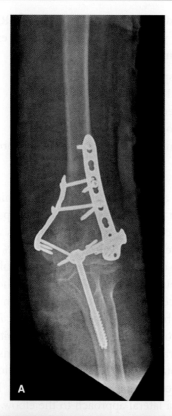

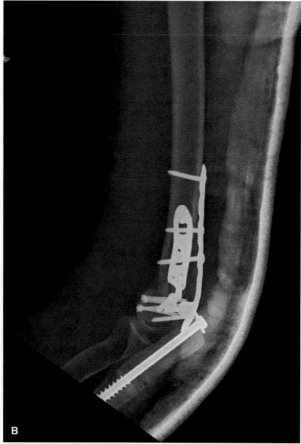

Figure 6–12 **A–B**

Symptomatic hardware is common as well, especially with an olecranon fracture or osteotomy. In this case, however, the olecranon osteotomy was fixed with a cancellous screw and washer which requires hardware removal less frequently than other fixation methods such as tension band wiring, where wire back-out is a frequent issue. Another complication, specifically associated with an olecranon osteotomy, is nonunion of the osteotomy site.

Objectives: Did you learn...?

- Classification of distal humerus fractures?
- The expected articular exposure of the various approaches to the distal humerus?
- The expected loss of motion following ORIF of distal humerus fractures, in particular the loss of terminal extension?

CASE 12

Dr. James N. Foster

You are consulted to evaluate the right elbow of a 38-year-old female who was involved in a motor vehicle collision earlier in the day. History reveals that she is left-hand–dominant and that she works as a chemistry professor at a local university. Physical examination demonstrates significant swelling about the left elbow with abrasions posteriorly about the olecranon but no deep open wounds. She is unable to actively extend her elbow and has significant pain with passive elbow range of motion. Imaging shows a displaced transverse fracture of the olecranon. Pre- and postoperative lateral radiographs of the elbow are shown in Figure 6–13A and B, respectively.

What is the mechanical basis for this method of fracture fixation?

A. Absolute stability of the fracture is achieved through multiple points of rigid fixation.
B. There is controlled distraction of the fracture at the articular surface with elbow extension.
C. The construct acts as an internal splint providing relative stability of the fracture at the articular surface allowing for secondary bone healing.
D. Conversion of the triceps extensor force to a dynamic compressive force at the articular surface during elbow flexion.

Discussion

The correct answer is (D). A tension band wire (TBW) construct achieves static fixation dorsally with dynamic

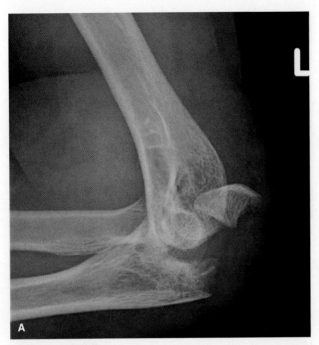

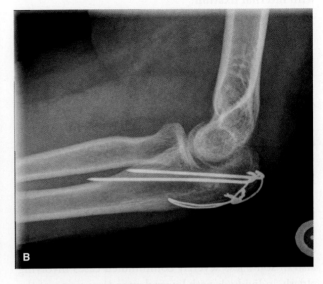

Figure 6–13 **A–B**

compression at the articular surface allowing for primary bone healing. Tension band wiring can be done where there are clear tension and compression surfaces of a bone, such as the olecranon or the patella and can use either K-wires or screws in combination with wire or a robust suture. The concept involves tensioning the wire (or suture) over the tension surface of a bone such that the distracting forces exerted on that surface are then converted to compressive forces on the opposite side.

What is the most important technical factor in preventing K-wire migration (backing out) when using a TBW construct?

A. Ensuring proximal bent wire ends are buried beneath the triceps fibers
B. Proper tensioning of the wire knots on either side of the construct
C. Achieving bicortical purchase with the K-wires
D. The quality of the articular surface reduction

Discussion

The correct answer is (A). While bicortical purchase does improve fixation, the most important factor is burying the proximal wire ends beneath the triceps. There is also risk associated with overpenetration of the anterior ulnar cortex, where the AIN and ulnar artery are in close proximity, and the proximal radioulnar articulation

is potentially violated. While TBW constructs are very successful in achieving fracture union, with rates higher than 90% reported in the literature, they are frequently irritating and require removal of hardware for this reason after fracture healing as often as 33% to 80% of the time.

Which of the following would be a contraindication to using a tension band wire (TBW) construct to fix an olecranon fracture?

A. A transverse fracture pattern
B. The presence of fracture comminution
C. An open fracture of the olecranon
D. A short oblique fracture which does not extend past the midpoint of the trochlear notch

Discussion

The correct answer is (B). Comminution is a contraindication for the use of a tension band wire construct due to the potential to overcompress and cause narrowing of the greater sigmoid notch. A TBW also risks inadequate stabilization of the fracture in the setting of comminution. Mild to moderate comminution is an indication for plate fixation, as is the presence of articular fragment impaction. Another indication for plate fixation is a long oblique fracture which extends past 50% of the greater sigmoid notch, as these fractures are poorly controlled with a TBW construct.

What is the preferred treatment of a severely comminuted fracture of the olecranon where achieving a congruent joint surface is unlikely to be achieved with internal fixation?

A. Splinting or casting in 45 to 90 degrees of flexion and neutral forearm rotation until early fracture consolidation
B. A bridge plate construct over the defect/comminution to promote secondary bone healing
C. Total elbow arthroplasty with reattachment of the triceps to the implant
D. Fragment excision with triceps advancement

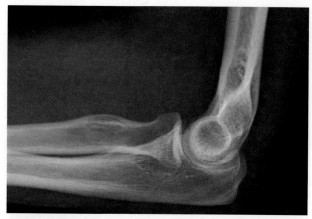

Figure 6–14

Discussion

The correct answer is (D). The primary goal in fixation of an olecranon fracture is to achieve a congruent joint surface. When this is not possible due to severe comminution of the fracture or due to bone loss, and also in some less severely comminuted cases involving elderly individuals with lower demands, excision of the proximal olecranon fragment with advancement of the triceps tendon is an acceptable treatment option. It has been suggested in the literature that as much as 50% to 75% of the olecranon articular surface can be excised without leading to gross elbow instability, provided that the coronoid process remains intact. Even when the triceps tendon is reattached in a dorsal position on the remaining olecranon to maximize triceps extension strength, it is reported that at least 24% of extension strength is lost.

Objectives: Did you learn...?

- Indications for and potential complications with the use of tension band wiring?
- Technical considerations in creating a tension band wire construct?
- When the use of plate and screw fixation or fragment excision is appropriate?

CASE 13

Dr. James N. Foster

A 43-year-old, active man presents to your clinic with a chief complaint of elbow pain. He tells you that he came down awkwardly onto an extended arm the previous evening in a soccer game. He denies dislocating his elbow and says he was able to finish the game but also says that his arm felt strange, and he had to repeatedly "shake out" the elbow through the remainder of the game. Following the game he went to a local emergency department because of persistent pain, where x-rays were taken (Fig. 6–14). He was told by the Emergency Physician that there was only a very small fracture of his ulna and likely nothing to worry about. He was given a sling and told to follow-up with you.

Multiple plain radiographic views of the elbow were reviewed and there appears to be a small fracture of the coronoid with no other fractures identified. His elbow examination in clinic is difficult to interpret due to swelling and pain with stability examination, although there is slight laxity noted with varus stress despite his guarding.

What injury are you concerned about and what would be an appropriate imaging workup at this point?

A. Coronoid tip fracture; no further imaging as plain films are sufficient
B. Anteromedial facet fracture; order a CT of the elbow
C. MCL injury; order an MRI of the elbow
D. Coronoid tip fracture; order a CT of the elbow

Discussion

The correct answer is (B). The plain radiograph shows a fracture line through the tip of the coronoid process, however a fracture of the coronoid tip and one involving the anteromedial facet of the coronid can occasionally be difficult to differentiate on plain radiographs alone. The lack of a dislocation event in the clinical history and the varus laxity on clinical examination should raise suspicion for a fracture of the anteromedial facet of the coronoid. A fracture of the coronoid tip is more frequently associated with an elbow dislocation and

Table 6–2 O'DRISCOLL CORNOID FRACTURE CLASSIFICATION

Fracture	Subtype	Description
Tip	1	≤2 mm of cornoid height
	2	>2 mm of cornoid height
Anteromedial	1	Anteromedial rim
	2	Anteromedial rim and tip
	3	Anteromedial rim and sub-lime tubercle (± tip)
Basal	1	Cornoid body and base
	2	Transolecranon basal coronoid fracture

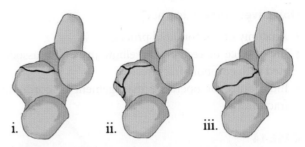

Figure 6–15 (Illustrated by David Beavers.)

arthritis when left untreated. Figure 6–15 depicts the three types of coronoid fractures as described by O'Driscoll, with "ii" outlining the various fractures of the anteromedial facet.

Which of the coronoid fracture patterns listed warrants surgical fixation?

A. Transversely oriented tip fracture measuring 2 mm in height which is associated with posterolateral rotatory instability of the elbow (PLRI)
B. Base fracture involving approximately 60% of the coronoid height
C. Anteromedial facet fracture associated with varus instability
D. Fracture of the tip which measures 5 mm in height on plain radiographs which also show slight anterior elbow subluxation
E. All of the above fracture patterns warrant surgical fixation

Discussion

The correct answer is (E). Historically it was suggested that the coronoid process only needed to be addressed surgically if a fracture involved at least 50% of the process, however the importance of the coronoid as a contributor to elbow stability is now more understood. Any fracture of the coronoid, if associated with elbow instability, warrants surgical fixation. This includes very small tip fractures, which can be fixed with a suture lasso technique if they are too small to accept screw fixation. The only coronoid fractures which have acceptable outcomes with nonsurgical management are small fractures without associated elbow subluxation and without radiocapitellar joint opening on stress radiographs. This change in practice with respect to coronoid fractures is due to the high percentage of unacceptable clinical outcomes including chronic instability and early arthritis seen with nonsurgical management of coronoid fractures.

valgus instability. It is suggested that a CT of the elbow be ordered to further characterize all coronoid fractures in order to determine an appropriate treatment plan. Above is a summary of the O'Driscoll classification of coronoid fractures in Table 6–2. The O'Driscoll system differs from the classic Regan and Morrey system in that it focuses on the importance of the anteromedial facet rather than classifying strictly based on the level of the coronoid process fracture.

What type of elbow instability is associated with fractures of the anteromedial facet of the coronoid?

A. Varus posteromedial rotatory instability
B. Recurrent posterior elbow dislocations
C. Anteromedial instability
D. Posterolateral rotatory instability

Discussion

The correct answer is (A). The various types of coronoid fractures are associated with predictable elbow instability patterns. Coronoid tip fractures are frequently seen as part of a terrible triad elbow injury (LCL rupture, radial head fracture, and coronoid fracture), which often results in posterolateral rotatory instability (PLRI). Anteromedial facet fractures are seen when there is a varus force on the extended elbow, leading to failure of the LCL and impingement of the anteromedial coronoid under the trochlea. As up to 60% of the anteromedial facet is unsupported by the ulnar metaphysis, it is prone to fracture under strong varus force. It is important to recognize the sometimes subtle anteromedial facet fracture and accompanying varus instability, as this has been shown to progress to ulnohumeral

Objectives: Did you learn...?

- Anatomy of the coronoid process?
- Importance of recognizing elbow instability associated with coronoid fractures?
- Indications for operative management of coronoid fractures?

CASE 14

Dr. James N. Foster

A 36-year-old, right-hand-dominant male presents to the emergency department with right arm and elbow pain after he fell over his handle bars while mountain biking. Physical examination finds the right upper extremity to be an isolated injury with the exception of some abrasions and ecchymosis about his face and bilateral upper extremities. Examining his elbow reveals tenderness about the radial head and marked pain with flexion, extension, pronation, and supination. There does not appear to be any mechanical block to motion although crepitation is appreciated with forearm rotation. Radiographs are shown in Figure 6–16A and B.

Which of the following would be an indication for operative treatment of this radial head fracture?

A. Severe pain which limits passive range of motion on examination of the elbow in the emergency department
B. Fracture involvement of 30% of the radial head articular surface
C. 2 mm of fracture displacement at the articular surface
D. Restricted forearm supination with mechanical block to motion

Discussion

The correct response is "D." The included images show a partial radial head fracture with displacement. While 2 mm of articular displacement is a relative indication for operative management, the only choice listed which is an agreed-upon surgical indication for partial radial head fractures is a fracture which produces a block to motion. Severe pain limiting a complete range of motion examination is not uncommon in the acute injury setting. Aspiration of elbow hematoma with or without injection of local anesthetic can assist with pain control and allow for a more accurate range of motion examination to determine whether or not the fracture is creating a mechanical block to motion. Other indications

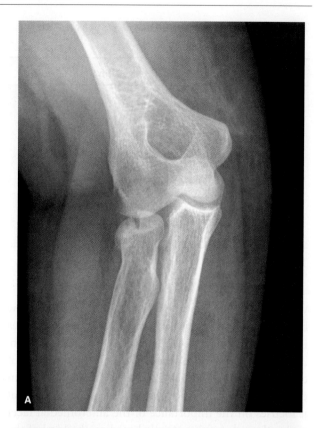

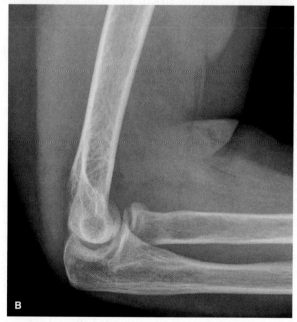

Figure 6–16 **A–B**

for operative treatment of a radial head fracture include comminuted fractures and those associated with complex injuries such as elbow dislocations, Monteggia fractures, or distal radioulnar joint (DRUJ) disruption.

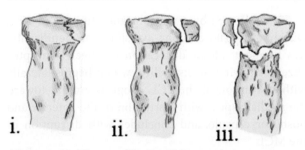

Figure 6–17 (Illustrated by David Beavers.)

Figure 6–17 demonstrates the Mason classification of radial head fractures.

The patient follows up in your clinic and is noted to have pain with pronation and supination which is greater than would be expected 1 week out from injury. He is also exquisitely tender about the distal radius and ulna.

Which possible missed injury are you most concerned for?

A. Triangular fibrocartilage complex (TFCC) tear
B. Distal radius fracture
C. Distal radioulnar joint (DRUJ) disruption
D. Triquetral avulsion fracture

Discussion

The correct answer is (C). When treating patients acutely who have traumatic musculoskeletal injuries, it is not uncommon for injuries of the hand or wrist to go initially undiagnosed. Concomitant injuries to the elbow and wrist are found in approximately 30% of radial head fractures. Of the listed wrist injuries above, a disruption of the DRUJ is of particular importance when accompanying a radial head or neck fracture. This injury combination is known as the Essex-Lopresti lesion and constitutes not only a radial head fracture and DRUJ injury, but also a disruption of the interosseous membrane of the forearm. It is important to recognize this injury early as it is associated with significantly worse outcomes when treated nonoperatively, or with radial head resection, as compared to these treatments in the setting of an isolated radial head fracture. A retrospective review on 20 patients with this injury pattern showed good to excellent elbow outcomes in 80% of those whose injury was recognized prior to initial surgical intervention, and in only 27% of those whose Essex-Lopresti injury was discovered at a later date.

You plan to perform open reduction with internal fixation of this radial head fracture.

When using plate and screw fixation for radial head or neck fractures, where should the plate be placed?

A. Anteriorly (volar) with the forearm in supination
B. Directly lateral with the forearm in supination
C. Directly lateral with the forearm in neutral position
D. As dorsal as possible with the forearm in pronation
E. 180 degrees from the radial styloid

Discussion

The correct answer is (C). Anatomic studies of the proximal radioulnar joint have found there to be an approximately 90- to 110-degree arc of the radial head which does not articulate with the ulna during pronation or supination. This is known as the "safe zone" and it can be identified intraoperatively by placing the forearm into neutral position, where this zone is then centered about the equator of the radial head. This nonarticulating region is the desired location to position hardware for internal fixation. Figure 6–18 demonstrates this "safe zone" with the forearm in neutral position, supination, and pronation.

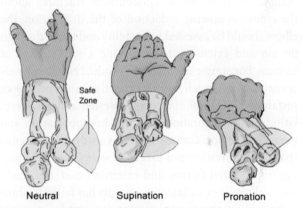

Figure 6–18 (Illustrated by David Beavers.)

Objectives: Did you learn…?

- Assess for associated injuries with radial head fractures?
- Indications for operative management?
- "Safe zone" for hardware placement on the radial head and/or neck?

CASE 15

Dr. James N. Foster

You receive a call from an emergency department physician informing you that she has a patient who will need follow-up for an elbow dislocation. She tells you that she reduced and splinted the patient's elbow, which was dislocated on her physical examination, but that she does not yet have any imaging of the elbow. The patient is currently at radiology waiting for postreduction plain radiographs to be taken.

What is the most appropriate initial treatment for a simple dislocation of the elbow which reduces concentrically?

A. Splint immobilization or long arm cast for 3 to 4 weeks followed by passive ROM exercises

B. Splint at 90 degrees for 3 weeks followed by active and passive ROM exercises

C. Splinting with early MRI to assess the degree of ligamentous injury about the elbow

D. Early operative treatment to repair the injured collateral ligaments of the elbow

E. Immobilization less than 2 weeks followed by early active and passive ROM exercises

Discussion

The correct answer is (E). An elbow dislocation is termed "simple" if there are no concomitant fractures about the elbow. Following reduction of the dislocation, the elbow should be assessed for stability and taken through flexion and extension to determine a stable range of motion. For simple dislocations, residual elbow stiffness is encountered much more frequently than is persistent instability. Mehlhoff et al. demonstrated a direct correlation between duration of elbow immobilization and persistent flexion contracture. This study recommends that immobilization not exceed 2 weeks before initiating unprotected flexion and extension exercises. Early surgical repair of collateral ligaments has failed to show improved outcomes over early motion and nonoperative treatment for simple elbow dislocations.

In elbow dislocations, what is the most common mechanism of failure of the LCL?

A. Midsubstance rupture

B. Soft tissue avulsion off the humeral attachment

C. Bony avulsion off the humeral attachment

D. Bony avulsion off the ulnar attachment

Discussion

The correct answer is (B). McKee et al. evaluated 62 consecutive elbow dislocations and fracture dislocations requiring surgical treatment and injury to the LCL. The most common injury pattern was a soft tissue avulsion from the lateral condyle of the humerus

in 52%, followed by a midsubstance rupture in 29%. Distal soft tissue or bony avulsion was significantly less frequent. Elbow dislocation has been conceptualized as a "ring of instability" which begins laterally with disruption of the LCL, progress around toward the medial aspect with disruption of the anterior and posterior capsule, and concludes with disruption of the MCL.

The ED physician calls you back after plain radiographs and a subsequent CT of the elbow showing fractures of the coronoid and the radial head (Fig. 6–19A–C).

How does the presence of these fractures change your treatment plan for this elbow dislocation?

A. It does not affect the treatment, which should still consist of brief splinting and early ROM.

B. This is an elbow injury which should be treated operatively with repair of the LCL, ORIF of the coronoid, and ORIF or radial head arthroplasty for the radial head fracture.

C. This is an elbow injury which should be treated with operative management only after the patient has worked with physical therapy and regained near full elbow ROM.

D. This represents a more significant injury which should be treated with a longer period of immobilization to allow for fracture healing prior to beginning ROM exercises with PT.

E. This is an elbow injury which should be treated operatively with repair of the LCL, ORIF of the coronoid, and resection of the fractured radial head.

Discussion

The correct answer is (B). This injury represents a "terrible triad," which consists of an elbow dislocation (LCL rupture) with concomitant radial head fracture and coronoid fracture. It is important to recognize this injury pattern for prognostic reasons, as these injuries are frequently associated with fair to poor outcomes even when treated appropriately by experienced surgeons. A standardized surgical approach to the Terrible Triad injury has been established by Pugh et al. This sequential approach involves addressing the coronoid fracture first, followed by radial head ORIF or replacement depending on the nature of the radial head fracture, and then repair of the LCL rupture or avulsion. After addressing these three components of the injury, elbow stability is then reassessed. If instability persists, repair of the MCL and/or placement of a hinged external fixator is performed as necessary.

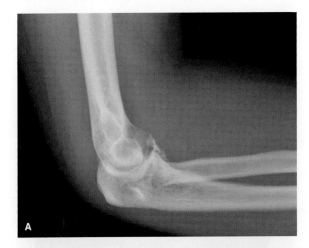

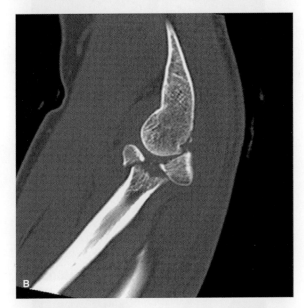

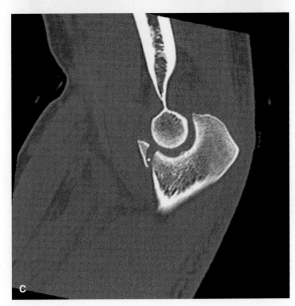

Figure 6–19 **A–C**

The injury is treated operatively and the post-op radiographs are shown in Figure 6–20A and B. The MCL was found to be competent on intraoperative examination.

At the conclusion of the procedure, in what position should the elbow be splinted?

A. Flexion and pronation
B. Flexion and supination
C. Extension and pronation
D. Extension and supination
E. Flexion and neutral forearm position

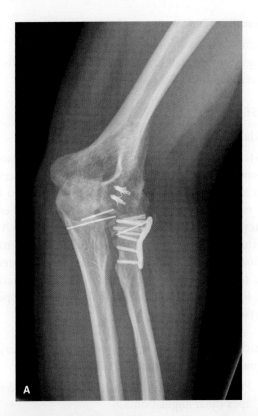

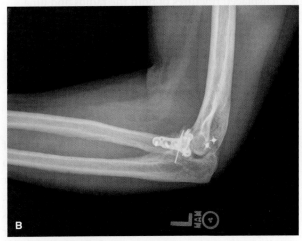

Figure 6–20 **A–B**

Discussion

The correct answer is (A). There is increased bony congruity about the elbow as flexion increases. Pronation tightens the LUCL and holds the radiocapitellar joint reduced. Mathew et al. suggest that if the LCL has been repaired and the MCL is intact, the arm should be splinted at 90 degrees of flexion at the elbow and pronation of the forearm. They suggest that if both ligaments have been repaired, the forearm be positioned in neutral and to consider splinting in supination if the MCL has not been securely fixed.

Objectives: Did you learn...?

- Simple versus complex elbow dislocations?
- Ligamentous stabilizing structures about the elbow?
- Terrible Triad injury and treatment?

CASE 16

Dr. James N. Foster

A 54-year-old, right-hand-dominant, industrial worker is brought to your hospital after his left arm was caught in a machine at work. He sustained fractures to both the radius and ulna, which were imaged in the emergency department and are shown in Figure 6–21A and B. This is a closed injury and the extremity remains neurovascularly intact with moderate swelling present. The plan is for operative fixation of these fractures, and the patient is prepped for transport to the operating room.

Which of the following are indications for surgical management of forearm fractures in an adult?

A. Fracture of the radius with 75% translation and slight apex ulnar angulation
B. Displaced fractures of both the radius and ulna
C. Fracture of the ulna with an associated radial head dislocation
D. Fracture of the radius with an associated DRUJ disruption
E. All of the above

Discussion

The correct answer is (E). In adults, the restoration of anatomic alignment of the radius and ulna is critical to forearm function, to include the proximal radioulnar joint, distal radioulnar joint (DRUJ), and the radial bow. Treatment of adults with displaced forearm fractures or complex injuries such as those listed in the answer choices is associated with unsatisfactory outcomes as

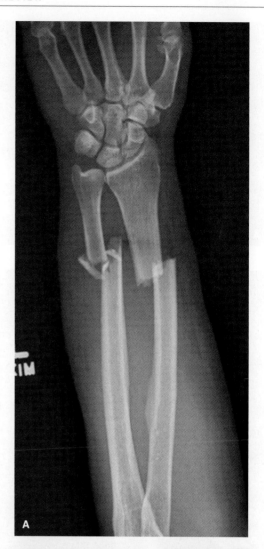

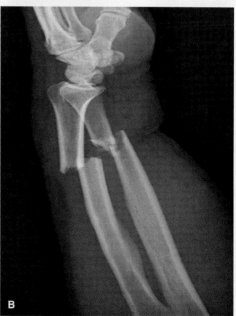

Figure 6–21 **A–B**

often as 92% of the time. These poor outcomes are due to a variety of reasons including malunion, nonunion, or radioulnar synostosis. Forearm fractures in adults are almost exclusively treated surgically with the exception of minimally or nondisplaced fractures of the ulnar shaft, which in isolation can be managed with casting or fracture bracing with satisfactory outcomes.

Once the patient is prepped and draped in the operating room, you draw out your planned incisions on the forearm.

What is the primary reason for using two incisions as opposed to one incision when performing ORIF of both bones of the forearm?

A. Higher rates of fracture union
B. Lower risk of infection
C. Improved accuracy with restoration of the native radial bow
D. Lower risk of synostosis formation

Discussion

The correct answer is (D). Using a single incision to address both the radius and ulna for ORIF has been shown to lead to a significantly higher incidence of radioulnar synostosis thereby severely limiting forearm rotation. Since the loss of forearm rotation can be quite disabling, surgical excision of the synostosis is recommended. The restoration of the radial bow has not been correlated with one versus two incisions, however it is of critical importance when fixing a radial shaft fracture. The native bow of the radial diaphysis has been found to average 9.3 degrees apex lateral and 6.4 degrees apex posterior in coronal and sagittal planes, respectively. The lack of adequate restoration of the bow has been shown to result in a significant decrease in both forearm rotation and grip strength.

What neurovascular structure is at high risk of injury and must be protected when approaching a proximal one-third radius fracture from either the volar (Henry) or dorsal (Thompson) approach?

A. Posterior interosseous nerve (PIN)
B. Anterior interosseous nerve (AIN)
C. Radial artery
D. Ulnar artery
E. Median nerve

Discussion

The correct answer is (A). The ulna lies subcutaneously throughout its length and is approached almost exclusively through a direct approach between the FCU and ECU. The

radius is more often approached via the Henry approach, which utilizes the interval between brachioradialis and pronator teres proximally and between brachioradialis and FCR more distally, however it can also be approached dorsally via the Thompson approach. The Thompson approach utilizes the interval between ECRB and EDC. In either approach, the PIN lies in precarious proximity to the proximal aspect of the radius and is at risk for injury both during surgical dissection as well as during retraction. To protect the PIN when using the Henry approach, the forearm should be supinated and the supinator should be dissected subperiosteally and handled with care to avoid excessive traction on the nerve. With the Thompson approach, the PIN is most easily identified exiting the supinator, and once identified it should be protected.

Objectives: Did you learn…?

- The importance of the radial bow?
- Indications for surgical treatment?
- Surgical approaches and at-risk structures during exposure?

CASE 17

Dr. James N. Foster

A 34-year-old, right-hand-dominant male is brought to the emergency department by his friends with a chief complaint of right arm pain and deformity. Earlier in the day he was thrown from his dirt bike during an amateur race and attempted to break his fall with his arm. Your examination finds that he is nontender about his elbow but has significant pain and deformity about the forearm and wrist. His radiographs are shown in Figure 6–22A and B.

Which of the following is not a radiographic indicator of possible distal radioulnar joint (DRUJ) instability?

A. Shortening >5 mm of the radius
B. Apex dorsal angulation of the radial shaft fracture
C. Widening of the DRUJ on an AP radiograph
D. DRUJ incongruity on a true lateral radiograph
E. Fracture of the base of the ulnar styloid

Discussion

The correct answer is (B). Choices A, C, D, and E are all radiographic signs of possible DRUJ instability. The injury shown here is a radial shaft fracture with concomitant DRUJ injury, also known as a Galeazzi fracture. This fracture is treated surgically with ORIF of

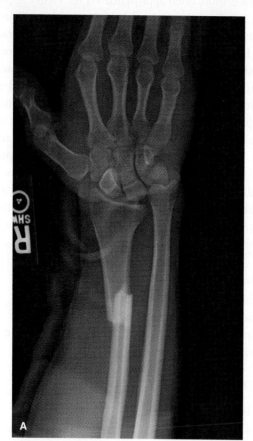
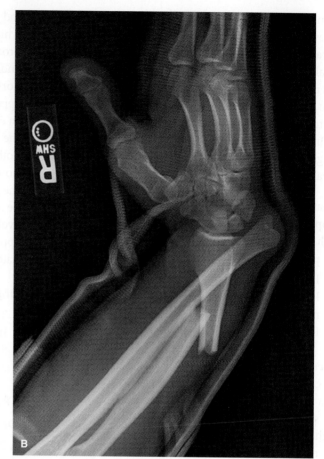

Figure 6-22 **A–B**

the radial shaft fracture followed by reassessment of the DRUJ with intraoperative fluoroscopy. If the DRUJ is found to be irreducible by closed means, it is possible that the ECU tendon is interposed between the radius and ulna. An unreducible DRUJ warrants open reduction and removal of any interposed tissue.

Following anatomic reduction and rigid fixation of the radial shaft fracture, which of the following fracture patterns are most likely to be associated with a persistently unstable DRUJ?

A. Radius fracture 4 cm proximal to the distal radius midarticular surface
B. Radius fracture at the apex of the radial bow
C. Radial shaft 9 cm proximal to the distal radius midarticular surface
D. Fracture of the radius just distal to the radial tuberosity

Discussion

The correct answer is (A). Following ORIF of the radial shaft fracture, the DRUJ must be assessed for stability.

Rettig and Raskin in their series of 40 Galeazzi fractures found that after fixation of the radius fracture, those fractures located less than 7.5 cm from the distal radius midarticular surface required fixation of a persistently unstable DRUJ 55% of the time, whereas fractures greater than 7.5 cm from the midarticular surface were persistently unstable at the DRUJ only 6% of the time.

After ORIF of the radius, the distal ulna is still able to be translated dorsally out of the sigmoid notch with the forearm held in supination.

What is the appropriate next step in management?

A. Short arm thumb spica cast for 6 weeks to allow the TFCC to heal
B. Long arm immobilization with the forearm in supination for 6 weeks
C. Sugar tong splint with the forearm in neutral position for 4 to 6 weeks
D. K-wire fixation of the DRUJ and long arm immobilization with the forearm in supination for 6 weeks

E. K-wire fixation of the DRUJ and long arm immobilization with the forearm in pronation for 6 weeks

Discussion

The correct answer is (D). After fixation of the radius, the DRUJ is reassessed. At this point there are several possibilities: A stable DRUJ, a reducible but persistently unstable DRUJ, and a nonreducible DRUJ. If the DRUJ is stable, some suggest that no further immobilization is required and early motion should be initiated, whereas others suggest that the forearm should still be splinted in supination for 6 weeks. If the DRUJ remains unstable but is reducible, the ulna should be transfixed to the radius in supination just proximal to the sigmoid notch using one or two K-wires and the forearm then splinted in supination for 6 weeks. If the DRUJ is not able to be anatomically reduced by closed means, it should be opened and any interposed tissue removed. The TFCC should then be repaired and the forearm pinned in supination for 6 weeks.

Objectives: Did you learn...?

- The radiographic signs suggesting DRUJ instability on injury radiographs?
- The predictive value of fracture location as it relates to a persistently unstable DRUJ following radius fixation?
- When the DRUJ warrants splinting versus pinning versus open surgical fixation?

CASE 18

Dr. James N. Foster

You are called to the emergency department to evaluate the right arm of a 26-year-old female who fell approximately 15 ft off of an apartment balcony. She appears to have a deformity about the proximal right forearm and is markedly swollen. She also has several rib and facial fractures but is alert and oriented and does not have any open wounds, and she has no neurovascular deficits on examination. The lateral radiograph on initial presentation is shown in Figure 6–23.

What treatment plan will provide this patient the best chance for a successful outcome?

A. Open reduction of the radial head dislocation with K-wire fixation of the proximal radioulnar joint and long arm immobilization with the forearm in supination
B. Closed reduction of the ulna fracture and radial head dislocation with long arm casting for 4 to 6 weeks
C. ORIF of the ulna fracture with closed reduction of the radial head dislocation and brief immobilization

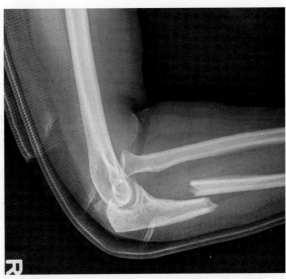

Figure 6–23

D. ORIF of the ulna and closed reduction of the radial head dislocation with long arm casting for 4 to 6 weeks

Discussion

The correct answer is (C). The depicted injury is an ulna fracture with associated dislocation of the proximal radius, known as a Monteggia injury. Whereas in children the treatment is most often closed reduction with long arm cast immobilization, in adults these injuries are almost exclusively treated surgically. The mainstay of surgical treatment is anatomic reduction and fixation of the ulna, which usually leads to reduction of the proximal radius. "D" is an incorrect choice here because immobilizing the adult elbow for a prolonged period leads to increased loss of motion, and in this injury pattern, is unnecessary after ORIF of the ulna fracture. The Bado classification is used to classify Monteggia fractures. In Type I, the radius is dislocated anterior, in Type II, the dislocation is posterior, in Type III, the dislocation is lateral, and in Type IV, there is a fracture of both the radius and ulna shaft with proximal radius dislocation.

After anatomic reduction and fixation of the ulna fracture, the radial head remains unable to be reduced by closed means.

What is most likely to be interposed and preventing reduction?

A. The annular ligament
B. The lateral ulnar collateral ligament
C. An osteochondral fragment
D. Anterior joint capsule
E. The posterior interosseous nerve (PIN)

Discussion

The correct answer is (A). Anatomic reduction of the ulna must first be confirmed as a malreduction, can prevent reduction of the radial head. If the ulna is anatomically reduced, and the radial head remains dislocated, the annular ligament can in some cases remain intact and prevent reduction of the radial head. In this situation, the annular ligament should be divided and subsequently repaired after reduction of the radiocapitellar joint. In more rare circumstances, the PIN can become interposed and prevent anatomic reduction as well, although this is less common than the annular ligament.

Which of the following structures do not play a significant role in the stability of the proximal radioulnar joint (PRUJ)?

A. The annular ligament
B. The radial fossa of the ulna
C. The LCL complex
D. The MCL complex
E. The interosseous membrane (IOM)

Discussion

The correct answer is (D). The PRUJ has relatively little bony contribution to its stability, with only approximately 18% of the radial head circumference articulating with the radial fossa of the ulna at a given time. The annular ligament and LCL complex contribute to the stability of the PRUJ, but the central band of the IOM provides the most significant longitudinal stability when sectioned in anatomic studies. The critical importance of the IOM in maintaining radioulnar alignment in the setting of a radial head fracture is exemplified in an Essex-Lopresti injury.

Objectives: Did you learn...?

- The Bado classification for Monteggia fracture dislocations?
- Operative versus nonoperative management?
- Anatomy of the proximal radioulnar joint?

CASE 19

Dr. James N. Foster

A 67-year-old, left-hand-dominant, retired female sustained a left distal radius fracture when she tripped in her garden and fell onto her outstretched hand. She underwent closed reduction in the emergency department and was placed into a short arm cast on the day of injury. Her injury radiographs are shown in Figure 6–24A and B.

In addition to analgesic medications, what adjunctive medication should the patient be started on as part of her treatment for this injury?

A. Vitamin E
B. Vitamin C
C. Estrogen replacement
D. Bisphosphonate

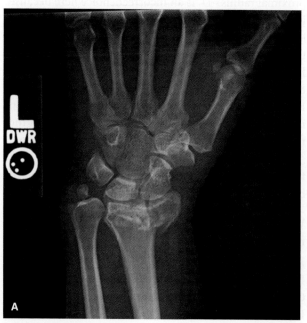
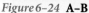
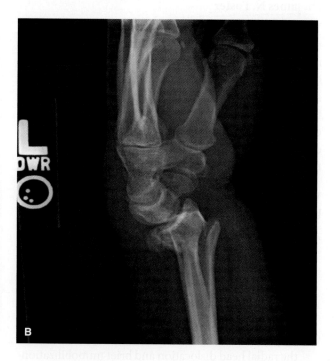

Figure 6–24 **A–B**

Discussion

The correct answer is (B). As part of the latest AAOS Clinical Practice Guidelines (CPG), approved in December of 2009, it is suggested that patients with distal radius fractures be treated with adjuvant vitamin C as a preventative therapy aimed at reducing the likelihood of developing a complex regional pain syndrome (CRPS). While the studies cited in the CPG statement are limited, CRPS can be quite debilitating and there is some data showing a decreased frequency of developing CRPS with supplemental daily vitamin C after injury.

At her first follow-up appointment, 1 week after her initial fracture reduction and cast placement, repeat radiographs in clinic show that she has lost both radial height and volar tilt.

Which of the following is known to be a predictor of fracture instability with closed treatment?

A. Age greater than 50
B. Initial dorsal angulation >20 degrees
C. Open fracture
D. Difficulty in obtaining initial reduction
E. Female sex

Discussion

The correct answer is (B). Acceptable results with closed reduction are generally accepted as radial inclination of at least 15 degrees on PA view, less than 5 mm of radial length shortening, less than 15 degrees of dorsal radial tilt, or less than 20 degrees of volar tilt, and less than 2 mm of articular step-off. Factors predicting failure of closed reduction and immobilization have been studied many times, and one predictive factor that is referenced often is the amount of initial fracture angulation. Also frequently shown to have significant predictive value is increasing patient age (over 58 to 65 years old depending on the study) and the presence of dorsal comminution.

You decide to treat her fracture surgically with a volar plate after she has failed nonoperative management. Her post-op radiographs are shown in Figure 6–25A and B.

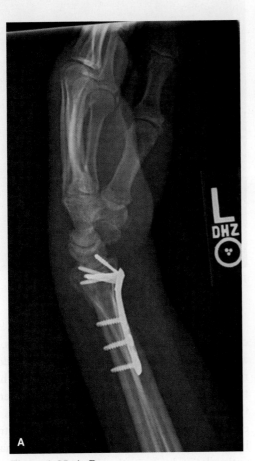

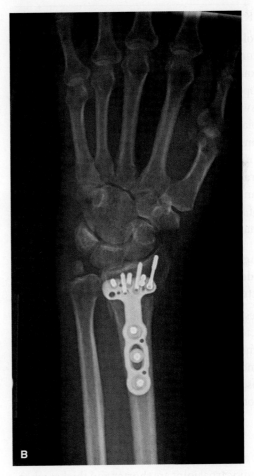

Figure 6–25 **A–B**

Which of the following is not an indication for surgical fixation of distal radius fractures?

A. Postreduction radial shortening >3 mm
B. Intra-articular displacement >2 mm
C. Postreduction dorsal tilt >10 degrees
D. Concomitant ulnar styloid fracture

Discussion

The correct answer is (D). Choices A, B, and C are the indications for surgical fixation of distal radius fractures according to the latest CPG. Other relative indications for surgical treatment include predicted or established metaphyseal instability, bilateral fractures, or other impairment of the contralateral extremity.

Objectives: Did you learn...?

• Indications for operative management of distal radius fractures?
• Predictors of loss of reduction in patients with distal radius fractures?

CASE 20

Dr. Bryan K. Lawson

A 42-year-old, right-hand-dominant police officer sustains an injury to his right wrist in a motor vehicle collision. On examining him in the emergency department he has no open wounds but has obvious deformity and moderate swelling. He also complains of dysesthesias over his volar thumb, index, and long fingers. Sensory examination finds that his two-point discrimination is intact to 5 mm throughout all digits of the right hand. His radiographs are shown in Figure 6–26A and B.

After hanging traction in finger traps he regains nearly all of his radial height on AP fluoroscopic imaging but remains slightly dorsally tilted on a lateral view.

Why is longitudinal traction unlikely to restore the native 12-degree volar tilt in this displaced distal radius fracture?

A. The presence of dorsal comminution
B. Insufficient muscle relaxation
C. Differences in strength and orientation between the volar and dorsal extrinsic ligaments
D. Interposed flexor pollicis longus impeding anatomic reduction of the volar cortex

Discussion

The correct answer is (C). The volar extrinsic ligaments about the radiocarpal joint are shorter and thicker when

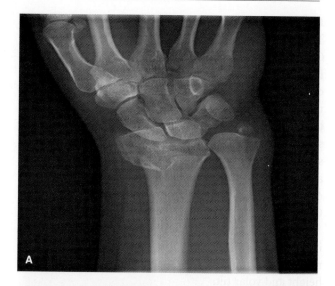

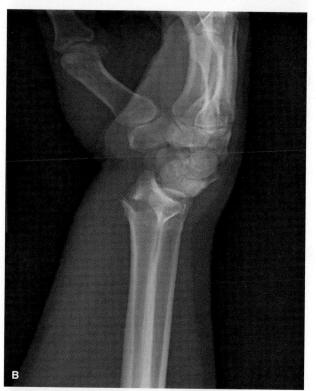

Figure 6–26 **A–B**

compared to the dorsal extrinsic ligaments. They are also oriented more vertically than are the dorsal ligaments, which have a relative "z" orientation. The orientation of the dorsal ligaments allows for more lengthening than is allowed by the volar ligaments. This results in earlier tensioning of the short, straight, and strong volar ligaments with the application of longitudinal traction with relative laxity in the dorsal ligaments, preventing the restoration of volar tilt at the distal radius articular surface.

Following reduction and application of a plaster splint, the patient is sent to radiology for postreduction radiographs. Upon his return to the emergency department he complains that his pain is increasing in the wrist and hand. Two-point discrimination now is worsened to 9 mm in the thumb, index, and long fingers.

What is the most appropriate treatment at this stage?

A. Urgent carpal tunnel release

B. Elevation above the level of the heart and application of an ice pack

C. Administration of oral corticosteroids and re-evaluation in 4 to 6 hours

D. Serial measurement of the pressure within the carpal tunnel with a Stryker needle

Discussion

The correct answer is (A). The development of progressive median nerve dysfunction in the setting of a distal radius fracture is a form of acute carpal tunnel syndrome. This has been a recognized complication of distal radius fractures for many years, and the treatment is surgical release of the carpal tunnel. While acute carpal tunnel syndrome is known to occur more frequently with high-energy distal radius fractures than low-energy fractures, Dyer et al. showed that the amount of translation of the fracture was the most significant radiographic parameter in predicting acute carpal tunnel syndrome in the setting of distal radius fractures.

He is taken to the operating room urgently where a carpal tunnel release is performed. He also undergoes ORIF of the distal radius using a volar plate. Postoperative radiographs are shown in Figure 6–27A and B.

Which of the following is true regarding differences in volar and dorsal plating for distal radius fractures?

A. Radiocarpal articular exposure is improved with the volar approach compared to dorsal.

B. Extensor tendon irritation and rupture is seen in dorsal plating but not in volar plating.

C. The dorsal aspect of the distal radius provides a more congruent surface than the volar surface for situating a plate for ORIF.

D. The volar fixed angle plates allow for improved fixation of osteopenic bone or those fractures with metaphyseal defects.

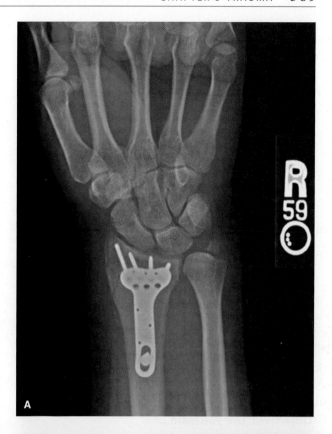

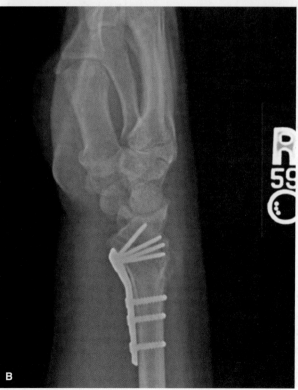

Figure 6–27 **A–B**

Discussion

The correct answer is (D). While classically the distal radius was approached and plated dorsally, there has been a transition in the recent past to performing a large number of distal radius fracture ORIF procedures through a volar approach. Choice A is incorrect because the radiocarpal joint is visualized more easily from the dorsal approach due to the presence of the volar wrist ligaments. Extensor tendon, as well as flexor tendon, irritation and rupture is seen with both dorsal and volar plating. Lister's tubercle can be deceiving on the lateral view when performing volar plating, and exposed screw tips dorsally is a risk for tendon irritation. Placing the volar plate too distal on the radius, past the "watershed line," increases the risk of plate contact with the flexor tendons and subsequent development of irritation and potentially rupture. In addition to the benefit of being able to provide stable fixation to osteopenic bone and fractures with metaphyseal defects, Ruch and Papadonikolakis recently found volar locked plating to have less frequent volar collapse and fewer complications when compared with dorsal plating.

Objectives: Did you learn...?

- Treatment of acute carpal tunnel syndrome in the setting of a distal radius fracture?
- Volar versus dorsal plating considerations?

CASE 21

Dr. Bryan K. Lawson

A 30-year-old male presents to your local trauma center following a motor vehicle collision. On arrival to the trauma bay his vital signs reveal a pulse of 127 with a manual blood pressure that is within normal limits. On your initial assessment you do not appreciate any gross deformity or open wounds to the extremities. The trauma team proceeds with the ATLS protocol.

All of the following radiographic views are recommended in the ATLS protocol for evaluation of the acutely traumatized patient EXCEPT:

A. Anteroposterior pelvic view
B. Lateral cervical spine view
C. Anteroposterior chest view
D. Single anteroposterior view of any perceived long bone deformity

Discussion

The correct answer is (D). After completion of the primary survey and AP chest, AP pelvis, and lateral C-spine, film are considered the most useful radiographic adjuncts at this very early stage of the trauma survey. Even in the setting of gross extremity deformity these three images remain the essential radiographic views to obtain.

The primary and secondary surveys are completed, and the patient is now tachycardic to the 140s with otherwise stable vitals. His pelvic examination is limited by his morbid obesity, however you note ecchymosis over the anterior abdomen and concomitant scrotal edema. His AP pelvis is shown in Figure 6–28.

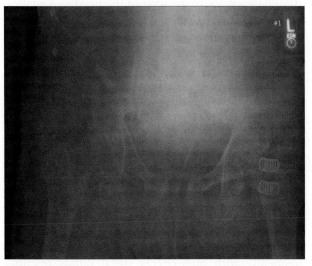

Figure 6–28

What is the next most appropriate step?

A. Obtain CT scan to classify extent of pelvic ring injury
B. Place pelvic binder after ruling out nonpelvic etiologies for the patients with tachycardia
C. Place pelvic binder centered over the iliac wings without delay
D. Place pelvic binder centered over the greater trochanters without delay

Discussion

The correct answer is (D). The patient remains tachycardic following the primary and secondary ATLS surveys. Furthermore, he displays cutaneous stigmata of a pelvic ring injury on examination with concomitant anterior diastasis of the pubic symphysis. The next most appropriate step as the consulting orthopedists will be appropriate placement of a pelvic binder, centered over the greater trochanters, prior to transfer for advanced imaging.

Which of the following is the most common associated injury with fractures of the pelvic ring?

A. Long bone fractures
B. Chest injuries
C. Abdominal injuries (liver, spleen, bladder, and urethral trauma)
D. Spine fractures

Discussion

The correct answer is (B). Chest injuries are present in up to 63% of patients who presents with pelvic fractures. Long bone fractures, abdominal injuries, and spine fractures are also commonly found in these multiply injured patients (50%, 40%, and 25%, respectively).

Objectives: Did you learn...?

- ATLS principles in the workup and management of a pelvis fracture?
- Injuries commonly associated with pelvic fractures?

CASE 22

Dr. Bryan K. Lawson

A 45-year-old cyclist arrives to the trauma bay after being hit by a motor vehicle while crossing a highway earlier in the evening. The patient is awake but somnolent in the trauma bay. Your examination does not reveal any open wounds or gross deformity about the extremities. An AP pelvis and CT imaging reveal a lateral compression Type II (LC-II) pelvic ring injury. Based on the mechanism of injury and described Young–Burgess injury classification type.

Which answer best describes the radiographic finding most likely associated with this patient's injury?

A. Impacted sacral alar fracture and ipsilateral superior and inferior ramus fractures
B. Pubic symphysis diastasis greater than 2.5 cm with external rotation of either hemipelvis and anterior sacroiliac joint widening
C. Superior and inferior ramus fractures with ipsilateral posterior ilium fracture
D. Superior and inferior ramus fractures with ipsilateral sacral compression fracture and external rotation of the contralateral hemipelvis

Discussion

The correct answer is (C). The described LC-II injury involves ipsilateral ramus and ilium crescent fractures as described above. Choices A, B, and D represent Young–Burgess LC-I, APC-II, and LC-III type injuries, respectively.

The decision is made to stabilize the patients pelvic ring injury with a temporary external fixator.

Which construct will is best suited to resist further internal rotation of the patient's hemipelvis?

A. Anterior external fixator with dual 4-mm pins placed in bilateral iliac crests
B. Anterior external fixator with parallel supra-acetabular pins
C. Anterior hybrid construct (supra-acetabular and iliac crest pins)
D. Anterior external fixator with single 5-mm pins placed in bilateral iliac crests

Discussion

The correct answer is (B). Archdeacon et al. demonstrated in their 2009 biomechanical analysis that despite the superior resistance to flexion and extension provided by hybrid frames, supra-acetabular constructs were superior in resisting internal/external rotation of the hemipelvis.

What is the most likely cause of mortality due to an associated injury given this patient's pelvic ring fracture morphology?

A. Pelvic and abdominal visceral injury
B. Thoracic injury
C. Distal extremity vascular injury
D. Closed head injury

Discussion

The correct answer is (D). Closed head injury is the most common cause of death with this patient's injury pattern. Pelvic and abdominal viscera injuries are related to patient mortality following APC type injuries.

Objectives: Did you learn...?

- The Young–Burgess classification of pelvic ring injuries (LC)?
- Associated injuries in patients with pelvic ring injuries?

CASE 23

Dr. Bryan K. Lawson

A 65-year-old male presents to the trauma bay with Young–Burgess APC type II pelvic ring injury.

This specific injury pattern includes which of the following pelvic ligaments?

A. Iliolumbar
B. Sacrospinous
C. Posterior Iliosacral
D. Inguinal

Discussion

The correct answer is (B). The APC II injury pattern will include pubic diastasis >2.5 cm with anterior widening of the sacroiliac joints. Anatomically this correlates with injury to the pubic symphyseal ligaments, pelvic floor ligaments (sacrotuberous and sacrospinous), and the anterior sacroiliac ligaments. The iliolumbar ligaments are primarily involved in vertical shear or Tile C type injury patterns. Posterior iliosacral ligaments are involved in APC III type injuries. Inguinal ligament injury is not classically described in any of the Young–Burgess fracture patterns.

Approximately what percentage of patients who undergo preperitoneal packing for hemodynamic instability in the setting of pelvic ring fracture (without another obvious hemorrhage source) will require subsequent angiography for continued hemorrhage?

A. 3%
B. 17%
C. 35%
D. 50%

Discussion

The correct answer is (B). Cothren et al. describe the efficacy of preperitoneal packing for recalcitrant hemorrhage in pelvic trauma in their 2007 JOT series. All patients with hemodynamic instability in the setting of pelvic fracture underwent external fixation with concomitant preperitoneal packing. Only 16.7% of patients temporized with these measures required further intervention.

The decision is made to stabilize the patients posterior pelvic ring injury with percutaneous instrumentation.

What radiographic landmark on the lateral pelvic view represents the anterior margin of the "safe zone" for percutaneous sacroiliac screw placement?

A. Iliac wing cortical density
B. Anterior cortex of S1
C. Superior endplate of S1
D. Anterior cortex of S2

Discussion

The correct answer is (A). Miller et al. describe the radiographic safe zones for percutaneous sacroiliac screw placement in their 2012 JAAOS review article. The anterior iliac cortical density (seen in Fig. 6–29) represents the anterior extent of the safe zone to ensure appropriate hardware location within the SI articulation. These images must still be correlated with AP, outlet, and inlet views to ensure no other forms of dysmorphism prior to screw placement.

This patient has up to a 90% chance of developing which long-term sequelae following his displaced APC type pelvic ring injury?

A. Fecal incontinence
B. Ipsilateral abductor weakness
C. Dyspareunia
D. Erectile dysfunction

Discussion

The correct answer is (D). Collinge et al. describe increasing age and APC-type fracture patterns as significant risk factors for recalcitrant postinjury erectile dysfunction in males. Choices A to C are all associated with APC type injuries however with lower reported prevalence rates.

Objectives: Did you learn...?

• The Young-Burgess classification of pelvic ring injuries (APC)?

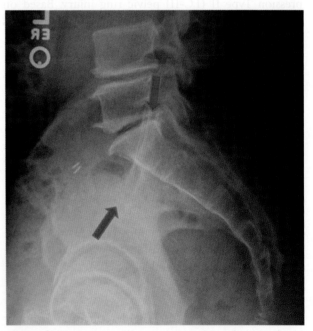

Figure 6–29

- Anatomic landmarks associated with safe percutaneous iliosacral screw placement?
- Long-term complications associated with APC pelvic ring injuries?

CASE 24

Dr. Bryan K. Lawson

A 38-year-old female presents to your clinic now 1 year after diagnosis with an APC Type I pelvic ring injury that was managed nonoperatively. The patient remains neurovascularly intact with a primary complaint of continued groin pain with activity.

Which radiographic view is most effective at elucidating residual pelvic instability?

A. Standing obturator oblique pelvic view
B. Supine AP, inlet, and outlet pelvic series
C. Weight-bearing double leg iliac inlet pelvic view
D. Standing single leg AP pelvic view

Discussion

The correct answer is (D). Seigel et al. describe the utility of single-leg stance AP pelvic radiographs in evaluating for pelvic instability. These standing films were able to elucidate pelvic instability (defined as ≥0.5 cm vertical translation of the symphyseal bodies). This study directly compared the single-leg views to a supine pelvic series. The views described in choices A through C were not included in this evaluation.

What percentage of patients presenting with unstable SI injury or symphyseal disruption will have concomitant displaced acetabular fracture?

A. 1% to 3%
B. 5% to 7%
C. 15% to 20%
D. >30%

Discussion

The correct answer is (B). Letournel and more recently Suzuki et al. have described the rate of displaced acetabular fractures in the setting of a displaced pelvic ring injury at 6.7% and 5.1%, respectively.

Objectives: Did you learn...?

- Radiographic examination to diagnose residual pelvic instability?

CASE 25

Dr. Bryan K. Lawson

A 24-year-old male presents following a motor vehicle collision. His primary complaint is of lower back pain. No focal neurological deficits are noted on his examination. An axial cut of his CT scan is shown in Figure 6–30.

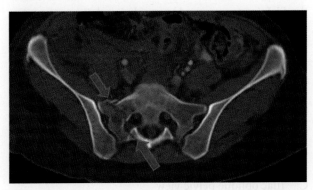

Figure 6–30

Given the location of the vertical component of this patients sacral fracture; what is the rate of neurological deficit (either lower extremity symptoms or bowel, bladder, or sexual dysfunction) associated with this injury pattern?

A. 6%
B. 28%
C. 45%
D. 57%

Discussion

The correct answer is (B). The rate of neurologic injury associated with Denis Type II sacral fractures (through the sacral foramen) is 28%. The rate for Type I (lateral to the foramen) and Type III (medial to the foramen) injuries are 6% and 57%, respectively.

Nonsurgical treatment of sacral fractures is considered a reasonable option in all of the following scenarios, EXCEPT which of the following?

A. Neurologically intact patient with a displaced transverse fracture at the level of the S4 foramen.
B. A neurologically intact patient with a unilateral nondisplaced Denis Type II fracture involving the ventral sacral cortex.
C. A neurologically intact patient with a unilateral displaced Denis Type I fracture involving both the ventral and dorsal cortices.

D. A neurologically intact elderly patient with bilateral nondisplaced Denis Type II fracture involving only the ventral cortex.

Discussion

The correct answer is (C). Nonsurgical management is typically reserved for patients with a sacral fracture morphology that does not compromise spinopelvic stability. As such nondisplaced fractures that are below the SI Joint (response A) or only involving one cortex (responses B and D) may undergo these conservative treatment modalities.

The decision is made to treat the patient's sacral fracture with percutaneous sacroiliac screws.

Which view will minimize the risk of iatrogenic foot drop due to aberrant hardware placement?

A. Inlet pelvic view
B. Obturator outlet pelvic view
C. Iliac oblique pelvic view
D. Outlet pelvic view

Discussion

The correct answer is (A). The pelvic inlet view will allow visualization of the anterior to posterior trajectory of the sacroiliac screw, thus allowing the surgeon to avoid anterior breach and lower lumbar root injury, which drapes over the ventral surface of the sacral ala.

All are radiographic findings that represent varying presentations of sacral dysmorphism EXCEPT which of the following?

A. The sacral alae are at the same level as the iliac crest on the outlet view
B. Recession of the anterior alar cortex on the axial CT view
C. Residual disc space between the upper two sacral segments on the outlet view
D. Paradoxical inlet view of the upper sacral segments on the AP or outlet views

Discussion

The correct answer is (D). This represents occult sacral fracture dislocation or U-type sacral fracture. Sacral dysmorphism is a collective term to describe multiple aberrations in sacral osteology that may preclude safe hardware placement if not recognized preoperatively. The sacral alar anatomy and slope are variable. Upper sacral segment abnormalities are common. Predictable

dysplastic patterns can be easily identified using pelvic outlet and true lateral sacral plain radiographs along with CT scans and include:

1. The sacrum is not recessed within the pelvis on the outlet image.
2. Mammillary processes are seen on the outlet image.
3. The upper sacral foramen is dysmorphic on the outlet image.
4. The alar slope is acute on the lateral view.
5. A residual disc space between the upper two sacral segments is seen on the outlet image.
6. "Tongue-in-groove" SI articulations are noted on the CT scan.

Objectives: Did you learn...?

- Denis classification of sacral fractures and corresponding frequency of neurologic injury?
- Complications associated with the placement of percutaneous iliosacral screws?
- Characteristics of sacral dysmorphism?

CASE 26

Dr. Bryan K. Lawson

A 67-year-old female presents to your clinic with pelvic and groin pain for 5 days after a low-impact fall from sitting height. On examination she has full asymptomatic hip ROM and remains ambulatory with the above symptoms. Radiographs films are negative for fracture, and you decide to send her for nuclear imaging, of which a representative image is shown in Figure 6–31.

What is the name of the radiographic finding pictured below and what pathology does this represent?

A. H-sign, iliac crescent fracture
B. H-sign, sacral insufficiency fracture
C. Lambda-sign, sacroiliitis
D. Lambda-sign, iliac crescent fracture

Discussion

The correct answer is (B). The image below displays an H-sign as seen with sacral insufficiency fractures. Lambda is a fracture morphology seen in complex sacral fractures. Iliac crescent fractures are a component of the LC-II type pelvic ring injury. Sacroiliac joint pathology would likely not have the central uptake within the sacrum on this imaging modality.

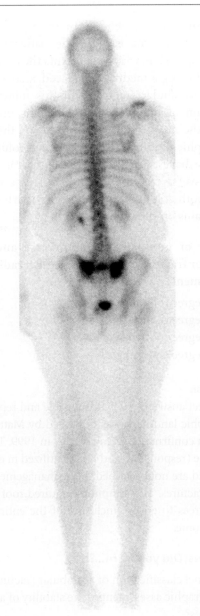

Figure 6–31

What is the estimated incidence of this specific form of pathology in women over 55 years of age, and what is the most common cause?

A. 1%, postmenopausal osteoporosis
B. 5%, low-energy trauma
C. 10%, postmenopausal osteoporosis
D. 25%, low-energy trauma

Discussion

The correct answer is (A). Commonly these postmenopausal females will present with no history of acute trauma. The mainstay of treatment is conservative with bedrest/early mobility.

Objectives: Did you learn...?

• Diagnosis of sacral insufficiency fracture?
• Incidence and most common cause of sacral insufficiency fracture?

CASE 27

Dr. Bryan K. Lawson

A 24-year-old male presents to the trauma bay as a transfer from a level 3 facility. On report EMS states that the transfer diagnosis is a displaced acetabular fracture. You initiate your musculoskeletal evaluation.

Approximately what percentage of patients presenting with acetabular fracture will have clinically apparent or occult associated orthopaedic diagnoses?

A. 2%
B. 10%
C. 35%
D. 55%

Discussion

The correct answer is (D). Matta reported a 56% incidence of associated injuries in patients presenting with acetabular fracture.

On your evaluation the patient displays significant ecchymosis over his lateral thigh with a palpable fluid collection. On further investigation, he appears to have diminished sensation over this area of his thigh.

Approximately what percentage of patients with this pathology will have positive culture results on aspiration or open debridement and irrigation?

A. 5%
B. 20%
C. 45%
D. 60%

Discussion

The correct answer is (C). Hak et al. describe a 46% culture positive rate among these closed degloving injuries associated with pelvic and acetabular fractures. This soft tissue diagnosis must be considered and mitigated prior to any plan for operative fixation.

Which radiographic view will allow clear evaluation of the posterior wall when evaluating suspected acetabular fracture?

A. Inlet view
B. Iliac oblique view

C. False profile view

D. Obturator oblique view

Discussion

The correct answer is (D). The obturator oblique view allows further evaluation of the posterior wall and anterior column. The iliac oblique view will allow visualization of the anterior wall and posterior column. The inlet view is useful in evaluation of pelvic ring injury and during sacroiliac screw placement. The false profile view is used in the evaluation of femoral acetabular impingement and has not been described for classifying acetabular fracture.

Objectives: Did you learn...?

- Frequency of positive cultures associated with Morel-Lavallée/degloving lesions?
- Optimal radiographic view for visualization of the posterior wall of the acetabulum?

CASE 28

Dr. Bryan K. Lawson

A 45-year-old female presents following a motor vehicle collision where she was a restrained passenger. She remains awake and alert with stable vital signs. The primary and secondary surveys are completed with a primary finding of left hip pain. Initial plain radiographs and CT imaging reveal breaks in the iliopectineal and ilioischial lines without a fracture of the obturator ring.

Based on the Letournel classification system, how would the acetabular fracture described be classified?

A. Transverse

B. Both column

C. Anterior column plus anterior hemitransverse

D. T-type

Discussion

The correct answer is (A). The transverse fracture pattern will violate the ilioischial and iliopectineal radiographic lines without an obturator ring injury. All other response options will require a fracture of the obturator ring.

If the above fracture pattern has a fracture line exiting the obturator ring and no portion of the joint surface is attached to the intact ilium, what is the new classification of this acetabular fracture pattern?

A. Transverse plus posterior wall

B. T-type

C. Posterior hemitransverse

D. Both column

Discussion

The correct answer is (D). The patient's imaging reveals a spur sign, which represents the cortex of the ilium following a medially displaced, associated both column acetabular fractures. In this injury pattern no portion of the acetabulum remains in continuity with the intact ilium, thus producing this reliable radiographic finding. In general any column fracture must have a fracture of the obturator ring, and any transverse fracture (including T-type fractures) involve both columns, but a portion of articular surface remains on the ilium.

Stability of nondisplaced transverse and T-type acetabular fractures are based on which radiographic measurement?

A. 60-degree roof arc angle

B. 20-degree center edge

C. 45-degree roof arc angle

D. 20-degree alpha angle

Discussion

The correct answer is (C). This reliable and reproducible radiographic landmark was described by Matta in 1986 and again confirmed by Vrahas et al. in 1999. The center edge angle (responses B and D) are utilized in evaluation of FAI and are not described in the management of acetabular fractures. The minimum required roof arc angle is 45 degrees to ensure inclusion of the entire weight-bearing dome.

Objectives: Did you learn...?

- Letournel classification of acetabular fractures?
- Radiographic assessment of the stability of acetabular fractures?

CASE 29

Dr. Bryan K. Lawson

You are consulted by the general surgery trauma team for further evaluation of a 35-year-old male with a displaced acetabular fracture. The patient's radiographs reveal fracture lines extending through both the iliopectineal and ilioischial lines with dissociation of the acetabulum from the intact ilium.

Which surgical approach will allow direct visual and/or indirect tactile assessment of this entire fracture pattern during operative fixation?

A. Stoppa

B. Kocher–Langenbeck

C. Watson–Jones

D. Ilioinguinal

Discussion

The correct answer is (D). The ilioinguinal approach will allow direct visualization of the entire inner table of the ilium, pelvic brim, and anterior column, with concomitant tactile access to the outer table of the ilium and posterior column.

All are indications for interval skeletal traction in this patient while awaiting definitive fixation EXCEPT which of the following?

A. Unstable hip joint

B. Associated both column fracture pattern

C. Incarcerated intra-articular fragment

D. Recalcitrant medial subluxation of the femoral head

Discussion

The correct answer is (B). Reponses A, C, and D are all indications for skeletal traction in a patient presenting with a displaced acetabular fracture. Associated both column fracture is not an indication in isolation.

All are considered absolute operative indications for acetabular fractures EXCEPT which of the following?

A. Irreducible fracture-dislocation

B. Intra-articular bone fragments

C. Associated both column fracture

D. Associated femoral head fracture

E. Transverse acetabular fracture with 20 degree roof arc angle

Discussion

The correct answer is (C). Nonoperative management of associated both column acetabular fracture is a reasonable management option assuming secondary articular congruence of the distal anterior and posterior column fragment (secondary articular congruence).

Objectives: Did you learn...?

• Operative indications for acetabular fractures?

• Surgical approaches for acetabular fractures?

CASE 30

Dr. Bryan K. Lawson

A 68-year-old, active male presents to the emergency department after being struck by a motor vehicle while riding his bicycle. Radiographic assessment reveals weight-bearing dome impaction as demonstrated in Figure 6–32.

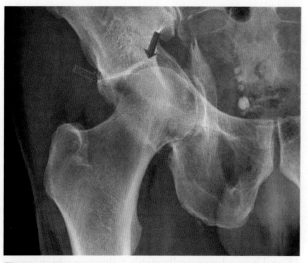

Figure 6–32

What is the ideal treatment for this patient?

A. Extensile approach (iliofemoral) for ORIF of both columns

B. ORIF of both columns with acute total hip arthroplasty

C. Kocher-Langenbeck approach for direct reduction and fixation of the posterior column and percutaneous anterior column fixation

D. Nonoperative management with skeletal traction

Discussion

The correct answer is (B). The patient's radiographs reveal significant superior medial impaction of the acetabulum associated with this patient's acetabular fracture. This "gull-sign" was originally described in the 60s as a radiographic representation of severe medial joint impaction. Anglen et al. evaluated this geriatric population with these specific radiographic findings and determined overall outcomes were poor despite open reduction and internal fixation. In this setting (patient >65 with significant medial joint impaction) acute total hip arthroplasty should be considered after open reduction and fixation of the acetabular fracture.

Which radiographic view is optimal for evaluation of the superomedial joint impaction that is characteristic of a geriatric acetabular fracture?

A. Inlet view

B. Iliac oblique view

C. False profile view

D. Obturator oblique view

Discussion

The correct answer is (D). The obturator oblique view is most useful for the evaluation of superomedial joint impaction in this patient population.

Objectives: Did you learn…?

- Indications for considering ORIF and acute THA for an acetabular fracture?
- The optimal radiographic view to visualize superomedial joint impaction in geriatric acetabular fractures?

CASE 31

Dr. David J. Tennent

A 53-year-old male arrives in the trauma bay with a GCS 15 and hemodynamically stable following a high-speed motor vehicle crash. He is complaining of severe right hip pain and is unable to move his right lower extremity. You note that his leg is shortened, slightly flexed, internally rotated, and adducted. He has symmetric pulses, and he is neurologically intact throughout his extremity. He has a normal examination otherwise. As part of the standard Advanced Trauma Life Support algorithm, an an AP pelvis is obtained seen in Figure 6–33.

What do you do next?

A. Obtain a CT scan to evaluate for incarcerated fragments and acetabular fracture pattern
B. Emergent hip reduction prior to further pelvic imaging
C. Obtain ABI

D. Proceed directly to OR for open reduction of hip and internal fixation of acetabulum
E. Admit the patient to the floor for closed reduction under anesthesia in the morning

Discussion

The correct answer is (B). This presentation is classic for a posterior hip dislocation occurring during a motor vehicle crash and is often called a "dashboard injury" due to the axially directed force that is transmitted from the dashboard of a vehicle through the knees with the hips flexed and adducted as is normal while sitting in a vehicle. As a result, ipsilateral knee injuries are common. In an otherwise stable patient without associated femoral neck fracture, closed reduction of the dislocated hip should be attempted urgently regardless of acetabular fracture. This is performed in order to decrease the incidence of avascular necrosis, which can be as high as 15%, and chondral damage to the femoral head. However, if vascular injury is suspected, obtaining prereduction ABIs should be performed as part of a thorough neurovascular examination. Due to the high trait of sciatic nerve injuries (more commonly the peroneal division), a thorough neuro examination should be conducted pre- and postreduction. Furthermore, an attempt at closed reduction should be performed prior to proceeding to the OR for open reduction.

After completing the remainder of the ATLS protocol, you reduce the hip and obtain the AP pelvis seen in Figure 6–34.

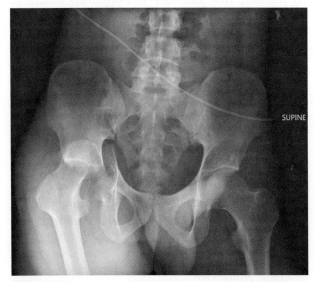

Figure 6–33

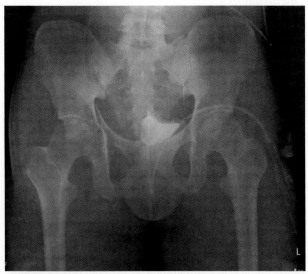

Figure 6–34

What is the next appropriate step?

A. MRI of hip
B. CT pelvis with intravascular contrast
C. CT pelvis without contrast
D. Repeat reduction attempt
E. Judet views of pelvis to evaluate acetabulum fracture

Discussion

The correct answer is (C). Following closed reduction of a hip with an associated acetabulum fracture, a CT pelvis without contrast should be ordered in order to evaluate for incarcerated fragments, malreduction, impaction of the acetabulum and/or femoral head, and overall fracture pattern. Doing so will also allow you to better evaluate the acetabulum fracture pattern. MRI or ultrasound of the hip is not indicated in this situation and, although Judet views are needed, these should be ordered following evaluation for incarcerated fragments. IV contrast is not needed in this situation as the patient has no evidence of vascular injury and will not provide you with meaningful information.

During the CT scan, a small subdural hematoma is also discovered and the patient is taken to the ICU for further care. You notice on the CT pelvis without contrast that his hip is not concentrically reduced. You subsequently repeat the reduction attempt and are unable to adequately obtain a well-reduced hip due to the continued posterior subluxation of the hip. You then place a distal femoral traction pin and apply traction, which keeps the hip concentrically reduced.

What structure is most at risk with distal femoral traction pin placement?

A. Peroneal nerve
B. Femoral artery
C. Medial geniculate artery
D. Popliteal artery
E. Sciatic nerve

Discussion

The correct answer is (C). When placing a distal femoral traction pin, one must be aware of surrounding neurovascular structures. Traditional teaching has stated that the femoral artery at Hunter's canal is most at risk when placing a distal femoral pin; however, anatomic studies have shown that the medial geniculate artery is most at risk when placing this pin at a distance between 9 and 12 mm. The femoral artery can be found at approximately 29 to 35 mm from the course of the traction pin.

Five months after open reduction and internal fixation of his posterior acetabulum fracture, the patient presents to clinic with continued right hip pain deep in his groin that is worse with internal rotation and walking up stairs. Repeat radiographs of his hip reveal a well-healed acetabular fracture and sclerosis of his femoral head.

What is the most likely etiology of his hip pain?

A. Posttraumatic osteoarthritis
B. Avascular necrosis of the femoral head
C. Femoroacetabular impingement
D. Missed ligamentum teres avulsion fracture
E. A or B

Discussion

The correct answer is (E). Commonly associated injuries following a posterior hip dislocation include posttraumatic osteoarthritis (PTOA), femoral head osteonecrosis, sciatic nerve injury, ipsilateral knee injuries, and recurrent dislocations. PTOA has been noted to occur between 20% and 40% of hip dislocations with a higher incidence occurring with associated acetabular fractures. A time-dependent association has been noted with AVN of the femoral head in both animal and human models with times to reduction greater than 6 to 8 hours and 12 hours, respectively, showing increased incidence of AVN of up to 40%. This is primarily due to disruption of the blood supply to the femoral head, primarily the medial femoral circumflex artery.

Objectives: Did you learn...?

- Diagnostic and treatment considerations in posterior hip dislocations?
- Anatomic considerations of distal femoral traction pin placement?
- Complications of traumatic hip dislocations?

CASE 32

Dr. David J. Tennent

A 47-year-old male was a restrained driver in a motor vehicle crash while on his way to work. He was transferred from an outside hospital with a reduced, prior left hip dislocation and pelvic fractures. On arrival to the trauma bay he was a GCS 15 and hemodynamically stable complaining of left hip pain. His physical examination was significant for a painful logroll, tenderness in his hip flexion crease, weak dorsiflexion, and toe extension in his left lower extremity. Tertiary examination is otherwise negative. Radiographs of his pelvis display a concentrically reduced hip.

What is your next step in management?

A. Obtain Judet and inlet/outlet views
B. Obtain a noncontrast CT scan
C. Obtain a CT scan with contrast
D. Proceed to OR for nerve exploration
E. Obtain nerve conduction studies for complete evaluation of nerve deficit

Discussion

The correct answer is (B). This patient sustained a posterior hip dislocation following a motor vehicle crash. This frequently occurs when a posteriorly directed force is axially translated through the knee with a flexed hip in what is commonly called a "dashboard injury." When this injury occurs, immediate closed reduction should be attempted. Following appropriate reduction, a postreduction CT scan should be obtained to evaluate for associated fractures and/or incarcerated fractures. Additional pelvic views show appropriate postreduction but may not be sensitive enough for associated pathology. Routine use of contrast post reduction is unnecessary and exposes the patient to unnecessary contrast. Exploration of the sciatic nerve and nerve conduction studies are inappropriate at this time as the patient most likely has a sciatic neuropraxia that resolves in 60% to 70% of all injuries. Knee ligamentous injuries are common in these injuries.

On complete review of the postreduction CT scan you find a reduced hip with an intact posterior acetabulum with a fracture line extending through the femoral head above the level of the fovea with 3 mm of articular step-off and no femoral neck fracture.

How would you classify this fracture?

A. Pipkin I
B. Pipkin II
C. Pipkin III
D. Pipkin IV

Discussion

The correct answer is (B). The Pipkin classification (Table 6–3) is used to describe femoral head fractures and their associated conditions. This classification system has been found to correlate with functional outcomes with higher Pipkin classification resulting in worse functional outcomes. A Pipkin I fracture is a femoral head fracture below the level of the fovea. Although

Table 6–3   PIPKIN CLASSIFICATION

Type I	Fracture below fovea not involving weight-bearing surface of femoral head
Type II	Fracture above fovea involving weight-bearing surface of femoral head
Type III	Type I or Type II with associated femoral neck fracture
Type IV	Type I or Type II with associated acetabulum fracture

these are frequently treated nonsurgically as they do not involve the weight-bearing surface, there is some literature that suggests that those patients undergoing fragment excision may do better than those treated nonoperatively. A Pipkin II fracture is a fracture of the femoral head that is above the fovea. These fractures do involve the weight-bearing surface. Nondisplaced fractures may be treated nonoperatively with restricted weight bearing and range of motion restrictions; however, those fractures with >1 to 2 mm of intra-articular step-off require open reduction and internal fixation in order to restore articular integrity. Pipkin III fractures are femoral head fractures with associated femoral neck fractures. These fractures have a high rate of AVN associated with them due to disruption of the femoral head blood supply and require operative fixation. Pipkin IV fractures are fractures of the femoral head associated with acetabular fractures. These fractures also frequently require operative management due to the associated joint instability and incongruity.

Following completion of appropriate ATLS workup, the patient is taken to the operative room for open reduction and internal fixation of his femoral head.

What approach is best suited for this procedure?

A. Kocher–Langenbeck (posterior)
B. Smith–Petersen (anterior)
C. Direct lateral
D. Ludloff (Medial)
E. Anterolateral (Watson-Jones)

Discussion

The correct answer is (B). Optimal surgical approach to the femoral head fracture is dependent of fracture pattern and associated injuries. This patient has a Pipkin II fracture that is most appropriately assessed using the Smith–Petersen direct anterior approach. The Smith–Petersen approach utilizes the internervous plane between the femoral and superior gluteal nerves. Studies have found that this approach has decreased rates of AVN, less blood loss, decreased operating, but increased rates of heterotopic ossification for Pipkin I and II fractures. In Pipkin III and IV fractures, the associated injuries also need to be appropriately addressed via single- or dual-incision techniques.

Objectives: Did you learn...?

• Fracture classification of femoral head fractures?
• Surgical approaches for femoral head fractures?

CASE 33

Dr. David J. Tennent

A 23-year-old male presents to the emergency department following a hard landing while skydiving. He is unable to ambulate secondary to pain in his right hip. He has pain with logroll and while conducting a straight leg raise. His leg is shortened and externally rotated. Pulses and neurologic examination is symmetric to his contralateral side. An AP radiograph of the right hip is shown in Figure 6–35.

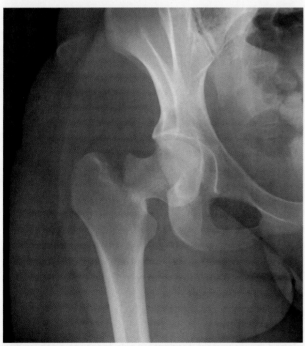

Figure 6–35

What treatment option is most reasonable for this patient?

A. Closed reduction and protected weight bearing for 3 months

B. Closed reduction and percutaneous screw fixation
C. Total hip arthroplasty
D. Hemiarthroplasty
E. Open reduction and internal fixation

Discussion

The correct answer is (E). This is a young patient with a displaced femoral neck fracture. The Garden classification and Pauwels classification are most commonly used to classify these fractures. The Garden classification (Table 6–4) is based on the degree of displacement and fracture orientation. Garden 1 fractures are incomplete/valgus impacted fractures. Due to the valgus impaction, this is considered a stable fracture. Garden 2 fractures are complete, nondisplaced fractures. This is also considered a stable fracture pattern. Although stable fractures in young patients who comply with weight-bearing restrictions for a minimum of 6 to 8 weeks can be treated nonoperatively; due to potential complications with displacement, the majority are treated surgically with ORIF. Garden 3 and 4 fractures are unstable fractures with incomplete displacement and complete displacement respectively. These require prompt open reduction and internal fixation in the young patient due to concern for AVN, which can be as high as 40% in displaced femoral neck fractures. In high-energy injuries with a vertical fracture line, the Pauwels classification (Table 6–5) can be used to describe the fracture stability based on

Table 6–4   GARDEN CLASSIFICATION (LOW ENERGY)

Type I	Incomplete, valgus impacted fracture
Type II	Complete, nondisplaced fracture
Type III	Complete fracture with <50% displacement
Type IV	Completely displaced fracture

Table 6–5   PAUWELS CLASSIFICATION (HIGH ENERGY)

Type I	Vertical fracture line <30 degrees from horizontal
Type II	Vertical fracture line 30–50 degrees from horizontal
Type III	Vertical fracture line greater than 50 degrees from horizontal

the amount of vertical shear force across the fracture. Higher Pauwels classification correlates with increased instability and higher rates of nonunion and AVN, as weight transmission across the fracture site creates higher shear forces at a higher Pauwels angle. In young patients with femoral neck fractures, the standard of care is open reduction and internal fixation of displaced femoral neck fractures in order to obtain an anatomic reduction and decrease postoperative complications. Cephalomedullary nailing is not indicated in this fracture pattern. Arthroplasty in a young patient is also not indicated as a primary surgical option.

The patient returns to clinic 3 months postoperatively following open reduction and internal fixation with a sliding hip screw and antirotation screw. He now complains of hip pain. He states that his pain originally improved but has now been increasing over the last month. He is otherwise doing well and denies any repeat trauma.

What is the patient's most likely diagnosis?

A. Avascular necrosis
B. Nonunion
C. Posttraumatic arthritis
D. Symptomatic hardware
E. Malunion

Discussion

The correct answer is (A). Urgent anatomic reduction and internal fixation is required in displaced femoral neck fractures in order to preserve the blood supply to the femoral head. The medial femoral circumflex artery supplies the majority of the blood supply to the femoral head with the lateral femoral circumflex, the ascending cervical branches, and the artery of the ligamentum teres providing a lesser degree of blood. Disruption of these vessels with increasing displacement is presumed to increase the risk of avascular necrosis which studies have shown occur in 10% to 40% of displaced fractures. Although increased intracapsular pressure due to hematoma formation has been theorized to increase AVN rates, this has not been proven. Fracture nonunion is a common complication following open reduction and internal fixation of femoral neck fractures occurring 10% to 30% of cases in multiple studies. Nonunion is related to the degree of initial displacement and more commonly associated with a varus malreduction.

Repeat radiographs taken in clinic demonstrate loss of fracture reduction with varus malposition.

What is the next treatment option?

A. Total hip arthroplasty
B. Hemiarthroplasty
C. Revision open reduction and internal fixation with screw fixation
D. Valgus intertrochanteric osteotomy with blade plate fixation
E. Revision open reduction and internal fixation with dynamic hip screw and iliac crest bone graft

Discussion

The correct answer is (D). Treatment of failed open reduction and internal fixation of a femoral neck fracture in a young patient requires a valgus intertrochanteric osteotomy with a blade plate. The valgus intertrochanteric osteotomy converts the shear forces across the nonunion site into a compressive force, which improves the potential for progressing to union. Revision open reduction and internal fixation with screws or blade plate with bone grafting are not preferred revision options. Furthermore, arthroplasty options in young patients are not preferred due to complications and longevity concerns associated with these implants.

Objectives: Did you learn...?

- Classification of femoral neck fractures?
- Treatment options for primary and revision femoral neck fractures?
- Complications of femoral neck fractures?

CASE 34

Dr. David J. Tennent

A 70-year-old female fell from standing while leaving church. She was brought to the emergency department due to her inability to bear weight on her left lower extremity. She complains of pain in her left hip and has pain with hip motion. She denies pain elsewhere. On further questioning she states she has had pain with ambulation in bilateral hips for several years and is a community ambulator without assistive devices. She is in good health otherwise with minimal medical comorbidities. Radiograph of her hip shows a displaced basicervical femoral neck fracture with varus malalignment.

What is her best treatment option?

A. Percutaneous screw fixation
B. Open reduction and internal fixation

C. Hemiarthroplasty
D. Total hip arthroplasty
E. Protected weight bearing

Discussion

The correct answer is (D). This is an elderly patient with prior hip pain and without significant comorbidities that would preclude her from undergoing a total hip arthroplasty. Furthermore, in active elderly patients with prior hip arthropathy, total hip arthroplasty is preferred due to decreased revision rates, improved Harris Hip scores, and improved quality of life scores compared to open reduction and internal fixation and hemiarthroplasty. Hemiarthroplasty would be more appropriate in a patient without prior hip pain, a patient in poor medical health, neurologic condition that increases dislocation risk, or a more inactive patient. Protected weight bearing in an otherwise healthy patient is not indicated for treatment of a displaced femoral neck fracture.

In discussion with the family and patient preoperatively, they are concerned about what her postoperative function will be as she was previously a very active individual. They are also worried that she will not be able to survive this injury.

What is the patient's predicted mortality at 1 year following a femoral neck fracture?

A. No difference at 1 year
B. 0% to 15%
C. 16% to 35%
D. 36% to 55%
E. >55%

Discussion

The correct answer is (C). The predicted 1-year mortality rate for an elderly patient following a femoral neck fracture is between 14 and 36. The predicted loss of independence for an elderly individual following a femoral neck fracture at 1 year is 50%. When looking at surgical timing of femoral neck fractures in elderly individuals, it is important to perform surgery as quickly as medically feasible. Previous studies have shown that when surgery was delayed more than 4 days in otherwise healthy patients, mortality risk increased significantly. Furthermore, in patients who required medical management of an acute comorbidity prior to surgery, 30-day mortality increased by 2.5 times that of those healthy patients.

The patient was indicated for total hip arthroplasty. Prior to undergoing surgery, the family states that the patient was recently diagnosed with early Parkinson's and has a history of alcoholism.

Which surgical approach would increase the risk of postoperative dislocation?

A. Posterior
B. Direct anterior
C. Anterolateral
D. Lateral
E. Equivalent risk of dislocation

Discussion

The correct answer is (A). Risk of dislocation following total hip arthroplasty occurs in 1% to 3% of all patients and most commonly occurs in the first month. Risk factors for postoperative dislocation include: prior hip surgery, female sex, greater than 70 years of age, posterior approach, component malposition, neuromuscular disorder (i.e., Parkinson's), drug or alcohol abuse, decreased offset, and decreased head–neck ratio. This patient has multiple risk factors for postoperative dislocation and, as such, a posterior approach should be avoided if possible.

Objectives: Did you learn...?

- Treatment options in elderly femoral neck fractures?
- Dislocation risks in elderly following THA?
- Importance of surgical approach on hip dislocation?

CASE 35

Dr. David J. Tennent

A 65-year-old male was struck by a car at low speed while crossing the street. Upon evaluation in the trauma bay he was found to have pain in his left hip with painful range of motion about his hip. He had strong, symmetric, palpable dorsalis pedis and posterior tibialis pulses and had full sensation in all dermatomal distributions in his bilateral lower extremities. His AP and lateral radiographs of his hip are shown in Figure 6–36A and B.

What is the most indicative sign of stability of this fracture nondisplaced intertrochanteric femur fracture seen in Figure 6–36A and B?

A. Intact posteriomedial cortex
B. Degree of metadiaphyseal comminution
C. No subtrochanteric extension of fracture
D. Displacement of greater trochanter less than 5 mm
E. Reverse obliquity fracture pattern

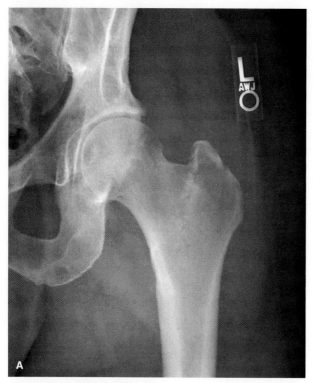

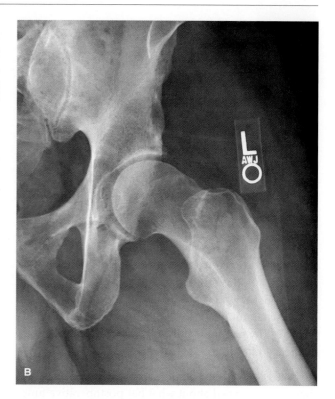

Figure 6–36 **A–B**

Discussion

The correct answer is (B). This patient sustained an intertrochanteric femur fracture. When evaluating these fractures it is paramount that the posterior medial cortex be examined in order to determine fracture stability as this impacts implant choice and fixation options, as does the presence of an intact lateral wall. An intact posterior medial cortex allows for resistance of compressive loads and resistance of varus collapse postoperatively. Unstable patterns include those fractures with reverse obliquity, comminuted posterior medial cortex, comminuted lateral wall, subtrochanteric extension, and displacement of the lesser trochanter. Stable fracture patterns allow the use of a sliding hip screw or cephalomedullary nail. However, unstable fractures preclude the use of a sliding hip screw due to high failure rates and collapse into varus and retroversion.

What fracture pattern presents an increased risk of intraoperative malreduction due to flexion of the proximal fragment when using a dynamic hip screw?

A.   Right-sided reverse oblique fracture
B.   Left-sided unstable intertrochanteric femur fracture
C.   Right-sided subtrochanteric femur fracture
D.   Left-sided basicervical femoral neck fracture
E.   All intertrochanteric fractures

Discussion

The correct answer is (B). Left-sided, unstable intertrochanteric femur fractures are at increased risk of malreduction interoperatively while placing the dynamic hip screw due to the rotational torque imparted on the fracture when positioning the implant. This causes clockwise rotation and proximal segment flexion due to the overall decrease in fracture stability. Right-sided fractures do not exhibit this phenomenon because this rotational torque is converted into a compressive force. A second antirotational screw can be placed prior to the compressive dynamic screw in order to assist with decreasing the incidence of malreduction when placing the dynamic hip screw.

When placing a dynamic hip screw, what is predictive of screw pullout postoperatively?

A.   Degree of peri-implant stability
B.   Associated femoral head fracture
C.   Age greater than 65
D.   Tip-apex distance
E.   Use of an additional (antirotation) screw

Discussion

The correct answer is (D). The tip-apex distance (TAD) is the summation of the distance between the femoral

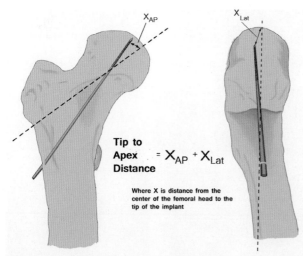

Figure 6–37 (Illustrated by David Beavers.)

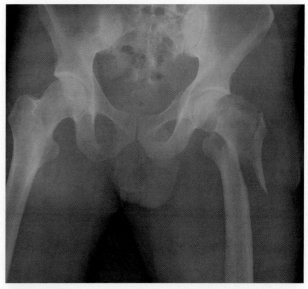

Figure 6–38

head and the tip of the screw (Fig. 6–37). It has been shown to be predictive of screw cutout. The other factors listed above likely contribute to screw cutout but have not yet been proven. A TAD >25 mm is indicative of increased screw pullout.

Objectives: Did you learn...?

- Radiographic indicators of stability?
- Predictors of fixation failure?
- Risks for malreduction?

CASE 36

Dr. David J. Tennent

A 34-year-old, male bull rider is brought to the emergency department after being bucked from his bull. He has abrasions over his left upper and lower extremities with exquisite tenderness over his left hip, pain with longroll, and tenderness in his left groin. An AP pelvis radiograph is shown in Figure 6–38.

What treatment is most appropriate in this injury?

A. Lateral entry long intramedullary nail
B. Piriformis entry long intramedullary nail
C. Sliding hip screw
D. Short cephalomedullary nail
E. Long cephalomedullary nail

Discussion

The correct answer is (E). When choosing an implant for fixation of an intertrochanteric femur fracture, it is most important to consider the fracture stability. The above fracture is a comminuted, reverse oblique frac-

ture. Due to the reverse oblique nature of the fracture, a sliding hip screw, short intramedullary nail, and standard femoral intramedullary nail are not appropriate implant choices when considering the risk of excessive collapse with use of these implants.

When using an intramedullary nail for fixation of the above fracture, what factor can cause peri-implant failure at the time of placement?

A. Lateral starting point
B. Varus malreduction
C. Use of smaller diameter interlocking screws
D. Tip-apex distance equal to 16 mm
E. Nail radius of curvature equal to 300 degrees

Discussion

The correct answer is (E). Larger nail radius of curvature is associated with higher rate of anterior cortex penetration at the time of implant placement. The average femoral anatomic radius of curvature is approximately 120 degrees. As such, femoral intramedullary implants with larger radii of curvatures (more straight) place increased stresses on the anterior cortex. This can cause an increased risk of anterior distal femoral cortex penetration. A tip-apex distance greater than 25 mm is associated with increased implant cutout. Varus malreduction and a lateral starting point have not been shown to have higher rates of peri-implant failures. Of note, peri-implant fractures are more common when using nails compared to plates.

What is predictive of mortality in patients greater than 65 following a hip fracture at 2 years post-injury?

A. Mechanism of injury
B. American Society of Anesthesiologist (ASA) classification
C. Length of surgery
D. Male sex
E. Type of fracture

Discussion

The correct answer is (B). Hip fractures in elderly patients are associated with higher rates of mortality at 6 months. However, in patients greater than 65, increased ASA classification at the time of surgery has been shown to have a mortality rate three times that of those with lower ASA scores. Other categories have not been shown to have higher rates of mortality at 2 years. Other predictors of mortality in the first year following a hip fracture include: male gender, intertrochanteric fracture, fixation delay greater than 4 days, age greater than 85, higher ASA classification, and increased number of medical conditions.

Objectives: Did you learn...?

• Fixation options for intertrochanteric femur fractures?
• Importance of implant design on fracture fixation?
• Predictors of mortality following hip fractures?

CASE 37

Dr. David J. Tennent

An 84-year-old female presents to her family practice physician with thigh pain for the past 3 months. On further discussion with her in clinic, she states that she has had pain in her thigh for approximately 3 months. She attributes this to beginning a new walking regimen in order to lose weight. Her medical history includes: significant osteoporosis (treated with alendronate for the past 8 years), hypertension, hyperlipidemia, and diabetes. She denies any history of trauma and only an upper respiratory infection approximately 2 weeks prior. Her last T score was −1.8. Radiographs reveal subtrochanteric sclerosis or cortical thickening as shown in Figure 6–39.

What is her most likely diagnosis?

A. Osteomyelitis
B. Insufficiency fracture
C. Osteomyelitis
D. Renal osteodystrophy
E. Stress reaction

Discussion

The correct answer is (E). This patient's clinical history and radiographs are consistent with a bisphosphonate-

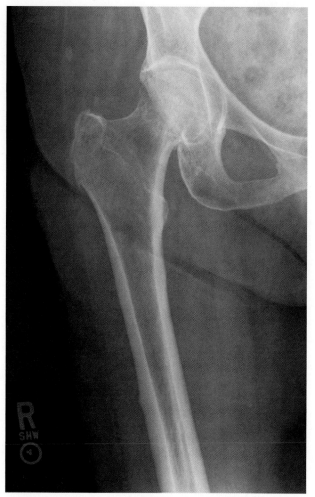

Figure 6–39

related fracture of her subtrochanteric region. This a relatively uncommon side effect of prolonged bisphosphonate use. The typical history consists of prolonged bisphosphonate use greater than 5 years, insidious onset of pain, and no trauma. Radiographs often display lateral cortical thickening progressing to a transverse fracture line with medial spike.

What is the mechanism of action of alendronate?

A. Farnesyl pyrophosphate inhibition
B. Formation of inappropriate ATP analogue
C. RANK ligand inhibition
D. Adenyl cyclase activation
E. Increased renal absorption of vitamin D

Discussion

The correct answer is (A). Nitrogen-containing bisphosphonates, such as alendronate, risedronate, zolendranate, and ibandronate, decrease osteoclast function via inhibition of the cholesterol pathway via farnesyl pyrophosphate synthase and GTPase prenylation. Formation of a toxic ATP analogue is the mechanism of action of non–nitrogen-containing bisphosphonates such as clodronate and etidronate. RANK ligand inhibitors, such as denosumab, inhibit RANKL binding to RANK via monoclonal Ig2. Parathyroid hormone analogues, such as teriparatide injections, given daily, increase bone density by increasing coupled bone remodeling.

The patient discontinues bisphosphonate use; however, 1 week later the patient presents to the emergency department with severe pain in her left thigh and inability to bear weight. Radiographs display a transverse fracture line with a medial cortical spike (Fig. 6–40).

What is the appropriate treatment for this fracture?

A. Short intramedullary nail
B. Long intramedullary nail
C. Dynamic hip screw
D. External fixator application
E. Tension band

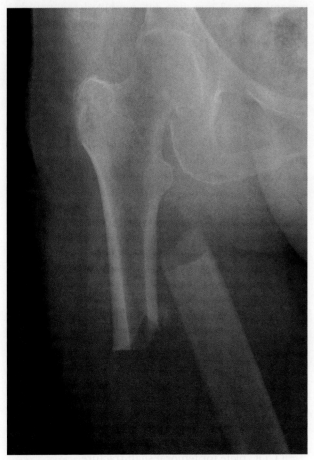

Figure 6–40

Discussion

The correct answer is (B). The use of a long intramedullary nail would be most appropriate for this fracture type. Subtrochanteric fractures are defined as fractures occurring within 5 cm of the lesser trochanter. The use of a short intramedullary nail in this region would be inappropriate due to the location of the distal interlocking screw. The use of a dynamic hip screw in this fracture would be inappropriate due to the high rate of nonunion and fixation failure. Use of a fixed-angle blade plate is possible, however, this can be associated with increased morbidity as weight bearing commonly must be restricted in the postoperative period.

How should the proximal fragment be manipulated to assist in reducing this fracture?

A. Adduction, internal rotation, and extension
B. Abduction, internal rotation, and extension
C. Adduction, external rotation, and flexion
D. Abduction, external rotation, and extension
E. Adduction, internal rotation, and flexion

Discussion

The correct answer is (A). The typical deformity associated with subtrochanteric femur fractures is flexion, abduction, and external rotation due to the pull of the iliopsoas, gluteus, and short external rotators. Consequently, internal rotation, extension, and adduction of the proximal fragment will help obtain the appropriate reduction. Lateral positioning can aid in fracture reduction by making it easier to bring the distal segment to the flexed proximal segment.

Objectives: Did you learn...?

- Mechanism and complications of common osteoporosis treatments?
- Treatment of subtrochanteric femur fractures?
- Common reduction technique for subtrochanteric femur fractures?

CASE 38

Dr. David J. Tennent

A 38-year-old male struck by a motor vehicle while crossing the street presented to the ED with a blood pressure of 156/92, an HR of 112, a lactate of 0.8, and Glasgow Coma Scale of 15. He was complaining of severe pain in his left lower extremity. He has brisk dorsalis pedis and posterior tibial pulses bilaterally. He has normal rectal tone and no spinal tenderness. His pelvic examination is stable to compression. He

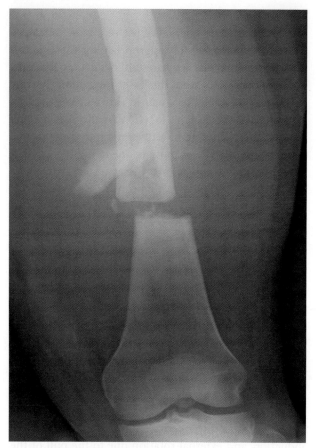

Figure 6–41

has pain over his left femur and left hip. An AP pelvis, an AP internal rotation view of the left hip, and left femur films were obtained displaying a transverse midshaft femur fracture (Fig. 6–41). After confirming the midshaft femur fracture with radiographs, a CT pelvis with 2-mm cuts through the femoral necks was obtained.

What is the incidence of concomitant extremity injury following a traumatic femoral shaft fracture?

A. 10% rate of contralateral distal femur fracture
B. 15% rate of ipsilateral femoral neck fracture
C. 15% rate of ipsilateral distal femur fracture
D. 5% rate of ipsilateral femoral neck fracture
E. 5% rate of contralateral femoral neck fracture

Discussion

The correct answer is (D). Concomitant proximal femur fractures occur in less than 10% of femoral shaft fracture cases. Furthermore, when they do occur, they are missed in up to 30% of cases. As such, it is

necessary to critically evaluate the femoral neck in all cases of femoral shaft fractures in order to fully evaluate the patient's injury patterns and corresponding treatment plan.

What additional intraoperative imaging should be obtained prior to surgery to fully evaluate for the presence of concomitant injuries prior to femoral shaft fixation?

A. Inlet/outlet pelvic views
B. Stress radiographs of knee
C. Judet views of pelvis
D. Traction views of proximal femur
E. Lateral of femoral neck

Discussion

The correct answer is (E). Concomitant femoral shaft and neck fractures are missed in up to 30% of cases due to the insensitivity of conventional imaging. As such, the femoral neck must be closely evaluated as this injury will dictate fracture fixation order and implant choice. Tornetta et al. have proposed a diagnostic algorithm consisting of an AP internal rotation view of the femoral neck, 2-mm fine-cut computed tomographic scan through the femoral neck, an intraoperative fluoroscopic lateral of the ipsilateral femoral neck prior to fixation, and AP/lateral hip radiographs following fracture fixation prior to waking the patient. This algorithm was found to decrease the incidence of missed femoral neck fractures by 91%.

If the patient is found to have a nondisplaced, ipsilateral femoral neck fracture on additional intraoperative imaging, what is the best order and method of surgical fixation of these fractures?

A. Open reduction and cephalomedullary nail fixation for treatment of femoral neck and shaft fractures
B. Closed reduction femoral neck with percutaneous screw fixation followed by retrograde intramedullary femoral nail for shaft fracture
C. Open reduction of femoral neck fracture with screw fixation followed by retrograde femoral nailing
D. Antegrade intramedullary nailing of femoral shaft followed by open reduction and percutaneous screw fixation of femoral neck
E. Open reduction and internal fixation using sliding hip screw of femoral neck fracture followed by open reduction and internal fixation using 4.5-mm LCDC plate for femoral shaft fracture

Discussion

The correct answer is (B). The order of ipsilateral femoral shaft and femoral neck fracture fixation is dictated by the urgency of femoral neck reduction in order to decrease the rates of avascular necrosis of the femoral head. As such, open reduction of the femoral neck should precede fixation of the femoral shaft. Following this, as the implant construct fixing the femoral neck will block antegrade intramedullary nailing and will cause increased stresses across the femoral neck, retrograde intramedullary nailing is the preferred implant choice for femoral shaft fixation.

How much femoral anteversion is acceptable following femoral intramedullary nailing when compared to the uninjured extremity?

A. 5 degrees
B. 10 degrees
C. 15 degrees
D. 20 degrees
E. 25 degrees

Discussion

The correct answer is (C). Anatomic studies have shown that in normal subjects differences in femoral anteversion are up to 15 degrees. Studies have also shown that increasing femoral malrotation is associated with increasing incidence of functional gait disturbances. There are several techniques that can be used to obtain appropriate femoral rotation in transverse femoral shaft fractures. A basic technique to establish appropriate femoral rotation includes assessing the cortical diameters across the fracture site. More complex techniques involve using the uninjured extremity to establish appropriate rotation. One technique uses the contralateral extremity to estimate femoral anteversion on the injured side. By using fluoroscopy prior to the case, the angular difference between a true lateral of the femoral neck and true lateral of the knee (femoral anteversion) can be obtained. This can then be used to "dial in" the injured extremity anteversion by ensuring the femoral anteversion has been restored. A second technique utilizing lateral-only imaging uses the neck-horizontal angle to determine anteversion. Using this technique, a true lateral of the knee is obtained. Following this, a lateral view of the proximal femur is obtained without changing the intensifier angle. The angle formed between the femoral neck and a horizontal line at the base of the monitor forms the neck horizontal angle. A third technique that can be used to asses rotation relies

on the profile of the lesser trochanter on a true AP of the hip. Again, the uninjured extremity must be imaged prior to initiating the case and the profile of the lesser trochanter obtained using the uninjured extremity is compared to the injured in order to obtain appropriate rotational alignment.

Objectives: Did you learn...?

- Association of femoral shaft and neck fractures?
- Important diagnostic imaging to obtain in femoral shaft fractures?
- Importance of the order of fixation in femoral neck/shaft fractures?

CASE 39

Dr. David J. Tennent

A 37-year-old, male motorcyclist was struck by another vehicle at highway speeds. He was intubated in the field. On arrival to the trauma bay his GCS is 3T, heart rate is 130 beats per minute, blood pressure is 90/58 mm Hg, lactate is 8, and his base deficit is 6. He is found to have a grade IV splenic laceration, multiple rib fractures, a pelvic ring injury, a closed left femur fracture, a comminuted Gustilo–Anderson 3C tibia fracture, and a small intraparenchymal hemorrhage (Fig. 6–42A–C). He is stabilized in the trauma bay and taken directly to the operating room by the general surgery team for exploratory laparotomy.

What is the best indicator of end-organ perfusion in this patient?

A. Blood pressure
B. Heart rate
C. Glasgow Coma Scale
D. Base deficit
E. Lactate

Discussion

The correct answer is (E). This patient is in Class III shock. However, the most sensitive marker for end-organ perfusion is lactate <2 mmol/L. While blood pressure, heart rate and base deficit are all important markers to consider when evaluating adequate resuscitation, these are most irregular in a state of uncompensated shock. Following initial resuscitation, when the above markers have normalized, adequate tissue perfusion may still be compromised and is most appropriately evaluated using lactate. The classes for shock can be reviewed in Table 6–6.

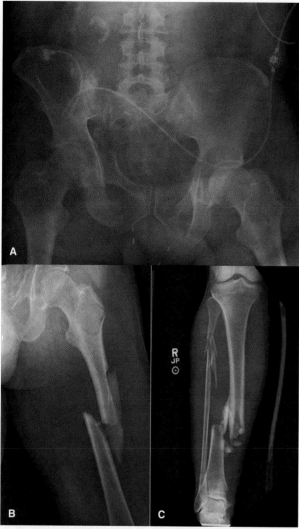

Figure 6-42 **A–C**

What is the most appropriate management of his extremity injuries?

A. Pelvic external fixator placement, irrigation and debridement, and external fixation of the tibia and of the femur

B. Pelvic external fixator placement, irrigation and debridement of the tibia followed by wound closure and intramedullary nail, external fixation of the femur

C. External fixator placement with irrigation and debridement of the tibia and skeletal traction of the femur

D. Pelvic external fixator placement, irrigation and debridement and external fixation of the tibia and open reduction and internal fixation of femur

E. Pelvic external fixator placement, irrigation and debridement of tibia with wound coverage and intramedullary nailing of tibia and retrograde intramedullary nailing of femur

Discussion

The correct answer is (A). This patient is inadequately resuscitated and should be treated via damage control orthopaedic principles. Stabilization of pelvis and long bones should be conducted expeditiously as to not provide an additional insult to the patient's physiologic state. This should be ideally completed in less than 2 hours. Furthermore, the patient is most susceptible to additional ischemic brain injury during the first 24 hours and, as such, additional insults should be minimized. Once fully stabilized, the patient's pelvis and long bone fractures should be addressed, ideally converting the external fixators of the tibia and femur to definitive fixation within the following 2 weeks.

What complication has been shown to increase as the interval between external fixator conversion and internal fixation increases?

A. Nonunion
B. Infection
C. Pulmonary embolism
D. Deep venous thrombosis
E. Wound necrosis

Table 6-6   CLASSIFICATION OF SHOCK

Class	Heart Rate (bpm)	Blood Pressure	Urine (mL/hr)	% Blood Loss	pH
I	Normal	Normal	>30	<15%	Normal
II	>100	Normal	20–30	15–30%	Normal
III	>120	Decreased	5–15	30–40%	Decreased
IV	>140	Decreased	Negligible	>40%	Decreased

Discussion

The correct answer is (B). Multiple studies have shown that infection rates increase with a longer conversion interval between external fixation and internal fixation of long bone fractures. Although low in closed femur fractures, increased infection rates have been shown after only 2 days of external fixation. In open tibia fractures, external fixation for greater than 2 weeks has been shown to have greater infection rates.

Objectives: Did you learn...?

- Basic principles of damage control orthopaedics?
- Determination of appropriate trauma resuscitation?
- Timing of external fixation to definitive fixation of long bone fractures?

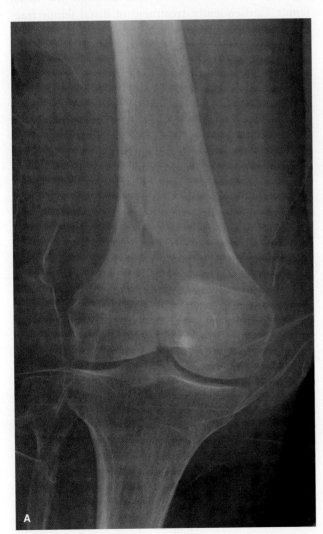

A

Figure 6–43 **A–B**

CASE 40

Dr. David J. Tennent

A 23-year-old rancher presents to the emergency department after being trampled by a bull. He complains of severe pain in his right leg with inability to flex or extend his knee and exquisite tenderness over his distal femur. He is neurovascularly intact otherwise and without open wounds. Radiographs are shown in Figure 6–43A and B.

What is the next step in evaluation of his injury?

A. CT with contrast
B. Ankle brachial index (ABI)

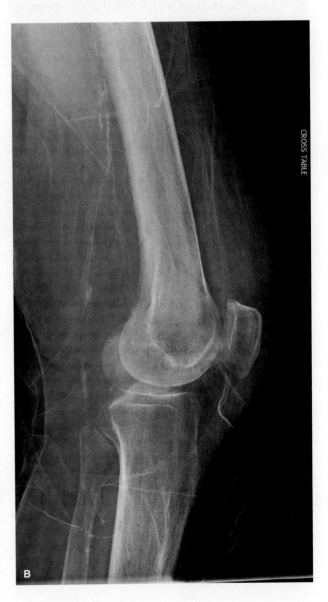

CROSS TABLE

B

C. MRI left knee
D. Ligamentous examination
E. CT without contrast

Discussion

The correct answer is (E). It is most important to evaluate for the presence of an associated coronal split fracture (Hoffa fracture) extending into the articular surface. These fractures are often missed on plain radiographs as they are not easily appreciated. The incidence of a Hoffa fracture is 38% and, if missed, can cause malreduction and failure of fixation.

What screw orientation is most commonly needed when a Hoffa fracture is present?

A. Oblique screw from lateral to medial into the lateral femoral condyle
B. Anterior to posterior screw in the medial femoral condyle
C. Oblique screw from medial to lateral into the medial femoral condyle
D. Anterior to posterior screw into the lateral femoral condyle
E. Anterior to posterior screws into the medial and lateral femoral condyles

Discussion

The correct answer is (D). A Hoffa fracture is a coronal split through the distal femoral condyle. These are often missed on plain radiographs. When present, the fracture most commonly involves the lateral femoral condyle alone 80% of the time. This fracture requires an anterior to posteriorly oriented screw through the lateral femoral condyle.

What view is needed to decrease the incidence of a common hardware complication following submuscular plating?

A. Anterior–posterior view of knee
B. 25-degree internal rotation view of knee
C. Lateral view of knee
D. Sunrise view of knee
E. 10-degree external rotation view of knee

Discussion

The correct answer is (B). The slope of the distal femoral metaphysis is 25 degrees medially and 10 degrees laterally in the sagittal plane. When using a laterally based submuscular distal femoral plate it is important to obtain a 25-degree internal rotation view of the knee. This allows for visualization down the slope of the medial femoral cortex that will show protruding screws causing pain and irritation if the screws are too long. The AP and lateral views of the knee are also important for proper plate position intraoperatively.

What precludes the use of a retrograde intramedullary nail following a stable fracture, without signs of implant loosening, around a PCL-sacrificing total knee arthroplasty that occurred 3 weeks postoperatively?

A. Proximity to the femoral component
B. PCL-sacrificing design
C. Aseptic loosening of femoral component
D. Proximity of primary surgery
E. Cruciate-retaining design

Discussion

The correct answer is (B). This design precludes passage of an intramedullary nail through the distal femur. Consequently, treatment of distal femur fractures with this construct is limited to open reduction and internal fixation via plate fixation and antegrade intramedullary nailing. This injury does not show evidence of aseptic loosening, and proximity to the index surgery does not play a role in implant choice. In fractures displaying hardware loosening or failure, the arthroplasty components must be exchanged for revision components. Cruciate-retaining designs do not have this same limitation.

Objectives: Did you learn…?

- Importance of Hoffa fragment in distal femur fractures?
- Importance of TKA design when treating periprosthetic distal femur fractures?
- Anatomic considerations of distal femur fractures?

CASE 41

Dr. Andrew Sheean

A 43-year-old male presents to the emergency department after falling approximately 15 ft while trimming tree branches. Per the report of emergency medical service personnel at the scene, the patient complained of excruciating right knee pain and was found to have a deformity of the right knee that improved when it "was pulled on" as the patient felt a "clunk." On examination, the patient complains of persistent pain about the right knee. The skin is intact and there appears to be no gross deformity. There is a palpable pulse over the dorsalis pedis artery; however, you are unable to palpate a pulse over the posterior tibial artery.

What is your next step in evaluating the injured extremity?

A. Perform a ligamentous knee examination
B. Obtain a computerized tomogram with intravenous contrast of the right leg
C. Obtain orthogonal radiographs of the right knee
D. Measure the ankle brachial index (ABI) of the right leg

Discussion

The correct answer is (D). The vignette describes a circumstance that should raise one's suspicion for a knee dislocation, and ABIs must be determined as approximately 40% of knee dislocations are associated with injuries to the popliteal artery. Of these injuries, anterior dislocations are most common and result in anterior translation of the tibia relative to the femur, stretching the popliteal vessels and causing intimal tears. An ABI of <0.9 has been shown to have 100% sensitivity, specificity, and positive predictive value for significant arterial injury. An abnormal ABI should prompt vascular surgery consultation.

Based upon your examination, you are also concerned about the possibility of a concomitant nerve injury.

Which nerve is most likely to be injured?

A. Peroneal nerve
B. Tibial nerve
C. Saphenous nerve
D. Sural nerve

Discussion

The correct answer is (A). The incidence of neurologic injury after knee dislocation has been documented to range from 16% to 40%. Of these injuries, the peroneal nerve is most commonly injured, occurring in approximately one-third of all knee dislocations. It is vulnerable to injury especially in lateral and posterolateral knee dislocations as it winds around the proximal fibula and courses into the anterior compartment of the leg.

Upon testing of the ligamentous stability of the involved knee, several ligaments are suspected to be injured. Figure 6–44 demonstrates an MRI typical of this injury.

Which of the following structure(s) is most likely to be injured if increased posterolateral rotation is noted on physical examination?

A. Anterior cruciate ligament (ACL)
B. Posterior cruciate ligament (PCL)

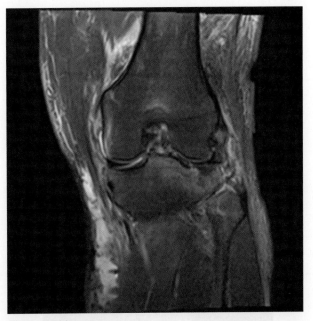

Figure 6–44

C. Popliteus and fibular collateral ligament
D. Semimembranosus and medial collateral ligament (MCL)

Discussion

The correct answer is (C). The finding of increased posterolateral rotation is suggestive of an injury to the posterolateral corner (PLC). The main static stabilizers of the PLC include the popliteus, fibular collateral ligament, and the popliteofibular ligament. Together, these structures restrain varus, external rotation, and coupled posterior translation and external rotation of the tibia on the femur.

Objectives: Did you learn...?

• The incidence of vascular injury and the evaluation in the setting of knee dislocation?
• The incidence of nerve injury in the setting of knee dislocation?
• The ligamentous anatomy about the knee and the description of multiligamentous knee injuries in the setting of dislocation?

CASE 42

Dr. Andrew Sheean

A 48-year-old woman presents to the emergency department complaining of acute left knee pain and inability to bear weight after falling on a flexed knee. She is unable to perform a straight leg raise. Figure 6–45A and B shows a lateral and AP radiographs of her left knee.

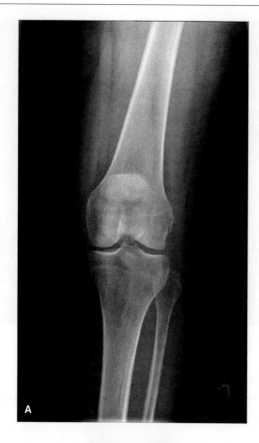

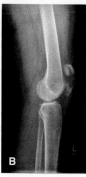

Figure 6–45 **A–B**

All of the following suggest disruption of the extensor mechanism EXCEPT:

A. With the knee flexed 90 degrees, the superior pole of the patella lies superior to the anterior surface of the femur

B. With the knee flexed 30 degrees, the inferior pole of the patella is aligned with the level of Blumensaat's line

C. An Insall–Salvati ratio of greater than 1.0

D. An Insall–Salvati ratio of less than 1.0

Discussion

The correct answer is (B). With the knee flexed 30 degrees, the inferior pole of the patella normally is

aligned to the level of Blumensaat's line. Thus answer B describes a normal anatomic relationship. With the knee flexed 90 degrees, the superior pole of the patella should normally lie inferior to the anterior surface of the femur. The Insall–Salvati ratio compares the height of the patella to the length of the patellar tendon. A ratio of less than 1.0 suggests patella alta and disruption of the patellar tendon, while a ratio of greater than 1.0 suggests patella baja and disruption of the quadriceps tendon.

Which of the following is NOT an indication for operative treatment of patellar fractures?

A. Stellate fracture pattern with 1 mm of intra-articular incongruity

B. Transverse fracture pattern with 3 mm of displacement

C. Osteochondral fracture associated with an intra-articular loose body

D. Compromised extensor mechanism function

Discussion

The correct answer is (A). Choices B, C and D all accurately describe relative indications for operative treatment of patellar fractures. A stellate fracture pattern with a relatively small amount of intra-articular incongruity, however, may be treated nonoperatively, provided that the extensor mechanism remains intact.

Regarding partial patellectomy, all of the following are true EXCEPT:

A. Partial patellectomy is indicated in the setting of comminuted superior or inferior pole fractures measuring less than 50% of the patella's height.

B. As the size of the resected inferior pole increases so too do the contact stresses increase across the patellofemoral joint.

C. Partial patellectomy has been demonstrated to offer superior clinical results compared to internal fixation for fracture patterns with extensive inferior pole comminution.

D. Repair of associated medial and lateral retinacular injuries may lead to altered patellofemoral mechanics and an increase in patellar subluxation.

Discussion

All are true except for answer "D." Partial patellectomy is a reasonable treatment approach for fractures of either the superior or inferior pole measuring less than 50% of the patellar height, especially in the setting of significant comminution. As the size of the resected portion of the inferior pole increases so too do the contact stresses across the patellofemoral joint. Partial patellectomy has been shown to offer superior outcomes in the setting of extensive inferior pole comminution. Repair of the medial and lateral retinacular injuries is a critical aspect of addressing associated soft tissue injuries to ensure optimization of patellofemoral mechanics.

Objectives: Did you learn...?

- Operative indications for fixation of patellar fractures?
- The role of partial patellectomy in the setting of comminuted superior or inferior pole fracture patterns?
- The importance of restoring extensor mechanism function?

CASE 43

Dr. Andrew Sheean

A 43-year-old woman presents to the emergency department after sustaining a twisting-type injury to her left knee. There is a ballotable effusion but the soft tissues around the knee are intact without significant ecchymosis or concern for impending compromise. ABIs are measured to be greater than 1.0. Radiographs demonstrate an isolated split fracture of the lateral tibial plateau.

What is the most common soft tissue injury associated with this fracture pattern?

A. Medial meniscus tear
B. Lateral meniscus tear
C. Posterolateral corner tear
D. Posterior cruciate ligament tear

Discussion

The correct answer is (B). While medial meniscal injuries are most commonly associated with bicondylar tibial plateau fractures, injury to the lateral meniscus has been shown to occur in up to 91% of tibial plateau fractures.

Which of the following statements is correct regarding the anatomy of the proximal tibia?

A. The lateral tibial plateau is distal to the medial tibial plateau.
B. The articular surface of the lateral tibial plateau is more concave compared to that of the medial tibial plateau.

C. The lateral tibial plateau is more resistant to failure than the medial tibial plateau.
D. The tibial plateau has a slight valgus orientation relative to the shaft.

Discussion

The correct answer is (A). The lateral tibial plateau is distal to the medial plateau, which accounts for the slight varus orientation of the plateau relative to the shaft. The articular surface of the lateral tibial plateau is more convex than that of the medial tibial plateau. The medial tibial plateau is more resistant to failure than the lateral tibial plateau, and this explains why medial tibial plateau fractures are generally thought of as denoting a higher-energy mechanism of injury.

Regarding the meniscal repair in the setting of a split lateral tibial plateau, which of the following statements is correct?

A. Failed meniscal repair requiring subsequent meniscectomy has been shown to accelerate the development of post-traumatic arthritis.
B. Peripheral longitudinal lesions of the posterior meniscus should be repaired in an "outside-in" suture technique.
C. Peripheral longitudinal lesions of the anterior meniscus should be repaired in an "all-inside" technique.
D. Complex meniscal tears within the inner area of the meniscus should be resected.

Discussion

The correct answer is (D). Complex meniscal tears in the avascular zone should be resected. Peripheral, posterior meniscal lesions should be repaired in an "all-inside" technique so as to avoid the popliteal neurovascular structures. Conversely, anterior meniscal lesions can be repaired in an "outside-in" fashion. Even if a meniscal repair fails and requires subsequent resection, there may be a protective effect on the articular cartilage of a temporary repair.

Regarding the meniscal repair in the setting of a split fracture of the lateral tibial plateau, which of the following statements is correct?

A. Failed meniscal repair requiring subsequent meniscectomy has been shown to accelerate the development of post-traumatic arthritis.
B. Peripheral longitudinal lesions of the posterior meniscus should be repaired in an "outside-in" suture technique.

C. Peripheral longitudinal lesions of the anterior meniscus should be repaired in an "all-inside" technique.

D. Complex meniscal tears within the inner area should be resected.

Discussion

The correct answer is (D). Complex meniscal tears in the avascular zone should be resected. Peripheral, posterior meniscal lesions should be repaired in an "all-inside" technique so as to avoid the popliteal neurovascular structures. Conversely, anterior meniscal lesions can be repaired in an "outside-in" fashion. Even if a meniscal repair fails and requires subsequent resection, there may a protective effect on the articular cartilage of a temporary repair.

Objectives: Did you learn...?

• The osseous anatomy of the proximal tibia?
• The associations between lateral tibial plateau fractures and the surrounding soft tissues?
• The surgical management of associated lateral meniscal injuries?

CASE 44

Dr. Andrew Sheean

A 37-year-old male presents to the emergency department after a fall from 20 ft. Figure 6–46 depicts an AP radiograph of the patient's right knee. The skin about the knee is intact, however, there is significant ecchymosis and evolving hemorrhagic blisters noted medially. ABI measures 1.1 and this appears to be an isolated injury.

Based upon the description of the patient's knee, what is the most appropriate next step in the management of this injury?

A. Closed reduction and application of a long leg cast in 30 degrees of knee flexion

B. Open reduction internal fixation using a lateral buttress plate and raft screws

C. Open reduction internal fixation using a lateral buttress plate and a separate posteromedial plate

D. Application of a knee-spanning external fixator

Discussion

The correct answer is (D). The vignette describes a bicondylar tibial plateau fracture with extensive injury to the surrounding soft tissues. Egol et al. describe their success in treating high-energy proximal tibia fractures

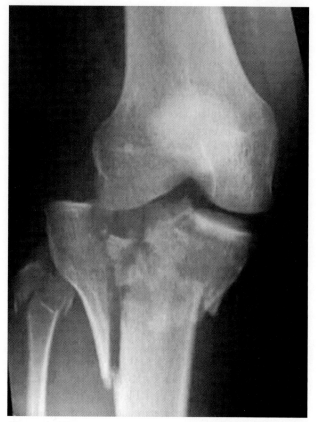

Figure 6–46

in temporizing knee-spanning external fixators, citing low infection rates, improved soft tissue access, and the mitigation of articular damage.

Regarding the surgical tactic used to address bicondylar tibial plateau fractures, which of the following statements is true?

A. Plating of both lateral and posteromedial fracture fragments can reliably be approached through one midline incision.

B. Coronal splits of the posterior aspect of the medial condyle can be stabilized by appropriately oriented lag screws that allow compression across fragments.

C. Heterotopic ossification is a frequent complication of high-energy tibial plateau fractures.

D. Posteromedial intra-articular fragments not properly stabilized tend to collapse into varus.

Discussion

The correct answer is (D). Posteromedial fragments tend to collapse into varus even with newer locking plate technology. When applying lateral and posteromedial plates, a two-incision approach significantly reduces the risk of nonunion and infection. If posteromedial coronal split fragments are to be addressed by laterally placed screws, a locked construct has been shown to be biomechanically superior to lag screws. Heterotopic ossification is an infrequent complication of high-energy tibial plateau fractures. The exception to this generalization being in the setting of a fracture-knee dislocation, which is more likely to be complicated by heterotopic ossification formation.

All of the following are true regarding complications and outcomes related to high-energy tibial plateau fractures EXCEPT:

A. Those fractures treated definitively with external fixators exhibit acceptable clinical outcomes in terms of range of motion when compared to the contralateral extremity.

B. The degree of residual articular step-off is a major determinant of the development of post-traumatic arthritis.

C. Extra-articular malunions are more common than intra-articular malunions.

D. The rate of septic arthritis related to external fixator placement can be mitigated by placing pins and wires at least 14 mm below the joint.

Discussion

The correct answer is (B). The degree of residual articular step-off has not reliably been shown to predict the development of post-traumatic arthritis. Weigel and Marsh demonstrated that patients treated definitively with a uniplanar external fixator have good prognosis with satisfactory knee function at 2- and 5-year follow-up. Nonunion typically occurs in the proximal tibial metaphysis. Reid et al. defined the "safe zone" for the placement of periarticular pins through a cadaver model showing the maximum distance between the reflected joint capsule and subchondral bone to be 13 mm.

Objectives: Did you learn...?

- Understand the advisability of a staged surgical approach to high-energy tibial plateau fractures?
- The surgical tactic is dependent upon the nature of the fracture. In general, better outcomes have been reported with a two-plate construct when addressing a posteromedial coronal split fragment?
- Outcomes of operatively treated tibial plateau fractures are often dictated by the restoration of the joint axis rather than the amount of residual articular incongruity?

CASE 45

Dr. Andrew Sheean

A 26-year-old man involved in a high-speed motor vehicle collision arrives to the emergency department with an obvious deformity of the right leg. Orthogonal radiographs of the right tibia/fibula are depicted in Figure 6–47A and B. An initial assessment deems the patient to be stable with no evidence of associated intrathoracic or intra-abdominal injuries. The skin is intact, there are palpable pulses distally, soft compartments, and the patient is deemed suitable for operative treatment.

All of the following are contained within the deep posterior compartment of the leg EXCEPT:

A. Tibialis posterior
B. Flexor digitorum longus
C. Plantaris
D. Flexor hallucis longus

Discussion

The correct answer is (C). All of the above are contained within the deep posterior compartment of the leg except for plantaris, which lies in the superficial posterior compartment. Additionally, the posterial tibial vessels and nerve lie within the deep posterior compartment. The superficial posterior compartment also contains the gastrocnemius and soleus. The anterior compartment contains the anterior tibial artery, deep peroneal nerve, tibialis anterior, extensor hallucis longus, and the extensor digitorum communis with accompanying peroneus tertius. The lateral compartment contains the superficial peroneal nerve, peroneus brevis, and peroneus longus.

The patient is indicated for intramedullary nailing of this closed fracture. The patient is positioned supine with the knee in a flexed position, and a medial parapatellar approach is used.

Which of the following statements regarding the operative management of this injury is false?

A. The starting guide wire is placed in line with the medial aspect of the lateral tibial spine on the AP radiograph, and just below the articular margin on the lateral view.

B. The use of a thigh tourniquet during reaming does not appear to increase the risk of thermal necrosis within the tibia.

C. There is no benefit to reamed versus unreamed intramedullary nailing of closed tibia fractures.

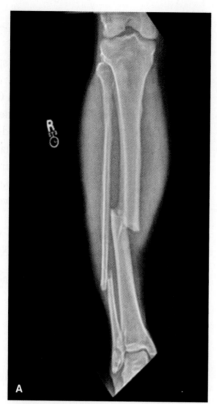

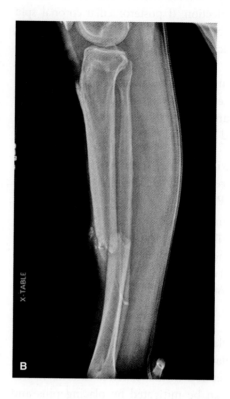

Figure 6–47 **A–B**

D. Anterior knee pain following intramedullary nailing of the tibia can be expected in up to 50% to 75% of patients.

Discussion

The correct answer is (C). In a large, prospective, randomized clinical trial, the SPRINT study demonstrated a benefit for reamed intramedullary nailing of closed tibia fractures. This same benefit was not shown for open fractures. Choice A accurately describes the optimal starting point for intramedullary nailing of tibia fractures. The generation of heat during reaming has been shown to be a function of reamer size and isthmus diameter more so than whether or not a tourniquet is used. Anterior knee pain is a common patient complaint (more than 70% of respondents in one series) following reamed intramedullary nailing of the tibia with the knee in the flexed position.

The patient undergoes successful intramedullary nailing and is transferred to the medical surgical floor. Six hours postoperatively, the patient begins to complain of progressively worsening anterior leg pain that is exacerbated by ankle motion. Palpable pulses are present distally. The patient's blood pressure is measured to be 107/66 mm Hg.

Which statement accurately describes the appropriate evaluation of the patient's condition?

A. As the patient's fracture has been definitively stabilized, the knee should be flexed and the leg elevated.

B. In order to completely evaluate the extent of underlying intracompartmental pressures, it is advisable to measure compartment pressures as remote from the original fracture as possible.

C. An intracompartmental pressure measured to be 25 mm Hg is an indication for urgent fasciotomies.

D. The presence of palpable pulses does not rule out the possibility of an evolving compartment syndrome.

Discussion

The correct answer is (D). Although the patient's pulses are palpable distally, this finding alone should not be used to rule out compartment syndrome. The fact that a tibia fracture has been stabilized definitively with an intramedullary implant does not preclude the possibility of compartment syndrome postoperatively. Compartment syndrome remains a clinical diagnosis and the presence of increased pain with passive stretch of the toes/ankles raises the clinical suspicion. Compartment pressures can be measured to provide additional information. When measuring compartment pressures, the pressure should be checked within 5 cm of the fracture. The decision to perform fasciotomies for treatment of compartment syndrome is based upon the difference (ΔP) between the diastolic pressure and the measured compartment pressure rather than an absolute measured compartment pressure. A ΔP value of 30 mm Hg or less warrants fasciotomies.

When assessing the adequacy of reduction of a tibia fracture, all of the following are considered acceptable parameters EXCEPT:

A. Less than 1 cm shortening
B. Less than 10 degrees of sagittal plane deformity
C. Less than 20 degrees of internal rotation
D. Less than 5 degrees of coronal plane deformity

Discussion

The correct answer is (C). All of the answer choices correctly describe appropriate parameters for alignment of the tibia with the exception of 20 degrees of internal rotation. No more than 10 degrees of rotational alignment is considered acceptable for tibia fractures.

Objectives: Did you learn...?

- The anatomy of the compartments of the leg?
- The appropriate guide wire start point for intramedullary nailing of the tibia with the knee flexed?
- The common deformity encountered in fractures of the proximal tibia?
- Incidence of anterior knee pain following intramedullary nailing of the tibia with the knee flexed?
- The diagnosis and management of compartment syndrome in the setting of closed tibia fracture?

CASE 46

Dr. Andrew Sheean

A 49-year-old male is brought to the emergency department after a high-speed motor vehicle collision. There is a significant soft tissue defect about the proximal left leg with gross contamination. The dorsalis pedis and posterior tibial arterial pulses are palpable. A single AP radiograph of the knee is shown in Figure 6–48. The patient is indicated for application of a knee-spanning external fixator. Figure 6–49 shows the left leg after debridement and irrigation.

Based upon the appearance of this wound, this open fracture is most appropriately described according to the Gustilo–Anderson classification as:

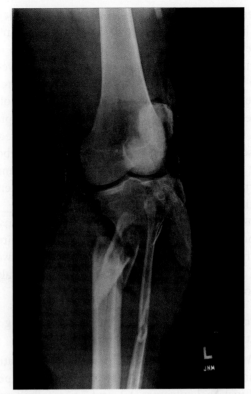

Figure 6–48

A. II
B. IIIA
C. IIIB
D. IIIC

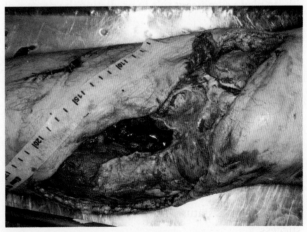

Figure 6–49

Discussion

The correct answer is (C). Type II injuries are relatively low energy and have soft tissue wounds greater than 1 cm but are not associated with significant soft tissue damage or periosteal stripping. Type IIIA injuries are associated with high-energy mechanisms with more significant soft tissue damage and periosteal stripping, although these injuries have adequate soft tissue for primary coverage. Type IIIB injuries are associated with more severe soft tissue damage and periosteal stripping. The extent of soft tissue damage necessitates soft tissue coverage procedure. Type IIIC injuries are open fractures that require a vascular repair. The patient is indicated for debridement and irrigation with application of a knee-spanning external fixator, which is appropriate given the extensive soft tissue damage and gross contamination.

Postoperatively, the patient is interested in discussing the prognosis of his left lower extremity. He inquires as to whether or not below-the-knee amputation would offer more of a clinical benefit versus a limb salvage approach.

Which of the following statements regarding amputation and limb salvage is correct?

A. When controlling for injury severity, patients undergoing primary amputation exhibit superior functional outcomes at 2- and 7-year follow-up.

B. The extent of soft tissue damage is most important factor in determining the viability of severely injured lower extremity.

C. The fact that the patient's plantar sensation was intact at the time of his presentation portends a favorable outcome with limb salvage.

D. The patient's socioeconomic status has been shown to play a significant role in predicting the success of limb salvage.

Discussion

The correct answer is (B). The most important determinant of whether or not a severely injured lower extremity should be amputated or salvaged is the extent of the associated soft tissue injuries. The LEAP study group demonstrated that patients who underwent amputation had functional outcomes similar to those patients treated with limb salvage. Neither the status of a patient's plantar sensation nor their socioeconomic status were predictors of limb salvage success.

Which of the following statements regarding the management of large soft tissue defects associated with open tibia fractures is correct?

A. The use of negative pressure wound dressings have not been shown to influence the need for free flap coverage.

B. The use of negative pressure wound dressings have been shown to lower infection rates in Type IIIB tibia fractures.

C. Deep infection rates significantly decrease when soft tissue coverage is delayed for at least 72 hours.

D. Initial debridement of large soft tissue wounds is best accomplished by high-flow, pulsatile lavage.

Discussion

The correct answer is (B). Bhattacharyya et al. demonstrated that the use of negative pressure wound dressings does not significantly allow for coverage delay for open tibia fractures. The use of negative pressure wound dressings have been shown to decrease the need for free flap coverage of large soft tissue defects. In a series of 84 Type IIIB and IIIC tibia fractures, a single-stage procedure involving fixation with immediate flap coverage demonstrated significantly lower infection rates compared to the group in which coverage was undertaken more than 72 hours after injury. There is concern that pulsatile lavage damages healthy tissues and has the potential to increase the deep penetration of gross and microscopic contamination when used in the management of contaminated open fractures, which has been corroborated in an animal model.

Objectives: Did you learn...?

- The Gustilo–Anderson classification system for open fractures?
- Prognostic factors associated with severe lower extremity injuries and the LEAP Study Group findings pertaining to functional outcomes amongst amputees and those treated with limb salvage?
- The infection rates for open fractures and strategies to manage large soft tissue defects?

CASE 47

Dr. Andrew Sheean

A 55-year-old man is involved in a high-speed motorcycle crash. Upon presentation to a level 3 trauma center, he is found to be hemodynamically unstable with a closed proximal third tibia fracture. He is indicated for an emergent exploratory laparotomy and application of an external fixator to the right leg. After a period of observation in the intensive care unit, he is transferred to a level 1 trauma center for definitive management. Radiographs of his right leg after application of an external fixator are shown in Figure 6–50A and B.

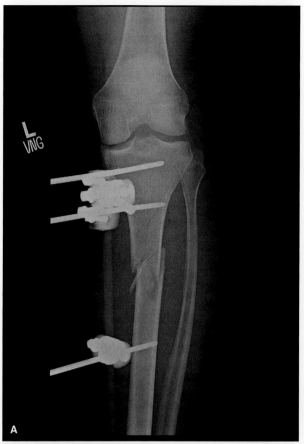
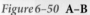
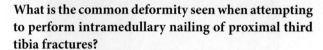
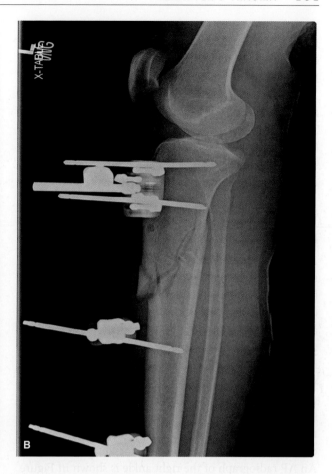

Figure 6–50 **A–B**

What is the common deformity seen when attempting to perform intramedullary nailing of proximal third tibia fractures?

A. Varus and apex anterior
B. Valgus and apex anterior
C. Varus and apex posterior
D. Valgus and apex posterior

Discussion

The correct answer is (B). The valgus and procurvatum deformity is seen commonly in proximal third tibia fractures and is secondary to several distinct factors. Apex anterior angulation occurs as a consequence of the extension moment induced by the patella tendon, which is exacerbated by knee flexion. Valgus deformity is often the result of a starting point that is too medial, resulting in eccentric direction of the nail in the proximal tibial metaphysis and the resulting lateral trajectory of the implant as it moves distally.

An adjunct to intramedullary nailing of proximal third tibia fractures involves the placement of blocking (poller) screws to prevent the predictable deformity of these fractures.

Which of the following accurately describes the appropriate position of two blocking screws when placed in the proximal segment?

A. Anterior and lateral to the nail
B. Anterior and medial to the nail
C. Posterior and lateral to the nail
D. Posterior and medial to the nail

Discussion

The correct answer is (C). In order to prevent the predictable valgus and apex anterior deformity seen with proximal third tibia fractures, blocking screws should be placed in the concavity of the deformity—posterior and lateral—to the nail in the proximal segment.

The patient is indicated for submuscular plating of the depicted fracture using a minimally invasive percutaneous plate osteosynthesis (MIPPO) technique.

Based upon the known complication of this technique for plating proximal third tibia fractures, which of the following physical examination findings might be expected in this patient who complains of a neurologic deficits postoperatively?

A. Weakness in great toe dorsiflexion
B. Numbness in the first web space
C. Numbness of the lateral plantar aspect of the foot
D. Numbness of the dorsum of the foot

Discussion

The correct answer is (D). Superficial peroneal nerve (SPN) injury, as manifested by numbness over the dorsum of the foot, is a described complication of percutaneous plating of proximal tibia fractures.

CASE 48

Dr. Andrew Sheean

A 29-year-old woman arrives to the emergency department after jumping from the second story of a burning building. Upon presentation, she is obtunded and hemodynamically unstable. Her condition, however, stabilizes after transfusion of two units of packed red blood cells and two units of fresh, frozen plasma. She is found to have a subdural hematoma and a splenic laceration, which compels transfer to the intensive care unit for observation. On secondary survey, significant ecchymosis, swelling, and evolving fracture blisters are noted of the right ankle. The right foot has dopplerable signals over both the posterior tibial and dorsalis pedis arteries. An AP radiograph of the right ankle is shown in Figure 6–51.

The Volkman fragment typically observed in this injury retains connections to which of the following ligaments?

A. Anterior tibiofibular ligament
B. Posterior tibiofibular ligament
C. Interosseous membrane
D. Deltoid ligament

Discussion

The correct answer is (B). The Volkman (posterolateral) fragment retains its connections via the posterior tibiofibular ligament. The Chaput (anterolateral) fragment retains its connections via the anterior tibiofibular ligament.

The most appropriate initial management of this injury is:

A. Closed reduction and splinting
B. Application of ankle-spanning external fixator
C. Definitive open reduction and internal fixation within 72 hours of injury
D. Primary below-knee amputation

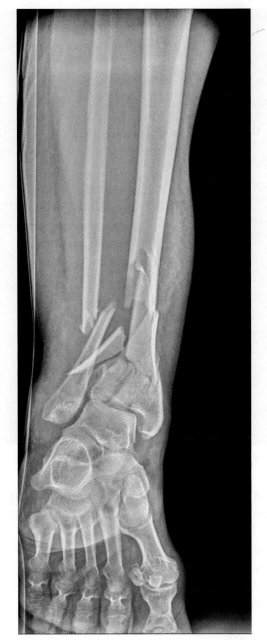

Figure 6–51

Discussion

The correct answer is (B). Attempts at early definitive fixation involving surgical approaches through a damaged soft tissue envelope have been fraught with complications including wound-healing problems and infection. As a consequence, staged protocols have been developed to address these injuries. Following closed, provisional reduction, application of temporary, ankle-spanning external fixation allows for provisional fixation and reestablishment of relative length and alignment. Definitive internal fixation of the tibia is approached once soft tissue swelling dissipates, which is commonly 7 to 14 days post-injury. Primary amputation in the setting of a well-perfused foot without gross significant soft tissue loss would be inappropriate.

According to the elements of successful pilon fracture management set forth by Ruëdi and Allgöwer, which of the following accurately describes the correct order of steps for fixation:

A. Restoration of fibular length, reconstruction of metaphyseal shell, metaphyseal–diaphyseal fixation, bone grafting

B. Reconstruction of metaphyseal shell, bone grafting, metaphyseal–diaphyseal fixation, restoration of fibular length

C. Restoration of metaphyseal shell, bone grafting, restoration of fibular length, metaphyseal–diaphyseal fixation

D. Restoration of fibular length, reconstruction of metaphyseal shell, bone grafting, metaphyseal–diaphyseal fixation

Discussion

The correct answer is (D). Ruëdi and Allgöwer's classic description of the operative approach to pilon fracture fixation advocated a sequential approach: restoration of fibular length, reconstruction of the metaphyseal shell, bone grafting, and metaphyseal–diaphyseal fixation.

All of the following factors have been shown to negatively impact outcomes of patients with pilon fractures treated operatively EXCEPT:

A. Lack of a college degree

B. Marital status

C. Workman's compensation

D. Annual income less than $25,000

Discussion

The correct answer is (C). Pollak et al. performed a retrospective analysis of 103 patients that underwent operative treatment of pilon fractures. Factors significantly related to poor results included: the presence of two or more comorbidities, being married, having an annual income less than $25,000, not having a high-school diploma, and having been treated with external fixation with or without limited internal fixation. Whether or not workman's compensation was involved was not shown to be a significant predictor of poor outcomes.

Objectives: Did you learn...?

- The staged management of pilon fractures?
- The anatomy associated with pilon fractures?
- The patient-specific factors shown to predict outcomes pertaining to pilon fractures?

CASE 49

Dr. Andrew Sheean

A 55-year-old man complains of right ankle pain and inability to bear weight after he fell down a hill while mowing his lawn. He was splinted at a local urgent care facility and was instructed to report to the emergency department for further evaluation. Upon examination, the patient's skin over the ankle is intact, albeit significantly swollen without skin wrinkles noted. AP and lateral radiographs of the right ankle demonstrate a spiral fracture of the fibula at the level of the plafond.

Regarding the anatomy of the ankle joint, all of the following are correct EXCEPT:

A. Cadaveric studies have demonstrated that as little as 1 mm of lateral talar shift within the mortise decreases the joint contact area by 42%.

B. The deep deltoid ligament is composed of two structures, the anterior talotibial ligament and the calcaneotibial ligament.

C. The syndesmosis is composed of four structures; the anterior inferior tibiofibular ligament, the posterior inferior tibiofibular ligament, the calcaneofibular ligament, the interosseous ligament.

D. The anterior neurovascular bundle lies lateral to the extensor hallucis longus tendon at the level of the ankle joint.

Discussion

The correct answer is (C). The syndesmosis is composed of the anterior inferior tibiofibular ligament, the posterior inferior tibiofibular ligament, transverse tibiofibular ligament, and the interosseous ligament. The calcaneofibular ligament is one of three lateral collateral ligaments along with the posterior and anterior talofibular ligaments.

In which of the following scenarios is nonoperative management appropriate?

A. An oblique fibula fracture at the level of the plafond and 8 mm medial clear space widening

B. A transverse fracture distal to the plafond

C. A trimalleolar ankle fracture with a posterior malleolar fracture that comprises approximately 40% of the joint surface

D. A comminuted fibula fracture at the level of the plafond with tibiofibular clear space of 7 mm

Discussion

The correct answer is (B). Answer B describes a Danis–Weber A ankle fracture, which can be managed effectively nonoperatively in a removable splint of some kind. The description in choice A describes radiographic findings suggestive of an associated deltoid ligament injury. Generally speaking, trimalleolar ankle fractures require operative fixation. Choice D describes radiographic findings suggestive of an associated syndesmotic injury.

Which of the following statements accurately describes the pattern of injury in one of the four types of ankle fractures as described in the Lauge–Hansen classification?

A. A supination–external rotation injury involves a lateral short oblique fibula fracture oriented from anterosuperior to posterosuperior.

B. A transverse fracture of the medial malleolus is a unique feature of a pronation–abduction injury.

C. An avulsion of the posterior malleolus is a unique feature of a pronation–external rotation injury.

D. A vertical medial malleolus fracture is a unique feature of the supination–adduction injury.

Discussion

The correct answer is (D). A vertical medial malleolus fracture is unique to supination–adduction injuries. The lateral short oblique fibula fracture observed with supination–external rotation injuries is oriented from anteroinferior to posterosuperior. A transverse fracture of medial malleolus may be observed in supination–external rotation, pronation–abduction, and pronation–external rotation injuries. Avulsions of the posterior malleolus can be observed in supination–external rotation and pronation–external rotation injuries.

Which of the following statements regarding the Danis–Weber classification system is correct?

A. Type A injuries frequently involve injury to the syndesmosis.

B. Type B injuries typically spare the syndesmosis.

C. Type C injuries typically involve pronation–adduction forces.

D. Type A injuries frequently involve supination–adduction forces.

Discussion

The correct answer is (B). Type B injuries do not typically involve injury to the syndesmosis. Type A injuries do not involve syndesmotic injury. Moreover, these injuries usually are the result of supination–adduction type forces. Type C injuries are commonly the result of pronation–external rotation forces.

A supination–adduction type injury should raise one's concern for which of the following associated findings that may significantly impact the patient's long-term functional outcome?

A. Syndesmotic disruption

B. Spring ligament avulsion

C. Marginal impaction of the anteromedial plafond

D. Fracture of the posterior process of the talus

Discussion

The correct answer is (C). In a series of 44 supination–adduction type ankle fractures, 19 patients had displaced vertical medial malleolus fracture patients. Eight of 19 (42%) were found to have marginal impaction of the anteromedial plafond. All eight patients underwent open reduction and internal fixation with elevation of the articular component, and all had good to excellent functional outcomes.

Objectives: Did you learn...?

- The ligamentous anatomy of the ankle joint?
- The common mechanisms and pathoanatomy of the Lauge–Hansen and Danis–Weber classification systems?
- Characteristics of ankle fractures that can be treated nonoperatively?
- The association of anteromedial marginal impaction of the plafond with supination–adduction ankle fractures?

CASE 50

Dr. Andrew Sheean

A 43-year-old woman complains of right ankle pain and inability to bear weight after she slipped and fell while walking down her driveway. AP and lateral radiographs of the right ankle are shown in Figure 6–52A–C.

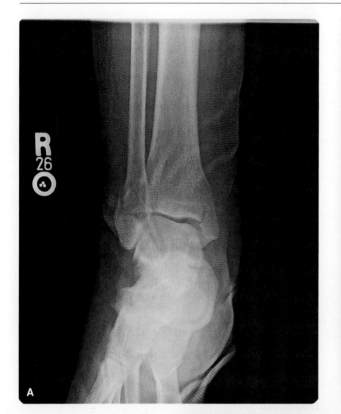

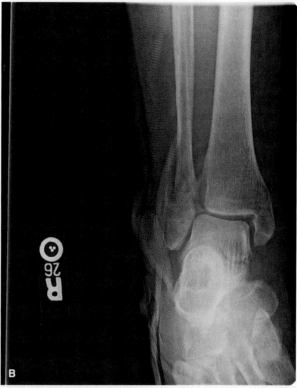

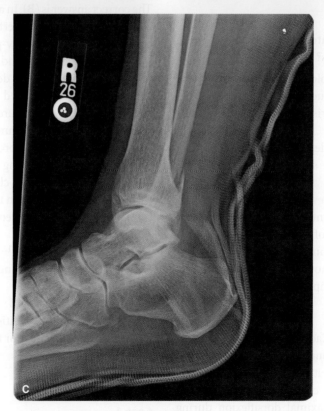

Figure 6–52 **A–C**

Which the following findings should raise one's suspicion of an associated syndesmotic injury?

A. Tibiofibular clear space measuring greater than 6 mm in both the AP and mortise views

B. Tibiofibular overlap of greater than 1 mm in the AP view

C. A spiral fracture of the proximal third of the fibula

D. Dynamic fluoroscopic views that demonstrate decreasing degree of tibiofibular overlap with progressive internal rotation

Discussion

The correct answer is (C). A spiral fracture of the proximal fibula (Maisonneuve fracture) is associated with a syndesmotic injury. In both the AP and mortise views, the tibiofibular clear space should measure less than 6 mm. The tibiofibular overlap should be greater than 1 mm in the mortise view. In the absence of injury, both the tibiofibular overlap and medial clear space decrease normally with internal rotation.

The patient is indicated for open reduction and internal fixation. After fixation of the fibula and medial malleolus, a stress test is performed and the syndesmosis is found to be unstable.

Which of the following statements is true regarding fixation of the syndesmosis?

A. Because of the morphology of the talus, the syndesmosis should be reduced with the ankle in dorsiflexion so as to not risk over tightening of the joint.

B. Cadaveric studies have demonstrated screws engaging four cortices to be stiffer compared to those engaging three cortices.

C. The trajectory of the screws should be oriented parallel to the tibiotalar joint in the coronal plane and parallel to the surface of the operating table with the leg in neutral rotation.

D. Syndesmotic screws should be inserted in a lag fashion to augment compression across the joint.

Discussion

The correct answer is (B). Cadaveric studies have demonstrated that engaging four cortices improves syndesmotic stability although it is unclear if this finding results in any difference in clinical outcome. Tornetta et al. demonstrated that maximal dorsiflexion during syndesmotic reduction is not necessary to avoid overtensioning of the syndesmosis. The trajectory of the syndesmotic screws should be 25 to 30 degrees obliquely

from posterolateral to anteromedial to account for the posterior position of the fibula relative to the tibia in the axial plane. Syndesmotic screws should be fully threaded and not inserted in a lag fashion to avoid overtensioning.

Which of the following statements is FALSE regarding the fixation of medial malleolar fragments?

A. Non-comminuted fractures of the anterior colliculus larger than 1 × 1 cm can typically be fixed with a screw.

B. Screws should be inserted posterior to the anterior colliculus so as to diminish the likelihood of injuring the posterior tibial tendon.

C. Regarding the competence of the deltoid ligament, the size of the medial malleolar fracture has been shown to be the most important variable in determining stability.

D. Screws placed with the lag by method technique have been shown to be biomechanically superior to partially threaded screws placed with the lag by design technique.

Discussion

The correct answer is (B). In a cadaveric model, Femino et al. showed that screws inserted posterior to the anterior colliculus resulted in screw-posterior tibial tendon contact in all the specimens and frank tendon injury in 50% of the specimens. Tornetta demonstrated that the deltoid ligament is typically spared in supramalleolar fractures and incompetent in fractures of the anterior malleolus measuring less than 17 mm in the sagittal plane. Biomechanical analysis and prospective series have shown fully threaded screws using a lag by technique method to be biomechanically and clinically superior to partially threaded screws inserted in the lag by technique method for fixation of medial malleolar fragments.

Objectives: Did you learn...?

• The radiographic findings suggestive of a syndesmotic injury?

• Current concepts and understanding related to proper syndesmotic fixation?

• The proper technique for fixation of medial malleolar fracture fragment?

BIBLIOGRAPHY

Case 1

American College of Surgeons. *Atls Student Course Manual: Advanced Trauma Life Support Student Course Manual*; 9th ed. 2012.

Case 2

Bartlett CS, Helfet DL, Hausman MR, Strauss E. Ballistics and gunshot wounds: effects on musculoskeletal tissues. *J Am Acad Orthop Surg.* 2000;8(1):21–36.

Dickey RL, Barnes BC, Kearns RJ, Tullos HS. Efficacy of antibiotics in low velocity gunshot fractures. *J Orthop Trauma.* 1989;3:6–10.

Geissler WB, Teasedall RD, Tomasin JD, Hughes JL. Management of low velocity gunshot-induced fractures. *J Orthop Trauma.* 1990;4:39–41.

Watters J, Anglen JO, Mullis BH. The role of débridement in low-velocity civilian gunshot injuries resulting in pelvis fractures: a retrospective review of acute infection and inpatient mortality. *J Orthop Trauma.* 2011;25(3):150–155.

Case 3

Hassinger SM, Harding G, Wongworawat MD. High-pressure pulsatile lavage propagates bacteria into soft tissue. *Clin Orthop Relat Res.* 2005;439:27–31.

Hauser CJ, Adams CA Jr, Eachempati SR, Council of the Surgical Infection Society. Surgical Infection Society guideline: prophylactic antibiotic use in open fractures: an evidence-based guideline. *Surg Infect (Larchmt).* 2006;7(4):379–405.

Owens BD, White DW, Wenke JC. Comparison of irrigation solutions and devices in a contaminated musculoskeletal wound survival model. *J Bone Joint Surg Am.* 2009;91 (1):92–98.

Case 4

Glass ER, Thompson JD, Cole PA, Gause TM II, Altman GT. Treatment of sternoclavicular joint dislocations: a systematic review of 251 dislocations in 24 case series. *J Trauma.* 2011;70(5):1294–1298.

Groh GI, Wirth MA. Management of traumatic sternoclavicular joint injuries. *J Am Acad Orthop Surg.* 2011;19(1): 1–7.

Higginbotham TO, Kuhn JE. Atraumatic disorders of the sternoclavicular joint. *J Am Acad Orthop Surg.* 2005;13(2): 138–145.

Rockwood CA Jr, Odor JM. Spontaneous atraumatic anterior subluxation of the sternoclavicular joint. *J Bone Joint Surg Am.* 1989;71(9):1280–1288.

Waters PM, Bae DS, Kadiyala RK. Short-term outcomes after surgical treatment of traumatic posterior SC fracture-dislocations in children and adolescents. *J Pediatr Orthop.* 2003;23:464–469.

Wirth MA, Rockwood CA Jr. Acute and chronic traumatic injuries of the sternoclavicular joint. *J Am Acad Orthop Surg.* 1996;4(5):268–278.

Case 5

Canadian Orthopaedic Trauma Society. Nonoperative treatment compared with plate fixation of displaced midshaft clavicular fractures. A multicenter, randomized clinical trial. *J Bone Joint Surg Am.* 2007;89(1):1–10.

Jeray KJ. Acute midshaft clavicular fracture. *J Am Acad Orthop Surg.* 2007;15(4):239–248.

McKee MD, Pedersen EM, Jones C, et al. Deficits following nonoperative treatment of displaced midshaft clavicular fractures. *J Bone Joint Surg Am.* 2006;88(1):35–40.

Oh JH, Kim SH, Lee JH, Shin SH, Gong HS. Treatment of distal clavicle fracture: a systematic review of treatment modalities in 425 fractures. *Arch Orthop Trauma Surg.* 2011;131(4):525–533.

Zlowodzki M, Zelle BA, Cole PA, Jeray K, McKee MD; Evidence-Based Orthopaedic Trauma Working Group. Treatment of acute midshaft clavicle fractures: systematic review of 2144 fractures: on behalf of the Evidence-Based Orthopaedic Trauma Working Group. *J Orthop Trauma.* 2005;19(7):504–507.

Case 6

Cote MP, Wojcik KE, Gomlinski G, et al. Rehabilitation of acromioclavicular joint separations: operative and nonoperative considerations. *Clin Sports Med.* 2010;29(2):213–228.

Oki S, Matsimura N, Iwamoto W, et al. Acromioclavicular joint ligamentous system contributing to clavicular strut function: a cadaveric study. *J Shoulder Elbow Surg.* 2013;22(10): 1433–1439.

Reid D, Polson K, Johnson L. Acromioclavicular joint separations grades I-III: a review of the literature and development of best practice guidelines. *Sports Med.* 2012;42(8):681–696.

Case 7

Althausen PL, Lee MA, Finkemeier CG. Scapulothoracic dissociation: diagnosis and treatment. *Clin Orthop Relat Res.* 2003;(416):237–244.

Clements RH, Reisser JR. Scapulothoracic dissociation: a devastating injury. *J Trauma.* 1996;40(1):146–149.

McGahan JP, Rab GT, Dublin A. Fractures of the scapula. *J Trauma.* 1980;20:880–883.

Van Noort A, van Kampen A. Fractures of the scapula surgical neck: outcome after conservative treatment in 13 cases. *Arch Orthop Trauma Surg.* 2005;123:696–700.

Zelle BA, Pape HC, Gerich TG, Garapati R, Ceylan B, Krettek C. Functional outcome following scapulothoracic dissociation. *J Bone Joint Surg Am.* 2004;86-A(1):2–8.

Case 8

Jia Z, Li W, Qi Y, et al. Operative versus nonoperative treatment for complex proximal humeral fractures: a meta-analysis of randomized controlled trials. *Orthopaedics.* 2014;37(6):e543–e551.

Lefevre-Colau MM, Babinet A, Fayad F, et al. Immediate mobilization compared with conventional immobilization for impacted nonoperatively treated proximal humerus fractures: a randomized controlled trial. *J Bone Joint Surg Am.* 2007;89:2582–2590.

Case 9

Ali E, Griffiths D, Obi N, Tytherleigh-Strong G, Van Rensburg L. Nonoperative treatment of humeral shaft fractures revisited. *J Shoulder Elbow Surg.* 2015;24(2):210–214.

Jia Z, Li W, Qi Y, et al. Operative versus nonoperative treatment for complex proximal humeral fractures: a meta-analysis of randomized controlled trials. *Orthopaedics*. 2014;37(6):e543–e551.

Ladermann A, Stimec BV, Denard PJ, Cunningham G, Collin P, Fasel JH. Injury ro the axillary nerve after reverse shoulder arthroplasty: an anatomical study. *Orthop Traumatol Surg Res*. 2014;100(1):105–108.

Sarris I, Weiser R, Sotereanos DG. Pathogenesis and treatment of osteonecrosis of the shoulder. *Orthop Clin North Am*. 2004;35(3):397–404, xi. Review.

Case 10

Ali E, Griffiths D, Obi N, Tytherleigh-Strong G, Van Rensburg L. Nonoperative treatment of humeral shaft fractures revisited. *J Shoulder Elbow Surg*. 2015;24(2):210–214.

Cadet ER, Yin B, Schulz B, Ahmad CS, Rosenwasser MP. Proximal humerus and humeral shaft nonunions. *J Am Acad Orthop Surg*. 2013;21(9):538–547.

Heineman DJ, Bhandari M, Poolman RW. Plate fixation or intramedullary fixation of humeral shaft fractures—an update. *Acta Orthop*. 2012;83(3):317–318.

Padhye KP, Kulkarni VS, Kulkarni GS, et al. Plating, nailing, external fixation, and fibular strut grafting for non-union of humeral shaft fractures. *J Orthop Surg (Hong Kong)*. 2013;21(3):327–331.

Case 11

Galano GJ, Ahmad CS, Levine WN. Current treatment strategies for bicolumnar distal humerus fractures. *J Am Acad Orthop Surg*. 2010;18:20–30.

McKee MD, Jupiter JB. Trauma to the adult elbow and fractures of the distal humerus. In: Browner BD, Levine AM, Jupiter JB, Trafton PG, Krettek C, eds. *Skeletal Trauma*. 4th ed. Philadelphia, PA: WB Saunders; 2009;vol 4:1503–1592.

Mehne DK, Jupiter JB. Fractures of the distal humerus. In: Browner BD, Jupiter JB, Levine AM, Trafton PG, eds. *Skeletal Trauma*. 2nd ed. Philadelphia, PA: WB Saunders; 1992;vol 2:1146–1176.

Morrey BF. Current concepts in the treatment of fractures of the radial head, the olecranon, and the coronoid. *J Bone Joint Surg [Am]*. 1995;77-A:316–327.

Müller ME, Nazareon S, Koch P, Schaftsker J. *Comprehensive Classification of Fractures of Long Bones*. Berlin, Germany: Springer-Verlag; 1990:330.

Wilkinson JM, Stanley D. Posterior surgical approaches to the elbow: a comparative anatomic study. *J Shoulder Elbow Surg*. 2001;10:380–382.

Case 12

Hak DJ, Golladay GJ. Olecranon fractures: treatment options. *J Am Acad Orthop Surg*. 2000;8:266–275.

Huang TW, Wu CC, Fan KF, Tseng IC, Lee PC, Chou YC. Tension band wiring for olecranon fractures: relative stability of Kirschner wires in various configurations. *J Trauma*. 2010;68:173–176.

Rouleau DM, Sandman E, Van Riet R, Galatz LM. Management of fractures of the proximal ulna. *J Am Acad Orthop Surg*. 2013;21:149–160.

Case 13

Budhoff JE. Coronoid fractures. *J Hand Surg*. 2012;37A: 2418–2423.

Doornberg JN, Ring D. Coronoid fracture patterns. *J Hand Surg*. 2006;31A:45–52.

Steinmann SP. Coronoid process fracture. *J Am Acad Orthop Surg*. 2008;16:519–529.

Tashjian RZ, Katarincic JA. Complex elbow instability. *J Am Acad Orthop Surg*. 2006;14:278–286.

Case 14

Hotchkiss RN: Displaced fractures of the radial head: internal fixation of excision? *J Am Acad Orthop Surg*. 1997;5:1–10.

Mathew PK, Athwal GS, King GJ. Terrible triad injury of the elbow: current concepts. *J Am Acad Orthop Surg*. 2009;17:1 37–151.

Ring D. Elbow fractures and dislocations. In: Bucholz RW, Court-Brown CM, Heckman JD, Tornetta P, eds. *Rockwood and Green's Fractures in Adults*. 7th ed. vol I, Section II. Philadelphia, PA: LWW; 2009:905–944.

Trousdale RT, Amadio PC, Cooney WP, Morrey BF. Radioulnar dissociation: a review of twenty cases. *J Bone Joint Surg [Am]*. 1992;74:1486–1497.

Case 15

Kuhn MA, Ross G. Acute elbow dislocations. *Orthop Clin N Am*. 2008;39:155–161.

Mathew PK, Athwal GS, King GJ. Terrible triad injury of the elbow: current concepts. *J Am Acad Orthop Surg*. 2009;17:137–151.

McKee MD, Schemitsch EH, Sala MJ, O'Driscoll SW. The pathoanatomy of lateral ligamentous disruption in complex elbow instability. *J Shoulder Elbow Surg*. 2003;12:391–396.

Mehlhoff TL, Noble PC, Bennett JB, Tullos HS. Simple dislocation of the elbow in the adult: results after closed treatment. *J Bone Joint Surg [Am]*. 1988;70:244–249.

O'Driscoll SW, Morrey BF, Korinek S, An KN. Elbow subluxation and dislocation: a spectrum of instability. *Clin Orthop*. 1992;280:186–197.

Pugh DM, Wild LM, Schemitsch EH, King GJ, McKee MD. Standard surgical protocol to treat elbow dislocations with radial head and coronoid fractures. *J Bone Joint Surg [Am]*. 2004;86:1122–1130.

Case 16

Bauer G, Arand M, Mutschler W. Post-traumatic Radioulnar Synostosis After Forearm Fracture Osteosynthesis. *Arch Orthop Trauma Surg*. 1991;110:142–145.

Chow SP, Leung F. Radial and ulnar shaft fractures. In: Bucholz RW, Court-Brown CM, Heckman JD, Tornetta P, eds. *Rockwood and Green's Fractures in Adults*. 7th ed. vol I, Section II. Philadelphia, PA: LWW; 2009:881–904.

Schemitsch EH, Richards RR. The effect of malunion on functional outcome after plate fixation of fractures of both bones of the forearm in adults. *J Bone Joint Surg Am*. 1992; 74:1068–1078.

Case 17

Chow SP, Leung F. Radial and ulnar shaft fractures. In: Bucholz RW, Court-Brown CM, Heckman JD, Tornetta P, eds. *Rockwood and Green's Fractures in Adults*. 7th ed. vol I, Section II. Philadelphia, PA: LWW; 2009:881–904.

Giannoulis FS, Sotereanos DG. Galeazzi fractures and dislocations. *Hand Clin*. 2007;23:153–163.

Rettig ME, Raskin KB. Galeazzi fracture-dislocation: a new treatment-oriented classification. *J Hand Surg Am*. 2001;26: 228–235.

Case 18

Konrad GG, Kundel K, Kreuz PC, Oberst M, Sudkamp NP. Monteggia fractures in adults. *J Bone Joint Surg [Br]*. 2007; 89:354–360.

Mathew PK, Athwal GS, King GJ. Terrible triad injury of the elbow: current concepts. *J Am Acad Orthop Surg*. 2009;17: 137–151.

Ring D, Jupiter JB, Simpson NS: Monteggia fractures in adults. *J Bone Joint Surg [Am]*. 1998;80:1733–1744.

Weiss AP, Hastings H. The anatomy of the proximal radioulnar joint. *J Shoulder Elbow Surg*. 1992;1:193–199.

Case 19

Lichtman DM, Bindra RR, Boyer MI, et al. AAOS Clinical Practice Guideline Summary: Treatment of Distal Radius Fractures. *J Am Acad Orthop Surg*. 2010;18:180–189.

Ruch DS, McQueen MM. Distal radius and ulna fractures. In: Bucholz RW, Court-Brown CM, Heckman JD, Tornetta P, eds. *Rockwood and Green's Fractures in Adults*. 7th ed. vol I, Section II. Philadelphia, PA: LWW; 2009:829–880.

Case 20

Dyer G, Lozano-Calderon S, Gannon C, Baratz M, Ring D. Predictors of acute carpal tunnel syndrome associated with fractures of the distal radius. *J Hand Surg*. 2008;33:1309–1313.

Ilyas AM, Jupiter JB. Distal radius fractures – classification of treatment and indications for surgery. *Hand Clin*. 2010;26:37–42.

Ruch DS, McQueen MM. Distal radius and ulna fractures. In: Bucholz RW, Court-Brown CM, Heckman JD, Tornetta P, eds. *Rockwood and Green's Fractures in Adults*. 7th ed. vol I, Section II. Philadelphia, PA: LWW; 2009:829–880.

Ruch DS, Papadonikolakis A. Volar versus dorsal plating in the management of intra-articular distal radius fractures. *J Hand Surg*. 2006;31:9–16.

Case 21

American College of Surgeons Committee on Trauma. *Advanced Trauma Life Support Program for Doctors*. 8th ed. Chicago, IL: American College of Surgeons; 2008.

Demetriades D, Karaiskakis M, Toutouzas K, Alo K, Velmahos G, Chan L. Pelvic Fractures: epidemiology and predictors of associated abdominal injuries and outcomes. *J Am Coll Surg*. 2002;195(1):1–10.

John MF. *Orthopaedic Knowledge Update 10*. Rosemont, IL: American Academy of Orthopaedic Surgeons, Copyright; 2011.

Mark DM, Stephen RT, Jennifer H. *Review of Orthopaedics*. 6th ed. Philadelphia, PA: Elsevier, Copyright; 2012.

Case 22

Archdeacon MT, Arebi S, Le TT, Wirth R, Kebel R, Thakore M. Orthogonal pin construct versus parallel uniplanar pin constructs for pelvic external fixation: A biomechanical assessment of stiffness and strength. *J Orthop Trauma*. 2009;23(2):100–105.

Burgess AR, Eastridge BJ, Young JW, et al. Pelvic ring disruptions: effective classification system and treatment protocols. *J Trauma*. 1990;30(7):848–856.

John MF. *Orthopaedic Knowledge Update 10*. Rosemont, IL: American Academy of Orthopaedic Surgeons, Copyright; 2011.

Mark DM, Stephen RT, Jennifer H. *Review of Orthopaedics*. 6th ed. Philadelphia, PA: Elsevier, Copyright; 2012.

Case 23

Burgess AR, Eastridge BJ, Young JW, et al. Pelvic ring disruptions: effective classification system and treatment protocols. *J Trauma*. 1990;30(7):848–856.

Collinge CA, Archdeacon MT, LeBus G. Saddle-horn injury of the pelvis: the injury, its outcomes, and associated male sexual dysfunction. *J Bone Joint Surg Am*. 2009;91(7):1630–1636.

Cothren CC, Osborn PM, Moore EE, Morgan SJ, Johnson JL, Smith WR. Preperitoneal pelvic packing for hemodynamically unstable pelvic fractures: a paradigm shift. *J Trauma*. 2007;62(4):834–842.

Langford JR, Burgess AR, Liporace FA, Haidukewych GJ. Pelvic fractures: Part 1. Evaluation, classification, and resuscitation. *J Am Acad Orthop Surg*. 2013;21(8):448–457.

Langford JR, Burgess AR, Liporace FA, Haidukewych GJ. Pelvic fractures: Part 2. Contemporary indications and techniques for definitive surgical management. *J Am Acad Orthop Surg*. 2013;21(8):458–468.

Case 24

Langford JR, Burgess AR, Liporace FA, Haidukewych GJ. Pelvic fractures: Part 2. Contemporary indications and techniques for definitive surgical management. *J Am Acad Orthop Surg*. 2013;21(8):458–468.

Letournel E, Judet R, Elson R. *Fractures of the Acetabulum*. 2nd ed. Berlin, Germany: Springer-Verlag; 1993.

Siegel J, Templeman DC, Tornetta P III. Single-leg-stance radiographs in the diagnosis of pelvic instability. *J Bone Joint Surg Am*. 2008;90(10):2119–2125.

Suzuki T, Smith WR, Hak DJ, et al. Combined injuries of the pelvis and acetabulum: nature of a devastating dyad. *J Orthop Trauma*. 2010;24(5):303–308.

Case 25

Denis F, Davis S, Comfort T. Sacral Fractures: an important problem. Retrospective analysis of 236 cases. *Clin Orthop Relat Res.* 1988;227:67–81.

Mehta S, Auerbach JD, Born CT, Chin KR. Sacral fractures. *J Am Acad Orthop Surg.* 2006;14(12):656–665.

Miller AN, Routt ML Jr. Variations in sacral morphology and implications for iliosacral screw fixation. *J Am Acad Orthop Surg.* 2012;20:8–16.

Phelan ST, Jones DA, Bishay M. Conservative management of transverse fractures of the sacrum with neurological features: A report of four cases. *J Bone Joint Surg Br.* 1991; 73(6):969–971.

Raj DR. *Orthopaedic Knowledge Update 4: Spine.* Rosemont, IL: American Academy of Orthopaedic Surgeons, Copyright; 2012.

Robles LA. Transverse sacral fractures. *Spine J.* 2009;9(1):60–69.

Routt ML Jr, Simonian PT, Agnew SG, Mann FA. Radiographic recognition of the sacral alar slope for optimal placement of iliosacral screws: a cadaveric and clinical study. *J Orthop Trauma.* 1996;10:171–177.

Schmidec HH, Smith DA, Kristiansen TK. Sacral fracture. *Neurosurgery.* 1984;15(5):735–746.

Case 26

Given CA. Sacral insufficiency. *Appl Radiol.* 2006;35(5):38–41.

Gotis-Graham I, McGuigan L, Diamond T, et al. Sacral insufficiency fractures in the elderly. *J Bone Joint Surg Br.* 1994;76: 882–886.

Mehta S, Auerbach JD, Born CT, Chin KR. Sacral fractures. *J Am Acad Orthop Surg.* 2006;14(12):656–665.

Weber M, Hasler P, Gerber H. Insufficiency fractures of the sacrum: twenty cases and review of the literature. *Spine.* 1993;18:2507–2512.

Case 27

Hak DJ, Olson SA, Matta JM. Diagnosis and management of closed internal degloving injuries associated with pelvic and acetabular fractures: The MOREL-Lavallee lesion. *J Trauma.* 1997;42(6):1046–1051.

Matta J. Fractures of the acetabulum: accuracy of reduction and clinical results in patients managed operatively within three weeks after the injury. *J Bone Joint Surg Am.* 1996;78 (11):1632–1645.

Case 28

Beaulé PE, Dorey FJ, Matta JM. Letournel classification for acetabular fractures: assessment of interobserver and intraobserver reliability. *J Bone Joint Surg Am.* 2003;85-A(9):1704–1709.

Durkee NJ, Jacobson J, Jamadar D, Karunakar MA, Morag Y, Hayes C. Classification of common acetabular fractures: radiographic and CT appearances. *AJR.* 2006;187:915–925.

John MF. *Orthopaedic Knowledge Update 10.* Rosemont, IL: American Academy of Orthopaedic Surgeons, Copyright; 2011.

Mark DM, Stephen RT, Jennifer H. *Review of Orthopaedics.* 6th ed. Philadelphia, PA: Elsevier, Copyright; 2012.

Case 29

John MF. *Orthopaedic Knowledge Update 10.* Rosemont, IL: American Academy of Orthopaedic Surgeons, Copyright; 2011.

Mark DM, Stephen RT, Jennifer H. *Review of Orthopaedics.* 6th ed. Philadelphia, PA: Elsevier, Copyright; 2012.

Matta JM et al. *Surgical Approaches to Fractures of the Acetabulum and Pelvis.* Copyright J.M. Matta; 1996.

Case 30

Anglen JO, Burd TA, Hendricks KJ, Harrison P. The "Gull Sign": A harbinger of failure for internal fixation of geriatric acetabular fractures. *J Orthop Trauma.* 2003;17(9):625–634.

Berkebile RD, Fischer DL, Albrecht LF. The Gull-Wing Sign: Value of the lateral view of the pelvis in fracture dislocation of the acetabular rim and posterior dislocation of the femoral head. *Radiology.* 1965;84:937–939.

Case 31

Foulk DM, Mullis BH. Hip dislocation: evaluation and management. *J Am Acad Orthop Surg.* 2010;18(4):199–209.

Kwon JY, Johnson CE, Appleton P, Rodriguez EK. Lateral femoral traction pin entry: risk to the femoral artery and other medial neurovascular structures. *J Orthop Surg Res.* 2010;5:4.

Case 32

Droll KP, Broekhuyse J, O'Brien P. Fractures of the femoral head. *J Am Acad Orthop Surg.* 2007;15(12):716–727.

Swiontkowski MF, Thorpe M, Seiler JG, Hansen ST. Operative management of displaced femoral head fractures: case-matched comparison of anterior versus posterior approaches for Pipkin I and Pipkin II fractures. *J Orthop Trauma.* 1992;6:437–442.

Case 33

Angelini M, McKee MD, Waddell JP, Haidukewych G, Schemitsch EH. Salvage of failed hip fracture fixation. *J Orthop Trauma.* 2009;23(6):471–478.

Dedrick DK, Mackenzie JR, Burney RE. Complications of femoral neck fracture in young adults. *J Trauma.* 1986; 26(10):932–937.

Swiontkowski MF. Intracapsular fractures of the hip. *J Bone Joint Surg Am.* 1994;76:129–138.

Case 34

Blomfeldt R, Törnkvist H, Ponzer S, Söderqvist A, Tidermark J. A randomized controlled trial comparing bipolar hemiarthroplasty with total hip replacement for displaced intracapsular fractures of the femoral neck in elderly patients. *J Bone Joint Surg Br.* 2007;89:160–165.

Egol KA, Koval KJ, Zuckerman JD. Functional recovery following hip fracture in the elderly. *J Orthop Trauma.* 1997; 11(8):594–599.

Case 35

Baumgaertner MR, Curtin SL, Lindskog DM, Keggi JM. The value of the tip-apex distance in predicting failure of fixation of peritrochanteric fractures of the hip. *J Bone Joint Surg Am*. 1995;77(7):1058–1064.

Browner BD, Jupiter JB, Levine AM, eds. *Skeletal Trauma*. 2nd ed. Philadelphia, PA: WB Saunders; 1998:1833–1881.

Lindskog DM, Baumgaertner MR. Unstable intertrochanteric hip fractures in the elderly. *J Am Acad Orthop Surg*. 2004;12(3):179–190.

Mohan R, Karthikeyan R, Sonanis SV. Dynamic hip screw: does side make a difference? Effects of clockwise torque on right and left DHS. *Injury*. 2000;31(9):697–699.

Case 36

Egol KA, Chang EY, Cvitkovic J, Kummer FJ, Koval KJ. Mismatch of current intramedullary nails with the anterior bow of the femur. *J Orthop Trauma*. 2004;18(7):410–415.

Moran CG, Wenn RT, Sikand M, Taylor AM. Early mortality after hip fracture: is delay before surgery important. 2005;87(3):483–489.

Ostrum RF, Levy MS. Penetration of the distal femoral anterior cortex during intramedullary nailing for subtrochanteric fractures: a report of three cases. *J Orthop Trauma*. 2005;19(9):656–660.

Richmond J, Aharonoff GB, Zuckerman JD, Koval KJ. Mortality risk after hip fracture. *J Orthop Trauma*. 2003;17(1):53–56.

Case 37

Lundy DW. Subtrochanteric femoral fractures. *J Am Acad Orthop Surg*. 2007;15(11):663–671.

Puhaindran ME, Farooki A, Steensma MR, Hameed M, Healey JH, Boland PJ. Atypical subtrochanteric femoral fractures in patients with skeletal malignant involvement treated with intravenous bisphosphonates. *J Bone Joint Surg Am*. 2011;93(13):1235–1242.

Case 38

Bennet FS, Zinar DM, Kilgus DJ. Ipsilateral hip and femoral shaft fractures. *Clin Orthop*. 1993;296:168–177.

Daffner RH, Riemer BL, Butterfield SL. Ipsilateral femoral neck and shaft fractures: an overlooked association. *Skeletal Radiol*. 1991;20(4):251–254.

Lindsey JD, Krieg JC. Femoral malrotation following femoral intramedullary nail fixation. *J Am Acad Orthop Surg*. 2011;19:17–26.

Peljovich AE, Patterson BM. Ipsilateral femoral neck and shaft fractures. *J Am Acad Orthop Surg*. 1998;6(2):106–113.

Tornetta P 3rd, Kain MS, Creevy WR. Diagnosis of femoral neck fractures in patients with a femoral shaft fracture. Improvement with a standard protocol. *J Bone Joint Surg Am*. 2007;89(1):39–43.

Case 39

Bhandari M, Zlowodzki M, Tornetta P III, Schmidt A, Templeman DC. Intramedullary, nailing following external fixation in femoral and tibial shaft fractures. *J Orthop Trauma*. 2005; 19:140–144.

Della Rocca GJ, Crist BD. External fixation versus conversion to intramedullary nailing for definitive management of closed fractures of the femoral and tibial shaft. *J Am Acad Orthop Surg*. 2006;14:S131–S135.

Porter JM, Ivatury RR. In search of the optimal end points of resuscitation in trauma patients: a review. *J Trauma*. 1998;44(5):908–914.

Roberts CS, Pape HC, Jones AL, Malkani AL, Rodriguez JL, Giannoudis PV. Damage control orthopaedics: evolving concepts in the treatment of patients who have sustained orthopaedic trauma. *Instr Course Lect*. 2005;54:447–462.

Case 40

Gwathmey FW Jr, Jones-Quaidoo SM, Kahler D, Hurwitz S, Cui Q. Distal femoral fractures: current concepts. *J Am Acad Orthop Surg*. 2010;18(10):597–607.

Nork SE, Segina DN, Aflatoon K, et al. The association between supracondylar-intercondylar distal femoral fractures and coronal plane fractures. *J Bone Joint Surg Am*. 2005;87(3):564–569.

Case 41

LaPrade RF, Ly TV, Wentorf FA, Engebretsen L. The posterolateral attachments of the knee: a qualitative and quantitative morphologic analysis of the fibular collateral ligament, popliteus tendon, popliteofibular ligament, and lateral gastrocnemius tendon. *Am J Sports Med*. 2003;31(6):854–860.

Mills WJ, Barei DP, McNair P. The value of the ankle-brachial index for diagnosing arterial injury after knee dislocation: a prospective study. *J Trauma*. 2004;56:1261–1265.

Rihn JA, Cha PS, Groff YJ, Harner CD. The acutely dislocated knee: evaluation and management. *J Am Acad Orthop Surg*. 2004;12:334–346.

Wascher DC. High-velocity knee dislocation with vascular injury. *Clin Sports Med*. 2000;19(3):457–477.

Case 42

Bedi A, Karunakar MA. Patella fractures and extensor mechanism injuries. In: Bucholz RW, Heckman JD, Court-Brown CM, Tornetta P, eds. *Rockwood and Green's Fractures in Adults*. Philadelphia, PA: Lippincott Williams & Wilkins; 2010:1752–1779.

Bostman O, Kiviluoto O, Nirhamo J. Comminuted displaced fractures of the patella. *Injury Br J Accid Surg*. 1981;13: 196–202.

Case 43

Gardner MJ, Yacoubian S, Geller D, et al. The incidence of soft tissue injury in operative tibial plateau fractures: an MRI imaging analysis of 103 patients. *J Orthop Trauma*. 2005;19:79–84.

Kobbe P, Pape HC. Lateral tibial plateau fractures. In: Wiesel SW, ed. *Operative Techniques in Orthopaedic Surgery*. Philadelphia, PA: Lippincott Williams & Wilkins; 2011:622–628.

Case 44

Egol KA, Tejwani NC, Capla EL, Wolinsky PL, Koval KJ. Staged management of high-energy proximal tibia fractures (OTA types 41): the results of a prospective, standardized protocol. *J Orthop Trauma.* 2005;19(7):448–455.

Reid JS, Van Slyke MA, Moulton MJ, Mann TA. Safe placement of prixmal tibial transfixation wires with respect to intracapsular penetration. *J Orthop Trauma.* 2001;15:10–17.

Weigel DP, Marsh JL. High-energy fractures of the tibial plateau. Knee function after longer follow-up. *J Bone Joint Surg Am.* 2002;84 A(9):1541–1551.

Case 45

Bhandari M, Guyatt G, Tornetta P 3rd, et al. Randomized trial of reamed and unreamed intramedullary nailing of tibial shaft fractures. *J Bone Joint Surg Am.* 2008;90(12): 2567–2578.

Giannoudis PV, Snowden S, Matthews SJ, et al. Friction burns within the tibia during reaming. Are they affected by the use of a tourniquet? *J Bone Joint Surg Br.* 2002;84(4):492–496.

Lefaivre KA, Guy P, Chan H, Blachut PA. Long-term follow-up of tibial shaft fractures treated with intramedullary nailing. *J Orthop Trauma.* 2008;22(8):525–529.

Case 46

Bhattacharyya T, Mehta P, Smith M, Pomahac B. Routine use of wound vaccumm-assisted closure does not allow coverage delay for open tibia fractures. *Plast Reconstruc Surg.* 2008;121(4):1263–1266.

Bosse MJ, MacKenzie EJ, Kellam JF, et al. An analysis of outcomes of reconstruction of amputation of leg-threatening injuries. *N Engl J Med.* 2002;347(24):1924–1931.

Dedmond BT, Kortesis B, Punger K, et al. The use of negative-pressure wound therapy (NPWT) in the temporary treatment of soft-tissue injuries associated with high-energy open tibial shaft fractures. *J Orthop Trauma.* 2007;21(1):11–17.

Gopal S, Majumder S, Batcherlor AG, Knight SL, De Boer P, Smith RM. Fix and flap: the radical orthopaedic and plast treatment of severe open fractures of the tibia. *J Bone Joint Surg Br.* 2000;82(7):959–966.

MacKenzie EJ, Bosse MJ, Kellam JF, et al.; LEAP Study Group. Factors influencing the decision to amputate or reconstruct after high-energy lower extremity trauma. *J Trauma.* 2002;52(4):641–649.

Case 47

Deangelis JP, Deangelis NA, Anderson R. Anatomy of the superficial peroneal nerve in relation to fixation of tibia fractures with the less invasive stabilization system. *J Orthop Trauma.* 2004;18:536–539.

Ricci WM, O'Boyle M, Borrelli J, Bellabarba C, Sanders R. Fractures of the proximal third of the tibial shaft treated with intramedullary nails and blocking screws. *J Orthop Trauma.* 2001;15(4):264–270.

Case 48

Pollak AN, McCarthy ML, Bess RS, Agel J, Swiontkowski MF. Outcomes after treatment of high-energy tibial plafond fractures. *J Bone Joint Surg Am.* 2003;85:1893–1900.

Ruëdi T, Allgöwer M. Fractures of the lower end of the tibia into the ankle joint. *Injury.* 1969;1:92–99.

Sirkin M, Sanders R, DiPasquale T, Herscovici D Jr. A staged protocol for soft tissue management in the treatment of complex pilon fractures. *J Orthop Trauma.* 1999;13(2):78–84.

Case 49

Carr JB. Malleolar fractures and soft tissue injures of the ankle. In: Browner B, Levine A, eds. *Skeletal Trauma.* 4th ed. Philadelphia, PA: Elsevier; 2009:2530–2536.

McConnell T, Tornetta P III: Marginal plafond impaction in association with supination adduction ankle fractures: a report of eight cases. *J Orthop Trauma.* 2001;15:447–449.

Case 50

Femino JE, Gruber BF, Karunakar MA. Safe zone for the placement of medial malleolar screws. *J Bone Joint Surg Am.* 2007;89(1):133–138.

Ricci WM, Tornetta P, Borrelli J. Lag screw fixation of medial malleolar fractures: a biomechanical, radiographic, and clinical comparison of unicortical partially threaded lag screws and bicortical fully threaded lag screws. *J Orthop Trauma.* 2012;26(10):602–606.

Tornetta P III, Spoo JE, Reynolds FA, Lee C. Overtightening of the ankle syndesmosis: is it really possible? *J Bone Joint Surg Am.* 2001;83:489–492.

Tornetta P. Competence of the deltoid ligament in bimalleolar ankle fractures after medial malleolar fixation. *J Bone Joint Surg Am.* 2000;82:843–848.

Zalavras C, Thordarson D. Ankle syndesmotic injury. *J Am Acad Orthop Surg.* 2007;15(6):330–339.

7

Reconstruction

Ayesha Abdeen

CASE 1

Dr. Valentin Antoci Jr.

An 82-year-old woman, with a BMI of 33.9 and history of total hip replacement performed 8 years ago, sustained a fall when attempting to walk to the bathroom. She has been unable to bear weight or ambulate since the fall. Radiographs and clinical picture of the implant in Figure 7–1 reveal a fracture of the femoral neck. This mechanism of implant failure likely occurred due to:

Based on biomechanical literature available, this fracture occurred due to:

A. Mismatch between the tensile strength of the stem and neck
B. Mechanical preparations and markings on the implant
C. Nonmodular nature of the component
D. Trunnionosis and interface wear
E. The increased interface stresses of cemented implants

Discussion

The correct answer is (B). This patient had a hybrid total hip arthroplasty with a cemented femoral component and a press-fit acetabular component. The fracture most

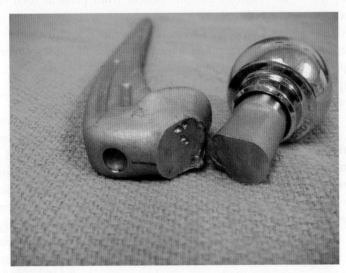

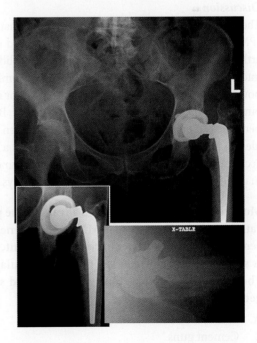

Figure 7–1

likely occurred due to mechanical etching/laser marking on the component during production. Multiple manufacturers have experienced similar failures with designs in the late 1990s and have withdrawn those devices off the market. Fractures of femoral stems at the modular head–neck junction have also been reported infrequently and are due to fretting fatigue. Risk factors for such fractures include: excessive body weight and inadequate proximal osseous support because of trochanteric osteotomy, reduced preoperative bone stock, osteolysis, loosening, and/or implant undersizing.

"Trunnionosis" is the phenomenon of wear debris generated at the modular junction between the femoral head and tapered femoral neck ("trunnion") of the stem. Implant generated metallic wear debris can be a concern when large femoral head sizes are used (greater than 40 mm in diameter) as well as metal-on-metal bearing surfaces. However in this case, radiographs demonstrate that a 32-mm head was used, and there was no clear indication of wear. The bearing surface in this implant is metal on polyethylene.

During cement mixing, the process of polymerization is started by:

A. Barium sulfate
B. Benzoyl peroxide
C. Dimethyl toluidine
D. Hydroquinone
E. Hylamer

Discussion

The correct answer is (B). Poly(methyl methacrylate) (PMMA) is a transparent Plexiglas typically used in joint arthroplasty. The material acts as a grout to solidify the interface between bone and the implant. During mixing, a powder of polymer, barium sulfate, and an initiator is combined with the liquid monomer and accelerator. Benzoyl peroxide is typically used as an initiator. Hydrogen peroxide can play a similar role. Dimethyl toluidine is a typical accelerator. Barium sulfate is usually used in cements to make the material radiodense and visible on x-rays.

Modern cement techniques have advanced the preparation and application of PMMA. First-generation cementing involved finger packing the cement, which is still the method often used on the acetabular side. The difference between third generation and second generation usually involves the use of:

A. Pressurization
B. Cement guns

C. Pulse lavage and drying the canal
D. Brushing the canal
E. Cement restrictor

Discussion

The correct answer is (A). Second-generation techniques introduced cement guns, restrictors, as well as better techniques of preparing the canal by pulse lavage, brushing, and drying. Third-generation techniques usually involve vacuum mixing, precoating the implant surface, and pressurization. The Swedish registry suggested that vacuum mixing may worsen long-term survival. Ideal cementing technique involves at least a 2-mm mantle in all seven Gruen zones. The stem should take at least ⅓ of the canal. The distal mantle should be at least one diameter. Barrack et al. have defined a grading system for cementing with grade A showing a uniform, even mantle around the entire prosthesis while grade D has 100% radiolucency at the interface. The quality of cementing has been shown to directly correlate with outcome.

During preparation the cement goes through multiple stages that include a "doughy" phase, working time, insertion time, and setting time. While setting, cement undergoes an exothermic reaction with 12 to 14 kcal released per 100-g cement. Rapid mixing, high humidity, and high temperature shorten the process.

The press-fit acetabular component is widely accepted as a standard in the United States. The Swedish registry data, though, show that:

A. Press-fit stems generally have less pain and less revision rate
B. Press-fit cups have higher failure rate and revisions
C. Younger patients benefit from press-fit total hip arthroplasty
D. Cemented femurs had a higher rate of fracture
E. In femoral neck fractures, press-fit implants generally have better survival

Discussion

The correct answer is (B). The Swedish Hip Arthroplasty Registry is an extensive, detailed National Quality database of outcomes following THR performed in Sweden since 1979. Results from the Swedish Registry data support the use of cemented total hip replacement for both the femur and acetabulum. Press-fit stems have a higher rate of fracture, subsidence, and thigh pain. No specific differences were seen per age group, even though the revision curve for both cemented and uncemented components seem to decline faster after

10 to 12 years. Some authors suggest that, in the setting of insufficiency fractures that are associated with worse bone quality, cemented total hip replacements provide more reliable results. Press-fit stems, especially with use of aggressively tapered designs, leads to higher risk of fractures.

Osteolysis is seen in Charnley zone 1 around the acetabulum and mild asymmetry in the position of the femoral head in the cup. The process through which osteolysis takes place in this design is driven by:

A. Lymphocytes
B. Macrophages
C. Osteoblasts
D. Eosinophils
E. Lymphoblasts

Discussion

The correct answer is (B). Metal-on-polyethylene hips lead to polyethylene particle wear. The subsequent osteolysis is usually driven by a macrophage mediated process. By comparison, the recently described metal particle wear is a lymphocytic process, termed ALVAL (aseptic lymphocyte-dominated vasculitis-associated lesions). Adverse local tissue reactions (ALTR) around metal-on-metal components is being increasingly recognized, initially due to the bearing surface, and more recently due to the process of trunnionosis.

The bearing surface used in this total hip replacement is metal-on-polyethylene. Alternative bearings include metal-on-metal, ceramic-on-ceramic, and ceramic-on-polyethylene. By comparison to first-generation ceramic bearing surfaces, third-generation ceramic-on-ceramic bearings show:

A. Higher incidence of osteolysis, squeaking, and head fractures
B. Higher incidence of pain and instability
C. Lower incidence of osteolysis, squeaking, and head fractures
D. Higher failure rate and need for revision
E. 100% survival at 10 years

Discussion

The correct answer is (C). Ceramic bearings have demonstrated significantly better wear characteristics compared to conventional metal-on-polyethylene bearing surfaces both clinically and in wear simulators. Squeaking, which has been documented previously with initial ceramic designs, is now reported at less than 1%.

Helpful Tip:

Both cemented and press-fit fixation techniques are associated with good results following total hip arthroplasty. Cementing technique is critical in determining long-term implant survival and should include canal preparation, pressurization, and a good cement mantle interface.

Objectives: Did you learn...?

• How to recognize bearing materials and associated complications?
• Implant fixation mechanisms and modern cementing techniques?
• Bearing surface wear and the biologic process involved?

CASE 2

Dr. Ayesha Abdeen

A 50-year-old female underwent metal-on-metal (MoM) total hip arthroplasty 1 year ago for osteoarthritis. Her pain initially resolved, however she is now experiencing new onset buttock and thigh pain as well as clicking of her hip. She comes to you with an x-ray performed at an outside hospital and has questions pertaining to whether or not she is at risk of developing cancer and whether the hip implant should be revised to a non-MoM device (Fig. 7–2).

Which of the following is TRUE regarding MoM bearing surfaces?

A. Unlike polyethylene-on-metal bearing surfaces, MoM surfaces do not create particulate debris
B. MoM bearing surfaces do generate particulate debris. These particles are larger but fewer in number than

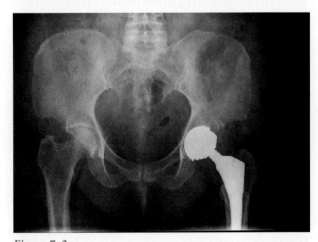

Figure 7–2

those created with polyethylene-on-metal bearing surfaces

C. MoM bearing surfaces are characterized by higher wear during a "running-in" period that occurs during the first 1 to 2 years following MoM THR

D. Serum metal ions generated with MoM devices correlates directly with the patient's level of activity

Discussion

The correct answer is (C). MoM bearing surfaces have been approved for use in the United States since 1999. The results regarding second-generation MoM implants have been promising and suggestive that there may be less failure due to osteolysis and wear as seen with conventional polyethylene and metal. Although MoM implants are considered a low-wear alternative bearing surface, MoM does generate particulate debris. These particles are smaller but more numerous than polyethylene particles. Hip simulator tests have demonstrated a higher wear rate of MoM implants during a "running-in" period that corresponds to the first million cycles in a simulator or the first 1 to 2 years in vivo which is then followed by steady-state wear. The amount of wear debris in MoM devices has not been found to correlate with a patient's level of activity.

Which of the following tests should be performed on this patient?

A. Plain radiographs of the pelvis and hip
B. ESR and CRP
C. Blood cobalt and chromium ions levels
D. Cross-sectional imaging (MARS MRI)
E. All of the above

Discussion

The correct answer is (B). In any painful THR a plain film should be obtained to rule out mechanical failure, loosening, or periprosthetic fracture. Deep prosthetic joint infection must also be ruled out, and therefore ESR and CRP are indicated. Blood Co and Cr ion levels should be obtained to determine whether the patient may be experiencing any of the potential reactions to metal ion particulate debris generated from the MoM bearing surface. Possible sequelae of increased serum metal ions include local tissue reactions, pseudotumors, and hypersensitivity. MRI imaging reveals a region of lymphocytic reaction next to a metal-on-metal prosthesis. MR imaging with "metal artifact-reducing sequences" (MARS) has been used to identify lymphocytic responses manifesting as aseptic lymphocyte-dominated vasculitis-

associated lesions (ALVAL). Contrast enhancement can occur in bone, synovial tissue, joint capsule, and at the periphery of a soft tissue mass. A relationship between MRI findings and pain has not been found.

Variations in cobalt/chromium serum levels following MoM THR are associated with all of the following EXCEPT:

A. Femoral head size
B. T-cell counts
C. Lymphocytic changes
D. Retroverted femoral component
E. Cup abduction angle

Discussion

The correct answer is (D). Variations in cobalt/chromium levels following THR are associated with excessive cup abduction angles as well as excessive cup anteversion which results in the contact zone of the bearing surface near or on the rim of the cup. Rim contact increases the rate of wear. Clinically, malposition of the cup has been associated with increased generation of metal ion debris resulting in increased serum metal ion levels. MoM bearings of large diameter result in greater systemic exposure of metal ions than smaller-diameter heads. In addition, lymphocyte reactivity has been found to correlate with increased metal ion exposure.

What is the recommended course of action in patients with asymptomatic MoM implants according to the Food and Drug Administration (FDA)?

A. Revision to a conventional bearing surface if serum cobalt level is greater than 2 μg/L
B. Serial MARS imaging
C. Serial measurement of serum metal ion levels
D. If the implant is functioning properly, the FDA does not recommend serial routine soft tissue imaging or serum ion levels be performed

Discussion

The correct answer is (B). Although the vast majority of MoM implants have been successful, the Medicines and Healthcare Products Regulatory Agency (MHRA) in the UK issued a medical device alert in April 2010 for all MoM hip replacements base upon a trend of early failures. Subsequently on May 6, 2011 the United States Food and Drug Administration issued a postmarket surveillance study of all MoM hip implants. In February 2011 the FDA launched an MoM hip webpage indicating that MoM hip implants pose additional risks in comparison to all other hip implants. On January 17, 2013 the FDA issued an updated public health Safety Communication on MoM hip implants with detailed information regarding the recommended course of action before and after implantation of an MoM hip device. The FDA is currently not recommending revision arthroplasty based upon a specific threshold serum metal ion level and asserts that the decision to revise should be based upon overall clinical assessment and active symptoms.

The FDA has identified risk factors for developing adverse local tissue reactions (ALTR) following MoM hip implantation. These risk factors include all of the following EXCEPT:

A. Corticosteroid use
B. Malalignment of the acetabular or femoral components
C. Renal insufficiency
D. Excessively low BMI
E. Patients with suspected metal allergies

Discussion

The correct answer is (D). The FDA webpage on MoM implants suggests the following risk factors for ALTR following MoM hip replacements:

• Patients with bilateral implants
• Patients with resurfacing systems with small femoral heads (44 mm or smaller)
• Female patients
• Patients receiving high doses of corticosteroids
• Patients with evidence of renal insufficiency
• Patients with suppressed immune systems
• Patients with suboptimal alignment of device components
• Patients with suspected metal sensitivity (e.g., cobalt, chromium, nickel)
• Patients who are severely overweight
• Patients with high levels of physical activity

According to the FDA, the following systemic problems can occur as a result of MoM implants EXCEPT:

A. A general hypersensitivity/rash
B. Thyroid dysfunction
C. Cardiomyopathy
D. Cognitive impairment
E. Multiple myeloma

Discussion

The correct answer is (E). The FDA webpage regarding MoM implants lists a number of clinical sequela of

increased serum metal ions including general hypersensitivity, thyroid dysfunction, cardiomyopathy, cognitive impairment, auditory or visual impairment, and psychological disturbance. Specific neoplasms have not been linked to increased metal ions in the bloodstream according to the FDA.

Helpful Tip:

Metal ion testing may be indicated in patients with symptomatic MoM bearing hips. Not all testing laboratories can accurately detect more than trace levels (more than 10 μg/L) of cobalt or chromium. Many laboratories use different techniques and normal ranges, and therefore it can be difficult and inaccurate to compare results from one laboratory to another. Metal ion concentration values should be interpreted in conjunction with blood urea nitrogen (BUN) and creatinine to concurrently evaluate the patient's renal function. There is no threshold level of cobalt or chromium that indicates revision arthroplasty.

Objectives: Did you learn...?

• The recommended evaluation of a patient with symptomatic and asymptomatic MoM bearing surfaces?
• The possible local and system reactions to increased metallic debris as generated by MoM hip implants?

CASE 3

Dr. Valentin Antoci Jr.

A 51-year-old male presents with a chief complaint of left hip pain that has been progressively worsening for the past 6 months. He has groin pain and describes radiation to his knee. He has been taking a nonsteroidal anti-inflammatory medication with some relief but continues to limp and experience severe pain after walking to clinic.

Patient states a history of anxiety and COPD with inhaled corticosteroids treatment more than 10 years ago. Three years ago the patient was diagnosed with myelodysplasia and underwent a bone marrow transplant. He smokes half a pack of cigarettes per day and uses alcohol occasionally. He previously used heroin.

An x-ray is obtained (Fig. 7–3). What further studies would be recommended next in his management?

A. Ultrasound
B. Frog-leg lateral hip radiograph
C. CT pelvis and hip
D. Bone scan
E. Arthrogram

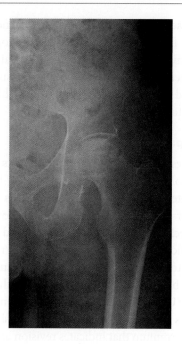

Figure 7–3

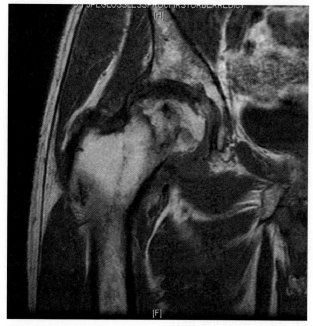

Figure 7–4

Discussion

The correct answer is (B). Based upon clinical history, the differential diagnosis in this patient may include stress fracture, femoroacetabular impingement, avascular necrosis, and tumor. While this patient's AP hip x-ray reveals osteonecrosis/avascular necrosis (AVN) of the left hip, this diagnosis is often missed on initial AP and shoot-through lateral radiographs. A frog-leg lateral visualizes the anteromedial part of the joint where collapse is initially observed. The Ficat–Arlet classification for osteonecrosis is based upon the following radiographic criteria:

I. Normal radiographs
II. Diffuse sclerosis and cysts
III. Subchondral fracture (crescent sign with or without collapse)
IV. Femoral head collapse, acetabular involvement, and arthritis

Ficat/Arlet stage I and II involve the precollapse period and are associated with the best prognostic value. Early disease can be detected on MRI imaging. Bilateral hip disease occurs in 50% of cases of osteonecrosis in which the cause is systemic (i.e., in most etiologies with the exception of unilateral hip trauma), therefore an MRI of the pelvis is indicated to evaluate the asymptomatic contralateral hip (Fig. 7–4). The Steinberg classification of femoral head osteonecrosis has been adapted to include MRI findings.

The patient is quite anxious about his diagnosis and insists that since he has had no trauma and no family history of osteonecrosis the diagnosis must be incorrect. Which of these conditions in the patient's history has been linked directly to AVN?

A. Corticosteroid inhalers
B. Hematologic disorders and myelodysplasia
C. Heroin abuse
D. Advanced age

Discussion

The correct answer is (B). Avascular necrosis is not well understood. The thought that vascular compromise may be associated with the injury has provided the premise for some early treatments but outcomes are inconsistent.

Trauma, sickle cell disease, hematologic disorders, Caisson disease, and irradiation are associated with AVN. The condition though has also been linked to systemic corticosteroid medications, alcohol abuse, smoking, and viral diseases including CMV, HIV/ antiretroviral treatment, rubella, and varicella.

Radiation, hematologic disease, HIV, asthma, alcoholism, and sickle cell disease are associated with AVN. In sickle cell disease, asymptomatic patients with MRI-detectable femoral head osteonecrosis will develop femoral head collapse in more than:

A. 10% of cases
B. 30% of cases

C. 60% of cases

D. 70% of cases

E. 100% of cases

Discussion

The correct answer is (D). According to several studies, most patients with sickle cell and early symptoms of AVN diagnosed on imaging will progress to collapse. Hernigou et al. documented the natural history of osteonecrosis of the femoral head in 121 initially asymptomatic patients with sickle cell disease and showed 91% developed hip pain and 77% demonstrated collapse over a 10-year period.

The patient requests any possible treatment to improve his chances of keeping his native hip healthy and remain active through his older years. He inquires if he should either try crutches or the option for some kind of surgery to help the lesions heal. You suggest that the treatment algorithm that is currently recommended for stage I disease involves:

A. Crutches and nonweight bearing

B. Low-intensity pulsed ultrasound (LIPUS)

C. Statins and vasodilators to counteract the avascular process

D. Core decompression and percutaneous drilling

E. Total hip replacement

Discussion

The correct answer is (D). Nonweight bearing has not been a particularly successful treatment modality. LIPUS has been tried with similarly low success. Pharmacological treatment has also been attempted with statins, vasodilators, and anticoagulants showing no clear improvement in AVN.

Bisphosphonate treatment can be of benefit in early osteonecrosis. The inhibition of osteoclasts and the resorption process was thought to slow weakening of the femoral head and collapse. Some studies have shown no change in progression of disease with a need for arthroplasty while other studies have shown a benefit.

The current algorithms for AVN involve core decompression for stage I or II (precollapse) disease. Over 80% of stage I diseases and 60% of stage II diseases have been shown to be successfully managed with decompression or drilling. Once collapse has occurred, the overall outcomes worsen significantly. Bone grafting is an option but patients often progress to require a total hip replacement.

The patient continues to have pain following nonoperative treatment. He has read about hip resurfacing and despite your caution of metal-on-metal bearings, he would like to proceed with hip resurfacing. You further caution him that he is at higher risk of failure due to:

A. His young age

B. Male gender

C. Osteonecrosis of the femoral head

D. Arthritis

E. Comorbidities

Discussion

The correct answer is (C). Even though currently out of favor due to increasing concerns regarding the systemic and local sequelae of metal ions, the results of hip resurfacing have been most successful in patients under 55 years of age, male, with a diagnosis of osteoarthritis. Resurfacings in patients with AVN have higher risk of failure due to presence of osteonecrosis into the femoral neck. Total hip arthroplasty yields more reproducible results in this setting.

Nevertheless, total hip replacement in younger patients and patients with AVN has been shown to have a higher failure rate compared to the older population.

Helpful Tip:

Groin pain in a younger patient with risk factors for AVN should be evaluated closely. Frog lateral will show collapse, but in the absence of those findings an MRI should be obtained to rule out a fracture or early stages of AVN. Based on the degree of disease, bisphosphonates, core decompression and drilling, bone grafting, limited replacements including hemiarthroplasty, and total hip replacements can be performed. Hip preservation techniques are recommended for precollapse disease, and arthroplasty is recommended for postcollapse. Younger patients with more advanced disease have overall worse outcomes in the long term.

Objectives: Did you learn...?

• Recognize AVN, x-ray, and MRI findings?

• Know the comorbidities associated with AVN and their direct or indirect risk?

• Understand the treatment algorithm?

CASE 4

Dr. Valentin Antoci Jr.

A 52-year-old postmenopausal female presents with progressive hip pain. She points to the pain in "C-clamp" distribution around the hip, mostly localized

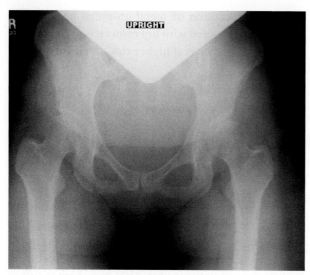

Figure 7–5

in her groin. She likes to run, but has not been able to do so over the last year. She describes start-up thigh pain and pain with putting her shoes on, getting in and out of cars, and deep flexion. The primary care physician was concerned with the possibility of femoroacetabular impingement and obtained an MRI that shows cartilage thinning and focal defects, as well as degenerative labral tear. A radiograph is also obtained (Fig. 7–5). The patient asks about her labral tear and the possibility of repair. Her pain persists despite anti-inflammatory medication, physical therapy, and activity modification.

When discussing the options for management, based on available data, the best intervention would be:

A. Observation
B. Hip arthroscopy with labral repair
C. HemiCAP partial arthroplasty
D. Hip resurfacing
E. Total hip arthroplasty

Discussion

The correct answer is (E). In the setting of ongoing pain despite nonsurgical treatment measures, total hip arthroplasty is indicated. Hip arthroscopy for debridement and labral repair is very successful in addressing isolated labral tears in younger patients but in the setting of arthritis the results are limited. HemiCAP partial arthroplasty is possible in a patient with a focal posttraumatic osteochondral defect or AVN but not in generalized arthritis. This patient does not fit the indications for hip resurfacing.

The Tonnis angle is a usual measurement used in the setting of acetabular dysplasia. This is measured by evaluating the angle created by:

A. A vertical line and the line connecting the center of femoral head to edge of acetabulum
B. A line along the ileum and another line along the acetabular roof
C. A horizontal line and the line along the acetabular roof
D. A horizontal line and the line from the teardrop to the acetabular edge
E. A line along the femoral axis and the line from the center of the femoral head to the center of knee

Discussion

The correct answer is (C). The angle of the sourcil was defined by Tonnis in the setting of dysplasia, with measurements greater than 10 to 12 being concerning. Other authors will also use the acetabular edge angle, the alpha angle, and acetabular angle of sharp.

The Crowe classification of acetabular dysplasia measures:

A. The degree of arthritis in dysplastic acetabuli
B. The amount of migration of the femoral head
C. The degree of lateralization of the femoral head
D. The amount of deformity of the femoral head
E. The degree of deformity of the acetabulum

Discussion

The correct answer is (B). Crowe classification quantifies the superior migration of the femoral head with respect to the true acetabulum. This is calculated by dividing the distance from the inferior tear drop to the inferomedial head–neck junction by femoral head size as a percentage of proximal migration of the femoral head.

Crowe I: less than 50% subluxation
Crowe II: 50% to 75% subluxation
Crowe III: 75% to 100% subluxation
Crowe IV: More than 100% superior migration

In contrast, the Tonnis classification evaluates the severity of arthritic changes:

Tonnis 0: No signs of degenerative joint disease
Tonnis I: Increased sclerosis and slight narrowing of joint space, normal femoral head
Tonnis II: Cysts, moderate narrowing, and femoral head deformity
Tonnis III: Cysts, severe narrowing, and severe femoral head deformity

The patient then inquires about treatment options other than joint replacement. You state that a pelvic osteotomy is an option, but she is not a candidate because of her:

A. Advanced arthritis
B. Young age
C. Good range of motion
D. Skeletal maturity
E. Female gender

Discussion

The correct answer is (A). The goal of an osteotomy is to reestablish normal hip biomechanics and delay degenerative change progression and the need for arthroplasty. Periacetabular osteotomies are possible in:

1. Younger patient
2. Minimal arthritis
3. Good preoperative range of motion
4. Skeletally mature
5. With dysplasia

Advanced dysplasia with significant superior migration of the femoral head requires work to bring the cup into its anatomic position. Lengthening of more than 4 cm is sometimes required which puts the sciatic nerve at high risk for traction neurapraxia. To avoid that, the surgeon can:

A. Use increased offset components to lateralize the hip
B. Perform an extended trochanteric osteotomy and advance the abductors
C. Use modular femoral components which allow surgeon to dial version appropriately
D. Perform a subtrochanteric osteotomy and shortening
E. Perform a neurolysis at the time of surgery

Discussion

The correct answer is (D). The risk of sciatic nerve palsy in hip dysplasia is 10 times the risk in a typical total hip arthroplasty and can top 15%. Even though several techniques are used in dysplastic hip, more than 4 cm of lengthening has a high risk of complications and should be considered for a femoral osteotomy and shortening. Depending on the case, some surgeons will also choose to maintain a superior position of the acetabulum, which is not ideal but acceptable.

Increased offset and modular femoral components are helpful in increasing stability, improving the overall version and decrease risk of dislocation. An extended

trochanteric osteotomy is sometimes necessary to address the contracted abductors.

Helpful Tip:

Hip dysplasia is a complex problem which may lead to severe degenerative joint disease requiring arthroplasty. In young patients, a periacetabular or femoral osteotomy is an option in the absence of degenerative changes and arthritis. Once arthritic changes and loss of cartilage has occurred, the results of osteotomy are significantly worse, with arthroplasty being the only option that would allow reproducible outcomes. Nevertheless, options for acetabular bone loss and femoral version correction should be available, including augments, and modular stems.

Objectives: Did you learn...?

- Diagnose dysplasia based on x-rays and geometric measurements?
- Classify dysplasia based on Crowe or other classification?
- Understand the associated complications possible after addressing dysplasia?

CASE 5

Dr. Valentin Antoci Jr.

A 57-year-old female presents to the office with atraumatic knee pain. Her pain is worse at the beginning of activities as well as the end of the day. She has trouble ascending and descending stairs. She uses anti-inflammatories intermittently with mild relief. On examination she has pain along the medial joint line but full range of motion. X-rays show characteristic medial joint space narrowing, subchondral sclerosis, and cysts.

All of the following are modifiable risk factors for knee osteoarthritis, except:

A. Patient weight
B. Hard labor
C. Trauma
D. Gender
E. Muscular weakness

Discussion

The correct answer is (D). Modifiable risk factors associated with arthritis include obesity, trauma, occupations involving hard labor, and overall deconditioning. Women are at higher risk for arthritis. White and Hispanics have higher rates of arthritis compared to African-American males and some Asian populations.

All the following are viable initial management options recommended by the AAOS, except:

A. Weight loss and diet control for BMI >25
B. Physical therapy for quadriceps/hamstring strengthening/stretching
C. Hyaluronic acid injections
D. Corticosteroid injections
E. Activity modification

Discussion

The correct answer is (C). The recent AAOS guidelines on osteoarthritis of the knee endorse the use of self-management programs, strengthening, low-impact aerobic exercises, and neuromuscular education. They also recommend weight loss for knee osteoarthritis patients with BMI >25 and activity modification. The committee could not recommend for or against the use of steroids due to inconclusive data, but the guidelines advise against the use of hyaluronic acid.

The patient asks regarding other modalities or intervention for her knee before considering total knee replacement. The following modalities have been ruled inconclusive except:

A. Acupuncture
B. Electrostimulation
C. Chondroitin sulfate
D. Tylenol
E. Valgus directing sports brace

Discussion

The correct answer is (C). The committee has found inconclusive evidence to recommend for or against acupuncture, electrostimulation, Tylenol and pain patches, as well as a valgus directing sports brace. Nevertheless, they have had a strong recommendation against the use of chondroitin sulfate due to the limited support in the literature for its use.

When comparing knee arthroscopy and lavage to placebo in the setting of knee arthritis, knee arthroscopy results in:

A. Complete reversal of symptoms
B. Improved symptom control and no progression to total knee arthroplasty
C. 50% improved symptoms at 3 months that remained consistent at 1 year
D. Significant improvement over 1 year followed by recurrence
E. No improvement of arthritis pain

Discussion

The correct answer is (E). The AAOS guidelines strongly recommend against the use of either needle lavage or arthroscopic lavage. No significant benefit has been documented. Nevertheless, the guidelines could not recommend for or against meniscectomy.

You explain to the patient that a total knee replacement is an elective procedure and that she should decide when her symptoms are negatively affecting her quality of life. The patient inquires about outcomes and any predisposing factors. You tell her that:

A. Preoperative range of motion typically determines postoperative range of motion
B. The risk of infection goes up the longer they wait for surgery
C. The improvement and patient satisfaction is worse if symptoms are worse
D. The sooner they have the replacement the higher the satisfaction rate
E. Recovery takes 6 weeks with return to full mobility

Discussion

The correct answer is (A). Total knee arthroplasty is a complex procedure with overall functional outcomes reported lower compared to the total hip. Even though patients report overall good outcomes, most studies have shown some patient bias in reported higher perceived outcomes compared to their actual functional status. It takes patients at least 6 months to regain their mobility and sustain full relief of symptoms. The overall improvement and patient satisfaction is better the worse their scores are before the surgery, with patients with minimum symptoms being most unsatisfied with overall outcomes. No link with infection and delay in surgery has been documented, even though complex surgery and the operative time may have a correlation. Preoperative range of motion and stiffness is linked to the postoperative range of motion, even if full range of motion is achieved intraoperatively in an anesthetized patient.

The AAOS guidelines show inconclusive support for or against a tibial osteotomy. Compared to a total knee arthroplasty, a high tibial osteotomy:

A. Has shorter recovery compared to a total knee arthroplasty
B. Works better in obese, inactive patients in which TKA has higher risk
C. Works better in older males compared to total knee arthroplasty

D. Can provide significantly improved symptom relief compared to TKA

E. Works similarly to TKA in thin, active individuals

Discussion

The correct answer is (E). Recommendation 14 of the AAOS guidelines suggests "The practitioner might perform a valgus producing proximal tibial osteotomy in patients with symptomatic medial compartment osteoarthritis of the knee." Classic indications include a younger, active, thin patient with a stable knee examination in whom the outcomes may approach the outcomes of a total knee replacement.

Osteoarthritis is a disease of cartilage. The matrix disruption and subchondral sclerosis results in:

A. Decreased water content

B. Increased collagen content

C. Decreased proteoglycan quantity

D. Decreased chondrocyte activity

E. Loss of chondrocytes

Discussion

The correct answer is (C). Osteoarthritis (OA) is a process that is pathophysiologically distinct from normal physiologic aging. In osteoarthritis, collagen changes include: increased water content, decreased collagen content, increased enzymatic activity, and increased chondrocyte numbers. There is also a decreased proteoglycan content in OA. Conversely in normal aging, cartilage changes include: decreased water content, normal collagen content with increased cross-linking, and decreased chondrocyte numbers.

The patient returns to you a year later stating worsening symptoms, associated instability, and decreased range of motion. Anti-inflammatory medication has provided minimal pain relief. X-rays show progressive medial as well as patellofemoral arthritis. The most reliable intervention in this case is:

A. Corticosteroid injection

B. Hyaluronan injection

C. High tibial osteotomy

D. Unicondylar knee replacement

E. Total knee replacement

Discussion

The correct answer is (E). In a patient with multicompartmental knee arthritis who has failed nonoperative treatment, a total knee replacement would provide the most reliable and reproducible results. Osteotomy or unicondylar knee replacements provide limited benefit in multicompartmental knee arthritis with associated instability.

Helpful Tip:

In 2013 the American Academy of Orthopaedic Surgeons (AAOS) published the second edition of clinical practice guidelines on the treatment of osteoarthritis of the knee. This evidence-based guideline indicated that anti-inflammatories, weight loss, and aerobic low-impact exercise have a strong support in the initial treatment of osteoarthritis. Acupuncture, other modalities, Tylenol, steroid injections, and bracing were found to be inconclusive. In contrast, the guidelines could not recommend the injection of hyaluronan or the use of arthroscopic lavage. Meniscectomies and tibial osteotomies have inconclusive and limited results, respectively.

Objectives: Did you learn...?

- Recognize arthritis?
- Follow AAOS guidelines for nonoperative management?
- Follow AAOS guidelines for early operative management?

CASE 6

Dr. Forrest H. Schwartz

A 67-year-old woman who is scheduled to undergo primary total hip arthroplasty for end-stage arthritis of the right hip calls your office to inform you that she just remembered that 15 years ago she had a blood clot after a long plane flight. She asks if this event will affect her scheduled surgery or expected postoperative course. You inform her that based on the 2011 AAOS guideline on preventing venous thromboembolic disease in patients undergoing elective total hip and knee arthroplasty:

A. There is strong evidence to support increasing the duration of her postoperative pharmacologic prophylaxis to at least 6 weeks because of her history of DVT

B. Her history of DVT makes her too "high risk" to undergo elective surgery and the procedure will have to be cancelled

C. She will be placed on warfarin postoperatively because it is more effective at preventing VTED than other forms of pharmacologic prophylaxis

D. A personal history of DVT does not increase the risk of VTED following elective hip and knee arthroplasty

E. She will receive both pharmacologic and mechanical prophylaxis in the postoperative period because of her history of prior deep venous thrombosis

Discussion

The correct answer is (E). Determining appropriate VTED prophylaxis remains a challenge in the setting of elective total hip and knee arthroplasty. There is no evidence regarding the optimal duration of pharmacologic prophylaxis in patients with a prior history of DVT and this remains an area of controversy that must be addressed on a case-by-case basis after discussion of the potential risks and benefits with the patient (choice A). The relative efficacy of different types of prophylaxis has been investigated, and there is not strong evidence to support the use of one pharmacologic agent over another (choice C). A personal history of DVT is the only risk factor known to increase the likelihood of VTE following total hip or knee arthroplasty (choice D); however, the relative increase in risk is not great enough to make proceeding with surgery unsafe (choice B). It is a consensus opinion in the 2011 AAOS guideline on preventing VTE that patients with a history of DVT be treated with both pharmacologic and mechanical prophylaxis (choice E).

Which of the following interventions are not supported by either consensus opinion or moderate scientific evidence in the 2011 AAOS guideline on preventing venous thromboembolic disease in patients undergoing elective total hip and knee arthroplasty?

A. Patients should discontinue antiplatelet agents (e.g., aspirin, clopidogrel) 5 to 7 days prior to elective total hip or knee arthroplasty
B. Early mobilization is an important adjunct in the prevention of VTED in patients undergoing elective total hip or knee arthroplasty
C. The use of neuraxial anesthesia decreases the risk of VTED when compared to the use of general anesthesia in elective total hip or knee arthroplasty
D. Routine postoperative screening duplex ultrasonography is not indicated in patients undergoing elective total hip or knee arthroplasty

Discussion

The correct answer is (C). The optimal time for discontinuation of antiplatelet agents has not been studied specifically in arthroplasty patients, but among nonarthroplasty patients there are multiple studies demonstrating increased operative blood loss in patients that did not stop antiplatelet agents prior to elective surgery (choice A). Early mobilization is a low-cost, low-risk intervention that promotes regional blood flow, so despite a lack of strong evidence, it is supported by AAOS consensus opinion (choice B). Studies comparing screening with venous ultrasonography with no screening do not show a significant difference in the rate of pulmonary embolus or hospital readmission for DVT in those patients who underwent routine screening (choice D). Multiple moderate/high-quality studies demonstrate no significant difference between the rates of VTED between neuraxial and general anesthesia (choice C).

Objectives: Did you learn...?

• The consensus opinion of the 2011 AAOS guidelines on preventing VTE?

CASE 7

Dr. Ayesha Abdeen

A 78-year-old female with a history of diabetes mellitus, hypertension, and tertiary syphilis presents with severe knee pain. Knee radiographs reveal extensive bone loss and neuropathic arthropathy. Conservative treatment measures (cortisone injections, activity modification, use of a cane) did not provide long-term relief and the patient seeks definitive management of her pain.

The surgical treatment should involve:

A. Unicompartmental knee arthroplasty
B. Posterior cruciate retaining knee arthroplasty
C. Cemented posterior stabilized knee arthroplasty
D. Long stemmed cemented condylar constrained knee arthroplasty
E. Hinged design knee arthroplasty

Discussion

The correct answer is (D). Neuropathic or Charcot arthropathy in patients with diabetes or neurosyphilis is associated with significant instability due to secondary ligamentous laxity. There can be profound bone loss and deformity in addition to ligamentous imbalance. In those patients, a high failure rate has been observed with primary knee designs, and a revision stemmed constrained condylar design has been recommended. The technical challenges in total knee arthroplasty in the setting of a neuropathic joint can require complex revision-type techniques and implants. A rotating hinge prosthesis can be required in very severe cases of instability if both collateral ligaments have been rendered insufficient. Careful balancing is important for overall outcome.

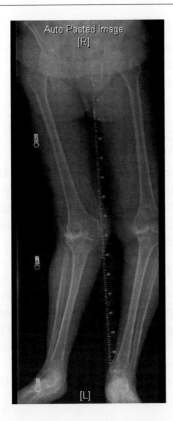

Figure 7–6

A standing hip to ankle 3 foot AP radiograph of the patient's lower extremities is shown in Figure 7–6.

What is the definition of mechanical axis?

A. A line drawn from the center of the pelvis to the center of the ankle

B. A line drawn from the center of the femoral head to the center of the talus

C. The angle subtended by a line drawn through the diaphysis of the femur and diaphysis of the tibia

D. The angle subtended by a line drawn from the ASIS to the center of the knee and a line from the center of the knee to the center of the ankle

Discussion

The correct answer is (B). Mechanical axis is the line drawn from the center of the femoral head to the center of the ankle/talus and should pass through the center of the knee. It can also be measured as an angle formed from a line drawn from the center of the femoral head to the center of the knee and from the center of the knee to the center of the ankle/talus. This should measure 0 degrees. The anatomic axis, on the other hand, is the angle formed by the diaphysis of the femur and tibia that measures approximately 5 to 7 degrees. The reason for

the difference between the anatomic and femoral axes is the presence of femoral offset whereby the center of the femoral head is offset laterally from the diaphysis of the femur. Mechanical axis is important when templating for total joint replacement surgery because postoperative malalignment (particularly varus malpositioning) has been shown to be associated with early component failure due to loosening.

Diabetes mellitus increases surgical risks in patients who undergo total knee replacement surgery. Which of the following is FALSE regarding TKR in diabetic patients?

A. The risk of DVT is higher in patients with DM compared to those without

B. Poorly controlled hyperglycemia may increase the incidence of superficial wound infection following TKR

C. Hemoglobin A1C should be less than 7.0% before any diabetic patient undergoes total knee replacement

D. Diabetes does not affect short-term outcomes as measured by functional outcome scores such as the Oxford Knee Score and Short Form-12

Discussion

The correct answer is (C). Diabetes mellitus is associated with increased perioperative risk including venous thromboembolism and infection. There is thought to be a linear increase in risk of complication following TKR as hemoglobin A1C increases, rather than a surge at a threshold of 7%. It has been shown that a large percentage (41%) of diabetic patients whose surgery was postponed due to poor long-term glycemic control were unable to achieve a goal hemoglobin A1C of 7% or less preoperatively.

Objectives: Did you learn...?

• The definition of mechanical axis?
• The increased risks associated with TKR in the diabetic patient?

CASE 8

Dr. Forrest H. Schwartz

A 63-year-old, Caucasian woman with a past medical history significant for obesity (BMI 41), chronic obstructive pulmonary disease, and hypertension asks you about her risk of a complication following total knee arthroplasty.

Which patient characteristic increases her risk of an adverse event in the perioperative period?

A. Age
B. Female gender
C. Obesity
D. Chronic obstructive pulmonary disease
E. Hypertension

Discussion

The correct answer is (C). Current data demonstrates a statistically significant increase in risk of perioperative complications in arthroplasty patients with a BMI >40, age >80, and diabetes mellitus. Although other medical comorbidities may require close monitoring in the perioperative period, they have not been shown to influence the risk of perioperative complications.

Which of the following factors will increase the likelihood of lower extremity malalignment in this patient following TKR?

A. Obesity
B. Preoperative deformity
C. Female gender
D. A and B

Discussion

The correct answer is (D). Both obesity and preoperative alignment have been identified as factors which correlate with postoperative malalignment. In a study by Estes et al. the effects of gender, side preoperative mechanical alignment, and BMI on alignment were analyzed, and it was found that preoperative mechanical limb alignment and BMI both had a significant effect on postoperative limb alignment following TKR.

Obesity is associated with all of the following TKR EXCEPT:

A. Wound infection
B. Mortality
C. Postoperative malalignment
D. Risk of DVT/PE

Discussion

The correct answer is (B). Obesity has not been proven to be associated with increased mortality or implant failure following total joint replacement surgery. Wallace et al. showed that there was an increased risk of wound infection and DVT/PE observed in obese patients undergoing THR or THR surgery, however an association between obesity and mortality was not observed in patients undergoing total joint replacement surgery.

Objectives: Did you learn...?
- The increase in risk of perioperative complications with obesity?
- Causes of malalignment in TKR?

CASE 9

Dr. Forrest H. Schwartz

A 56-year-old man who is hepatitic C and HIV positive and currently taking HAART presents to your clinic to discuss total hip arthroplasty. He states that he is concerned that being HIV positive will increase his risk of complications after total hip arthroplasty.

You inform him that:

A. HIV-positive status is an independent risk factor for complication after total joint arthroplasty
B. He has a higher risk of prosthetic joint infection
C. He has a higher risk of superficial wound infection requiring irrigation and debridement
D. Patient satisfaction after total hip arthroplasty is lower in patients with HIV

Discussion

The correct answer is (C). Historical studies of arthroplasty in HIV-positive patients showed an increased risk of perioperative complication, but these data tend to come from smaller series that focused on patients with a history of hemophilia or intravenous drug use, which have been shown to play a larger role in complication rates than HIV itself. Recent studies show that there is no difference in the overall rate of perioperative complication in HIV-positive patients undergoing total hip or knee arthroplasty. HIV-positive status does put patients at higher risk for certain complications including acute renal failure and superficial wound infection requiring irrigation and debridement.

What is the most likely source of hip arthropathy in this patient?

A. HAART related AVN of the femoral head
B. Hepatitis C–related AVN of the femoral head
C. CAM impingement
D. Trauma

Discussion

The correct answer is (A). There is a well-established association between long-term antiretroviral use and osteonecrosis of the femoral head in patients with a diagnosis of HIV. The exact mechanism by which these medications cause AVN remains unknown. In cases in which there is a systemic cause of AVN, 50% to 80% can be bilateral therefore an MRI should be performed on the asymptomatic side to rule out precollapse disease. In patients in whom the femoral head has not collapsed, core decompression is recommended. Those that have femoral head collapse are best treated with arthroplasty.

There is a higher likelihood of mechanical failure and infection in this patient due to which of the following reasons?

A. Male gender
B. Tall height
C. HIV infection
D. Hepatitis C infection
E. Antiretroviral use

Discussion

The correct answer is (D). In a study by Pour et al. a group of patients with Hepatitis C who underwent THR were found to have an increased incidence of implant loosening, dislocation, fractures, wound complications, and deep infection. The reason for this is unknown. Patients with hepatitis C were also found to have longer hospital stays and higher rates of reoperation and revision. As mentioned above, contemporary studies regarding patients with HIV who undergo THR have not shown a difference in infection and mechanical failure rates in patients with HIV in comparison to controls. Tall height and male gender have not been linked to mechanical failure or infection following THR.

Objectives: Did you learn...?

- The risks associated with TKR in patients with HIV and hepatitis C?
- Increase in wound complications in the HIV patient?
- The causes of AVN in the HIV-infected patient?

CASE 10

Dr. Ayesha Abdeen and Dr. Valentin Antoci Jr.

A 72-year-old female presents with a 2-year history of progressive knee pain. She has tried braces and anti-inflammatories with limited benefit. Her primary care physician prescribed a course of physical therapy and corticosteroid injections which did not provide pain relief. The patient is now dependent on a cane, has been gaining weight due to difficulty ambulating, and has trouble sleeping. X-rays of the knee show moderate arthritis, and physical examination reveals joint-line tenderness and knee pain that is exacerbated by range of motion of the hip.

The next step in management would involve:

A. Another series of corticosteroid injections
B. Since steroids failed, a series of hyaluronan injections
C. Additional x-rays of the hip
D. Arthroscopy to address the likely meniscus tear
E. Total knee replacement

Discussion

The correct answer is (C). Since the patient complains of knee pain and intra-articular injections did not provide relief, it is possible that her severe pain is referred pain such as from an ipsilateral arthritic hip or radicular pain originating from the spine. Examination of the hip and spine should be performed, and additional radiographs of the hip should be considered in order to rule out referred pain.

Upon further questioning it is revealed that the patient had trauma 30 years ago following a motor vehicle crash whereby she sustained a comminuted patellar fracture and underwent patellectomy. If conservative measures fail to provide pain relief, the recommended surgical treatment of her knee pain is:

A. Unicompartmental knee arthroplasty
B. Posterior cruciate retaining knee arthroplasty
C. Posterior stabilized knee arthroplasty
D. Constrained knee arthroplasty
E. Hinged design knee arthroplasty

Discussion

The correct answer is (C). In the absence of a fully functioning extensor mechanism, including patients with previous patellectomies, the use of a posterior stabilized prosthesis is indicated to prevent anterior tibial instability that would typically be constrained by the presence of the patella and a tighter extensor mechanism. A cruciate retaining device can be performed, however, studies suggest a higher failure rate in those patients.

The patient inquires regarding the possibility of press-fit components for her knee replacement as she has heard that bone cement is toxic. Cementless knee replacements have:

A. Increased infection risk
B. Increased polyethylene wear

C. Increased risk of fracture and notching

D. Increased risk for revision

E. Increased satisfaction and outcomes

Discussion

The correct answer is (D). Cementless knee replacements are associated with increased tibial loosening and associated need for revision. There is no established difference in infection, polyethylene wear, or patient satisfaction.

The patient has seen an advertisement about total knee replacements and has questions about an all-polyethylene tibial component. You tell her that these components result in:

A. Easier customization during the case

B. Increased rates of osteolysis

C. Decreased backside wear

D. Increased range of motion

E. Increased rate of revision

Discussion

The correct answer is (C). All-polyethylene tibial components appear to be superior to metal backed components in terms of wear and revision rates. Modular components are associated with increased backside wear due to micromotion between the insert and the metal base plate. Nevertheless, metal backed components allow for modularity and thus increased customization during the case, while monoblock tibial components require determination of size before cementing.

The patient undergoes primary posterior stabilized TKR. Intraoperatively after performing the tibial and femoral cuts including chamfers and PS box cut, while balancing the knee you notice that the knee is balanced in flexion, but she continues to have a flexion contracture. What is the next most logical step to correct this imbalance?

A. Resect more proximal tibia

B. Resect more distal femur

C. Downsize the femoral component to gain more range of motion

D. Remove posterior osteophytes and release posterior capsule

Discussion

The correct answer is (D). When balancing a primary total knee replacement with a gap technique, it is important to create a rectangular space that is symmetric

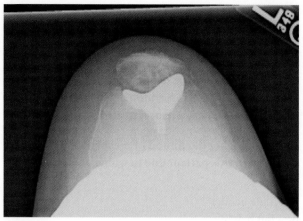

Figure 7–7

from medial to lateral and in flexion and extension. If there is sufficient range of motion in flexion, but there remains a "flexion contracture", this means that the knee cannot fully extend and the "extension" gap is tight while the flexion gap is appropriate. This means that the space between the femur is smaller when the knee is in 0 degrees of flexion in comparison to when the knee is at 90 degrees of flexion (see Fig. 7–7). In order to increase the extension gap, one must either remove posterior osteophytes and release posterior capsule (the osteophytes tent the capsule and create a tighter extension gap), recess the PCL in a PCL retaining knee, or remove more distal femoral bone. In this patient who has a PCL sacrificing knee, it is not an option to recess the PCL. Resecting more distal femoral bone is an option to correct the imbalance but requires applying the cutting jig again and recutting the chamfers if these have already been cut. The most simple next step at this stage of the total knee replacement would be to carefully remove the posterior femoral osteophytes and release the posterior capsule from the distal femur using electrocautery.

The patient subsequently healed uneventfully following posterior stabilized primary total knee replacement. She returns to clinic 8 months following her surgery with anterior knee pain associated with a clunking sensation when she gets up from a seated position, ascends stairs, or straightens her knee. What is likely the source of this problem?

A. Component malrotation

B. Excessively thick polyethylene insert

C. Early polyethylene wear

D. Fracture of the post on the polyethylene insert

E. Patella clunk syndrome

Discussion

The correct answer is (E). Due to the design of the posterior stabilized knee replacement with a large box cut in the femoral component, patella clunk syndrome can sometimes be observed wherein a nodule along the quadriceps surface catches over the trochlear notch when the knee is moving from an extended position to 30–45 degrees of flexion. Symptoms can be reproduced with resisted extension.

The recommended treatment for this patient is:

A. Observation
B. Manipulation under anesthesia
C. Arthroscopic synovectomy
D. Revision to a CR knee
E. Revision to stemmed constrained components

Discussion

The correct answer is (C). As discussed above, patella clunk is thought to be due to soft tissue constrained onto the femoral component. Arthroscopic synovectomy, excision of the scar tissue, and synovial fold above the patella result in improvement of symptoms. Further revision is not indicated at this time in the setting of well-aligned components.

When evaluating a painful total knee replacement, if there is concern for malrotation of the components, the radiographic modality of choice is:

A. Standing 3-ft x-rays
B. Flexion x-ray of the knee
C. Skyline view of the knee
D. CT imaging
E. MRI imaging

Discussion

The correct answer is (D). Although, axial radiographs may be used to detect axial rotation of the femoral component, CT is most commonly used for the purpose of measuring component rotation. MRI is also acceptable but would not typically be the first line in an otherwise normal patient.

Helpful Tip:

Cruciate retaining and posterior stabilized knee designs are competing trends with no significant difference in long-term outcome, range of motion, and stability in the hands of a good technician. Nevertheless, comfort with the design and understanding of degree of constraint and associated modularity is imperative in a successful total knee arthroplasty.

Objectives: Did you learn...?

• Recognize various prosthesis designs and their indications?
• Understand the spectrum of constraint in TKR?
• Understand how to balance a primary TKR?

CASE 11

Dr. Ayesha Abdeen

A 48-year-old female patient presents with anterior left knee pain. She has had a history of recurrent patellofemoral dislocations as an adolescent that was treated with multiple soft tissue procedures as well as tubercle osteotomy in the past. She underwent patellofemoral arthroplasty 2 years ago (Fig. 7–8) and continues to have anterior knee pain.

Which of the following is FALSE regarding patellofemoral arthroplasty?

A. The procedure is best performed in patients with anterior knee pain who have rheumatoid arthritis
B. PF arthroplasty should be avoided in patients with patellar maltracking or malalignment problems

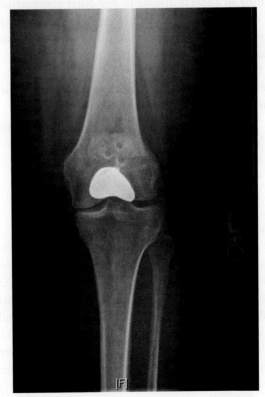

Figure 7–8

unless these problems are corrected preoperatively

C. External rotation of the trochlear component such that it is parallel to the epicondylar axis will improve patellar tracking

D. In the setting of medial or lateral joint-line pain, PF arthroplasty should be avoided

Discussion

The correct answer is (A). Inflammatory arthropathy, which typically affects the joint globally in all three compartments, is a contraindication to unicompartmental knee replacement. Patellofemoral arthroplasty will fail in the setting of patellar maltracking and therefore should be avoided or the malalignment/malrotation corrected prior to arthroplasty. Newer-generation "onlay" designs of PF arthroplasty have addressed some of the design concerns of the "inlay" implants whereby the trochlear component can be externally rotated to optimize patellar tracking and eliminate some of the concerns of patellar subluxation that occurred with first-generation PF arthroplasty designs. Patellofemoral arthroplasty should not be performed in the setting of medial and lateral disease in the knee as well as flexion contractions. It is possible to combine a medial or lateral UKA or autologous osteochondral grafting to address disease in one other compartment, but in general, the standard of care remains to be total knee arthroplasty if more than one compartment is affected.

The primary reason for failure and revision of first-generation patellofemoral replacement is:

A. Progression of disease in the medial and lateral compartments

B. Infection

C. Osteolysis/loosening

D. Patellofemoral catching and instability

Discussion

The correct answer is (D). The initial "inlay" style designs resulted in catching/subluxation of the patella and problems with patellar tracking. Contemporary improvements in trochlear component design with inlay implants implanted parallel to the epicondylar axis, improved radius of curvature, and tracking angles of the components have improved outcomes with respect to patellofemoral tracking. Long-term results of these contemporary designs have not yet been defined.

Which of the following techniques should be AVOIDED when performing patellofemoral arthroplasty?

A. Remove marginal osteophytes in the intercondylar notch

B. Restoration of anatomic patellar thickness

C. Lateralization of patellar component

D. External rotation of the trochlear/femoral component to be perpendicular to the AP axis of the femur

Discussion

The correct answer is (C). As in total knee replacement, the patellar component should be medialized to prevent lateral subluxation of the patella in PF arthroplasty. Other principles of patellar resurfacing should be adhered to including: attention to restoring the patient's own patellar thickness and external rotation of the femoral component to optimize patellofemoral tracking and to limit the potential for lateral catching and subluxation of the patella. Removal of osteophytes in the intercondylar notch will also improve tracking.

Objectives: Did you learn...?

- The indications for patellofemoral arthroplasty?
- The causes for revision of patellofemoral arthroplasty?

CASE 12

Dr. Ayesha Abdeen

A 59-year-old male with BMI 32 presents with severe medial knee pain corresponding to focal osteoarthritis of the medial compartment. He has undergone physical therapy, cortisone injections, and takes nonsteroidal anti-inflammatory medications with incomplete relief of his pain.

Which of the following is FALSE with respect to medial unicompartmental knee replacement in this patient?

A. UKA can be performed if he has a passively correctible varus deformity less than 10 degrees

B. UKA should be avoided if he has a fixed flexion contracture more than 5 degrees

C. An incompetent ACL is an absolute contraindication to UKA

D. Recent reports suggest UKA can be performed in the setting of mild obesity

Discussion

The correct answer is (C). Although historically an intact ACL has been included in the list of requisites for UKA, the absence of an ACL is not an absolute

CHAPTER 7 RECONSTRUCTION **431**

contraindication. UKA can be performed successfully in the ACL deficient knee as long there is not excessive instability of the knee. Excessive tibial slope should be avoided in the ACL deficient knee that undergoes UKA.

Which of the following concerning mobile-bearing unicompartmental knee replacement is TRUE?

A. There is a similar rate of dislocation of the bearing surface in comparison to fixed-bearing devices
B. Mobile-bearing UKA is recommended for both medial and lateral UKA procedures
C. Soft tissue balancing is critical in order to reduce the rate of spinout of the mobile-bearing insert
D. The results of mobile-bearing devices far exceed that of fixed bearing

Discussion

The correct answer is (C). One of the primary mechanisms of failure of a mobile-bearing UKA is spinout of the polyethylene insert. Meticulous soft tissue balancing is necessary to reduce the risk of this complication. Currently in the United States, mobile-bearing UKA is recommended for use only in the medial compartment. Data from the United Kingdom has shown a 10% rate of dislocation of the mobile-bearing insert when used in the lateral compartment.

Helpful Tip:

To accurately balance the mobile-bearing unicompartmental knee replacement, a leg holder that allows the leg to hang freely should be used to allow gravity to distract the knee in flexion so that the gap balancing can be appropriately assessed in order to select the appropriate bearing thickness.

Objectives: Did you learn...?

• The indications for unicompartmental knee replacement?
• The importance of soft tissue balancing and component position for the success of PF and unicompartmental knee replacements?

CASE 13

Dr. Ayesha Abdeen

A 65-year-old female presents with a painful, left total knee replacement that was performed 7 years ago. The pain began WITHOUT trauma several months ago and is progressively worsening. She has started to use a walker for ambulation and is becoming increasingly reliant on

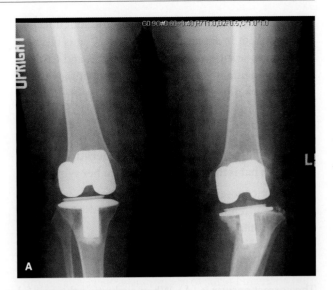

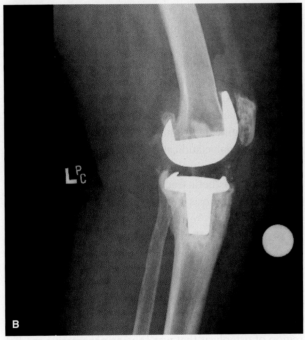

Figure 7–9 **A–B**

it. Examination shows a profound varus deformity with varus thrust. Radiographs are shown in Figure 7–9A and B.

What is the next step in evaluation of this patient?

A. ESR, CRP
B. Indium-labeled leukocyte scan
C. CT scan
D. Joint aspiration

Discussion

The correct answer is (A). In any painful knee replacement with loosening and mechanical failure, a diagnosis of infection should be ruled out. Prosthetic joint infection can be present in absence of overt clinical signs of infection such as redness, drainage, or fever. ESR and CRP are the most commonly used laboratory tests in the evaluation of the painful TKA. ESR less than 30 mm/h and CRP less than 10 mg/dL are consistent with a low likelihood of infection.

Serum inflammatory markers are negative in this patient. What is the most likely cause of her symptoms?

A. Aseptic loosening
B. Patellar tendinitis
C. Arthrofibrosis
D. Patellar clunk

Discussion

The correct answer is (A). When evaluating the painful total knee replacement, it is helpful to divide the etiology of the pain into either intra-articular/intrinsic or extra-articular/extrinsic knee pain. Intra-articular problems include aseptic loosening, malalignment, polyethylene wear, osteolysis, implant failure/breakage, arthrofibrosis, patellar clunk, and extensor mechanism dysfunction. Extra-articular problems include referred pain from the hip or spine, neuroma, complex regional pain syndrome, vascular claudication, soft tissue inflammation (pes anserine bursitis, patellar or quadriceps tendonitis), or periprosthetic fracture. It is always imperative to establish a diagnosis before embarking upon revision surgery as simply "re-doing" surgery without a diagnosis is not likely to lead to improvement of symptoms. This patient's x-rays demonstrate a periprosthetic fracture with loosening of the tibial component, medial bone loss, and collapse of the proximal medial tibia. This occurred without trauma and was progressive in nature, and thus the fracture likely occurred through a region of osteolysis that was causing progressive medial tibial collapse with concomitant aseptic loosening.

What other tests will be helpful in preoperative planning for this patient?

A. MRI
B. Bone scan
C. Metal allergy testing
D. 3-ft standing film

Discussion

The correct answer is (D). Since the patient has an abnormality of alignment, it is important to obtain a 3-foot standing view to measure mechanical and anatomic axis

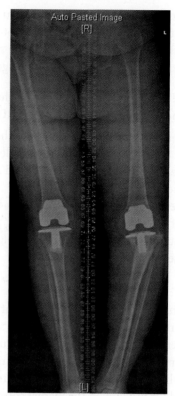

Figure 7–10

(Fig. 7–10). MRI is not helpful in the setting of most revision TKR. Bone scan is not indicated as the implants are clearly loose on plain films. Metal allergy testing is not likely to be the cause of the implant failure given that radiographs are consistent with aseptic loosening.

Which of the following is NOT considered a good reconstructive option to address the bone loss and loss of fixation in this case?

A. Fixation with long stems in the tibia and femur
B. Porous metal metaphyseal cones
C. Structural allograft
D. Metal augments
E. Morselized cancellous allograft

Discussion

The correct answer is (E). The x-rays demonstrate bone loss with an uncontained tibial defect and loosening of the components. Revision should include stemmed implants to improve fixation and a method to reconstruct the uncontained defect with either porous metal metaphyseal cones (such as Trabecular Metal™ cones), metal augments, or structural allograft. Cancellous graft can only be used in contained defects where there is

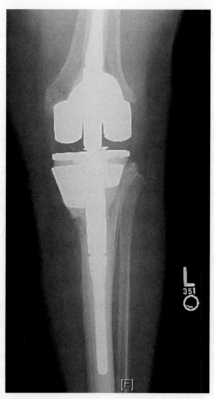

Figure 7–11

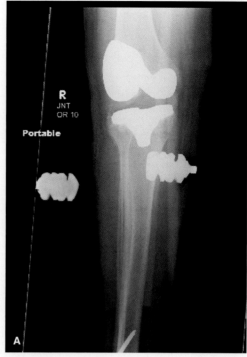

Figure 7–12 **A**

sufficient cortical bone to contain the defect. In this patient, porous metal cones were used to reconstruct the metaphyseal defect. Cemented stems were used for fixation, and a constrained implant was needed because of collateral ligament insufficiency (Fig. 7–11).

Objectives: Did you learn...?

- The evaluation for a painful knee in a patient with history of TKR?
- Causes for revision TKR?

CASE 14

Dr. Ayesha Abdeen

A 69-year-old woman underwent uncomplicated total knee replacement. She was being discharged from the rehabilitation center 3 weeks postoperatively. Her daughter, who was driving the car, sustained a seizure, and the patient sustained multiple injuries due to a motor vehicle crash as their car struck a light pole. She has an open wound and a painful, deformed right knee. She was seen at an outside hospital. Her leg wound was irrigated and debrided, and an external fixator was placed on her leg.

What is the best treatment strategy for this patient? A radiograph is shown in Figure 7–12A.

A. Closed treatment of the fracture with functional bracing
B. Irrigation and debridement of the open wound and revision TKR with open reduction, internal fixation of the fracture
C. Open reduction internal fixation of the fracture with retention of the components
D. Resection of the proximal tibia and reconstruction with a tumor prosthesis

Discussion

The correct answer is (B), (see Figure 7–12B). This periprosthetic fracture of the tibia with a loose tibial component requires revision because the tibial component is no longer well-fixed. The component cannot be retained with ORIF because it is unstable/loose. In the setting of a fracture around a well-fixed prosthesis, ORIF would be the treatment of choice but that does not pertain to this case since the implant is loose radiographically. Closed treatment is not an option for a displaced periprosthetic fracture with a loose component. Resection of the proximal tibia is not indicated as the fracture can be fixed and the tibial component revised.

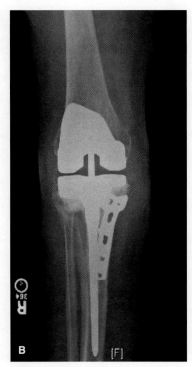

Figure 7–12 **B**

The patient presents with a draining wound and erythema 2 weeks after revision and ORIF of the tibial fracture. ESR and CRP are elevated as would be expected in the postoperative period. Aspiration reveals WBC 11,000. What is the best treatment option?

A. Irrigation and debridement and polyethylene liner exchange

B. One-stage exchange arthroplasty

C. Oral antibiotics

D. Intravenous antibiotics

Discussion

The correct answer is (A). The patient has an early prosthetic joint infection. She had an open fracture which increased the risk of prosthetic joint infection. Given that the infection is acute, a strategy of component retention is appropriate, however she should have operative irrigation and debridement and exchange of the polyethylene liner.

Helpful Tip:

Revision TKR requires careful resection of implants so as not to lose bone or cause fracture. Implants can be removed with a variety of techniques including stacked osteotomes, gigli saw, reciprocating saw, and extraction devices with slap hammer attachments. Soft tissues must be carefully respected, and revision

exposure techniques such as quadriceps snip, V-Y turndown, or tibial tubercle osteotomies may need to be performed in order to gain adequate exposure and reduce the risk of further soft tissue or bony damage.

Objectives: Did you learn...?

• The differential diagnosis for a painful total knee replacement?

• How to diagnose the etiology of the failed TKR?

• Revision techniques and treatment strategies for mechanical failure and periprosthetic fracture?

CASE 15

Dr. Forrest H. Schwartz

A 73-year-old man with a history of hypertension and hyperlipidemia presents to your office with right hip pain that he feels is a functional impairment and with radiographs demonstrating severe osteoarthritis of the right hip. During your discussion about total hip replacement, he states that he would like you to perform his surgery via an anterior approach because he has heard that it leads to a lower dislocation rate.

All of the following technical factors reduce the risk of dislocation in total hip arthroplasty except for:

A. Placing the acetabular component in 40 to 50 degrees of abduction

B. Use of a larger head size for a given neck diameter

C. Use of an implant with a skirted head

D. Use of an implant with a trapezoidal neck

E. Increasing the offset of the femoral component

Discussion

The correct answer is (C). The head-to-neck ratio of an implant plays a significant role in the risk of dislocation. The larger the head-to-neck ratio is for a given femoral component, the lower the risk for dislocation secondary to impingement. Increasing the size of the head for a given neck diameter (B) increases the head-to-neck ratio, whereas use of a skirted head (C) decreases the head-to-neck ratio. Correct component positioning (A) is fundamental to total hip arthroplasty and has been repeatedly demonstrated to play a crucial role in minimizing the risk of dislocation. Increasing the offset of the femoral component (E) lowers the risk of dislocation both by increasing the tension on the abductors and by decreasing the risk of impingement.

Which intervals are utilized to access the hip joint via an anterior approach?

A. Between sartorius and tensor fascia lata superficially/rectus femorus and gluteus medius deep
B. Between sartorius and rectus femorus superficially/tensor fascia lata and gluteus medius deep
C. Between gracilis and tensor fascia lata superficially/rectus femorus and gluteus medius deep
D. Between sartorius and tensor fascia lata superficially/rectus femorus and gluteus maximus deep
E. Between gluteus maximus and tensor fascia lata superficially/gluteus medius and gluteus minimus deep

Discussion

The correct answer is (A). The anterior (Smith–Peterson) approach to the hip utilizes the inter-nervous plane between sartorius (femoral nerve) and tensor fascia lata (superior gluteal nerve) superficially and rectus femorus (femoral nerve) and gluteus medius (superficial gluteal nerve) deep. The anterior approach to the hip is the only approach to the hip to utilize a true inter-nervous plane.

Which of the following choices correctly pairs the level of safety and the structures at risk with regard to acetabular screw placement during total hip arthroplasty?

A. Anterosuperior—safe—external iliac vessels
B. Anterosuperior—dangerous—obturator neurovascular bundle
C. Posterosuperior—safe—sciatic nerve and superior gluteal neurovascular bundle
D. Posterosuperior—safe—sciatic nerve and internal iliac vessels
E. Posteroinferior—safe—obturator neurovascular bundle

Discussion

The correct answer is (C). The acetabulum can be divided into quadrants by drawing a line from the anterior superior iliac spine through the center of the acetabulum and drawing a second line through the center of the acetabulum that runs perpendicular to the first. Radiographic and cadaveric studies have delineated the safety of, as well as the primary structures at risk of injury with, screw placement in each quadrant.

Quadrant	Level of Safety	Structures at Risk
Posterosuperior quadrant Superior gluteal neurovascular bundle	Safest	Sciatic nerve
Posteroinferior quadrant Inferior gluteal neurovascular bundle	Safe	Sciatic nerve
Anterosuperior quadrant	Dangerous	External iliac artery and vein
Anteroinferior quadrant	Dangerous	Obturator neurovascular bundle

After undergoing total hip arthroplasty via a posterior approach, the patient would be at the greatest risk of dislocation if he were to perform which of the following activities?

A. Putting on shoes and socks
B. Taking a seat on a low sofa
C. Sleeping on his back
D. Descending stairs
E. Walking at a brisk pace

Discussion

The correct answer is (B). Posterior hip precautions are to avoid flexion at the hip beyond 90 degrees, internal rotation at the hip past neutral, and adduction at the hip past neutral. Therefore, the patient would be at the highest risk of dislocation if he were to take a seat on a low sofa, resulting in hip flexion beyond 90 degrees. The other activities listed do not place the hip joint outside the range of motion dictated by posterior precautions.

Objectives: Did you learn...?

- The causes of hip dislocation after THR?
- Internervous plane of the anterior approach to the hip?
- Specifics of posterior hip precautions?

CASE 16

Dr. Ayesha Abdeen

A 64-year-old male with ankylosing spondylitis and history of prostate cancer undergoes THR for osteoarthritis

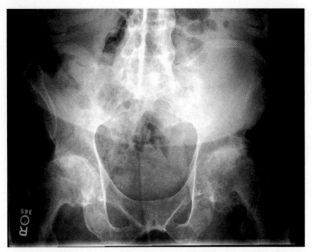

Figure 7–13

following total joint replacement. It has been shown to occur in patients that have had thrombolysis and full dose therapeutic anticoagulation for VTE following total hip arthroplasty. Although rare, it is important that this complication is recognized without delay so that emergent decompression can be performed to improve potential return of nerve function.

Six months following THR the patient's nerve function has returned and he presents with lateral-sided hip pain. Figure 7–14 reveals current films. What is the diagnosis?

A. Dermatomyositis
B. Soft tissue sarcoma
C. Heterotopic ossification
D. Metastatic disease

(Fig. 7–13). He has a history of atrial fibrillation and is on Coumadin. His immediate postoperative course is uneventful, and he is discharged from hospital on postoperative day 3. He resumed anticoagulation the evening after his surgery and has been on a Coumadin sliding scale. Ten days following surgery he returns with flank pain, dizziness, hypotension, and a foot drop that has been present for 24 hours. His INR is 4.3 and hematocrit is 20.

What is the LEAST likely cause of his symptoms?

A. Sciatic nerve injury during posterior approach
B. Retroperitoneal hematoma
C. Hip joint hematoma
D. Anemia

Discussion

The correct answer is (A). Given that the sciatic nerve palsy was not present immediately postoperatively but presented more than 1 week following surgery suggests that direct nerve injury at the time of surgery is unlikely. This patient has a supratherapeutic INR and likely has a hip hematoma that is causing a mass effect and irritation of the sciatic nerve. He has a concomitant retroperitoneal hematoma that can account for his flank pain.

What is the best course of action in this patient?

A. Reverse INR with FFP
B. Urgent evacuation of the hip hematoma
C. Observation of the retroperitoneal hematoma
D. All of the above

Discussion

The correct answer is (D). Sciatic nerve palsy as a result of an expanding hematoma is a rare complication

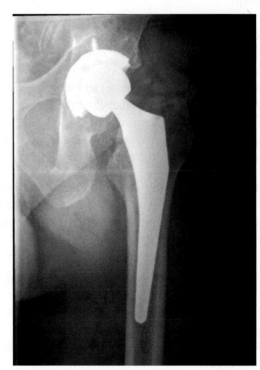

Figure 7–14

Discussion

The correct answer is (C). This x-ray reveals nonbridging heterotopic ossification.

What conditions are NOT associated with the formation of heterotopic ossification?

A. Ankylosing spondylitis
B. Diffuse idiopathic hyperostosis
C. Traumatic brain injury
D. Paget's disease of bone
E. Chronic Coumadin use

Discussion

The correct answer is (E). Heterotopic ossification occurs rarely following total hip replacement. The pathophysiology involves an unknown trigger that causes mesenchymal cells to differentiate into osteoprogenitor cells. Patients at risk of developing HO following THR include those with hypertrophic osteoarthritis, diffuse idiopathic hypertrophy, ankylosing spondylitis, and prior HO formation of the hip following THR. This condition is more common in men than in women following THR. Other causes of HO that forms in the body include Paget's disease and traumatic brain injury.

Given the patient has ankylosing spondylitis, what would have been an appropriate modality of prophylaxis for HO in this patient?

A. Indomethacin

B. External beam radiation

C. Bisphosphonates

D. Calcitonin

Discussion

The correct answer is (B). NSAIDs such as indomethacin and external beam radiation are the current prophylactic methods of preventing HO formation in patients that have high risk for developing HO following THR. However, this patient is chronically anticoagulated and therefore indomethacin would be contraindicated. The best modality in this patient would be external beam radiation. Ethylhydroxydiphosphonate is another agent that has been used and resulted in a delay of mineralization of osteoid, but clinical trials have shown that HO formation was not decreased, and the delay in mineralization did not significantly improve the range of motion of involved hips.

Objectives: Did you learn...?

• The causes of sciatic nerve palsy after THR?

• Diagnosis of hip joint hematoma?

• Treatment of hip joint hematoma?

• The risk factors for heterotopic ossification after THR?

CASE 17

Dr. Valentin Antoci Jr.

A 79-year-old female with a history of a left total hip replacement performed 10 years ago presents with worsening hip pain. The pain began 1 year ago when she noted progressive activity-related groin pain. She

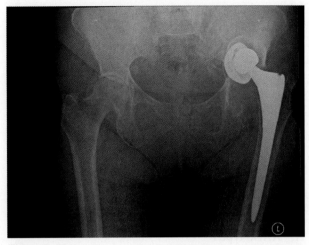

Figure 7–15

denies any trauma. The patient denies fever. She does not have night pain. A radiograph is shown in Fig 7–15 above. The patient has started using a walker.

What should be the next step in the evaluation of this patient?

A. Bone scan

B. Serum, ESR, and CRP

C. Metal ion testing including chromium levels

D. Physical therapy for abductor strengthening

E. Preoperative anesthesia evaluation before revision surgery

Discussion

The correct answer is (B). Despite the absence of fever and nocturnal pain, which if present would be associated with infection, infection should still be ruled out. A screening ESR and CRP helps determine the need for further aspiration.

The original Charnley hip replacements involved a cemented femoral component and cemented all-polyethylene acetabular cup with a 22-mm head. Recent 30-year follow-up data on the Charnley total hip replacement revealed that the leading reason for revision was:

A. Acetabular loosening

B. Femoral stem loosening

C. Both component loosening

D. Infection

Discussion

The correct answer is (A). Wroblewski et al. (2009) have reviewed 110 patients who underwent THR with the original Charnley prosthesis and have more than 30 years of follow-up; 11.8% (13 patients) required revision. The primary reason for revision in this series was acetabular component loosening. Both component loosening, infection, and loose stem followed in terms of prevalence for revision.

Based on the images above, the patient has superior acetabular bone loss with a combination of segmental and cavitary bone loss. According to the system designed by the American Academy of Orthopaedic Surgeon, this pattern of acetabular bone loss would be classified as:

A. AAOS type I
B. AAOS type II
C. AAOS type III
D. AAOS type IV
E. AAOS type V

Discussion

The correct answer is (C). The two most commonly used classification systems for the evaluation of acetabular bone loss following THR include the AAOS classification and the Paprosky classification for bone loss around the acetabulum. The classification systems are useful in providing some insight in further reconstruction options.

AAOS classification:

 I: Segmental bone loss involving part of the acetabular rim or medial wall
 II: Cavitary bone loss with preservation of good rim fit but volumetric loss
 III: Combination of segmental and cavitary bone loss
 IV: Pelvic discontinuity with separation between superior and inferior acetabulum
 V: Arthrodesis

Paprosky classification:

 I: Minimum deformity, intact rim
 II: A. Superior lysis but intact rim. B. Absent superior rim with superior migration. C. Medial wall destruction and migration
 III: A. Bone loss from 10 to 2 PM with superolateral migration. B. Bone loss from 9 to 5 PM with superomedial migration

This patient describes groin pain typically associated with acetabular component. In the case of a patient with extensive thigh pain and an x-ray showing metadiaphyseal bone loss with a minimum of 4 cm of intact cortical bone, this femoral lesion would be classified as:

A. Paprosky type I
B. Paprosky type II
C. Paprosky type IIIA
D. Paprosky type IIIB
E. Paprosky type IV

Discussion

The correct answer is (C). Similar to the AAOS classification for acetabular bone loss, the Paprosky classification allows for estimation of bone loss as well as reconstruction options available.

AAOS classification:

 I: Segmental—loss of cortical bone
 II: Cavitary—loss of endosteal bone with cortex intact
 III: Combination of segmental and cavitary bone loss
 IV: Malalignment due to previous trauma or disease
 V: Obliteration of canal due to trauma, fixation devices, or bone hypertrophy
 VI: Fracture or nonunion

Paprosky classification:

 I: Minimal metaphyseal bone loss
 II: Extensive metaphyseal bone loss with intact diaphysis
 IIIA: Extensive metadiaphyseal bone loss with a minimum of 4-cm diaphyseal bone
 IIIB: Extensive metadiaphyseal bone loss with more than 4-cm diaphyseal bone loss
 IV: Nonsupportive diaphysis

Surgical preparation involves evaluation of the clinical scenario and interpretation of all available results. In complex hip reconstruction such as this, additional studies may help with preoperative planning and preparation. If concerned, additional helpful imaging may involve:

A. Bone scan
B. MRI hip
C. CT of pelvis
D. Judet views
E. Arthrogram

Discussion

The correct answer is (C). Bone loss is often underestimated on typical x-rays. A CT allows for further understanding of the involved anatomy and appropriate preparation including the availability of augments, cages, jumbo cups, and any other reconstruction equipment necessary.

The reconstruction of the acetabulum involves an evaluation of the rim fit and the appropriate material

to be used for reconstruction. The use of structural bone allograft has been associated with:

A. High failure rate with component migration
B. Low failure rate with bone ingrowth
C. Decrease in the use of cages for pelvic discontinuity
D. Use in cups where rim is competent with good press-fit
E. Increased viral transmission

Discussion

The correct answer is (A). Until the recent introduction of trabecular metal augments and other reconstruction methods, structural allograft had been used extensively for acetabular reconstruction. When a good rim fit is obtained with the acetabular component, morselized bone graft and reamings can be used to pack any cavitary lesions behind the cup. Large structural/cortical allograft in the pelvis has been associated with most failures with subsequent resorption and cup migration.

The reconstruction options in this patient based on original x-rays involves:

A. Both component revision
B. Acetabular revision with allograft
C. Acetabular revision with augments
D. Liner exchange and retroacetabular bone grafting
E. Continue observation with repeat x-rays in 6 months

Discussion

The correct answer is (C). This patient requires acetabular revision at minimum. The femoral component appears in slight varus however no signs of osteolysis or component migration are seen.

On the acetabular side, the patient shows both segmental and cavitary losses but no suggestion of pelvic discontinuity. Further imaging may be helpful. In cases where the cup is in good position with signs of polyethylene wear and retroacetabular lysis, liner exchange and bone grafting through the screw wholes has been documented with good results. In this case, reconstruction with a jumbo cup, with or without augments to provide superior support, should reestablish normal cup position and geometry.

In cases of a Paprosky IIIA femur as discussed earlier, the viable reconstruction would involve:

A. A tapered stem with proximal ingrowth surface
B. A porous coated diaphyseal engaging implant
C. Extended trochanteric osteotomy with cemented long stem implant
D. Calcar replacing tapered stem
E. Megaprosthesis

Discussion

The correct answer is (B). A porous-coated diaphyseal engaging femoral stem is associated with over 95% survivorship at 10 years. Calcar replacing stems and megaprosthesis are each viable options in patients with calcar loss or loss of diaphyseal bone respectively, but are not the best option in the described defect.

Helpful Tip:

The initial evaluation of a painful total hip replacement should focus on all aspects of pain around the hip including infection and referred pain due to spinal pathology. The duration of symptoms may help delineate between progressive failure of the THA versus infection or new fracture. Components should be evaluated for position as well as radiographic signs of lucency. A determination of stability should be made based on extent of lysis and migration.

Once the decision for revision has been made, a clear plan should be outlined regarding the methods of reconstruction as well as alternatives in case more extensive pathology is noted. AAOS or Paprosky classifications help categorize the pathology and define a plan of action. The surgeon should be prepared to revise both components if intraoperative findings including component position require it.

Objectives: Did you learn...?

- Evaluate a painful total hip replacement and consider a differential?
- Identify lysis around components and classify the degree of bone loss?
- Produce a viable management approach for reconstruction including an understanding of structural bone graft, augments, cages, and use of jumbo cups?

CASE 18

Dr. Ayesha Abdeen

An 83-year-old female with a history of THR performed 14 years ago presents after an acute fall. She has a 2 year history of increasing thigh pain that initially began atraumatically. Figure 7–16 reveals a hip radiograph taken 1 month prior to the fall when she returned to her orthopaedic surgeon complaining of thigh pain. She has been unable to ambulate since the fall and presents to the emergency department for evaluation with new radiographs as seen in Figure 7–17.

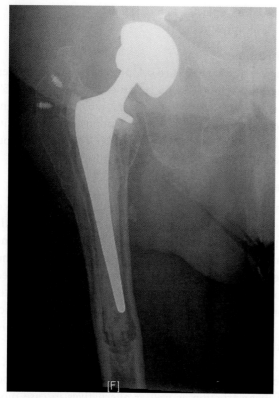

Figure 7–16

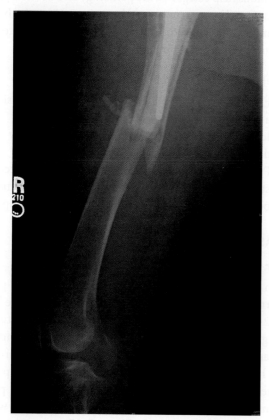

Figure 7–17

How is this fracture classified?

A. Vancouver A
B. Vancouver B1
C. Vancouver B2
D. Vancouver B3
E. Vancouver C

Discussion

The correct answer is (C). Periprosthetic femoral fractures around a total hip replacement are classified based upon location and whether or not the femoral stem is loose. According to the Vancouver classification, type A fractures involve the greater or lesser trochanters and type B involve the region of the femoral stem or immediately below the tip of the stem. Subtypes of B include B1 (implant stable), B2 (implant unstable with good bone stock), and B3 (implant unstable with poor bone stock). Type C fractures are below the stem and cement mantle. In this patient, the fracture is just distal to the tip of the stem and the implant is loose, therefore it is a Vancouver B2 fracture.

What is the recommended treatment for this fracture?

A. Open reduction internal fixation with a proximal femoral trochanteric plate
B. Minimally invasive reduction and internal fixation with a LISS plate
C. Revision of the femoral stem and strut allograft
D. Nonoperative treatment
E. Revision of both acetabular and femoral components

Discussion

The correct answer is (C). The patient has a stem that is loose clinically and radiographically. Now that she has sustained a fracture, the recommended treatment is revision to a diaphyseal engaging stem that bypasses the fracture. This should be augmented with either a cable-plate construct or a strut allograft to obtain additional rotational stability (Fig. 7–18). Open reduction internal fixation can be performed only in the setting of a well-fixed implant. In this situation, the implant will be likely to subside if open reduction internal fixation is performed with retention of the loose femoral stem. Open reduction internal fixation is the treatment of choice in a Vancouver B1 fracture in which the stem is stable or in a type C when the fracture is distal and remote from the stem. Type B3 fractures in which the metadiaphyseal bone is insufficient, require the use of structural allograft or tumor-type endoprosthesis.

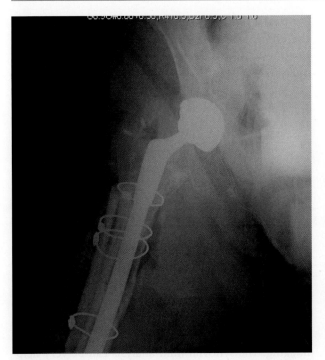

Figure 7–18

Objectives: Did you learn...?

• The classification and treatment of periprosthetic fractures?

CASE 19

Dr. Ayesha Abdeen

A 64-year-old patient with rheumatoid arthritis and seizure disorder presents to you for evaluation of a painful, dislocating LEFT total hip replacement. She reports that 3 days after her initial surgery performed 6 months prior, she fell due to a seizure and sustained a fracture dislocation of the hip. Her initial surgeon opted to treat this with closed reduction and observation for a greater trochanteric fracture. You were in the process of obtaining further operative reports and investigations while the patient was an outpatient. However, the patient had another fall and presented to the emergency department with inability to ambulate due to RIGHT hip pain. She underwent RIGHT total hip replacement 8 years prior and the hip was asymptomatic until the injury. Figure 7–19A reveals her pelvic x-ray at her first visit with you for evaluation of the left hip. Figure 7–19B is a pelvic x-ray performed in the ED after she fell onto the right hip.

What is the next best step in the course of this patients' treatment?

A. DEXA bone density test
B. MRI
C. Judet views
D. Bone scan

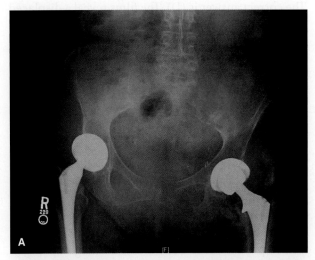

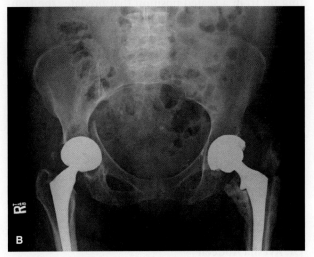

Figure 7–19 **A–B**

Discussion

The correct answer is (C). The patient has sustained a periprosthetic acetabular fracture. Judet views should be performed in order to further evaluate the fracture pattern.

What is the best treatment approach for this fracture?

A. Closed reduction and functional bracing
B. Open reduction and internal fixation with retention of the current components
C. Open reduction and internal fixation and revision of the femoral component only

D. Open reduction and internal fixation and revision of the acetabular component only

E. Open reduction and internal fixation and revision of both components

Discussion

The correct answer is (D). The films reveal a displaced periprosthetic acetabular fracture in which the acetabular component is unstable/loose. The fracture pattern is an anterior column fracture with a posterior hemitransverse fracture. This required removal of the loose acetabular component, anterior and posterior plate fixation, and revision of the acetabular component.

Helpful Tip:

Situations which are radiographically unclear whether an implant is loose in the setting of periprosthetic fracture, history taking can be very informative. In periprosthetic fractures of the femur, a history of "start-up" pain which occurred in the thigh upon getting up from a seated position that predates the traumatic event is suggestive of femoral loosening. In acute periprosthetic acetabular fractures, a history of prior groin or buttock pain can be suggestive of pre-existing acetabular cup loosening that was present at the time of the fall.

Objectives: Did you learn...?

• Identify and classify periprosthetic hip fractures?
• Recognize the appropriate treatment strategies for periprosthetic fractures based upon fracture pattern and stability of the components?

CASE 20

Dr. Ayesha Abdeen

A 72-year-old female with a history of diabetes mellitus underwent uncomplicated total knee replacement. She developed wound drainage 3 months postoperatively which was treated by her original surgeon with irrigation and debridement and liner exchange followed by intravenous antibiotics. Intraoperative cultures revealed MRSA. Her original surgeon eventually moved out of the country. She presents to you with recurrent drainage and erythema and distal wound dehiscence.

The patient had difficulty finding a new orthopaedic surgeon following the departure of her initial surgeon. Upon presentation in your clinic, the patient has had ongoing drainage and wound dehiscence for

the past 2 months. You perform a knee aspiration in the office. What are the diagnostic criteria for deep prosthetic joint infection based upon synovial fluid analysis?

A. 100,000 WBC, 80% neutrophils
B. 1,700 WBC, 65% neutrophils
C. 2,500 WBC, 75% neutrophils
D. 22,000 WBC, 60% neutrophils

Discussion

The correct answer is (B). In the setting of a chronically draining sinus, the diagnosis of prosthetic joint infection (PJI) is clear in this patient. However, in the absence of a draining wound the diagnosis of deep prosthetic joint infection can be difficult to make in many situations. When infection is not clinically obvious, the diagnosis is made based on a collaboration of data to include serum inflammatory markers and synovial fluid analysis as well as histopathologic analysis and imaging. The synovial fluid analysis can be very helpful in this setting. In the setting of the current patient, where infection is established based on the presence of a draining sinus communicating with the prosthesis, synovial fluid analysis is still helpful to confirm the diagnosis and to identify an organism and its antibiotic sensitivities. Synovial leukocyte count is much lower in prosthetic joint infection than it is in native joint infections. The diagnostic criterion for chronic PJI of the knee is a synovial leukocyte count of 1,700/cm^2 or 65% or more neutrophils.

The aspirate of the knee grows MRSA. What is the probability of MRSA eradication with irrigation and debridement and liner exchange/component retention?

A. 100%
B. 80%
C. 20% to 40%
D. 8%
E. Less than 1%

Discussion

The correct answer is (D). The treatment of PJI has been shown to be less successful with component retention than with two-stage exchange arthroplasty for the treatment of infected total knee replacements. In most reports, I and D with retention of the implant results in approximately 20% to 40% control of infection.

However, in patients with MRSA the success rate with component retention has been shown to be as low as 8%.

Two-stage exchange arthroplasty results in control of infection in approximately 90% of patients.

What is the standard of care treatment at this stage?

A. Repeat I&D and liner exchange
B. Wound VAC dressing over the region of dehiscence
C. IV antibiotics followed by long-term suppression
D. Two-stage exchange arthroplasty
E. One-stage revision arthroplasty

Discussion

The correct answer is (D). This patient has had a draining sinus over a total knee replacement for more than 3 weeks and thus by definition has a chronic infection. Furthermore, she has a virulent organism (MRSA). The standard of care in this setting is removal of the components, placement of an antibiotic spacer followed by intravenous antimicrobial therapy for 6 weeks followed by reimplantation if infection is eradicated at that time. In patients who have had symptoms of infection for less than 3 weeks, do NOT have a draining sinus, have an appropriate nonvirulent microorganism, or those with hematogenous spread and the prosthesis is well-fixed and functioning, these patients may be candidates for irrigation and debridement, exchange of the polyethylene liner and retention of the components.

Which of the following is FALSE as it pertains to antibiotic spacers?

A. Static spacers in the knee make exposure at the time of reimplantation difficult due to quadriceps shortening
B. Commercially available cement containing antibiotics should NOT be used for antibiotic laden cement spacers because they contain insufficient antibiotic concentration
C. The PROSTALAC has been shown to be superior to static spacers
D. There has been no appreciable difference in infection recurrence and functional outcomes in patient that have had static spacers in comparison to those that have had articulating spacers

Discussion

The correct answer is (C). Articulating spacers such as the PROSTALAC have not been shown to definitively improve function or infection rates in comparison to nonarticulating spacers. Articulating spacers have been found to offer no functional advantage over static spacers. Antibiotic laden cement spacers should contain 2 to 4 g of antibiotic per 40 g bag of cement, which is a higher dose than that available in commercially available cement containing antibiotics which is used for primary and revision joint replacement in absence of active infection.

Following debridement and removal of the components you notice that the extensor mechanism is disrupted at the site of the patellar tendon. What is the best method by which to reconstruct this?

A. Allograft extensor mechanism
B. Megaprosthesis—attach the quads tendon to the prosthesis
C. Suture the patellar tendon end-to-end
D. Gastrocnemius rotational flap

Discussion

The correct answer is (D). The best method of reconstruction of the extensor mechanism in the setting of wound dehiscence and prior infection is to use autologous tissue (not allograft due to the risk of recurrent infection). A gastrocnemius rotational flap will provide soft tissue coverage, can replace the missing/incompetent capsule to prevent ongoing soft tissue problems, and can also be connected to the remnant extensor mechanism and attached to the quads tendon to reconstruct the extensor mechanism. Suturing the patellar tendon end-to-end will not be successful as there is often significant retraction and the tissue tends to be too fragile to obtain a strong repair. A mega prosthesis is an option, however it is optimal to have a bony fragment of attachment (i.e., the tibial tubercle attached to the patellar tendon) to attach to the prosthesis to get bony ingrowth. In the setting of a midsubstance patellar tendon tear, this will not be the case. Furthermore, this option does not have the added benefit of soft tissue coverage to manage the defect in the capsule. A persistent defect in the joint capsule will result in subsequent drainage and wound problems.

Objectives: Did you learn...?

- The diagnostic criteria of an infected TKR?
- Treatment of infected TKR?

CASE 21

Dr. Ayesha Abdeen

A 77-year-old female with obesity undergoes left total hip arthroplasty at an outside hospital 14 days ago. She presents to your emergency department with a urinary tract infection, acute onset atrial fibrillation and hip pain. You are called by the emergency physician because he has noted that she has wound erythema in the hip incision in addition to new onset hip pain.

Which of the following is NOT considered a risk factor for infection following total joint replacement?

A. Morbid obesity
B. Postoperative atrial fibrillation
C. Postoperative urinary tract infection
D. Postoperative myocardial infarction
E. Bilateral surgery
F. Postoperative stroke

Discussion

The correct answer is (F). In a study by Pulido et al. prospective data was reviewed in over 9,000 total joint replacements in order to identify risk factors for prosthetic joint infection. The following were identified as independent risk factors: higher American Society of Anesthesiologists score, morbid obesity, bilateral arthroplasty, knee arthroplasty, allogeneic transfusion, postoperative atrial fibrillation, myocardial infarction, urinary tract infection, and longer hospitalization.

Prior to administration of antibiotics you suggest doing an image-guided aspiration of the hip. What is the LEAST common organism found in total joint replacement infections?

A. *Streptococcus*
B. *Staphylococcus aureus*
C. Peptostreptococcus
D. Enterococcus
E. Coagulase-negative staphylococcus

Discussion

The correct answer is (C). The most common causes of PJI are typically organisms that are on the skin that inoculate the joint at the time of surgery. Gram-positive cocci account for 65% of PJI including coagulase-negative staphylococci, *S. aureus*, streptococcus, enterococcus. Twenty percent of infections are polymicrobial. The next most common (6% of infections) include aerobic gram-negative bacilli including enterobacteriaceae, *Pseudomonas aeruginosa*. Anaerobes account for 4% of infections (propionibacterium and peptostreptococcus, finegoldia magna). Approximately 7% are culture negative and 1% are from a fungi.

What is the cutoff synovial fluid WBC and neutrophil count in a CHRONIC total hip replacement?

A. WBC 1,700 cells/cm^2; 65% neutrophils
B. WBC 2,500 cells/cm^2; 65% neutrophils
C. WBC 3,000 cells/cm^2; 80% neutrophils
D. WBC 4,200 cells/cm^2; 80% neutrophils

Discussion

The correct answer is (D). The synovial WBC and neutrophil count threshold for chronic PJI in the hip is slightly higher than that of the knee. Answer A is the threshold for the knee. In the hip, the WBC cutoff is 4,200 cells/cm^2 and 80% neutrophils.

All of the following are independent criteria for the diagnosis of PJI EXCEPT:

A. The presence of a sinus tract that communicates with the prosthesis is definitive evidence of PJI
B. The presence of acute inflammation as seen on histopathologic examination of periprosthetic tissue at the time of surgical debridement or prosthesis removal greater than 5 to 10 neutrophils per high powered field is diagnostic of PJI
C. Two or more intraoperative cultures or combination of preoperative aspiration and intraoperative cultures that yield the same organism.
D. Elevated ESR and CRP

Discussion

The correct answer is (D). ESR and CRP are expected to be elevated until 2 months and several months following joint replacement, respectively. The remaining answers (A through C) are all independent criteria of PJI as identified by the Infectious Diseases Society of America (IDSA) guidelines and published in 2012.

Helpful Tip:

There are no specific diagnostic imaging tests that are independently definitive for the diagnosis of PJI. Plain radiographs are often normal unless there is significant septic loosening of the components. Nuclear imaging with labeled leukocyte imaging or FDG-PET imaging may be an option in patients in whom the diagnosis of PJI is not established, but the strength of this recommendation is considered "weak" by the AAOS clinical practice guidelines for the diagnosis of PJI.

Objectives: Did you learn...?

- The diagnostic criteria for PJI?
- The synovial fluid cutoff values consistent with PJI?

- The utility of serum inflammatory markers in PJI?
- The treatment of early versus late PJI?

BIBLIOGRAPHY

Case 1

Amstutz HC, Campbell P, Kossovsky N, Clarke IC. Mechanism and clinical significance of wear debris-induced osteolysis. *Clin Orthop Relat Res.* 1992;(276):7–18.

Crites BM, Berend ME, Ritter MA. Technical considerations of cemented acetabular components: a 30-year evaluation. *Clin Orthop Relat Res.* 2000;(381):114–119.

Lakstein D, Eliaz N, Levi O, et al. Fracture of cementless femoral stems at the mid-stem junction in modular revision hip arthroplasty systems. *J Bone Joint Surg Am.* 2011;93(1): 57–65.

Malchau H, Herberts P, Eisler T, Garellick G, Söderman P. The Swedish total hip replacement register. *J Bone Joint Surg Am.* 2002;84-A (Suppl 2):2–20.

Moreau MF, Chappard D, Lesourd M, Monthéard JP, Baslé MF. Free radicals and side products released during methylmethacrylate polymerization are cytotoxic for osteoblastic cells. *J Biomed Mater Res.* 1998;40(1):124–131.

Willmann G. Ceramic femoral head retrieval data. *Clin Orthop Relat Res.* 2000;(379):22–28.

Case 2

Clarke MT, Lee PT, Villar RN. Dislocation after total hip replacement in relation to metal-on-metal bearing surfaces. *J Bone Joint Surg Br.* 2003;85(5):650–654.

De Haan R, Campbell PA, Su EP, De Smet KA. Revision of metal-on-metal resurfacing arthroplasty of the hip the influence of malpositioning of the components. *J Bone Joint Surg Br.* 2008;90(9):1158–1163.

Hallab NJ, Anderson S, Caicedo M, Skipor A, Campbell P, Jacobs JJ. Immune responses correlate with serum-metal in metal-on-metal hip arthroplasty. *J Arthroplasty.* 2004;19(8 Suppl 3): 88–93.

Müller GM, Månsson S, Müller MF, et al. MR imaging with metal artifact-reducing sequences and gadolinium contrast agent in a case-control study of periprosthetic abnormalities in patients with metal-on-metal hip prostheses. *Skeletal Radiol.* 2014;43(8):1101–1112.

Rieker C, Konrad R.Schön R. In vitro comparison of the two hard-hard articulations for total hip replacements. *Proc Inst Mech Eng H.* 2001;215(2):153–160.

Case 3

Chen CH, Chang JK, Lai KA, Hou SM, Chang CH, Wang GJ. Alendronate in the prevention of collapse of the femoral head in nontraumatic osteonecrosis: a two-year multicenter, prospective, randomized, double-blind, placebo-controlled study. *Arthritis Rheum.* 2012;64(5):1572–1578.

Hernigou P, Habibi A, Bachir D, Galacteros F. The natural history of asymptomatic osteonecrosis of the femoral head in adults with sickle cell disease. *J Bone Joint Surg Am.* 2006;88(12):2565–2572.

Lai KA, Shen WJ, Yang CY, Shao CJ, Hsu JT, Lin RM. The use of alendronate to prevent early collapse of the femoral head in patients with nontraumatic osteonecrosis: a randomized clinical study. *J Bone Joint Surg Am.* 2005;87(10): 2155–2159.

Mont MA, Ragland PS, Etienne G, Seyler TM, Schmalzried TP. Hip resurfacing arthroplasty. *J Am Acad Orthop Surg.* 2006;14(8):454–463.

Rosenwasser MP, Garino JP, Kiernan HA, Michelsen CB. Long term followup of through debridement and cancellous bone grafting of the femoral head for avascular necrosis. *Clin Orthop Relat Res.* 1994;(306):17–27.

Weinstein RS, Nicholas RW, Manolagas SC. Apoptosis of osteocytes in glucocorticoid-induced osteonecrosis of the hip 1. *J Clin Endocrinol Metab.* 2000;85(8):2907–2912.

Case 4

Argenson JN, Ryembault E, Flecher X, Brassart N, Parratte S, Aubaniac JM. Three-dimensional anatomy of the hip in osteoarthritis after developmental dysplasia. *J Bone Joint Surg Br.* 2005;87(9):1192–1196.

Dudkiewicz I, Salai M, Ganel A, Blankstein A, Chechik A. Total hip arthroplasty in patients younger than 30 years of age following developmental dysplasia of hip (DDH) in infancy. *Arch Orthop Trauma Surg.* 2002;122(3):139–142.

Feldman G, Dalsey C, Fertala K, et al. The Otto Aufranc Award: identification of a 4 Mb region on chromosome 17q21 linked to developmental dysplasia of the hip in one 18-member, multigeneration family. *Clin Orthop Relat Res.* 2010;468(2):337–344.

Gillingham BL, Sanchez AA, Wenger DR. Pelvic osteotomies for the treatment of hip dysplasia in children and young adults. *J Am Acad Orthop Surg.* 1999;7(5):325–337.

Nagoya S, Kaya M, Sasaki M, Tateda K, Kosukegawa I, Yamashita T. Cementless total hip replacement with subtrochanteric femoral shortening for severe developmental dysplasia of the hip. *J Bone Joint Surg Br.* 2009;91(9): 1142–1147.

Case 5

Anouchi YS, McShane M, Kelly F Jr, Elting J, Stiehl J. Range of motion in total knee replacement. *Clin Orthop Relat Res.* 1996;(331):87–92.

Hunter DJ, March L, Sambrook PN. Knee osteoarthritis: the influence of environmental factors. *Clin Exp Rheumatol.* 2002;20(1):93–100.

Ling SM, Joan MB. Pathophysiology of osteoarthritis.

Richmond J, Hunter D, Irrgang J, et al. American Academy of Orthopaedic Surgeons clinical practice guideline on the treatment of osteoarthritis (OA) of the knee. *J Bone Joint Surg Am.* 2010;92(4):990–993.

Case 6

Mont MA, Jacobs JJ. AAOS clinical practice guideline: preventing venous thromboembolic disease in patients undergoing elective hip and knee arthroplasty. *J Am Acad Orthop Surg.* 2011;19(12):777–778.

Case 7

Giori NJ, Ellerbe LS, Bowe T, Gupta S, Harris AH. Many diabetic total joint arthroplasty candidates are unable to achieve a preoperative hemoglobin A1c goal of 7% or less. *J Bone Joint Surg Am.* 2014;96(6):500–504.

Harris AH, Bowe TR, Gupta S, Ellerbe LS, Giori NJ. Hemoglobin A1c as a marker for surgical risk in diabetic patients undergoing total joint arthroplasty. *J Arthroplasty.* 2013;28(8 Suppl):25–29.

Moreland JR, Bassett LW, Hanker GJ. Radiographic analysis of the axial alignment of the lower extremity. *J Bone Joint Surg Am.* 1987;69(5):745–749.

Parvizi J, Marrs J, Morrey BF. Total knee arthroplasty for neuropathic (Charcot) joints. *Clin Orthop Relat Res.* 2003;416:145–150.

Case 8

Belmont PJ Jr, Goodman GP, Waterman BR, Bader JO, Schoenfeld AJ. 30-day postoperative complications and mortality following total knee arthroplasty: incidence and risk factors among a national sample of 15,321 patients. *J Bone Joint Surg Am.* 2014;96:20–26.

Estes CS, Schmidt KJ, McLemore R, Spangehl MJ, Clarke HD. Effect of body mass index on limb alignment after total knee arthroplasty. *J Arthroplasty.* 2013;28(8 Suppl):101–105.

Huddleston JI, Wang Y, Uquillas C, Herndon JH, Maloney WJ. Age and obesity are risk factors for adverse events after total hip arthroplasty. *Clin Orthop Relat Res.* 2012;470(2):490–496.

Wallace G, Judge A, Prieto-Alhambra D, de Vries F, Arden NK, Cooper C. The effect of body mass index on the risk of post-operative complications during the 6 months following total hip replacement or total knee replacement surgery. *Osteoarthritis Cartilage.* 2014;22(7):918–927.

Case 9

Lin CA, Kuo AC, Takemoto S. Comorbidities and perioperative complications in HIV-positive patients undergoing primary total hip and knee arthroplasty. *J Bone Joint Surg Am.* 2013;95:1028–1036.

Mazzotta E, Agostinone A, Rosso R, et al. Osteonecrosis in human immunodeficiency virus (HIV)-infected patients: a multicentric case–control study. *J Bone Miner Metab.* 2011;29(3):383–388.

Parvizi J, Sullivan TA, Pagnano MW, Trousdale RT, Bolander ME. Total joint arthroplasty in human immunodeficiency virus-positive patients: an alarming rate of early failure. *J Arthroplasty.* 2003;18:259–264.

Pour AE, Matar WY, Jafari SM, Purtill JJ, Austin MS, Parvizi J. Total joint arthroplasty in patients with hepatitis C. *J Bone Joint Surg Am.* 2011;93(15):1448–1454.

Case 10

Beight JL, Yao B, Hozack WJ, Hearn SL, Booth RE Jr. The patellar "clunk" syndrome after posterior stabilized total knee arthroplasty. *Clin Orthop Relat Res.* 1994;(299):139–142.

Bottros J, Gad B, Krebs V, Barsoum WK. Gap balancing in total knee arthroplasty. *J Arthroplasty.* 2006;21(4 Suppl 1):11–15.

Duffy GP, Berry DJ, Rand JA. Cement versus cementless fixation in total knee arthroplasty. *Clin Orthop Relat Res.* 1998;(356):66–72.

Jazrawi LM, Birdzell L, Kummer FJ, Di Cesare PE. The accuracy of computed tomography for determining femoral and tibial total knee arthroplasty component rotation. *J Arthroplasty.* 2000;15(6):761–766.

Mitchell B, McCrory P, Brukner P, O'Donnell J, Colson E, Howells R. Hip joint pathology: clinical presentation and correlation between magnetic resonance arthrography, ultrasound, and arthroscopic findings in 25 consecutive cases. *Clin J Sport Med.* 2003;13(3):152–156.

Paletta GA Jr, Laskin RS. Total knee arthroplasty after a previous patellectomy. *J Bone Joint Surg Am.* 1995;77(11):1708–1712.

Rand JA. Comparison of metal-backed and all-polyethylene tibial components in cruciate condylar total knee arthroplasty. *J Arthroplasty.* 1993;8(3):307–313.

Vernace JV, Rothman RH, Booth RE Jr, Balderston RA. Arthroscopic management of the patellar clunk syndrome following posterior stabilized total knee arthroplasty. *J Arthroplasty.* 1989;4(2):179–182.

Case 11

Leadbetter WB, Ragland PS, Mont MA. The appropriate use of patellofemoral arthroplasty: an analysis of reported indications, contraindications, and failures. *Clin Orthop Relat Res.* 2005;(436):91–99.

Lonner JH. Patellofemoral arthroplasty: the impact of design on outcomes. *Orthop Clin North Am.* 2008;39(3):347–354.

Lonner JH. Patellofemoral arthroplasty. *Orthopedics.* 2010;33(9):653.

Case 12

Engh GA, Ammeen D. Is an intact anterior cruciate ligament needed in order to have a well-functioning unicondylar knee replacement?. *Clin Orthop Relat Res.* 2004;(428):170–173.

Robinson BJ, Rees JL, Price AJ, et al. Dislocation of the bearing of the Oxford lateral unicompartmental arthroplasty a radiological assessment. *J Bone Joint Surg Br.* 2002;84(5):653–657.

Case 13

Ghanem E1, Parvizi J, Burnett RS, et al. Cell count and differential of aspirated fluid in the diagnosis of infection at the site of total knee arthroplasty. *J Bone Joint Surg Am.* 2008;90(8):1637–1643.

Haidukewych GJ1, Hanssen A, Jones RD. Metaphyseal fixation in revision total knee arthroplasty: indications and techniques. *J Am Acad Orthop Surg.* 2011 Jun;19(6):311–318.

Kamath AF1, Lewallen DG1, Hanssen AD1. Porous tantalum metaphyseal cones for severe tibial bone loss in revision knee arthroplasty: a five to nine-year follow-up. *J Bone Joint Surg Am.* 2015 Feb 4;97(3):216–223.

Case 14

Brandt CM, Sistrunk WW, Duffy MC, et al. *Staphylococcus aureus* prosthetic joint infection treated with debridement and prosthesis retention. *Clin Infect Dis*. 1997;24(5):914–919.

Rorabeck CH, Taylor JW. Classification of periprosthetic fractures complicating total knee arthroplasty. *Orthop Clin North Am*. 1999;30(2):209–214.

Case 15

McCollum DE, Gray WJ. Dislocation after total hip arthroplasty causes and prevention. *Clin Orthop Relat Res*. 1990;(261):159–170.

Rachbauer F, Kain MS, Leunig M. The history of the anterior approach to the hip. *Orthop Clin N Am*. 2009;40:311–320.

Wasielewski RC, Cooperstein LA, Kruger MP, Rubash HE. Acetabular anatomy and the transacetabular fixation of screws in total hip arthroplasty. *J Bone Joint Surg Am*. 1990;72(4):501–508.

Case 16

Iorio R, Healy WL. Heterotopic ossification after hip and knee arthroplasty: risk factors, prevention, and treatment. *J Am Acad Orthop Surg*. 2002;10(6):409–416.

Kjaersgaard-Andersen P, Ritter MA. Prevention of formation of heterotopic bone after total hip arthroplasty. *J Bone Joint Surg Am*. 1991;73(6):942–947.

Lewallen DG. Heterotopic ossification following total hip arthroplasty. *Instr Course Lect*. 1994;44:287–292.

Weil Y, Mattan Y, Goldman V, Liebergall M. Sciatic nerve palsy due to hematoma after thrombolysis therapy for acute pulmonary embolism after total hip arthroplasty. *J Arthroplasty*. 2006;21(3):456–459.

Case 17

Campbell DG, Garbuz DS, Masri BA, Duncan CP. Reliability of acetabular bone defect classification systems in revision total hip arthroplasty. *J Arthroplasty*. 2001;16(1):83–86.

Jasty M, Harris WH. Salvage total hip reconstruction in patients with major acetabular bone deficiency using structural femoral head allografts. *J Bone Joint Surg Br*. 1990;72(1):63–67.

Moyad TF, Thornhill T, Estok D. Evaluation and management of the infected total hip and knee. *Orthopedics*. 2008;31(6):581.

Puri L, Wixson RL, Stern SH, Kohli J, Hendrix RW, Stulberg SD. Use of helical computed tomography for the assessment of acetabular osteolysis after total hip arthroplasty. *J Bone Joint Surg Am*. 2002;84-A(4):609–614.

Wroblewski BM, Siney PD, Fleming PA. Charnley low-frictional torque arthroplasty follow-up for 30 to 40 years. *J Bone Joint Surg Br*. 2009;91(4):447–450.

Case 18

Sledge JB 3rd, Abiri A. An algorithm for the treatment of Vancouver type B2 periprosthetic proximal femoral fractures. *J Arthroplasty*. 2002;17(7):887–892.

Case 19

Laird A, Keating JF. Acetabular fractures a 16-year prospective epidemiological study. *J Bone Joint Surg Br*. 2005;87(7):969–973.

Masri BA, Meek RM, Duncan CP. Periprosthetic fractures evaluation and treatment. *Clin Orthop Relat Res*. 2004;(420):80–95.

Case 20

Brandt CM, Sistrunk WW, Duffy MC, et al. *Staphylococcus aureus* prosthetic joint infection treated with debridement and prosthesis retention. *Clin Infect Dis*. 1997;24(5):914–919.

Burger RR, Basch T, Hopson CN. Implant salvage in infected total knee arthroplasty. *Clin Orthop Relat Res*. 1991;(273):105–112.

Busfield BT, Huffman GR, Nahai F, Hoffman W, Ries MD. Extended medial gastrocnemius rotational flap for treatment of chronic knee extensor mechanism deficiency in patients with and without total knee arthroplasty. *Clin Orthop Relat Res*. 2004;(428):190–197.

Deirmengian C, Greenbaum J, Stern J, et al. Open debridement of acute gram-positive infections after total knee arthroplasty. *Clin Orthop Relat Res*. 2003;(416):129–134.

Durbhakula SM, Czajka J, Fuchs MD, Uhl RL. Antibiotic-loaded articulating cement spacer in the 2-stage exchange of infected total knee arthroplasty. *J Arthroplasty*. 2004;19(6):768–774.

Haddad FS, Masri BA, Campbell D, McGraw RW, Beauchamp CP, Duncan CP. The PROSTALAC functional spacer in two-stage revision for infected knee replacements. *J Bone Joint Surg Br*. 2000;82(6):807–812.

Fehring TK, Odum S, Calton TF, Mason JB. Articulating versus static spacers in revision total knee arthroplasty for sepsis. *Clin Orthop Relat Res*. 2000;(380):9–16.

Leone JM, Hanssen AD. Management of infection at the site of a total knee arthroplasty. *J Bone Joint Surg Am*. 2005;87(10):2335–2348.

Pozo J, Patel R. Infection associated with prosthetic joints. *N Engl J Med*. 2009;361:787–794.

Trampuz A, Hanssen AD, Osmon DR, Mandrekar J, Steckelberg JM, Patel R. Synovial fluid leukocyte count and differential for the diagnosis of prosthetic knee infection. *Am J Med*. 2004;117(8):556–562.

Zimmerli W, Widmer AF, Blatter M, Frei R, Ochsner PE, Foreign-Body Infection(FBI) Study Group. Role of rifampin for treatment of orthopedic implant-related staphylococcal infections: a randomized controlled trial. *JAMA*. 1998;279:1537–1541.

Case 21

Bilgen O, Atici T, Durak K, Karaeminoğullari, Bilgen MS. C-reactive protein values and erythrocyte sedimentation rates after total hip and total knee arthroplasty. *J Int Med Res*. 2001;29(1):7–12.

Del Pozo JL, Patel R. Infection associated with prosthetic joints. *N Engl J Med*. 2009;361(8):787–794.

Fink B, Makowiak C, Fuerst M, Berger I, Schäfer P, Frommelt L. The value of synovial biopsy, joint aspiration and C-reactive protein in the diagnosis of late peri-prosthetic infection of total knee replacements. *J Bone Joint Surg Br*. 2008;90(7):874–878.

Greidanus NV, Masri BA, Garbuz DS, et al. Use of erythrocyte sedimentation rate and C-reactive protein level to diagnose infection before revision total knee arthroplasty: a prospective evaluation. *J Bone Joint Surg Am.* 2007;89(7): 1409–1416.

Muller M, Morawietz L, Hasart O, Strube P, Perka C, Tohtz S. Diagnosis of periprosthetic infection following total hip arthroplasty—evaluation of the diagnostic values of pre- and intraoperative parameters and the associated strategy to preoperatively select patients with a high probability of joint infection. *J Orthop Surg.* 2008;3:31.

Osmon DR, Berbari EF, Berendt AR, et al. Diagnosis and management of prosthetic joint infection: clinical practice guidelines by the Infectious Diseases Society of America. *Clin Infect Dis.* 2013;56(1):e1–e25.

Parvizi J, Della Valle CJ. AAOS Clinical Practice Guideline: diagnosis and treatment of periprosthetic joint infections of the hip and knee. *J Am Acad Orthop Surg.* 2010; 18(12): 771–772.

Pulido L, Ghanem E, Joshi A, Purtill JJ, Parvizi J. Periprosthetic joint infection: the incidence, timing, and predisposing factors. *Clin Orthop Relat Res.* 2008;466(7):1710–1715.

Schinsky MF, Della Valle CJ, Sporer SM, Paprosky WG. Perioperative testing for joint infection in patients undergoing revision total hip arthroplasty. *J Bone Joint Surg Am.* 2008; 90:1869–1875.

8

Orthopaedic Oncology

John A. Abraham, Christina Gutowski, William Morrison, and Wei Jiang

CASE 1

A 10-year-old male presents to the emergency room complaining of right shoulder pain after falling during a soccer game. He denies history of pain in the shoulder or arm prior to the injury. X-rays taken in the emergency room are shown in Figure 8–1A and B.

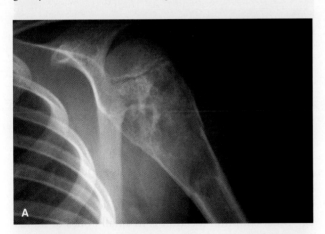

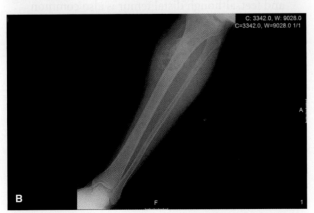

Figure 8–1 **A–B**

Which of the following is true of the lesion shown in the x-ray image?

A. Most common location is mid-diaphyseal in long bones
B. It is commonly filled with blood
C. It is usually associated with a soft-tissue mass
D. The natural history of this lesion is to fill in with bone as patient reaches skeletal maturity

Discussion

The correct answer is (D). The lesion shown in the x-rays is a unicameral bone cyst (UBC), which is a common, serous fluid-filled bone lesion that usually occurs in patients younger than 20 years of age. The natural history is that these lesions fill in with bone over time and may be asymptomatic unless the patient develops pathologic fracture. Unlike aneurysmal bone cysts, which are often filled with blood, a UBC rarely includes blood unless fracture is present. Cortical thinning may be seen on x-ray, but bone remodeling does not exceed the width of the physis and these lesions do not have associated soft-tissue masses.

What is the most appropriate emergency room management of this patient?

A. Admission to the hospital for immediate surgical treatment
B. Sling and nonweight bearing on the extremity now, with potential surgical management once fracture is healed
C. CT and MRI to evaluate extent of soft-tissue mass
D. Bone biopsy to document osteomyelitis and obtain culture, and IV antibiotics

Discussion

The correct answer is (B). Unicameral bone cysts with pathologic fracture do not routinely require cross-sectional imaging, as their radiographic characteristics allow them to be easily diagnosed on plain radiograph. A minimally displaced fracture such as this generally does not require surgical stabilization in the acute period. This fracture should be allowed to heal prior to treatment of the lesion. The x-ray shows characteristics more consistent with UBC than osteomyelitis.

In the absence of pathologic fracture, what is the first line of surgical treatment?

A. Curettage with bone grafting
B. Internal fixation
C. Aspiration and injection with methyl prednisolone acetate
D. Wide resection and reconstruction with humeral endoprosthetic implant

Discussion

The correct answer is (C). The initial surgical treatment of UBC is with aspiration and injection with methylprednisolone acetate. Internal fixation is generally not indicated except in high stress areas likely to undergo pathologic fracture. Curettage and bone grafting can be used in cases in which aspiration and injection fails. Wide resection and reconstruction is reserved for malignant tumors.

If found in the proximal femur, management of this lesion with or without pathologic fracture would consist of:

A. Wide resection and proximal femur reconstruction
B. Wide resection, reconstruction, and postoperative radiation
C. Curettage, bone grafting, and internal fixation
D. Percutaneous screw fixation alone

Discussion

The correct answer is (C). When a UBC is found in the proximal femur, curettage, bone grafting, and internal fixation are recommended to prevent pathologic fracture. In other locations where the risk of pathologic fracture is lower, standard treatment is generally intralesional injection of methylprednisolone acetate. Wide resection and radiation therapy are not necessary, as UBC is a benign lesion.

Objectives: Did you learn...?

• Characteristic features of simple, or unicameral, bone cysts, and features that distinguish UBC from aneurysmal bone cyst (ABC)?

• Acute and overall management of simple bone cysts?
• Indications of surgery for simple bone cysts?

CASE 2

A 20-year-old female presents to the office complaining of pain and swelling in the elbow. She denies any recent trauma and reports these symptoms have been progressing over the past year. She denies fever, chills, or recent weight changes. X-ray is shown in Figure 8–2.

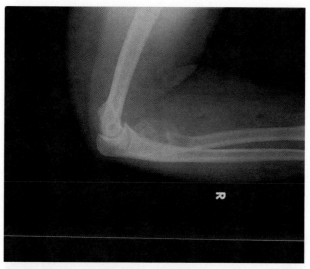

Figure 8–2

Which of the following x-ray findings is most consistent with this lesion?

A. Eccentric, radiolucent lesion that has expanded greater than the width of the epiphysis
B. Central lesion with loss of thin periosteal rim around the lesion
C. Most often accompanied by pathologic fracture
D. Most common location is in small bones of hands and feet, although distal femur is also common

Discussion

The correct answer is (A). Aneurysmal bone cysts are destructive, reactive bone lesions filled with multiple blood-filled cavities. They are eccentric on x-rays and cause bone remodeling which has the appearance of an expanded bone and can be beyond the width of the physis, unlike UBC. They occur most often in the distal femur, proximal tibia, pelvis, and posterior elements of the spine. Unlike giant cell tumors of bone, ABCs usually retain a thin periosteal rim. Unlike UBCs, these lesions cause pain and swelling, and pathologic fracture as a presenting symptom is relatively rare.

The following figure (Fig. 8–3A and B) show a low and high power histologic slide of the lesion. Which of the following best describes the histologic appearance of this lesion?

A. Woven bone, Aneurysmal blood vessels, osteoid producing cells

B. Sheets of small round blue cells with pleiomorphoism and nuclear atypia

C. Cavernous, blood-filled spaces without a true endothelial lining. Multinucleated giant cells within a fibrohistiocytic stroma are noted, without cellular atypia

D. Dense fibrous stroma with storiform pattern and limited nuclear atypia

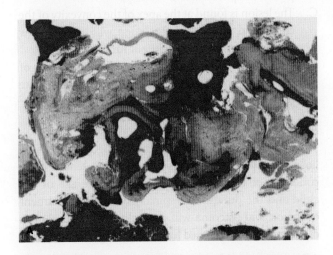

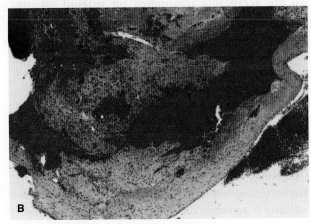

B

Figure 8–3 **A–B**

Discussion

The correct answer is (C). The histologic appearance seen in Figure 8–3A and B is best described as a cavernous, blood-filled spaces without a true endothelial lining. Multinucleated giant cells within a fibrohistiocytic stroma are noted, without cellular atypia are seen. This is a classic description of Aneurysmal Bone Cyst.

The patient brings an MRI of the elbow to the office that was ordered by her primary care physician a week prior. What findings would you expect to see that would confirm your diagnosis of ABC?

A. Large soft-tissue mass extending out of the proximal radius bone

B. Skip lesions throughout the radius

C. Fluid–fluid levels

D. Extensive edema within surrounding bone and soft tissue

Discussion

The correct answer is (C). Fluid–fluid levels are commonly seen on T2-weighted MRI, as this finding represents the separation of serum and blood products within the cyst. Skip lesions are metastases of a malignant process. ABCs can remodel the cortex and into surrounding soft tissue but retain their reactive periosteal rim and will not cause a large soft-tissue mass. Edema in the surrounding tissues is not a common finding on MRI in the absence of pathologic fracture.

When imaging is encountered that suggests ABC, which malignancy must also be considered in the differential?

A. Ewing sarcoma

B. Telangiectatic osteosarcoma

C. Periosteal osteosarcoma

D. Giant cell tumor

Discussion

The correct answer is (B). While rare, telangiectatic osteosarcoma can mimic ABC radiographically. Histologically, a malignant tumor is seen. Cartilage tumors (enchondroma, chondrosarcoma) will show radiographic characteristics of cartilage: arc-and-ring calcification or an expansile mass on imaging and/or cartilaginous matrix on histology. Periosteal osteosarcoma has a characteristic juxtacortical cloud-like density, and will not show blood-filled spaces on histology. Ewing sarcoma is characterized by periosteal elevation in an "onion-skinning" pattern and on histology is characterized by sheets of small, round blue cells.

Objectives: Did you learn...?

- Imaging characteristics of ABC?
- Histologic features of ABC?
- Important differential diagnosis of telangiectatic osteosarcoma and its features?
- Treatment of ABC?

CASE 3

A 23-year-old male presents to your office complaining of progressive low back pain for the past 6 months. The pain is at its worst at night. He, in addition, notes that he has been taking ibuprofen, because this medication works well to relieve his pain. He denies history of trauma or history of back pain before this year. He has no radicular symptoms. Physical examination reveals negative straight-leg raise, and he has full flexion and extension of the lumbar spine without increase in pain. X-rays taken in the office are negative.

What is the next step in evaluation and management of this patient?

A. Obtain oblique x-rays to reveal pars defect
B. Prescription for physical therapy
C. Electromyography and nerve conduction velocity studies
D. Thin-cut CT scan of the lumbar spine

Discussion

The correct answer is (D). The patient's history is most consistent with an osteoid osteoma, which is a benign osteoblastic bone tumor that involves a radiolucent nidus surrounded by a ring of sclerotic bone, and can occur in the vertebral arch. Nocturnal pain is a classic finding, as is good relief with NSAIDs since high prostaglandin and cyclooxygenase levels within the lesion are thought to play a role in pain generation. They are usually <1 cm in diameter and frequently missed on plain radiographs, therefore thin-cut CT scan is often the key to diagnosis because it will identify the radiolucent nidus. A pars defect is less likely, since he has no pain with flexion and extension. Physical therapy is not appropriate without a diagnosis at this time, and it is unlikely that EMG/NCV testing will be helpful since he has no neurologic symptoms.

Which of the following is true regarding the natural history of osteoid osteoma?

A. Benign lesion with rare lung metastases
B. Self-limiting which generally resolves in 2 to 4 years
C. Rarely require treatment when found in long bones, but aggressive treatment when present in vertebrae is always recommended
D. Benign lesion, with recurrence rate of 30% to 50% after treatment

Discussion

The correct answer is (B). Unlike osteoblastomas, the growth characteristics of osteoid osteoma are self-limited.

Pain may be an indication for treatment, but if given time these lesions will resolve with no malignant potential (average 3 years). Recurrence rates after radiofrequency ablation are <10%.

Which of the following is true regarding an osteoid osteoma causing a painful scoliosis?

A. The lesion is found at the center of the concavity of the curve, and removal of the lesion will usually allow resolution of the curve without further treatment
B. The lesion is found at the center of the concavity of the curve, and correction of the curve will require posterior spinal fusion
C. The lesion is found at the apex of the convexity of the curve, and removal of the lesion will usually allow resolution of the curve without further treatment
D. The lesion is found at the apex of the convexity of the curve, and correction of the curve will require posterior spinal fusion

Discussion

The correct answer is (A). When causing a painful scoliosis, an osteoid osteoma is usually at the center of the concavity of the curve. Depending on the age of the child and the duration of spinal asymmetry, treatment of the osteoid osteoma will generally lead to resolution of the curve without need for further surgical correction.

All are acceptable treatments for osteoid osteoma except:

A. Percutaneous radiofrequency ablation with CT-guided probe
B. Surgical resection
C. Long-term medical management with NSAIDs or aspirin
D. Intralesional injection of methylprednisolone acetate

Discussion

The correct answer is (D). The standard of care for osteoid osteoma is percutaneous radiofrequency ablation (RFA) of the lesion, where a CT-guided probe is inserted into the lesion and heated to 90°C for 4 to 6 minutes. This produces a 1-cm area of necrosis. Surgical resection or curettage is also acceptable treatment when the lesion is close to the spinal cord or nerve roots, other sensitive areas, or if RFA is not available. Patients who opt for nonsurgical management can control symptoms with long-term NSAIDs or aspirin, and usually after an average of 3 years these lesions cease to be painful as they have self-limited growth.

Objectives: Did you learn...?

- Clinical and imaging features of osteoid osteoma?
- To differentiate osteoid osteoma and osteoblastoma?
- Treatment of osteoid osteoma?

CASE 4

A 31-year-old male is seen in the emergency room after sustaining a knee injury. He reports he was playing pickup football this morning when he twisted his knee awkwardly. He felt a pop, and his knee swelled within 20 minutes. He was able to bear weight without much pain, but reports his knee felt unstable. X-rays taken in the emergency room are negative for fracture but demonstrate a lesion in the distal femur (Fig. 8–4).

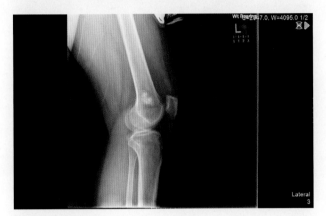

Figure 8–4

What is the most likely statement regarding this lesion?

A. It caused weakening of the bone and he likely sustained a nondisplaced pathologic fracture in this area that is not visible on x-ray

B. This is likely an incidental finding, and his pain is unrelated to the lesion

C. Extensive calcification of the lesion is concerning for malignant transformation

D. A skeletal survey is required to evaluate extent of disease

Discussion

The correct answer is (B). X-rays reveal many classic characteristics of an enchondroma, which is a benign tumor comprised of hyaline cartilage located in the medullary canal. Over time, the lobules of cartilage calcify, giving it the stippled, "arcs and rings" appearance on x-ray. Calcification implies a slow-growing or latent process, and areas of lucency are more concerning than calcified areas: either for sites of necrosis or more rapidly proliferating and spreading cartilage that may be aggressive. Enchondromas are rarely symptomatic and

rarely cause pathologic fracture, and furthermore the patient's history is more consistent with an intra-articular ligamentous injury than a distal femur fracture. This enchondroma represents an incidental finding on an x-ray performed for another reason, which is often the way these lesions are diagnosed.

The patient goes on to obtain an MRI of the knee, which reveals a tear of his anterior cruciate ligament. He is put in a knee immobilizer, nonweight bearing on the extremity, and is instructed to follow-up in the office within a week. What further management should be recommended regarding the lesion in his distal femur?

A. Follow with serial radiographs to ensure stability

B. Needle biopsy on elective basis to differentiate between enchondroma and chondrosarcoma

C. Curettage and bone graft at time of ACL reconstruction

D. Referral to medical oncology for workup of visceral malignancy

Discussion

The correct answer is (A). Asymptomatic enchondromas require no treatment, but should be followed with serial x-rays to monitor size, calcification, and other characteristics. If radiographs are suspicious for chondrosarcoma, further workup and possible surgery is necessary. Important to note regarding cartilage tumors is that pathologic examination is not reliable to differentiate between a benign enchondroma and a low-grade chondrosarcoma; instead, radiographic appearance is more accurate and important in this differentiation. Curettage and bone grafting is reserved for symptomatic enchondromas, but this patient has a reason for his pain (the ACL tear) and was asymptomatic prior to his acute injury. Surgical treatment for the enchondroma is not indicated.

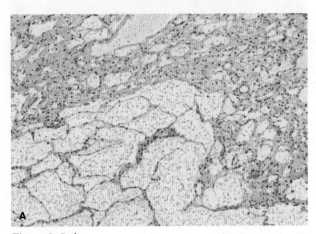

Figure 8–5 **A**

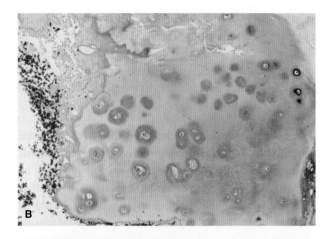

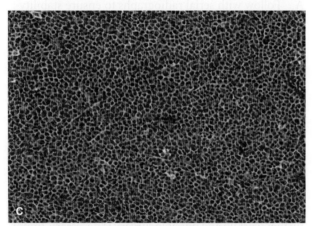

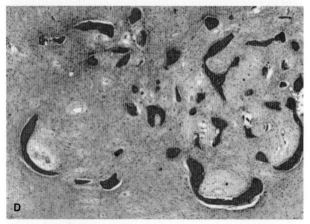

Figure 8–5 **B–D**

Which of the following histologic slides (Fig. 8–5A–D) represents this patient's lesion?

A. Figure 8–5A
B. Figure 8–5B
C. Figure 8–5C
D. Figure 8–5D

Discussion

The correct answer is (B). Enchondromas are composed of hyaline cartilage demonstrating a lobulated pattern. They have variable cellularity characterized by large, round chondroblasts surrounded by purple or blue matrix on hematoxylin and eosin (H&E) staining. Chondroblasts can be recognized by a typical "fried egg" appearance with a high proportion of cytoplasm. Nuclei can have mild atypia, with bean-shaped or even binucleate appearance, making grading of cartilage tumors by histology alone difficult. A high-power slide is shown in Figure 8–6 demonstrating these features.

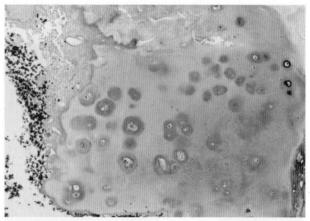

Figure 8–6

If the patient reported to you that he also had enchondromas in bilateral humeri and his contralateral femur, you become concerned about related conditions that involve multiple enchondromas. Which of the following is true?

A. Ollier disease is characterized by pancytopenia and multiple enchondromas, while Maffucci syndrome does not involve hematologic abnormalities

B. Maffucci syndrome involves vascular malformations and increased rate of visceral malignancy, while Ollier disease involves increased risk of malignant transformation of an enchondroma to a low-grade chondrosarcoma

C. Patients with Maffucci syndrome have an increased risk of fracture through their enchondromas, while patients with Ollier syndrome do not

D. A critical complication of both Ollier and Maffucci syndrome is hypercalcemia due to extensive bone destruction by the enchondromas

Discussion

The correct answer is (B). Ollier disease is characterized by multiple enchondromas with a 25% to 30% risk of malignant transformation to a low-grade chondrosar-coma. Maffucci syndrome involves multiple enchondro-mas, vascular malformations, and a high risk of developing a visceral malignancy. Hematologic abnormalities or elec-trolyte disturbances are rarely associated with these con-ditions. The risk of pathologic fracture in these patients is no greater than those with solitary enchondromas.

Objectives: Did you learn...?

- To recognize cartilage tumors on imaging?
- To recognize cartilage on a histology slide?
- The management of benign cartilage lesions?
- Syndromes of multiple enchondromas and their relevance?

CASE 5

A 20-year-old female presents to your office with a com-plaint of leg pain and mechanical symptoms. She has recently started running and reports a painful snapping sensation in her leg, and states she can feel a hard mass in her calf. X-ray is shown in Figure 8–7.

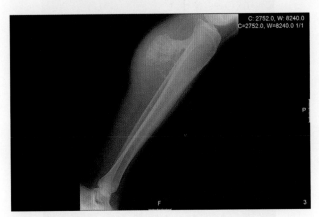

Figure 8–7

What type of lesion is this?

A. Chondromyxoid fibroma
B. Chondroblastoma
C. Pedunculated osteochondroma
D. Osteofibrous dysplasia

Discussion

The correct answer is (C). The imaging shows an oste-ochondroma. Osteochondromas can be either sessile, meaning having a broad origin from the underlying bone (looks like a mountain) or pedunculated, meaning having a stalk (looks like broccoli). The imaging is characteris-tic and usually diagnostic. Chondromyxoid fibroma and osteofibrous dysplasia both demonstrate a soap-bubble appearance within the bone, osteofibrous dysplasia is a tibial anterior cortical lesion, whereas CMF is eccentric and displays expansive remodeling. Chondroblastoma is predominantly a radiolucent epiphyseal lesion.

Which of the following imaging characteristics defines this lesion?

A. Corticomedullary continuity between host bone and the mass
B. Juxtacortical appearance, with mass sitting on top of uninterrupted cortex
C. Growth pointing towards the growth plate or joint
D. A cartilage cap that grows well after skeletal maturity

Discussion

The correct answer is (A). Osteochondromas are benign bone lesions in which histologically normal bone grows transversely away from the host bone. The lesion grows away from the growth plate or neighboring joint, and is covered with a cartilage cap. If this cap continues to grow after skeletal maturity, malignant transformation is a concern. A key diagnostic characteristic of osteo-chondroma on imaging studies is the presence of cor-ticomedullary continuity between the underlying bone and the lesion; a juxtacortical appearance where the underlying cortex is uninterrupted or is saucerized is more concerning for parosteal osteosarcoma or other periosteal lesions.

Multiple hereditary exostoses (MHE) is associated with a gene mutation within which loci?

A. p53
B. NF1
C. CD99
D. EXT1

Discussion

The correct answer is (D). The EXT1, EXT2, and EXT3 genetic loci are associated with this disorder. They are tumor suppressor genes, and the risk of malignant trans-formation of one of the osteochondromas is higher in patients with this condition. Mutations in p53 are asso-ciated with other malignancies, such as osteosarcoma. NF1 mutations are associated with neurofibromatosis, and CD99 is associated with Ewing sarcoma.

Which of the following clinical scenarios is most con-cerning for potential malignant transformation?

A. Twelve-year-old male with a similar lesion of lateral distal femur, experiencing popping and snapping during stair-climbing

B. Eight-year-old female with enlarging similar lesion of proximal fibula, with radiation of numbness and tingling down anterolateral lower leg

C. Forty-five-year-old male with a similar lesion on posterior scapular spine, that is now enlarging and is starting to become uncomfortable

D. Twenty-nine-year-old female with a similar lesion of her proximal femur, that has fractured after sustaining a mechanical fall

Discussion

The correct answer is (C). Osteochondromas are benign lesions that should not grow or begin to become painful after skeletal maturity. If they do, one must be concerned for malignant transformation into an osteosarcoma and further workup is required: an MRI should first be ordered to evaluate the thickness of the cartilage cap, which if greater than 1.5 cm is concerning for, but not diagnostic of, malignancy. The patients described in choices A and B are demonstrating common presentations of osteochondromas about the knee: snapping of muscles or tendons over the lesion, as well as peroneal nerve irritation. The patient in choice D has sustained a fracture of her osteochondroma, which can occur with trauma, but is not concerning for malignancy.

Objectives: Did you learn...?

• To recognize osteochondromas on imaging?
• When to be concerned about an osteochondroma clinically?
• The relevant genetics of osteochondroma and related syndromes?

CASE 6

A 14-year-old male presents to your office with a chief complaint of swelling about the left knee and decreased range of motion. His parents have read about pediatric orthopaedic malignancy and are extremely anxious about this possibly being due to a malignant process.

Which of the following is the most common malignant bone tumor in children?

A. Ewing sarcoma
B. Chondroblastoma
C. Osteosarcoma
D. Metastatic neuroblastoma

Discussion

The correct answer is (C). Osteosarcoma is the most common malignant bone tumor in children, with 1,000 to 1,500 new cases per year in the United States. It is most common in the second decade of life, with a bimodal age distribution and a second peak in the sixth decade of life. While Ewing sarcoma and metastatic neuroblastoma are also seen frequently in children, they are not as common as osteosarcoma. Chondroblastoma is another lesion of childhood, however, it is not malignant.

The imaging finding in Figure 8–8 represents:

A. Aggressive periosteal reaction
B. Normal bone growth within the tumor
C. Calcification of soft-tissue mass associated with parosteal osteosarcoma
D. Healing callus at previous site of pathologic fracture

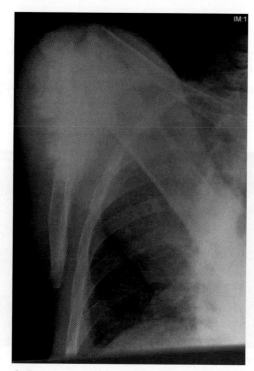

Figure 8–8

Discussion

The correct answer is (A). This characteristic imaging finding is termed "hair on end" periosteal reaction, which represents the periosteum's reaction to an aggressive, cortically destructive lesion. The imaging finding is seen in many malignant bone tumors and is not diagnostic of any one particular entity but is usually associated with a highly malignant tumor. The malignant bone production seen in parosteal osteosarcoma is more "cloudlike" in appearance and does not demonstrate the "hair on end" or "sunburst" pattern seen here, which can be seen in more aggressive osteosarcomas. An "onion-skinning" pattern can also be seen in which wisps of bone parallel to the cortex are seen in layers. This usually represents an intermediate-aggressive process which can be thought of as the bone making attempts to wall off the process repeatedly. Ewing sarcoma can often display this appearance. Healing callus at a fracture site has the appearance of mature normal bone.

Which of the following is true regarding the imaging findings in osteosarcoma?

A. Classic osteosarcomas are cortically based and extend radially

B. In skeletally immature individuals, most osteosarcomas do not extend past the epiphyseal plate

C. When they extend into the soft tissues, this mass is not visible on x-ray

D. Osteosarcomas are characterized by direct extension, and skip lesions are not seen

Discussion

The correct answer is (B). While osteosarcomas may approach the physis in skeletally immature patients, they rarely violate it and extend into the epiphysis, although this is possible. Classic osteosarcomas originate in the medullary canal and are not cortically based. There is also a category of juxtacortical osteosarcomas, which includes both periosteal and parosteal subtypes. Osteoid matrix appears as "fluffy" or "cloud-like" opacification within the tumor's soft-tissue mass. It is important to image the entire bone involved in osteosarcoma because skip lesions often exist which can change management significantly.

Objectives: Did you learn…?

- To recognize the appearance and significance of different types of radiographing findings on malignant bone imaging?
- To recognize and differentiate the subtypes of osteosarcoma?

CASE 7

An adolescent female complains of pain and swelling in her ankle. This is giving her deep pain which she can no longer tolerate. She has constant pain which does not necessarily worsen with weight bearing. Imaging and workup is performed. NSAIDs have not helped her pain.

X-rays are shown in Figure 8–9. What kind of lesion is this?

A. Osteochondroma

B. Clear cell chondrosarcoma

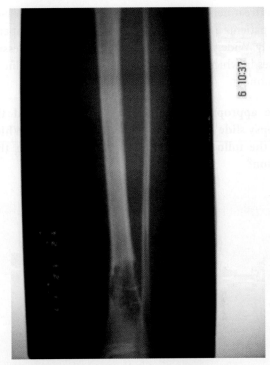

Figure 8–9

C. Chondromyxoid fibroma

D. Chondroblastoma

Discussion

The correct answer is (C). Chondromyxoid fibroma is a rare, benign bone tumor that can be locally aggressive. It appears on radiographs as a lobulated lesion demonstrating expansive remodeling with areas of thinned cortex. Generally, a thin rim of cortex can be seen at the periphery of the lesion, but in aggressive cases this may not be so. Stippled calcification can be seen suggesting a cartilaginous matrix. It tends to be central when in short tubular or flat bones, and eccentric in the metaphyseal portion of long bones. Feet are a common location. Osteochondromas project outward from the bone. Chondroblastomas are typically epiphyseal lesions. Clear cell chondrosarcoma is a rare epiphyseal cartilaginous malignancy.

What is the most appropriate treatment?

A. Wide resection and reconstruction

B. Curettage and bone grafting

C. Observation

D. Bisphosphonates

Discussion

The correct answer is (B). Curettage and bone grafting is the standard treatment for chondromyxoid fibroma.

This treatment is associated with a 25% recurrence risk, so patients must be monitored routinely postoperatively. Wide resection can be performed in aggressive cases in which curettage fails but is not the first line of treatment.

The appropriate operation is performed and the biopsy slide is shown in Figure 8–10A and B. Which of the following statements is true regarding this lesion?

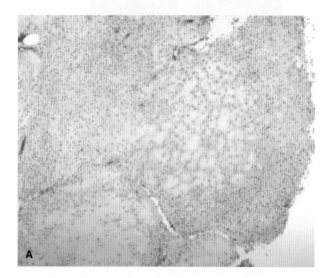

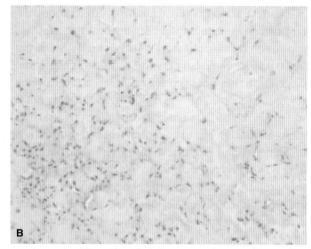

Figure 8–10 **A–B**

A. Sheets of giant cells are seen
B. The lesion demonstrates a high mitotic index
C. Chondroid, myxoid, and fibrous regions can all be seen
D. Bland fibrous cells in a storiform pattern are characteristic

Discussion

The correct answer is (C). Microscopically, the lesions consist of prominent lobular areas of cartilage with surrounding fibrous and myxoid stroma. That is, chondroid, myxoid, and fibrous areas can all be seen on one low-power slide. The bland spindle cells arrange at the periphery of the cartilage matrix. Scattered giant cells may be seen, but sheets of giant cells are more indicative of a giant cell tumor. Atypia, mitotic figures or a high mitotic index, and necrosis are not seen here but are suggestive of a malignant tumor. Bland fibrous cells in a storiform pattern suggest a nonossifying fibroma.

Objectives: Did you learn...?

• To recognize imaging and clinical features of chondromyxoid fibroma (CMF)?
• To recognize histologic features of CMF?
• The appropriate treatment of CMF?
• How to differentiate this lesion from other benign bone lesions?

CASE 8

A 40-year-old male presents with complaint of pain and swelling at the right wrist for 3 months. He works as a painter and uses his hands all day. He has been unable to paint due to decreased range of motion and severe pain in the wrist. Aspiration of the wrist is negative for infection. X-rays taken are shown in Figure 8–11A and B.

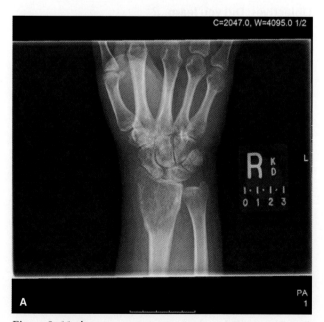

Figure 8–11 **A**

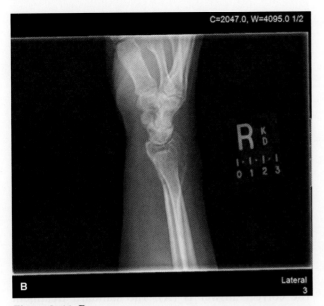

Figure 8–11 **B**

Which of the following histopathologic images (Fig. 8–12A through D) is most consistent with the lesion shown in Figure 8–11A and B?

Discussion

The correct answer is image (B). Sheets of osteoclast-like giant cells mixed with background mononuclear stromal cells are the key characteristics of giant cell tumor. The nuclei of the stroma cells are similar in size and appearance to the nuclei in the giant cells. This is typical histology of a giant cell tumor of bone.

Which of the following is a true statement regarding this lesion?

A. Despite its benign designation, a small percentage of patients develop lung metastases
B. Curettage and bone grafting is a reliable treatment, and local recurrence rate is close to zero
C. The extent of soft-tissue mass correlates with the tumor's malignancy potential
D. Fluid–fluid levels evident on MRI within the tumor suggest malignant transformation

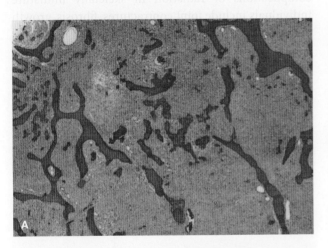

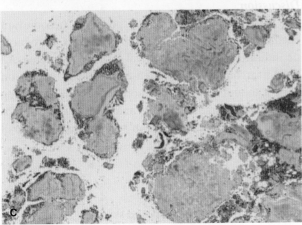

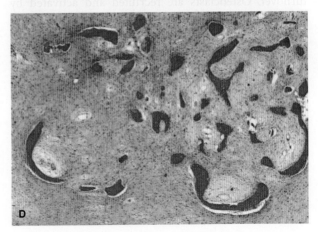

Figure 8–12 **A–D**

Discussion

The correct answer is (A). This is considered a benign but locally aggressive tumor with high rate of local recurrence. A small percentage of patients (fewer than 2%) will develop lung metastases, which are known as "benign pulmonary metastases" because they have a benign histology and generally do not compromise the patient survival as much as malignant metastases. After curettage with high-speed burr, a local adjuvant such as hydrogen peroxide, liquid nitrogen, or sterile water should be used to reduce the high local recurrence rate. These tumors can demonstrate areas of secondary intralesional aneurysmal bone cyst, evident by fluid–fluid levels on cross-sectional imaging and seen on histology.

What is the mechanism of bone destruction in this tumor?

A. Direct destruction of the bone by giant cells
B. pH imbalance caused by tumor cells resulting in alkaline phosphatase dysfunction
C. Secretion of factors by stromal cells which stimulates osteoclast recruitment and subsequent bone resorption
D. Recruitment of tumor cells by high number of giant cells which cause mechanical erosion of bony trabeculae

Discussion

The correct answer is (C). The mechanism of bone destruction in giant cell tumor is an example of a microsystem in which normal bone remodeling via the RANKL signaling pathway is upregulated causing locally increased bone resorption. That is, it is a stimulation by tumor cells of the normal mechanism of bone turnover. Osteoclasts are recruited and activated by cytokines secreted by tumor cells, and osteoclastic bone resorption is mediated by the RANKL pathway. For this reason, agents inhibiting RANKL signaling have been studied in treatment of giant cell tumor. Denosumab, an anti-RANK ligand antibody, has been recently approved for use in the treatment of this tumor.

Objectives: Did you learn…?

• To recognize the imaging and histology of giant cell tumor?
• Mechanism of tumor-mediated bone destruction?
• Treatment of giant cell tumor of bone?

CASE 9

A 15-year-old female is diagnosed with Ewing sarcoma of the tibia.

Which of the following is true regarding the treatment and prognosis of Ewing sarcoma?

A. Local control of the primary tumor can be achieved by either wide resection or external beam radiation
B. There is no role for chemotherapy in treatment of small, round blue cell tumors
C. Five-year survival for patients with isolated extremity Ewing sarcoma is 10% to 15%
D. Ewing sarcoma is one of the few musculoskeletal malignancies that can metastasize via lymph nodes

Discussion

The correct answer is (A). The standard treatment algorithm for Ewing sarcoma includes neoadjuvant chemotherapy followed by either resection or radiation therapy. Most isolated extremity lesions are treated with surgical resection rather than radiation, because complications of radiation in skeletally immature individuals include joint contractures, fibrosis, growth arrest, fracture, and secondary malignancy. Patients with isolated extremity Ewing sarcoma have a 5-year survival of 65% to 70%, and when it does metastasize, it does via hematogenous spread to the lungs, bone, or bone marrow.

Which of the following is a prognostic indicator for overall survival in Ewing sarcoma?

A. Periosteal reaction
B. Percent of necrosis after chemotherapy
C. Patient age
D. Intensity of radiotracer uptake on bone scan

Discussion

The correct answer is (B). Response to neoadjuvant chemotherapy (percent necrosis) is used as a prognostic indicator for overall survival in Ewing sarcoma. All Ewing sarcomas display intense radiotracer uptake on bone scan, and periosteal reaction is a nonspecific finding that appears in radiographs of many aggressive tumors. Patient age has not been shown to correlate with overall prognosis.

Objectives: Did you learn…?

• Ewing sarcoma treatment?
• Ewing sarcoma prognosis and staging?

CASE 10

A 24-year-old male presents to your office with a complaint of progressive dull, aching pain in his neck. Recently, he has developed sharp pain that radiates from his neck down his arm. He denies history of trauma. He denies fever or chills. X-rays of the spine are within normal limits. MR and CT are performed (Fig. 8–13).

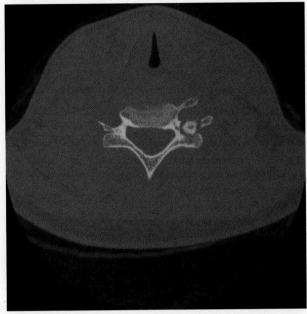

Figure 8–13

All of the following are characteristics of this lesion except:

A. Located in posterior elements of the spine

B. Can cause a painful scoliosis

C. Marked bone expansion can be seen

D. Large soft-tissue mass can impinge on exiting nerve roots

Discussion

The correct answer is (D). Osteoblastoma is a benign but locally aggressive osteoid-producing tumor. It is most common in the spine, especially the posterior elements. It is typically larger than 2 cm in diameter and on CT scan, can have central mineralization and marked bone expansion. This can cause spinal cord and nerve root impingement, as well as a painful scoliosis. Soft-tissue mass accompanying this bone-forming lesion is not typically seen.

The patient asks about surgical intervention versus nonoperative management. Is surgery indicated for this lesion, and why or why not?

A. Yes, because it has relatively high rate of malignant transformation

B. Yes, because this is an aggressive lesion that is not self-limiting

C. No, because pain is well controlled with aspirin and it is a self-limiting process that resolves spontaneously in approximately 3 years

D. No, because the lesion rarely if ever causes pain, or fracture and does not undergo malignant transformation

Discussion

The correct answer is (B). Unlike osteoid osteomas, osteoblastomas are not self-limiting and are actually quite locally aggressive. Especially in the spine, they usually cause symptoms of pain and sometimes a neurologic deficit. Treatment is curettage or marginal excision. They do not possess the potential for malignant transformation, therefore choice A is incorrect. Choice C describes a strategy for medically managing osteoid osteomas, which is not effective management of osteoblastomas.

The patient agrees to surgery. The most appropriate treatment for his osteoblastoma in the posterior elements of his spine is:

A. Wide resection alone

B. Wide resection with postoperative radiation therapy

C. Intralesional curettage with bone grafting or cementation

D. Neoadjuvant chemotherapy, then curettage and adjuvant therapy with phenol

Discussion

The correct answer is (C). Given the tumor has a predilection for the spine, the lesion is frequently found in a difficult anatomic location, often making surgery challenging. Curettage of osteoblastoma with bone grafting, or sometimes cementation, is the first-line surgical treatment. There is no role for systemic chemotherapy or radiation in first-line treatment. Wide resection is usually not necessary except in cases of recurrence, which can occur in 10% to 20% of cases.

Objectives: Did you learn...?

• To recognize clinical and imaging features of osteoblastoma?

- How to manage osteoblastoma?
- The differences between osteoid osteoma and osteoblastoma?

CASE 11

A 66-year-old man with history of retinoblastoma presents with right knee pain. AP and lateral radiographs are shown in Figure 8–14A and B.

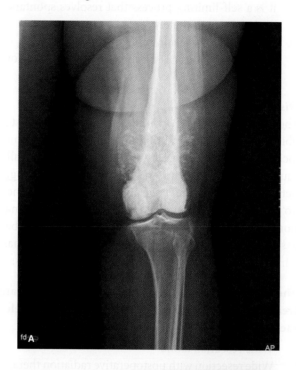

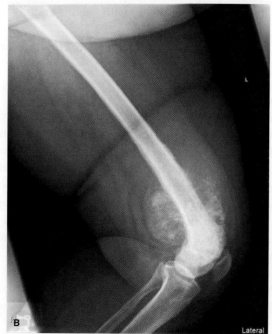

Figure 8–14 **A–B**

What is the most likely diagnosis?

A. Ewing sarcoma
B. Osteonecrosis
C. Osteomyelitis
D. Osteosarcoma

Discussion

The correct answer is (D). These x-rays reveal a bone-producing lesion in the distal femoral metadiaphysis. There is periosteal elevation and soft-tissue mass, consistent with osteosarcoma. The patient's history of retinoblastoma represents predisposition to osteosarcoma.

The patient asks about treatment recommendations. Which of the following is an accurate statement regarding management of his condition?

A. The standard treatment is neoadjuvant chemotherapy, followed by surgical resection, followed by additional adjuvant chemotherapy
B. The lesion is exquisitely radiosensitive, and management is therefore centered around radiation therapy only
C. Bone biopsy must be performed to isolate the infectious organism, and then targeted IV antibiotic therapy must be administered for 6 to 8 weeks
D. External beam radiation therapy should be performed prior to surgery, to minimize radiation dose and size of the field

Discussion

The correct answer is (A). The standard of care of classic osteosarcoma is chemotherapy, surgical resection (either limb-sparing surgery or amputation) followed by adjuvant chemotherapy. There is no role for radiation in the standard treatment of osteosarcoma. Choice C would be appropriate for osteomyelitis of the distal femur, however, x-rays shown are more consistent with malignancy as opposed to an infectious process.

Among other chemotherapeutic agents, doxorubicin is selected by the medical oncologist. What is the major toxic side effect of this drug?

A. Renal failure
B. Mucositis
C. Cardiotoxicity
D. Encephalopathy

Discussion

The correct answer is (C). Doxorubicin is a critical agent in the chemotherapeutic treatment algorithm for osteosarcoma. However, the potential for cardiotoxic side effects must be monitored. Methotrexate is associated with mucositis, ifosfamide is associated with renal failure and encephalopathy, and cisplatin is associated with neuropathy, hearing loss, and renal failure. Depending on the medical status of the patient, these drugs are commonly used individually or in combination for adjuvant chemotherapy for osteosarcoma.

Objectives: Did you learn...?

- Treatment and clinical/radiographic identification of osteosarcoma?

CASE 12

A 56-year-old male is referred to your office by his primary physician, with concern for metastatic disease. He has lytic lesions found throughout his skeleton, including in the left iliac crest and proximal femur. The iliac crest lesion is biopsied for diagnosis confirmation. Histology image is shown in Figure 8–15.

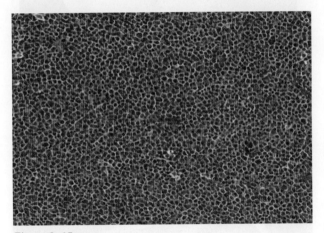

Figure 8–15

What is the correct diagnosis?

A. Ewing sarcoma
B. Metastatic prostate cancer
C. Metastatic renal cell carcinoma
D. Multiple myeloma

Discussion

The correct answer is (D). This slide shows typical features of multiple myeloma. On histopathologic examination, multiple myeloma consists of sheets of pleomorphic plasma cells with eccentric nuclei and abundant eosinophilic cytoplasm. The loose chromatin within the nucleus is arranged in the periphery, in a "clock-faced" pattern. Metastatic carcinomas have the appearance of the primary organ and can often be recognized in bone by the presence of glands, not seen in this slide. Ewing sarcoma is a small, round blue cell tumor, in which the cells have very little cytoplasm, as opposed to the abundant cytoplasm is myeloma cells.

Which immunohistochemistry stain is diagnostic for multiple myeloma?

A. CD-99
B. S-100
C. CD-28
D. Keratin

Discussion

The correct answer is (C). CD-28 is the immunohistochemistry stain associated with multiple myeloma. Ewing sarcoma is associated with CD-99 positivity, S-100 is a marker for malignant nerve sheath tumors and melanocytes, and keratin staining is nonspecific for many carcinomas.

The patient has a lytic lesion in the left proximal femur which is shown in Figure 8–16. He has pain with

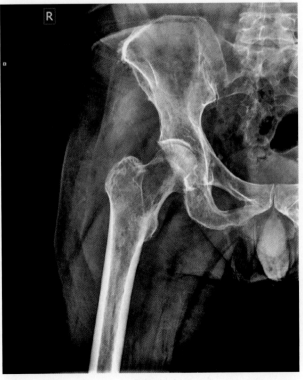

Figure 8–16

weight bearing and resultant ambulatory dysfunction. What would you recommend at this time regarding this finding?

A. Prophylactic fixation of femur with long cephalomedullary device

B. Prophylactic fixation of femur with dynamic hip screw construct

C. Cytotoxic chemotherapy in combination with dexamethasone

D. Bisphosphonate therapy

Discussion

The correct answer is (A). The patient's lytic lesion represents an impending pathologic fracture of the proximal femur, and he meets the criteria for undergoing prophylactic stabilization with a long cephalomedullary device. This is preferred to a dynamic hip screw because it provides stabilization to the entire femur, so that if a second lesion were to develop in the future in the same bone, it would not require any further surgery. If there were involvement of the femoral head, an arthroplasty procedure would be more appropriate. While multiple myeloma lesions are also treated with chemotherapy, bisphosphonates, and radiation, these treatment strategies should not replace surgical fixation of an impending fracture.

Objectives: Did you learn…?

• Histology of myeloma?

• Treatment of myeloma bone disease?

CASE 13

A 61-year-old female with several months of deep pain in the right shoulder is referred to you by her primary care physician. She presents to your office with the radiographs and an MRI is obtained (Fig. 8–17A–C).

Which of the following is true regarding the lesion shown in Figure 8–17A–C.

A. Needle biopsy is not as accurate in determining the grade as in other tumors

B. Lesions within the pelvis should be treated with neoadjuvant chemotherapy prior to resection

C. Lesions of the extremities should be treated with wide resection or amputation, regardless of their grade, because of high instance of skip lesions

D. When this lesion arises in the hand, it is especially concerning for metastasis

Discussion

The correct answer is (A). Chondrosarcoma is a malignant cartilage-producing tumor. Three grades exist, in addition to a dedifferentiated form, and histopathologic examination of these lesions is not as reliable predictor of grade as in other lesions. For this reason, evaluation of the imaging is critical in determining the appropriate management. Location is important to the diagnosis of these

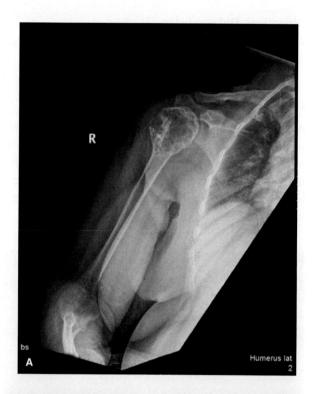

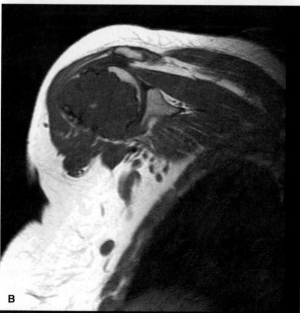

Figure 8–17 **A–B**

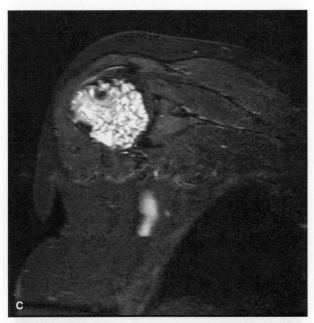

Figure 8–17 **C**

lesions; for example, lesions in the hand are most commonly benign enchondromas, while those in the scapula are more commonly malignant. These tumors have little or no sensitivity to chemotherapy and radiation; therefore surgical resection is the primary treatment. For grade 1 lesions of the extremities, which are locally aggressive but have limited, if any, potential to metastasize, intralesional curettage and bone grafting is an accepted treatment with low recurrence rate. Pelvis lesions of any grade generally have a poorer prognosis, so wide resection is preferred in the pelvis even for grade 1 chondrosarcoma.

An open surgical biopsy is performed. Biopsy slide is shown in Figure 8–18A and B. Treatment for this patient should consist of:

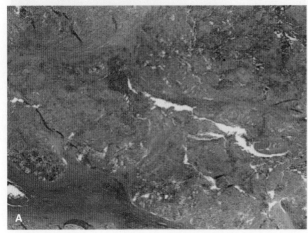

Figure 8–18 **A**

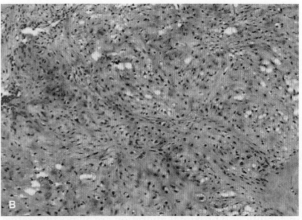

Figure 8–18 **B**

A. Preoperative radiation and wide resection with reconstruction
B. Postoperative radiation and wide resection with reconstruction
C. Preoperative chemotherapy and amputation
D. Wide resection and reconstruction

Discussion

The correct answer is (D). This is a chondrosarcoma. Figure 8–18A shows tumor surrounding all bony trabeculae, and the higher power view seen in Figure 8–18B demonstrates a very cellular tumor with pleiomorphism. Chondrosarcoma is treated with wide resection and if applicable, reconstruction. Preoperative radiation and/or chemotherapy have no usefulness in treatment of chondrosarcoma.

Postoperative x-ray is shown in Figure 8–19. Which of the following complications is seen more commonly

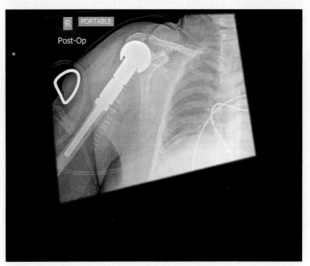

Figure 8–19

in allograft osteoarticular reconstruction than after this type of reconstruction?

A. Aseptic loosening
B. Fracture
C. Shoulder instability
D. Proximal migration

Discussion

The correct answer is (B). Allograft reconstructions of the proximal humerus have a higher rate of postoperative fracture than endoprosthetic reconstructions. However, aseptic loosening, abductor dysfunction leading to instability, and proximal migration are all postoperative problems that can be seen with endoprosthetic reconstructions of the humerus.

Objectives: Did you learn...?

- To recognize chondrosarcoma imaging?
- To recognize chondrosarcoma histology?
- Treatment of chondrosarcoma?
- Reconstructive options and pros and cons of various long bone reconstructions for malignant tumors?

CASE 14

A 34-year-old man presents to your office complaining of increasing pain in his hip and thigh. He reports that as a child, he was diagnosed with a bony growth in the area of his hip, but it never gave him trouble so no intervention was undertaken. For the past 3 months, he has been experiencing increasing deep-seated pain in this area, without history of trauma. He has had some mechanical symptoms as well with clicking and a gradual decrease in motion of his hip. He denies weakness, numbness, and tingling distally. X-rays of the femur are shown in Figure 8–20A and B.

What is particularly concerning about this patient's history and imaging?

A. Potential for malignant transformation
B. Potential for osteonecrosis
C. Potential for infection
D. Potential for permanent compressive neuropathy

Discussion

The correct answer is (A). The patient's radiographs reveal evidence of a proximal femur osteochondroma. After years of being symptom-free from this lesion, he has started to develop pain. This finding is concerning

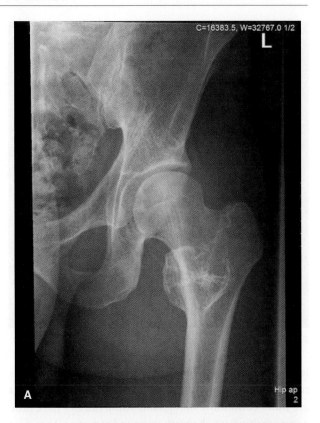

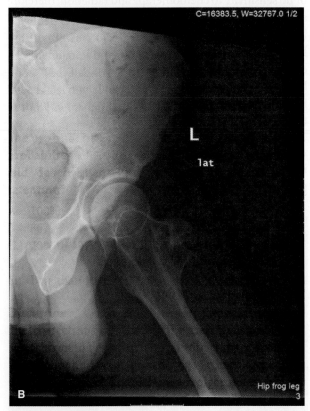

Figure 8–20 **A–B**

for malignant transformation of the lesion, which should not become painful or grow after skeletal maturity. There is no indication of osteonecrosis or infection, and he denies numbness, tingling, and weakness indicating that the lesion is likely not compressing nerves in the area. Malignant transformation of osteochondroma, although rare, is usually to a low-grade chondrosarcoma and must be monitored for.

Clear-cell chondrosarcoma is a rare subtype that has predilection for which location?

A. Flat bones: ilium and scapula
B. Pelvis and sacrum
C. Posterior elements of the spine
D. Epiphysis of long bones

Discussion

The correct answer is (D). Clear-cell chondrosarcoma is a rare subtype of chondrosarcoma, a malignant cartilage tumor. It occurs in the epiphysis of long bones, most commonly in the proximal humerus and proximal femur. It occurs in a slightly younger age group than conventional chondrosarcoma. On x-ray, a radiolucent, round, epiphyseal lesion is seen which can sometimes be mistaken for a benign chondroblastoma. Chondroblastomas usually are associated with pain, and significant bony edema around the lesion seen on T2-weighted images that are generally not seen with clear-cell chondrosarcoma.

You are seeing a patient in postoperative follow-up after hemipelvectomy and reconstruction for grade 2 chondrosarcoma. What is true regarding her long-term survival and prognosis?

A. If the tumor recurs locally, it will always increase in grade
B. Survival rate is improved with postoperative radiation therapy
C. The possibility of late progression of the disease requires long-term follow-up
D. Dedifferentiated tumors have similar survival rates and prognosis when compared with lower grade tumors

Discussion

The correct answer is (C). Long-term surveillance for both local recurrence and metastases to the lungs is recommended after chondrosarcoma resection, due to its propensity for late progression. When chondrosarcoma recurs locally, about 10% to 30% of the time the tumor increases in grade. Radiation therapy plays no role in traditional chondrosarcoma management. Overall survival depends on the grade of the tumor, with rates listed below.

Grade	Overall Survival Rate (%)
1	90
2	60–70
3	30–50
Dedifferentiated	10

Objectives: Did you learn...?

• Subtypes of chondrosarcoma?
• Staging and prognosis of chondrosarcoma?

CASE 15

A 13-year-old male presents to your clinic with 2 to 3 months of progressive pain in the elbow, as well as swelling and loss of range of motion. He also has had low-grade fevers. X-rays are shown in Figure 8–21A and B. Of note, ESR, LDH, and WBC counts are elevated on laboratory studies.

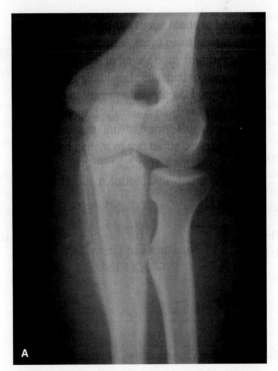

A

Figure 8–21 **A**

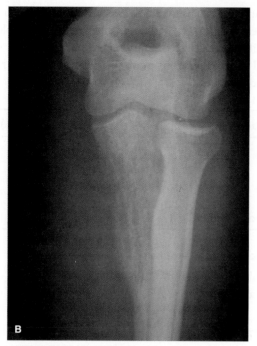

Figure 8–21 **B**

What is the likely diagnosis?

A. Osteomyelitis
B. Chondrosarcoma
C. Ewing sarcoma
D. Osteosarcoma

Discussion

The correct answer is (C). Ewing sarcoma is a malignant bone tumor composed of small, round blue cells and is the second most common primary bone tumor in children. Pain is the most common symptom, sometimes accompanied by limp, swelling, and fever. Since laboratory abnormalities (elevated WBC, ESR, and LDH) are often seen, this can be mistaken for infection. Radiographs reveal a permeative bone lesion with layered periosteal reaction, sometimes called "onion skinning." It is poorly margin-ated and permeative, accompanied often by an extensive soft-tissue mass that requires MRI to fully characterize.

What is the chromosomal translocation associated with this lesion?

A. t(11;22)
B. t(x;18)
C. t(12;16)
D. t(2;13)

Discussion

The correct answer is (A). The classic chromosomal translocation associated with Ewing sarcoma is t(11;22)

which results in the EWS/FLI1 fusion gene. This fusion can be identified by polymerase chain reaction and dif-ferentiates Ewing sarcoma from other round cell lesions. The other answers are incorrect: t(x;18) is seen in syno-vial sarcoma, t(12;16) is associated with myxoid liposar-coma, and t(2;13) is seen in alveolar soft parts sarcoma.

Which of the following histologic slides (Fig. 8–22A–D) is most consistent with this diagnosis?

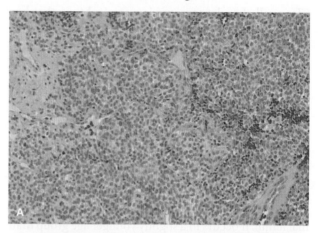

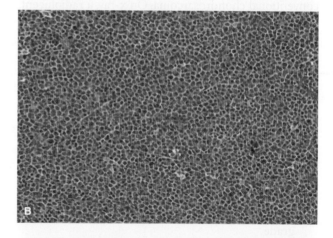

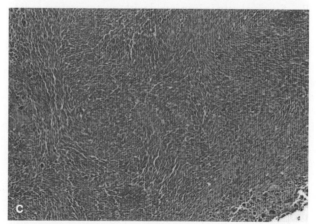

Figure 8–22 **A–C**

Figure 8–22 **D**

A. A
B. B
C. C
D. D

Discussion

The correct answer is slide (A). Histopathologic examination of Ewing sarcoma reveals small, round blue cells with prominent round or oval nuclei, and minimal cytoplasm. Slide B showed plasma cells, which in contrast to Ewing sarcoma cells, have abundant cytoplasm with eccentric clock faced nuclei. Slide C demonstrates a highly cellular synovial sarcoma, while slide D represents desmoid fibromatosis.

Which immunohistochemical stain is helpful to histologically differentiate this tumor from other marrow tumors?

A. CD31
B. CD99
C. CD34
D. S100

Discussion

The correct answer is (B). CD99 is a cell surface marker that is seen in Ewing sarcoma.

Objectives: Did you learn...?

• To recognize Ewing sarcoma imaging?
• To recognize Ewing sarcoma histology and genetics?

CASE 16

A 36-year-old female is referred to your office by her primary care physician. She has been complaining of progressive left knee pain and stiffness for the past 5 months, and an x-ray ordered by her PCP shows a lesion in the distal femur. Biopsy demonstrates a giant cell tumor of bone.

All of the following radiographic characteristics are consistent with giant cell tumor except:

A. These lesions arise in the metaphysis and can extend into the epiphysis to subchondral bone, crossing the physeal scar
B. Bone scan can be negative in approximately 30% of giant cell tumors
C. Giant cell tumor of bone can destroy the cortex and extend into the surrounding soft tissues, without maintaining a thin peripheral rim of bone
D. When involving the spine, they are located in the anterior vertebral body

Discussion

The correct answer is (B). Giant cell tumor demonstrates increased uptake on bone scan. Multiple myeloma is a case where bone scan can be falsely negative in up to 20% to 30% of cases. Giant cell tumors are eccentrically located, radiolucent lesions in the metaphysis and epiphysis of long bones that can extend to the subchondral surface with loss of a peripheral rim of bone. MRI is helpful in defining the extent of soft-tissue involvement. They are found in the anterior vertebral body when involving the spine.

Which of the following is true regarding the pathogenesis of giant cell tumor?

A. Giant cells secrete RANK ligand, which activates both the stromal cells and the neighboring osteoclasts to resorb bone
B. Recurrence rate and long-term results are similar whether local adjuvant or bone graft only is applied to curetted cavity
C. Benign metastasizing giant cell tumor commonly metastasizes to local and regional lymph nodes
D. The stromal cells represent the neoplastic cell in this lesion

Discussion

The correct answer is (D). The pathogenesis of giant cell tumor involves the secretion of RANK ligand by stromal cells, which in turn activates giant cells which possess the RANK receptor, to increase bone resorption. Denosumab, an anti-RANK ligand antibody which blocks this RANK–RANK ligand interaction, has been approved for use in treatment of this tumor. After extended curettage with high-speed burr, a local adjuvant such as hydrogen peroxide, sterile water, or liquid nitrogen has been shown to decrease the local recurrence rate. Rarely, giant cell tumor spreads hematogenously to the lungs, called benign pulmonary metastases, but is not known to metastasize to local or regional lymph nodes.

Objectives: Did you learn...?

• Clinical features and pathogenesis of giant cell tumor of bone?

CASE 17

A 62-year-old, African-American male is seen by his primary care physician. He complains of progressive soreness in his right hip, left thigh, and left proximal humerus.

What is the most common primary malignant bone tumor?

A. Osteosarcoma
B. Multiple myeloma
C. Giant cell tumor of bone
D. Chondrosarcoma

Discussion

The correct answer is (B). Multiple myeloma is a neoplastic proliferation of plasma cells producing a monoclonal protein. It is the most common primary malignancy of bone and commonly affects patients over 40 years old. It is also nearly twice as prevalent in African Americans when compared to Caucasians.

What are the common laboratory findings in multiple myeloma?

A. Normochromic, normocytic anemia, mildly elevated ESR, and hypercalcemia
B. Elevated white blood cell count, positive urine culture
C. Hypocalcemia and hyperphosphatemia
D. Abnormal iron studies and thyroid studies

Discussion

The correct answer is (A). Laboratory signs of multiple myeloma can include normochromic, normocytic anemia due to replacement of normal bone marrow by malignant plasma cells, an elevated ESR, and hypercalcemia secondary to osteoclast-mediated bone resorption at the sites of the multiple lytic areas throughout the skeleton. In addition to osteoclastogenesis that is mediated by RANKL, IL-6, and macrophage inflammatory protein-1α, osteoblastic activity is also suppressed by TNF and Dickkopf-1 (Dkk-1).

X-Rays are taken which reveal multiple sites of disease. Which of the following X-Rays (Fig. 8–23A–D) demonstrates a lesion most characteristic of myeloma?

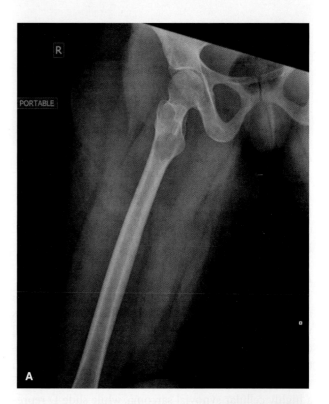

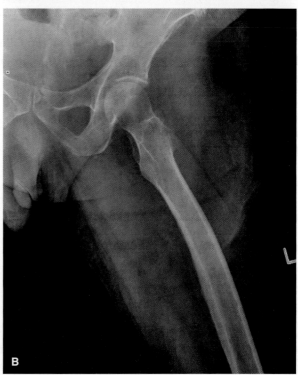

Figure 8–23 **A–B**

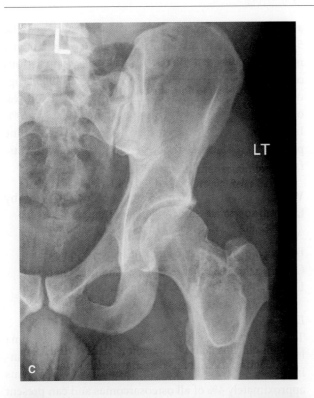

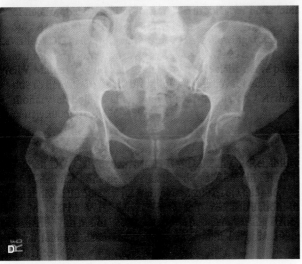

Figure 8–23 **C–D**

Discussion

The correct answer is Figure (B). On radiographs the classic appreareance of multiple myeloma is described as multiple punched out lytic lesions throughout the skeleton. Although there is a large lucent lesion in the intertrochanteric region of Figure A, the borders of this lesion are more well defined than one would expect for myeloma. The Xray in figure B shows multiple small punched out lesions particularly in the distal diaphysis that are characteristic of myeloma. Figure C had a sclerotic rim

which is more consistent with a benign tumor. Figure D represents a blastic lesion which is more consistent with a prostate or breast metastasis. Skeletal survey is the screening tool of choice to evaluate for other areas of concern, since bone scan may be negative in multiple myeloma. This is due to the minimal osteoblastic response in myeloma.

Objectives: Did you learn...?

- Clinical features, and radiology of multiple myeloma?

CASE 18

A 12-year-old patient with osteosarcoma of the proximal tibia undergoes image-guided biopsy for confirmation of diagnosis.

Which of the following histopathologic slides (Fig. 8–24A–D) is most consistent with osteosarcoma?

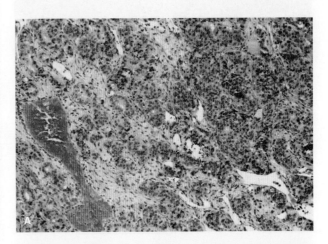

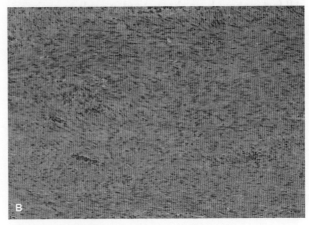

Figure 8–24 **A–B**

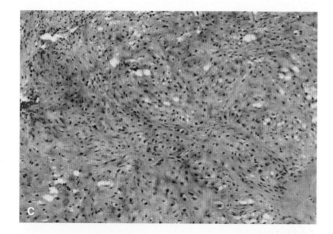

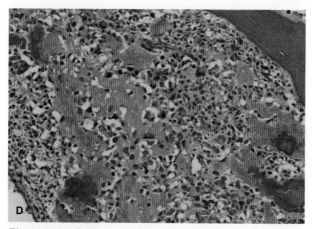

Figure 8–24 **C–D**

Discussion

The correct answer is slide (D). Histologic examination of osteosarcoma reveals "lace-like" pink osteoid formed by malignant osteosarcoma cells. The degree of pleomorphism and atypia is considerable. Areas of necrosis with few viable cells (if any) are often seen.

All factors have been shown to play a role in prognosis in osteosarcoma <u>except</u>:

A. Tumor grade
B. Dose of immediate postoperative radiation
C. Presence of skip lesions
D. Percent of necrosis after neoadjuvant chemotherapy

Discussion

The correct answer is (B). Radiation plays no role in the standard treatment of osteosarcoma. Tumor grade is the most prognostic indicator in osteosarcoma. In addition, the percentage of necrosis after adjuvant chemotherapy is related to overall survival, with >90% necrosis

associated with significantly increased survival. The 5-year survival of patients with localized osteosarcoma in an extremity is 65% to 70%, however, skip lesions occur in 10% of patients and represent a similar prognostic indicator as lung metastases. The 5-year survival of patients who present with metastatic disease is 20%. In addition, elevated lactate dehydrogenase and alkaline phosphatase have been reported to be poor prognostic factors.

Which variant of osteosarcoma is characterized by large, blood-filled cavities?

A. Parosteal osteosarcoma
B. Telangiectatic osteosarcoma
C. Periosteal osteosarcoma
D. High-grade surface osteosarcoma

Discussion

The correct answer is (B). Telangiectatic osteosarcoma is a rare histologic variant of osteosarcoma containing large, blood-filled cavernous spaces. It represents approximately 4% of all osteosarcomas and can present with pathologic fracture in 25% of cases. It appears on radiographs as a purely lytic lesion with cortical erosion, and MRI often shows fluid–fluid levels. Differential diagnosis therefore includes aneurysmal bone cyst. Treatment is the same as classic osteosarcoma.

Objectives: Did you learn...?

• Histology of osteosarcoma?
• Grading, staging, prognosis, and subtypes of osteosarcoma?

CASE 19

A 61-year-old female with progressive functional right hip pain is brought to your office by her daughter. She has recently received the diagnosis of multiple myeloma and is seeing a medical oncologist for chemotherapy and radiation to multiple lesions throughout her skeleton. She has a known myeloma lesion in the right intertrochanteric region of the femur.

Mirel criteria for risk of pathologic fracture includes all of the following parameters except:

A. Size of lesion
B. Location of lesion
C. Characteristics of pain associated with the lesion
D. Primary site of malignancy

Discussion

The correct answer is (D). Mirel score is a useful tool in the management of bone tumors and is used to identify patients who would benefit from prophylactic fixation of their bone lesion due to high enough risk of pathologic fracture. There are four criteria utilized in the scoring system: site, size, lesion characteristics, and pain characteristics. The primary source of malignancy (breast, lung, thyroid, etc.) is not included, as this has not been shown to correlate with fracture risk.

Her daughter asks about autologous stem cell transplant and overall survival with the disease.

Which of the following is the most accurate response?

A. Autologous stem cell transplant is no longer performed, since newer chemotherapy agents have improved 10-year survival rate to nearly 90%

B. Autologous stem cell transplant improves survival overall; still, the overall 10-year survival rate is only about 10%

C. Renal failure precludes a patient's ability to receive an autologous stem cell transplant

D. Autologous stem cell transplant offers a cure for multiple myeloma

Discussion

The correct answer is (B). The overall 10-year survival rate for patients with this condition is about 10%. Median survival is 3 years and prognosis is worse with renal failure. Autologous stem cell transplant has been shown to improve survival and is currently a treatment option in addition to chemotherapy, bisphosphonates, and radiation therapy.

Objectives: Did you learn...?

• To utilize Mirel scoring system to predict risk of pathologic fracture?
• Medical myeloma treatment and prognosis?

CASE 20

A 38-year-old female is referred to your office by her primary physician for a mass on her neck. It is painless and nontender to palpation. It is very firm on examination, and she reports that it has been slowly growing over 2 years. She brings an MRI ordered by her primary physician for your review (Fig. 8–25A and B).

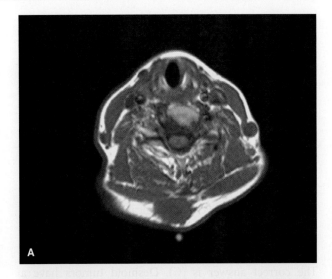

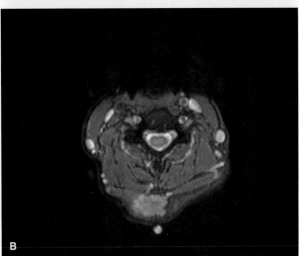

Figure 8–25 **A–B**

What is the most likely diagnosis?

A. Desmoid tumor
B. Lipoma
C. Intramuscular hemangioma
D. Heterotopic ossification

Discussion

The correct answer is (A). Desmoid tumor is a benign but locally aggressive fibrous neoplasm that is most likely located on chest wall/back, shoulder girdle, abdominal wall, and thigh. They are two to three times more common in females, and median age is in the third decade of life. They display low signal intensity on T1, low to medium signal intensity on T2, and enhancement on postgadolinium studies. The slow, benign-growing nature of this tumor, imaging studies, physical examination, and demographic of the patient all support this being a desmoid tumor over the other options. However, desmoid tumor cannot be distinguished from soft-tissue sarcoma by imaging alone, and biopsy is needed prior to resection to obtain a firm diagnosis.

What is the best description of a desmoid tumor in terms of its growth potential?

A. Self-resolving with time
B. Malignant
C. Benign but locally aggressive
D. Locally aggressive until surgical resection, then very low recurrence rate

Discussion

The correct answer is (C). Desmoid tumors have a highly infiltrative growth pattern but do not metastasize and have no risk of malignant transformation. In many cases, they may be observed. When surgical resection is necessary, these tumors are treated with wide resection. In recurrent cases, or cases where a recurrence would be particularly difficult to address, external beam radiation may be considered.

The patient undergoes resection of the desmoid tumor from her neck. A year later, the lesion begins to recur in the same area but deeper. She undergoes a second resection, but due to the concern for possible involvement of the nearby cervical spine if the tumor were to recur again, the patient is also given external beam radiation. The approximate dose of radiation to the area is:

A. 600 rad
B. 6 Gy
C. 60 Gy
D. 600 Gy

Discussion

The correct answer is (C). The total amount of postoperative radiation for soft-tissue tumors is approximately 60 Gy. The preoperative radiation dose is approximately 50 Gy, because the postoperative bed is more hypoxic and requires a higher dose of radiation to achieve the same effect. The daily dose of radiation therapy is delivered in fractions of 200 cGy per day. For heterotopic ossification prophylaxis, the dose is about 600 cGy. (1 cGy = 1 rad.)

Which of the following is associated with preoperative as opposed to postoperative radiation for soft-tissue tumors?

A. Higher dose and larger field
B. Decreased wound healing rates

C. Improved local control of tumor
D. Decreased functional outcome long term

Discussion

The correct answer is (B). Preoperative and postoperative radiation therapy are associated with equivalent local control rates for soft-tissue sarcomas. However, the side effects associated with each method differ. Preoperative radiation therapy is associated with a smaller field and lower dose, but the wound infection risk is much higher at approximately 35%. There is decreased local fibrosis seen after preoperative radiation, resulting in an improved long-term functional outcome. Postoperative radiation is associated with a much lower wound risk at approximately 15% but is associated with a higher dose over a larger field because the postoperative bed is hypoxic, and the entire incision and region of dissection must be treated. Since local control rates are the same, both delivery methods are acceptable and individual centers have established their own preferences as to which method they utilize under which circumstances.

Objectives: Did you learn...?

• Clinical and imaging features of desmoid tumor?
• Treatment options for desmoid fibromatosis?
• Differences between pre- and postoperative radiation treatment?

CASE 21

A 40-year-old male presents to your office with a chief complaint of pain and tingling down his left arm. He complains of some numbness at his fingertips. He notes that about 6 months ago, he noticed a growing lump in his upper arm. It has been growing slowly over time, and his symptoms have gotten worse. The area is relatively tender to palpation, and there is a positive Tinel sign with deep palpation of the mass, replicating his symptoms. MRI is shown in Figure 8–26A and B.

What is the likely diagnosis?

A. Angiosarcoma
B. Neurofibroma
C. Hemangioma
D. Schwannoma

Discussion

The correct answer is (D). The history suggests a nerve tumor based on the neurologic symptoms and the Tinel

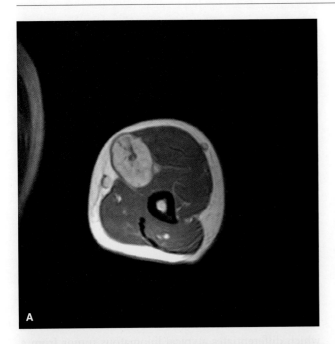

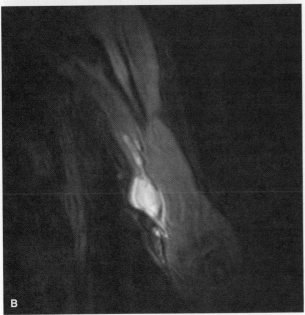

Figure 8–26 **A–B**

sign. The MRI shows characteristic findings of Schwannoma as discussed below.

Which of the following are not characteristic MRI findings?

A. Continuity with the affected nerve
B. "Split fat" sign with fat signal seen on either end of an oval mass
C. Central "target" seen on T1 images
D. Infiltrative pattern eroding into neighboring bone

Discussion

The correct answer is (D). Schwannoma is a benign soft-tissue tumor of Schwann cells. These tumors grow eccentrically from the nerve sheath and do not involve the nerve fibers themselves, therefore they can be surgically removed from the neighboring nerve, usually without causing any permanent nerve damage. Imaging studies reveal an oval mass which can often be seen to be continuous with a nerve fiber. A "split fat" sign is usually seen and can help make the diagnosis. These tumors demonstrate low signal intensity on T1 and high signal intensity on T2, with diffuse gadolinium enhancement. A central target may be seen on T1-weighted images, which is well demonstrated in this study. The tumor can produce peripheral nerve symptoms, and are generally firm and quite painful. Tapping the tumor with a finger can reproduce the nerve symptoms, which is called a Tinel sign. These tumors are benign and do not grow in an infiltrative pattern into neighboring bone.

Histologic examination performed on an incisional biopsy sample from the lesion reveals palisading and distinct Antoni A and Antoni B areas. What staining antibody could be used to support the diagnosis?

A. CD-28
B. S-100
C. CD-99
D. Schwann cells disintegrate with immunohistochemical staining, therefore no test is indicated

Discussion

The correct answer is (B). Schwannomas and other nerve tumors strongly stain positive for the S100 antibody. Although S-100 is not diagnostic of schwannoma, in the setting of appropriate imaging and histology, it is supportive of the diagnosis. CD-28 is used to aid in the diagnosis of multiple myeloma, and CD-99 is associated with Ewing sarcoma.

Objectives: Did you learn...?

• Clinical and imaging features of schwannoma?
• Histological features of schwannoma?

CASE 22

A 19-year-old female presents to your office complaining of an enlarging mass over her right anterolateral deltoid. On examination, she has a visible soft-tissue lump over the anterolateral aspect of her shoulder. It is relatively nontender to palpation and has some mobility with relation to the underlying muscle. There is no overlying skin problem. She denies numbness, tingling, or weakness distally. She has no complaints other than the mass is visible and would like it removed. MRI is shown in Figure 8–27.

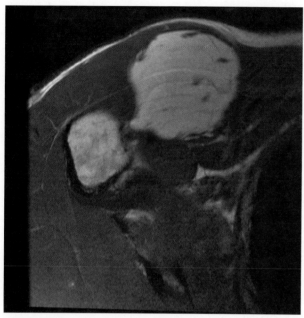

Figure 8–27

Based on the MRI result, which of the following is true?

A. She should have it removed, with histology and genetic testing of the specimen

B. Due to high recurrence rate, it should not be removed

C. She should get preoperative radiation followed by wide resection

D. Over time the lesion will regress on its own, and it should be treated with conservative symptomatic treatment

Discussion

The correct answer is (A). The MRI demonstrates a lipoma, which is a benign tumor of fat. In this case, the tumor is located in the deltoid musculature. There are fibrous septae and blood vessels within the lesion that could indicate an atypical lipomatous tumor (ALT). If any atypia is seen on histology, MDM-2 FISH testing should be performed, which is positive in ALTs. Since this is a large deep lesion, it should be removed and tested. Atypical lipomatous tumors do not metastasize but can recur. In a small percentage of cases, these tumors can dedifferentiate into a malignant tumor.

She proceeds with surgery, and the lesion is found on final pathology report to be MDM2-positive. What should you tell her at her follow-up visit?

A. She will need to return to the operating room for repeat wide resection

B. This is an atypical lipomatous tumor that has a higher recurrence rate than a typical lipoma, therefore should be watched with surveillance imaging more frequently and for longer duration than a typical lipoma

C. She will be referred to a medical oncologist to discuss this positive test

D. She should get radiation to the area since this test was positive

Discussion

The correct answer is (B). MDM2 is a marker that can be tested for by fluorescence in situ hybridization (FISH), which differentiates atypical lipomatous tumor from a plain lipoma. Atypical lipomas have a higher local recurrence rate, up to 50% at 10 years but do not metastasize. These tumors can be removed with marginal excision, however, patients should be followed more closely and for longer duration than lipoma patients due to the higher recurrence rate. These tumors do not require wide resection, chemotherapy, or radiation.

Objectives: Did you learn…?

• Clinical and imaging features of lipoma?

• To differentiate between lipoma and atypical lipomatous tumor, both clinically and genetically?

CASE 23

An athletic 24-year-old male is referred from his doctor's office for an abnormal finding on radiographs of his shoulder. His only recent history is that 6 weeks ago he sustained a direct blow to the shoulder by a pitch during a baseball game. The patient has noticed a firm mass in this area, which has been growing in size, and x-rays taken yesterday reveal a mass in the soft tissue of the shoulder. X-rays are shown in Figure 8–28A and B.

What is the most likely diagnosis, based on history, physical examination, and radiographs?

A. Intramuscular hemangioma

B. Ewing sarcoma

C. Parosteal osteosarcoma

D. Myositis ossificans

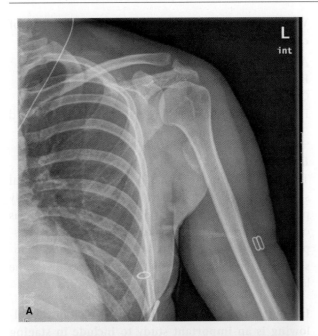

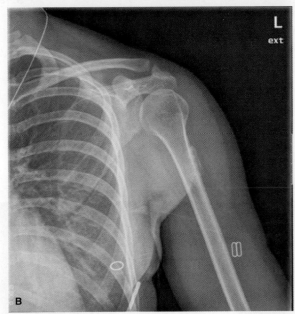

Figure 8–28 **A–B**

Discussion

The correct answer is (D). Myositis ossificans is a reactive process characterized by a well-circumscribed proliferation of fibroblasts, cartilage, and bone within a muscle, thought to be due to maturation and mineralization of a hematoma or bleeding into the muscle. It is a posttraumatic condition, and presents with pain, tenderness, swelling, and a growing firm mass within the soft tissues. Radiographic examination reveals an irregular, fluffy density in the soft tissues, which develops over time into increased peripheral mineralization

and a radiolucent center. This peripheral pattern of mineralization has been called to a "rose" pattern.

What is the natural history of this lesion?

A. It is a self-limited process
B. It is benign but locally aggressive and can erode nearby cortex or destroy nearby joints
C. It has high metastatic potential
D. It does have a low risk of benign metastasis to lungs

Discussion

The correct answer is (A). Myositis ossificans is a self-limited, benign process, so observation and physical therapy to maintain motion are indicated. This is a diagnosis that can be made on history, physical examination, and radiology studies most of the time, without need for biopsy.

Management at this point should consist of:

A. Biopsy followed by wide excision
B. Radiation followed by wide excision
C. Physical therapy and observation, with repeat radiographs
D. Chest CT and wide excision if CT is negative

Discussion

The correct answer is (C). Physical therapy and observation are the only necessary treatments indicated at this point. Physical therapy will maintain range of motion of the shoulder, as this lesion can be painful, and patients will self-limit their physical activity. Often, the size of the mass decreases after 1 year. Follow-up radiographs must be conducted to confirm maturation and stability of the lesion. Excision is only indicated once the lesion is mature (6–12 months) and only if the patient is symptomatic. Local recurrence rates increase if excision is performed in the initial stages.

Follow-up x-rays are obtained in 3-month intervals for the next 6 months. What would you expect to see?

A. Progressive mineralization of the periphery with a radiolucent center, followed by eventual mineralization of the center then resolution
B. Progressive growth and eventual destruction of the neighboring femoral cortex
C. Persistence of the mineralized mass without change over time
D. Pathologic fracture of the humerus

Discussion

The correct answer is (A). The radiographic characteristics of myositis ossificans evolve in a predictable pattern. The lesion initially appears as an irregular, fluffy density in the soft tissues. Over time, it organizes into a zonal pattern, displaying rimmed mineralization of the periphery with a radiolucent center. Eventually, the center will mineralize, and eventually the lesion will regress. Monitoring this predictable pattern gives reassurance that the lesion is indeed myositis ossificans.

Objectives: Did you learn...?

• To identify important tumor mimickers: infection, myositis ossificant?
• Imaging features of myositis ossificans?
• Treatment of myositis ossificans?

CASE 24

An 81-year-old female is brought to your office by her son. She has been treated for bilateral knee osteoarthritis for the past year by her primary care physician. A recent MRI was conducted and was concerning for an incidentally found 12-cm soft-tissue mass in her posterior thigh. She denies pain in this area but does admit to feeling a deep mass in the back of her thigh when she sits down. X-ray and MRI images are shown in Figure 8–29A and B.

Which soft-tissue sarcomas can exhibit areas of calcification?

A. Rhabdomyosarcoma and liposarcoma
B. Liposarcoma and synovial sarcoma
C. Fibrosarcoma and clear cell sarcoma
D. Malignant peripheral nerve sheath tumor and leiomyosarcoma

Discussion

The correct answer is (B). Liposarcoma and synovial sarcoma can show foci of calcification. In an elderly patient with a painless, enlarging soft tissue mass, areas of calcification on plain radiograph should raise suspicion for one of these two malignancies. Since liposarcoma is more common in this age group, this is the leading diagnosis for this patient based on imaging.

In addition to a standard chest CT, which of the following is an important study to include in staging workup of myxoid liposarcoma?

A. Lymph node biopsy
B. Head CT
C. Abdomen/pelvis CT
D. Renal function tests

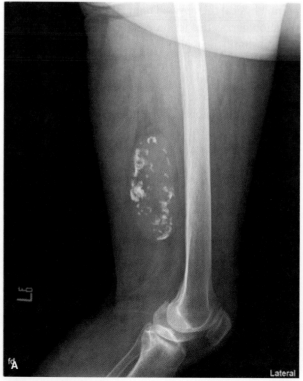

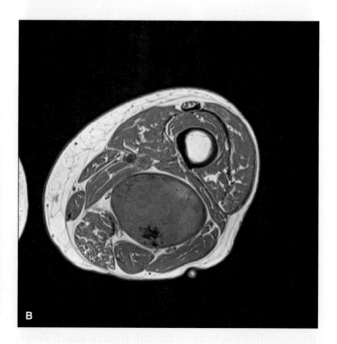

Figure 8–29 **A–B**

Discussion

The correct answer is (C). Myxoid liposarcomas have metastatic patterns that can differ from other sarcomas and have a propensity to metastasize to the retroperitoneum. Therefore, staging for this tumor should include a CT scan of the abdomen and pelvis in addition to a CT of the chest.

If staging workup does not show any evidence of metastases, what is the most appropriate treatment to recommend for the thigh lesion?

A. Chemotherapy and surgery, as these tumors are chemosensitive
B. Radiation only, as these tumors are extremely radiation-sensitive
C. Radiation and wide surgical resection
D. Chemotherapy and hip disarticulation

Discussion

The correct answer is (C). Wide surgical resection plus radiation is the treatment for large, deep extremity liposarcoma. If wide resection is not achievable, amputation can be considered. Due to the patients advanced age and the limited sensitivity of this tumor to chemotherapy, she is unlikely to benefit from chemotherapy.

After full laboratory and imaging workup, a biopsy is performed with image guidance. Pathology report confirms diagnosis of high-grade pleomorphic liposarcoma. It also reveals lesions in the lungs that are biopsied and shown to be metastasis. What stage does this represent, based on the American Joint Committee on Cancer (AJCC) Staging system for soft-tissue sarcoma?

A. III
B. IIA
C. IV
D. IIB

Discussion

The correct answer is (C). If distant metastases are present, this automatically categorizes the patient as stage IV. The presence of metastases is the most important prognostic factor in soft-tissue sarcoma staging. Other criteria important for AJCC staging include grade, size of the tumor, and regional lymph node involvement.

Objectives: Did you learn...?

• Clinical and imaging features of liposarcoma?
• Staging evaluation of liposarcoma?
• Treatment of liposarcoma?

CASE 25

A 33-year-old male presents to your office with a slow-growing area of swelling that he has noticed about the medial aspect of his ankle for the past 18 months. It is nontender, and he reports no history of trauma. He has received several injections into the ankle by his primary care provider, with no relief from the swelling. Extensive workup has been negative, and x-rays reveal small areas of calcification in the area anterior to the medial malleolus. MRI reveals a soft-tissue mass in the anteromedial ankle area, which is low intensity on T1-weighted images and high intensity on T2-weighted imaging.

You are concerned for a soft-tissue sarcoma. Which of the following is the most common soft-tissue sarcoma found in the foot and ankle region?

A. Epithelioid sarcoma
B. Synovial sarcoma
C. Angiosarcoma
D. Leiomyosarcoma

Discussion

The correct answer is (B). Synovial sarcoma is the most common soft-tissue sarcoma found in the foot and ankle region.

In addition to a staging workup you order an image-guided biopsy. The slide is shown in Figure 8–30. What is this patient's diagnosis?

A. Epithelioid sarcoma
B. Synovial sarcoma
C. Angiosarcoma
D. Leiomyosarcoma

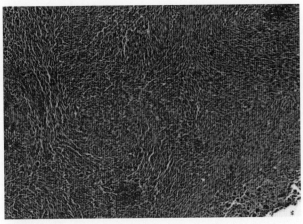

Figure 8–30

Discussion

The correct answer is (B). Histology of a synovial sarcoma shows a monophasic or biphasic pattern of cuboid epithelioid cells (lower right of slide and scattered areas) and fibrosarcoma-like spindle cells (remainder of slide). The epithelial cells are arranged in nests or chords, and the fibrous component involves plump, malignant spindle cells within minimal cytoplasm and dark nuclei.

Which of the following immunohistochemical stains is used to support this diagnosis?

A. Keratin
B. S-100
C. Intracellular melanin
D. Collagen

Discussion

The correct answer is (A). Synovial sarcoma stains positive with keratin. S-100 is positive in nerve tumors. With appropriate staining, intracellular melanin is noted in about 50% of patients with clear cell sarcoma.

What is the chromosomal translocation in synovial sarcoma, and what fusion products result from this translocation?

A. t(12;22); EWS-ATF1
B. t(12;16); CHOP-TLS
C. t(11;22); EWS-FLI1
D. t(x;18); SYT-SSX

Discussion

The correct answer is (D). The fusion product SYT-SSX1 or SYT-SSX2 is the result of a balanced chromosomal translocation t(x;18) in synovial sarcoma. Choice A represents the translocation associated with clear-cell sarcoma. Choice B represents the translocation in myxoid liposarcoma, and choice C represents the translocation in Ewing sarcoma.

Objectives: Did you learn...?

- To recognize synovial sarcoma imaging and histology?
- Synovial sarcoma genetics and immunohistochemical staining?

CASE 26

A 60-year-old male is diagnosed with a 6-cm deep high-grade undifferentiated pleomorphic sarcoma (UPS) of the soft tissue of his upper arm.

What is true about this malignancy?

A. It is the most common soft-tissue sarcoma in adults 55 to 80 years of age

B. It is derived from a neurovascular bundle, therefore neurologic symptoms are common
C. The balanced translocation associated with this malignancy is t(12;16)
D. Overall survival at 5 years is 95% if negative margins can be achieved

Discussion

The correct answer is (A). This diagnosis represents the most common soft-tissue sarcoma in adults 55 to 80 years of age. Although these tumors may involve nerves or vessels, UPS is not necessarily derived from a nerve or vessel, unlike MPNST or angiosarcoma. The translocation t(12;16) is associated with myxoid liposarcoma; there is no specific genetic defect associated with UPS, rather it is the category in which all sarcomas that are not otherwise specifically identified fall. Treatment is radiation and wide surgical resection, with chemotherapy in selected cases, and overall 5-year survival is 50% to 60%. UPS was formerly called MFH, or malignant fibrous histiocytoma, which is a term that is no longer used by modern sarcoma pathologists and is no longer acceptable nomenclature.

You recommend external beam radiation in conjunction with wide resection as treatment. Which of the following is true regarding external beam radiation therapy?

A. Postoperative radiation is associated with higher risk of wound-healing complications
B. Postoperative radiation is associated with a higher dose of irradiation
C. Preoperative radiation is associated with a higher risk of long-term fibrosis
D. Preoperative radiation is associated with a wider field of radiation

Discussion

The correct answer is (B). External beam radiation can be administered preoperatively or postoperatively with equivalent local control rates. Preoperative XRT followed by wide surgical resection is associated with a higher risk of wound-healing complications, a lower risk of long-term fibrosis, and a lower total dose of irradiation, administered to a smaller anatomical field.

Undifferentiated pleomorphic sarcoma (UPS) can develop as a secondary malignancy in each of the following except:

A. Fibrous dysplasia
B. Radiation to an area for treatment of a prior malignancy

C. Osteochondroma

D. Bone infarct

Discussion

The correct answer is (C). UPS of bone or soft tissue has been associated as a secondary lesion with fibrous dysplasia, bone infarcts, Paget sarcoma, and postradiation. Chondrosarcoma can develop as result of malignant transformation of osteochondroma.

Objectives: Did you learn...?

- Clinical features of undifferentiated pleomorphic sarcoma?

CASE 27

A 49-year-old female with several vertebral compression fractures presents to your office with an MRI of the spine concerning for metastatic disease. She is sent for CT of the chest, abdomen, and pelvis; whole-body bone scan; and several laboratory studies, and she returns today. CT scan and bone scan reveal several other concerning lesions, including one in the right iliac wing and left proximal humerus, but the CT fails to reveal any visceral masses. Laboratory studies are inconclusive.

What is the next best step in obtaining a diagnosis?

A. Image-guided needle biopsy from the iliac wing lesion

B. Open biopsy of vertebral body lesions, with decompression and fusion

C. Seeking medical oncology consultation

D. CT scan of the head

Discussion

The correct answer is (A). After appropriate imaging and laboratory studies have been conducted, an image-guided needle biopsy is indicated to achieve tissue diagnosis. Most studies document a greater than 90% yield and accuracy of guided needle biopsies. Although in some cases of primary bone and soft-tissue neoplasms, the diagnosis may require more tissue than can be obtained from a needle biopsy. For suspected metastatic disease, it is usually an effective way of obtaining a diagnosis without significant insult to the patients overall treatment. In this case, needle biopsy may be performed at the site of iliac wing metastases, as these are fairly superficial in location. An open biopsy of the spine is a far more invasive procedure, and decompression

and fusion is not indicated at this time as she has no cord compression and her primary malignancy is unknown.

Needle biopsy is performed by a musculoskeletal radiologist under CT guidance. The pathology report comes back as viable bone and cartilage, no evidence of malignancy. You suspect that the biopsy needle was in an inappropriate location, and you decide to perform an open biopsy of the iliac wing lesion. Which of the following is <u>not</u> a principle of open biopsy?

A. Use of drains in line with the incision, exiting the skin close to the incision

B. Intermuscular approach with complete exposure and protection of nearby neurovascular structures

C. Meticulous hemostasis with electrocautery

D. Limited longitudinal incision

Discussion

The correct answer is (B). While most orthopaedic operations are performed through an internervous interval, one of the principles of open biopsy is to perform the procedure in an area that can be subsequently resected to remove any contamination, which is more commonly an intramuscular approach. A limited longitudinal incision should be used, with attention paid to meticulous hemostasis. Exposure of neurovascular structures is avoided to prevent contamination of those structures. Drains are used to prevent hematoma formation and subsequent contamination.

Objectives: Did you learn...?

- The differences between needle biopsy and open surgical biopsy?
- The principles of open surgical biopsy?

CASE 28

A 27-year-old male patient presents to your office for a second opinion. He has been seen for left knee pain. For the past 6 months, his knee has been episodically swelling and giving him pain, with no antecedent traumatic event. He has had several aspirations which have been bloody. He has already had a diagnostic arthroscopy and was able to biopsy synovial tissue. The patient brings with him the pathology slides from this biopsy (Fig. 8–31).

What is the patient's diagnosis?

A. Synovial hemangioma

B. Synovial chondromatosis

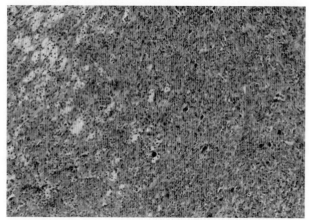

Figure 8–31

C. Rheumatoid arthritis
D. Pigmented villous nodular synovitis (PVNS)

Discussion

The correct answer is (D). This patient has PVNS of the knee. Histologic study of the synovium in PVNS on low-power view reveals rounded nodular aggregates and numerous finger-like, villous projections. Higher power reveals diagnostic mononuclear stromal cell infiltrate within the synovium: these cells are round with large nuclei and eosinophilic cytoplasm. There is prominent brown hemosiderin deposition, which differentiates this condition from others associated with synovitis. Hemosiderin-laden macrophages, multinucleated giant cells, and foam cells are also present but not required for diagnosis.

His arthroscopy revealed diffuse PVNS throughout the knee, and further surgery was recommended. He asks your recommendation in terms of treatment. What is the best response?

A. Treatment for diffuse PVNS is aggressive total synovectomy, using arthroscopic, open, or combined arthroscopic/open techniques
B. New chemotherapy regimens have made surgical resection obsolete
C. External beam radiation can be utilized as an alternative treatment to surgery, as PVNS is exquisitely radiosensitive
D. Aggressive synovectomy achieves virtually a zero recurrence rate

Discussion

The correct answer is (A). Arthroscopic or open treatment can be pursued for removal of a focal PVNS lesion.

The diffuse form requires aggressive total synovectomy using techniques that allow adequate exposure to the anterior and posterior knee; often an open approach is required posteriorly. High rates of recurrence exist, even with extensive synovectomy. Following multiple recurrences, external beam radiation is occasionally used and may lower the risk of further local recurrence. While some biologics are currently in clinical trial stages for PVNS, there is no definitive medical management that replaces surgical synovectomy.

If left untreated, which of the following will occur?

A. Eventual resolution
B. Metastasis
C. Bone and joint erosion and destruction
D. Development in contralateral knee

Discussion

The correct answer is (C). PVNS is a benign condition, although a few case reports have documented rare metastatic disease. PVNS is almost exclusively a monoarticular process and is generally not found in more than one joint, even over time. PVNS does not resolve on its own but rather progresses to eventual erosion of the bone and cartilage, with eventual joint destruction.

Objectives: Did you learn...?

• Natural history of PVNS?
• To recognize histologic features of PVNS?
• Treatment of PVNS?

CASE 29

A 45-year-old male presents to your office with right hip pain. The pain worsens with activity and started indolently about 2 years ago, without a preceding traumatic event. He also reports clicking and catching of the hip joint. He is worried that he has osteoarthritis and is anxious about getting a hip replacement at such a young age. X-rays are shown in Figure 8–32A and B.

Based on these x-rays, what is his most likely diagnosis?

A. PVNS
B. Destructive osteoarthritis
C. Chondrosarcoma
D. Synovial chondromatosis

Discussion

The correct answer is (D). Synovial chondromatosis is a metaplastic proliferation of hyaline cartilage nodules in

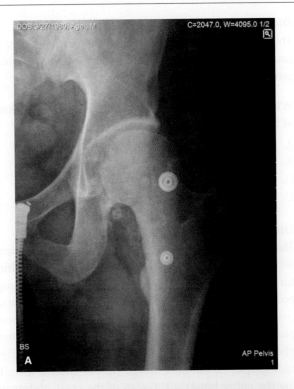

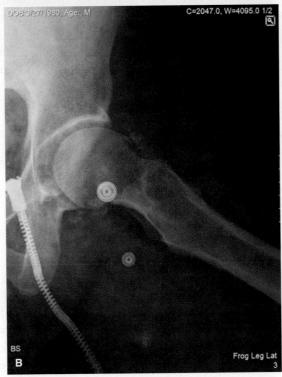

Figure 8–32 **A–B**

the synovial membrane. It causes pain and mechanical symptoms such as clicking, popping, and stiffness. It is most common in the hip and knee but has been reported in other joints. Initially the cartilage nodules are not visible on plain radiographs, and MR is required to visualize them. However, over time, the nodules calcify and become radiopaque. Erosions and joint destruction can occur over time.

What should you tell him about the natural history of his condition?

A. It is generally a benign process, but one that can damage the joint

B. It is a locally aggressive tumor that must be followed with serial radiographs and should be excised only if it appears suspicious for malignant transformation

C. The most common presentation of this condition is recurrent atraumatic hemarthroses, but it can occasionally present with these radiographic findings

D. Xanthine oxidase-inhibiting medications such as allopurinol should be started to prevent recurrence

Discussion

The correct answer is (A). Synovial chondromatosis is a benign metaplastic process. The calcified nodules within a tight joint space can be extremely destructive to the cartilage surfaces of the joint and therefore either open or arthroscopic synovectomy and loose body removal is recommended when this condition is diagnosed; for this reason, observation is not recommended. Malignant transformation has been reported, but is extremely rare. PVNS commonly presents with recurrent atraumatic hemarthroses. Xanthine oxidase inhibitors treat gout, not synovial chondromatosis.

Objectives: Did you learn...?

• To recognize clinical features and radiology of synovial chondromatosis?

• Natural history and etiology of synovial chondromatosis?

CASE 30

A left-hand-dominant, 66-year-old female is sent to your office for shoulder pain, possibly a rotator cuff tear. She has pain in her left shoulder and upper arm that is limiting her ability to use the extremity. It is exacerbated by weight bearing, although it does hurt her at night when she tries to sleep as well. She also reports a 30-lb weight loss in the past year. On examination, impingement signs are negative, although she does report pain in the upper arm when it is loaded or palpated.

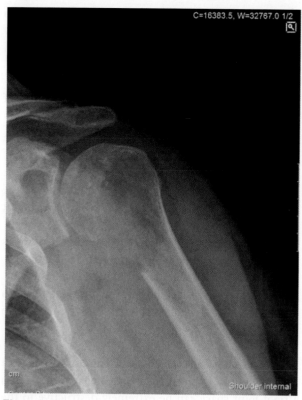

Figure 8–33

X-ray of her right shoulder is shown in Figure 8–33. What is the most likely cause of her shoulder pain?

A. Impending fracture through metastatic lesion in the proximal humerus
B. Osteoarthritis
C. Rotator cuff tear
D. Primary bone tumor of the proximal humerus

Discussion

The correct answer is (A). Metastatic bone disease is the most common reason for destructive bone lesions in adults. More than 1.4 million cases of cancer per year are diagnosed in the United States, and bone metastases develop in about 50% of patients. In this case, an impending fracture of the proximal humerus is responsible for the pain, based on the destructive imaging features.

Which of the following is unlikely to be the primary cancer site?

A. Breast
B. Kidney
C. Lung
D. Uterus

Discussion

The correct answer is (D). The most common primary cancer sites that metastasize to bone are breast, thyroid, prostate, lung, and kidney.

Which of the following is not included in the workup of an older patient with a destructive bone lesion?

A. CT scan of chest, abdomen, pelvis
B. Liver function tests
C. Electrolyte panel
D. Whole-body bone scan

Discussion

The correct answer is (B). The workup of an older patient with a destructive bone lesion includes a thorough history and physical examination (focusing on breast, lung, prostate, thyroid, and lymph nodes), electrolyte panel (with calcium), prostate-specific antigen, alkaline phosphatase, complete blood count, serum protein electrophoresis/urine protein electrophoresis, urinalysis, plain radiographs of the bone lesion (in two planes, including the entire bone), a CT scan of the chest, abdomen, and pelvis, and a whole-body bone scan. In up to 85% of patients, this workup will reveal the primary site of malignancy. Liver function tests are not routinely included in this workup, as hepatocellular cancer rarely metastasizes to bone.

Objectives: Did you learn...?

• To recognize metastatic bone disease on imaging?
• The workup of a patient who presents with a bone lesion?
• The common sites of primary disease which spreads to bone?

CASE 31

A 59-year-old male who has not seen a physician in 10 years reports to your office for ambulatory dysfunction secondary to right hip pain. It is related to activity and has been progressive for the past 4 months, to the point where it hurts whenever he walks. He is afraid he is developing osteoarthritis and will need a total hip replacement. X-rays reveal a blastic lesion in the right proximal femur.

What is the most likely diagnosis?

A. Metastatic renal cell carcinoma
B. Paget disease
C. Metastatic prostate cancer
D. Metastatic lung cancer

Discussion

The correct answer is (C). In a male patient over the age of 40 with blastic bone lesions, metastatic prostate cancer is the primary diagnostic consideration. For a male, the most common primary sites that result in blastic metastases are prostate and bladder. Especially since this patient hasn't been undergoing yearly prostate checks, his presentation is worrisome for metastatic prostate cancer.

In females, the most common primary malignancy resulting in mixed lytic and blastic bony metastases is:

A. Uterine
B. Ovarian
C. Lung
D. Breast

Discussion

The correct answer is (D). Breast cancer commonly develops lytic or mixed (lytic and blastic) bony metastases in females.

The patient denies history of malignancy, however, on further questioning he also reports progressive axial low back pain. Imaging is performed which demonstrates numerous spinal metastases. The presence of which anatomic structure results in a high frequency of metastatic lesions occurring in the spine?

A. Intervertebral discs
B. Batson venous plexus
C. Artery of Adamkiewicz
D. Cerebrospinal fluid

Discussion

The correct answer is (B). Baston venous plexus is a valveless plexus of veins around the spine that is believed to allow tumor cells easy access to the vertebral bodies.

Which of the following statements is true?

A. Lytic metastases have the same risk of fracture as blastic metastases
B. Blastic metastases have the same risk of fracture as normal bone
C. Mixed metastases are not at risk for fracture since the blastic areas strengthen the bone which cancels the effect of the lytic areas
D. Blastic metastases have a risk of pathologic fracture, but the risk is lower than lytic metastases

The correct answer is (D). Both lytic and blastic metastases can cause pathologic fracture. However, the risk is higher with lytic metastases, as demonstrated by the increased weighting in Mirel scoring system. Patients with blastic metastases and weight-bearing pain should be treated for impending fracture, in a similar fashion to patients with lytic mets.

Objectives: Did you learn...?

- Etiology of blastic metastases in men and women?
- Clinical features of blastic metastases?
- Anatomic considerations leading to metastatic bone disease?

CASE 32

A 49-year-old female with stage IV breast cancer presents to your office with worsening left hip pain. A recent bone scan ordered by her oncologist identifies multiple lesions in the spine, right humeral shaft, left clavicle, right ilium, and left proximal femur. She recently underwent radiation to the spine, left proximal femur, and right humeral shaft.

Which of the following is not included in Mirel scoring system?

A. Size of the lesion
B. Pain associated with the lesion
C. Lytic or blastic characteristics of the lesion
D. History of radiation to the lesion

Discussion

The correct answer is (D). Mirel scoring system is used to predict the risk of pathologic fracture in patients with metastatic bone lesions. The four criteria used to judge the risk are: radiographic appearance (blastic/mixed/lytic), size of the lesion (as a proportion of the shaft diameter), site, and characteristics of pain.

What is the mechanism behind bone destruction in a metastatic lesion, such as the one in these x-rays?

A. Tumor cells destroy the bone through direct extension into bone
B. Tumor cells stimulate osteoclasts to resorb bone
C. Tumor cells engulf cells comprising the bony trabeculae
D. an inflammatory response to tumor metastasis in the bone causes secretion of osteoclast-stimulating cytokines

Discussion

The correct answer is (B). Tumor cells secrete cytokines that stimulate the RANKL pathway; osteoclasts have RANK receptors for RANKL. Osteoblasts upregulate their secretion of RANKL within metastatic lesions, causing an upregulation in osteoclast precursors and eventually increased bone destruction.

What intervention would you recommend for her hip?

A.   Prophylactic fixation with long cephalomedullary nail

B.   Prophylactic fixation with short cephalomedullary nail

C.   Prophylactic fixation with dynamic hip screw device with two-hole plate

D.   Protected weight-bearing restriction and observation

Discussion

The correct answer is (A). The patient has an impending fracture, therefore she is indicated to have the lesion stabilized with a long cephalomedullary device. In prophylactic fixation, in cases of metastases, it is recommended to use an implant which protects the entire bone, such as a long intramedullary nail, in anticipation of potential development of another lesion elsewhere in the bone.

Objectives: Did you learn…?

•   Mirel scoring system?

•   RANKL pathway?

CASE 33

An 80-year-old female presents to your office with newly diagnosed lung cancer. She has multiple skeletal metastases. She complains of pain in the thoracic and lumbar spine as well as in the left tibia; she has several lytic lesions in these areas. She also complains of abdominal pain and some weakness.

What is the most likely metabolic abnormality that explains these symptoms?

A.   Anemia

B.   Hyponatremia

C.   Hyperkalemia

D.   Hypercalcemia

Discussion

The correct answer is (D). Hypercalcemia is present in 10% to 15% of cases of metastatic bone disease. It is especially common with lung and breast cancer. Symptoms include polyuria, polydipsia, anorexia, weakness, fatigue, and nausea/vomiting. Depression, irritability, coma, pruritus, and vision abnormalities are late symptoms.

She asks about bisphosphonate therapy. What is the mechanism of action of these agents?

A.   They induce osteoblastic activity

B.   They increase calcium and vitamin D uptake

C.   They inhibit osteoclastic activity

D.   They increase the thickness of cortical bone

Discussion

The correct answer is (C). Bisphosphonates inhibit osteoclastic activity by preventing the formation of microtubules at the cell's ruffled border, inducing apoptosis and preventing bone resorption. These agents are used in almost all cases of metastatic bone disease and can significantly decrease the risk of skeletal events.

What are the major concerns with utilization of bisphosphonates?

A.   Electrolyte abnormalities and cerebral edema

B.   Osteonecrosis of the jaw and atypical femoral stress fractures

C.   Increased risk of lymphoma and osteonecrosis of the femoral head

D.   Stress fractures in the lower extremity and cerebral edema

Discussion

The correct answer is (B). There is a small incidence of osteonecrosis as well as atypical proximal femur stress fractures described with long-term utilization of bisphosphonate therapy. No significant electrolyte abnormalities, risk of hematologic malignancy, osteonecrosis, or change in intracranial pressure has been described as a complication.

Objectives: Did you learn…?

•   Indications and side effects of bisphosphonates?

•   Metabolic abnormalities associated with metastatic bone disease?

CASE 34

A 71-year-old male with back pain has been referred to your office. His primary care physician ordered x-rays of the thoracic and lumbar spine, which revealed multiple compression fractures. An MRI was subsequently ordered, which was concerning for metastatic processes within the vertebral bodies. He also has had some right thigh pain and left shoulder pain. X-rays done in your office reveal lucencies in the mid-shaft of the right femur, and proximal left humerus. On questioning, he notes that his urine has been pink over the past several months.

Which of the following is <u>not</u> included in workup for this patient?

A. Urinalysis, urine protein electrophoresis
B. CT of chest, abdomen, and pelvis
C. Thyroid studies
D. MRI of the shoulder

Discussion

The correct answer is (D). The patient has several lytic lesions in the left humerus, right femur, and vertebral bodies causing symptomatic compression fractures. In a 71-year-old male, these are concerning for metastatic disease. He reports urinary symptoms, which are concerning for renal cell carcinoma, although he must be worked up for all common primary malignancies that metastasize to bone. These include breast, lung, prostate, thyroid, and renal cell. The workup includes a thorough history and physical examination, electrolyte panel (with calcium), alkaline phosphatase, CBC, PSA, serum and urine protein electrophoresis, CT scan of the chest/abdomen/pelvis, and total body bone scan.

His urinalysis is positive for gross blood, and CT scan of the abdomen reveals a fungating mass in his right kidney. Image-guided needle biopsy of the left humeral lesion is performed, which results in a

diagnosis of metastatic renal cell carcinoma. What is the next step in management of the shoulder?

A. An open biopsy of the left humeral lesion should be obtained, because needle biopsy is generally unreliable
B. Preoperative radiation to the right humerus, followed by fixation
C. Preoperative embolization of the humeral lesion
D. Total shoulder replacement

Discussion

The correct answer is (C). Embolization of the feeding vessels should be performed prior to prophylactic fixation of all renal cell metastases. Thyroid metastases and hepatocellular also tend to be highly vascular, and preoperative embolization should be considered in these cases as well to avoid catastrophic hemorrhage at the time of fixation.

Objectives: Did you learn...?

- Clinical features and workup of skeletal metastatic renal cell carcinoma?
- Management of renal cell carcinoma metastases to bone?

CASE 35

A 47 year old female with metastatic thyroid cancer has progressive left hip pain. X-rays are shown in Figure 8–34A–D.

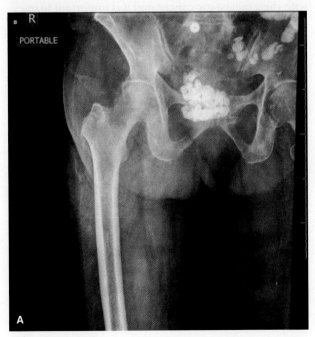

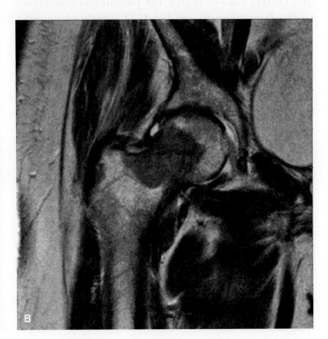

Figure 8–34 **A–B**

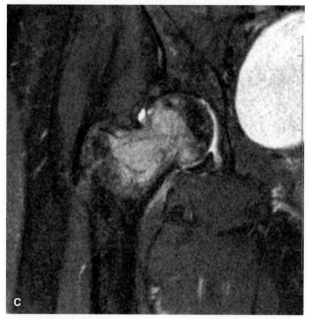

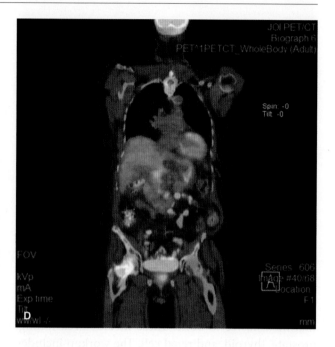

Figure 8–34 **C–D**

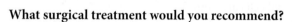

What surgical treatment would you recommend?

A. Hip arthroplasty

B. Cephalomedullary nailing with long intramedullary rod

C. Curettage and bone grafting of the lesion

D. Radiation therapy

Discussion

The correct answer is (A). The patient has metastases to the femoral neck and head. T1-weighted imaging shows a possible fracture line through the metastasis. Prophylactic stabilization of the femur with a cephalomedullary rod is not the best choice for this patient's condition. With the significant neck and head disease, arthroplasty is indicated. Curettage and bone grafting is an inappropriate treatment for a metastatic lytic lesion; this is generally used for benign lesions. Radiation therapy is used in conjunction with surgical stabilization but will not treat the mechanical symptoms associated with the nondisplaced fracture that has already occurred and can lead to arthrofibrosis of the hip joint.

He has a second lesion identified on bone scan that is located in the right sacrum. He has no significant pain in this area with sitting or standing. What other symptoms is it important to question him about?

A. Dizziness

B. Bladder/bowel dysfunction

C. Weakness in the hip flexors

D. Numbness in his fingertips

Discussion

The correct answer is (B). Sacral lesions often cause encroachment on the exiting sacral nerve roots. Patients may not associate changes in bladder or bowel habits with their metastatic cancer, and it is important to question patients specifically regarding these symptoms when they present with a sacral mass.

Objectives: Did you learn...?

• Management of difficult metastatic lesions?

CASE 36

A 30-year-old female presents to your office with a chief complaint of episodic right knee pain, swelling, and stiffness. She reports that over the past 6 months, she has been walking 3 miles per day as part of a new exercise program but does not report any history of acute trauma to the knee. Over the past 3 months, she has woken up to a swollen, stiff knee several times. She has had her knee aspirated twice during these episodes, and the aspirated fluid has been bloody in both cases. Other times, the process has self-resolved over about 5 days. She has never had issues with her knees before, denies fever and chills, and denies swelling or pain in any other joints. She has no family history of autoimmune or rheumatologic disease.

What is the most likely diagnosis?

A. Pigmented villonodular synovitis
B. Septic arthritis
C. Gout
D. Rheumatoid arthritis

Discussion

The correct answer is (A). PVNS is a proliferative synovial process that most commonly affects patients 30 to 50 years old. It presents clinically as recurrent atraumatic episodes of swelling, pain, and stiffness accompanied by hemarthrosis. Eighty percent of cases occur in the knee and usually it is monoarticular. The bloody aspirations, monoarticular presentation, and lack of family history of rheumatologic disease are support in favor of PVNS over rheumatoid arthritis in this patient.

What would you expect this patient's x-rays to reveal?

A. Chondrocalcinosis with a relatively preserved joint space
B. Well-defined erosions on both sides of the joint causing joint space collapse
C. A hypoplastic lateral femoral condyle and evidence of medial joint space narrowing
D. A well-aligned knee with preservation of joint space, no osteophytes, possible effusion

Discussion

The correct answer is (D). Early in the course of PVNS, x-rays are generally normal. After a long period of any untreated synovitis, erosions on both the femoral and tibial side can be seen; this signifies advanced, diffuse disease. Since this patient has only been having symptoms for 3 months, you would expect x-rays to be normal. MRI is the more sensitive test of choice for this lesion.

The patient brings an MRI to the office for your review. There is a focal nodule within the posterior aspect of the joint with low signal intensity on T1- and T2-weighted images. What does this low signal intensity represent?

A. Calcium urate deposition
B. Areas of fat within the lesion
C. Hemosiderin deposition
D. Blood vessels within the synovial fluid

Discussion

The correct answer is (C). PVNS is characterized on MRI as either focal or diffuse areas of low-signal on both T1- and T2-weighted images, due to hemosiderin deposits. There may also be fat present within the area, which is bright on T1 and T2.

Objectives: Did you learn...?

• Clinical and radiographic features of PVNS?

CASE 37

A 72-year-old female presents with progressive bilateral hip and pelvic soreness as well as back pain and headaches. X-rays of the pelvis and biopsy specimen are shown in Figure 8–35A and B.

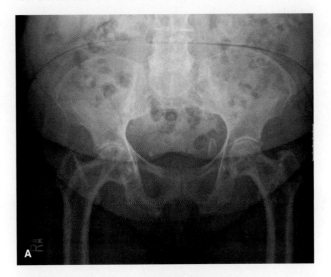

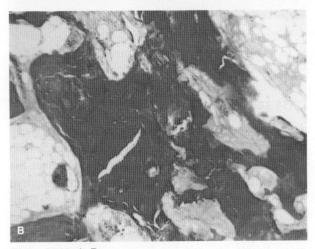

Figure 8–35 **A–B**

What is his most likely diagnosis?

A. Osteosarcoma of the pelvis
B. Osteopetrosis
C. Paget disease
D. Osteomyelitis

Discussion

The correct answer is (C). Paget disease is a remodeling disease characterized initially by osteoclast-mediated bone resorption and then disordered bone formation. On plain radiographs, coarsened trabeculae and cortical thickening are seen; there may be loss of distinction between the cortices and the medullary cavity and gross enlargement of the bone. Histologic appearance of this condition after bone biopsy reveals profound osteoclastic bone resorption with abnormal bone formation in a mosaic pattern. Prominent cement lines are seen. There is woven bone and irregular sections of thickened trabeculae.

What abnormal laboratory finding would you expect to find?

A. Increased thyroid-stimulating hormone
B. Increased alkaline phosphatase level
C. Decreased thyroid-stimulating hormone
D. Decreased alkaline phosphatase level

Discussion

The correct answer is (B). Increased alkaline phosphatase is a signal of increased bone turnover. These markers are also seen in the urine: N-telopeptide, hydroxyproline, and deoxypyridinoline. Calcium level is usually normal in Paget disease.

Objectives: Did you learn...?

• To recognize the clinical features of Paget disease?
• To recognize the histologic features of Paget disease?

CASE 38

A 52-year-old female is referred from her primary care physician's office. She has had vague lower back pain and constipation for the last 8 months, and over the past month she has experienced pain and tingling that radiates into her perineum. She has a history of a lumbar disc herniation when she was 20 years old and was in a motor vehicle collision. She was treated with microdiscectomy and has been asymptomatic since that time. Her primary care physician ordered an MRI

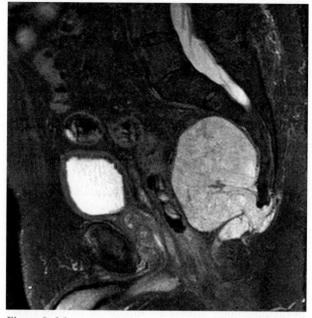

Figure 8–36

and refers her for concerning findings on this imaging (Fig. 8–36).

After appropriate workup, she obtains a needle biopsy of the lesion performed under image guidance. Biopsy specimens are shown in Figure 8–37A and B. What is the most likely diagnosis?

A. Metastatic adenocarcinoma
B. Metastatic renal cell carcinoma
C. Chondrosarcoma
D. Chordoma

Discussion

The correct answer is (D). The imaging and histology displayed are consistent with chordoma, which is

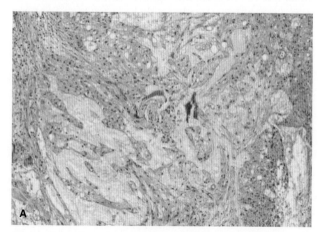

Figure 8–37 **A**

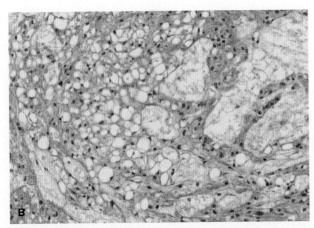

Figure 8–37 **B**

a slow-growing malignant bone tumor arising from notochordal nests and occurring in the spinal axis. Specifically, they arise in the base of the skull or in the sacrum. The histopathologic findings of myxoid and cartilaginous regions, with bubbly physaliferous cells that are distinguished by their abundant cytoplasm, are all suggestive of this diagnosis.

Which of the following statements is true regarding the immunohistochemical staining of chordoma and chondrosarcoma?

A. They both stain positively with S100, but chordoma stains with cytokeratin while chondrosarcoma does not

B. They both stain positively with cytokeratin, but chordoma stains with S100 while chondrosarcoma does not

C. They both stain positively with S100, but chondrosarcoma stains with cytokeratin while chordoma does not

D. They both stain positively with cytokeratin, but chondrosarcoma stains with cytokeratin while chordoma does not

Discussion

The correct answer is (A). Both of these lesions stain positively with S100, but cytokeratin is a valuable staining study to perform because it differentiates chordoma (which stains strongly positively) from chondrosarcoma (which does not stain with cytokeratin).

Which of the following immunohistochemical stains are specific for chordoma?

A. S100

B. CD34

C. Neurofibromin

D. Brachyury

Discussion

The correct answer is (D). Brachyury is an immunohistochemical test which helps confirm the diagnosis of chordoma. Brachyury staining is only positive in notochordal cell–derived tumors. The remaining stains are not specific for chordoma.

Objectives: Did you learn…?

• Imaging and clinical features of chordoma?
• Histologic features of chordoma?

CASE 39

A 45-year-old female with known metastatic breast cancer is referred to you by her oncologist. She has already previously undergone prophylactic nailing of her left humerus and right femur for impending fracture secondary to breast cancer metastases. She is now complaining of increasing pain in the left hip and thigh, and x-rays reveal a mixed blastic and lytic lesion in the intertrochanteric femur.

She asks about image-guided biopsy of this lesion. What is the best response?

A. It is absolutely necessary to biopsy this lesion prior to prophylactic fixation to confirm diagnosis

B. The lesion could be osteosarcoma or another primary bone malignancy, or a metastasis of a new primary tumor, therefore biopsy should be performed

C. Preoperative biopsy is not needed, as she has known metastatic disease to the skeleton and a mixed lesion is consistent with this diagnosis

D. Embolization should be performed prior to biopsy, since even needle biopsy of lucent lesions has relatively high risk of bleeding

Discussion

The correct answer is (C). Indications for biopsy include an unknown aggressive-appearing lesion, the first bone lesion in cancer that has not been documented as metastatic to the skeleton, and indeterminate lesions of unknown diagnosis based on less-invasive studies. This patient has known metastatic breast cancer to the skeleton, status post prior-prophylactic fixation of two long bones for breast cancer metastatic lesions. The fear of prophylactically fixing this lesion without a preoperative biopsy is the possibility that it could be a new malignancy; however, in this case, in particular because the mixed lytic and blastic picture is typical of breast metastasis, it is reasonable to assume these are additional breast metastases. Tissue can be sent to pathology from the operating room at the time of surgery, but a preoperative tissue biopsy is not necessarily needed. If this lesion appeared different from her prior mixed lesions in terms of imaging characteristics, or if the lesions were not consistent with her diagnosis, or any of the conditions initially mentioned, then a preoperative biopsy should be considered.

She asks about the options for surgical fixation. Her husband recently fell and broke his hip, and underwent ORIF with a sliding hip screw device. She requests a similar implant. What is your response?

A. A sliding hip screw/plate and screw construct is acceptable as long as acceptable fixation is achieved above and below the lytic lesion

B. A sliding hip screw/plate and screw construct is acceptable, however, she will have to limit her weight bearing after surgery, because it is a load-sharing device

C. A sliding hip screw/plate and screw construct is not the best implant in her setting, a long cephalomedullary device is preferred

D. A sliding hip screw/plate and screw construct is the fixation method of choice for her situation

Discussion

The correct answer is (C). In cases of prophylactic fixation of metastatic lesions to long bones, the fixation method of choice is almost always a long intramedullary nail (in extension into the head, in the humerus and femur.) This allows one procedure to achieve stable fixation of the entire length of the bone, in anticipation of future metastases developing in another area.

Objectives: Did you learn...?

• When it is critical to biopsy a bone lesion, and when it is not critical?

• What is the best treatment for long bone lesions?

CASE 40

A 78-year-old male is referred to your office by his general surgeon. Six years ago, he underwent surgery to remove a lipoma from his right upper back. The postoperative pathology report at that time showed

pleomorphic liposarcoma, and he therefore received radiation to the area. Over the past 4 months, he has been noticing a slowly enlarging mass in the area of his prior surgery.

After history, physical examination, and review of shoulder x-rays, what is the next best step?

A. Ultrasound of the shoulder

B. MRI of the shoulder with/without gadolinium, CT of the chest, abdomen, and pelvis

C. CT of the shoulder and CT of the head

D. Preoperative lab testing

Discussion

The correct answer is (B). The patient likely has recurrence of his liposarcoma. The mass must be evaluated with gadolinium-enhanced MRI, and in anticipation of recurrent malignancy, he should be evaluated for metastases. Pleomorphic liposarcoma usually metastasizes to the lungs or potentially the retroperitoneum, therefore a CT scan should be ordered in conjunction with the MRI.

Imaging reveals a large 9 cm × 5 cm × 4 cm intramuscular mass in the infraspinatus, consistent with liposarcoma. His chest CT is within normal limits. What is the most important prognostic factor in the AJCC classification system?

A. Size (< or >8 cm)

B. Nodal involvement

C. Discontinuous tumor within the same compartment

D. Presence of metastases

Discussion

The correct answer is (D). The AJCC staging system for soft-tissue sarcomas is based on the grade of the tumor, its size and depth, regional lymph node involvement, and presents of metastases. All other factors become irrelevant when metastases are present; the lesion is classified as stage IV in this case. Prognosis is based on stage, therefore the presence of metastases is the most highly correlated with overall prognosis.

What principle should be followed during your surgical treatment of his recurrent tumor?

A. The prior surgical scar and tract should be excised

B. The prior surgical scar and tract should be avoided

C. Incision is placed in the axillary fold, to reduce the visibility of the scar

D. A drain should be avoided

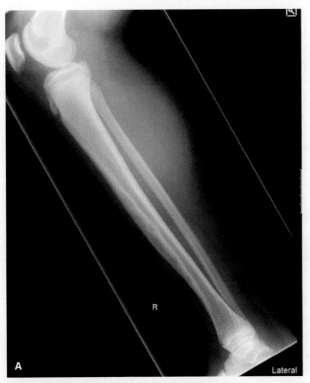

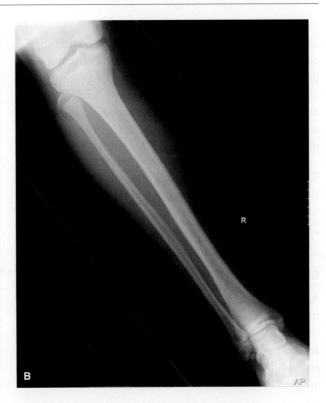

Figure 8–38 **A–B**

Discussion

The correct answer is (A). After an unplanned excision of a malignant tumor, you should assume that the tract used to gain access to the tumor and resect it is now contaminated with malignant cells. As part of your revision resection, the entire prior tract should be excised. Distant incisions are not used, regardless of cosmetics. Drains are often used in these cases to prevent hematoma formation. All drains should be placed in line with and close to the incision in the event the tract will need to be excised in the future.

Objectives: Did you learn…?

- To recognize a liposarcoma?
- Staging and workup of a soft-tissue sarcoma?
- Treatment of a soft-tissue sarcoma?

CASE 41

An 18-year-old male presents to your office with pain in his lower right leg and an enlarging mass over the anterior tibia. These symptoms have been worsening for the past 3 months. His pain waxes and wanes and tends to be associated with physical activity, and he is training for a marathon so he is quite anxious about this. He has tenderness over the subcutaneous border of the tibia,

and has a palpable mass there that is fixed to the bone. X-rays are shown in Figure 8–38A and B.

What is the most likely diagnosis?

A. Osteosarcoma
B. Enchondroma
C. Tibial stress reaction
D. Adamantinoma

Discussion

The correct answer is (D). Adamantinoma is a rare low-grade malignant bone tumor that occurs almost exclusively in the tibia. It can cause pain and tenderness in the anterior tibia and has a classic "soap-bubble" appearance on x-ray. A similar but benign lesion is osteofibrous dysplasia, and these tumors are considered to be on either end of a spectrum of disease of the same etiology.

Appropriate workup is performed and he is diagnosed with adamantinoma. What is the appropriate management of this patient?

A. Radiation therapy
B. Wide surgical resection
C. Radiation prior to wide surgical resection
D. Above-knee amputation

Discussion

The correct answer is (B). Standard of care is wide surgical resection with reconstruction. Given the diaphyseal location of most adamantinoma, intercalary grafting is commonly performed. Chemotherapy and radiation are not indicated in this condition, and local recurrence is associated with positive margins at the time of resection.

Objectives: Did you learn...?

- To recognize adamantinoma and its relative osteofibrous dysplasia?
- Treatment of adamantinoma?

CASE 42

A 60-year-old female with a history of breast cancer treated 5 years ago with mastectomy, chemotherapy, and radiation is seeing you for knee pain. X-rays of the knee are performed, which show moderate DJD. They also reveal a lesion in the distal femoral shaft. X-rays taken are displayed in Figure 8–39A and B.

Which of the following tests is <u>not</u> indicated at this time?

A. Bone scan
B. CT chest/abdomen/pelvis
C. Contralateral femur x-rays
D. Thyroid studies

Discussion

The correct answer is (C). The patient has a permeative lesion incidentally found on x-rays, with a remote history of nonmetastatic cancer. This lesion could represent the first metastasis of her breast cancer, metastasis of a different primary tumor, or a primary bone lesion. A workup must be started, which includes (but is not limited to) a bone scan, CT chest/abdomen/pelvis, and laboratory studies. Contralateral femur x-rays are not indicated at this point unless she is having pain in that area, or bone scan shows a lesion in that area.

Her extensive workup is negative for primary malignancy. A biopsy is performed and pathology report is consistent with metastatic breast cancer. An intramedullary nail is placed, and the specimens from the operating room are sent for biopsy. What other information can be obtained from the biopsy?

A. Estrogen and progesterone receptor expression
B. The duration of time the lytic lesion has been present

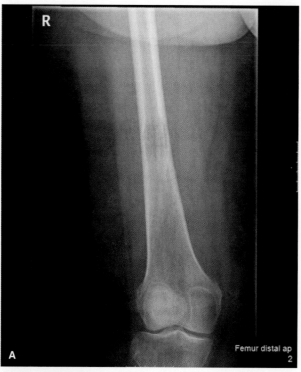

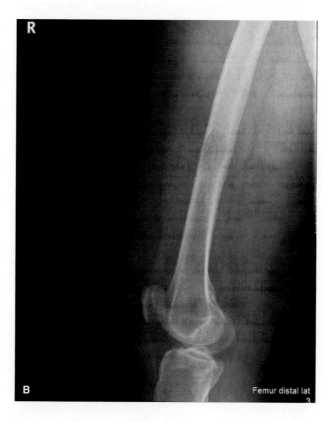

Figure 8–39 **A–B**

C. Risk of femoral shaft fracture

D. Potential response to radiation

Discussion

The correct answer is (A). In addition to identifying the primary site for this metastatic lesion, biopsy is specifically important in breast cancer metastases because the susceptibility to certain chemotherapeutic agents can be evaluated by testing for various receptor expressions by the tumor cells. For example, Herceptin is a chemotherapeutic agent that will only have an effect in patients with HER2+ breast cancer. Therefore, biopsy of the metastatic lesion can provide important information to drive medical oncologic treatment and prognosis. Importantly, the receptor status of any disease can change through the course of the disease as tumors continue to mutate, which may sometimes open new avenues for treatment. For this reason, any procedure done on a new metastatic bone lesion should include a biopsy of the tissue obtained at the time of surgery.

Objectives: Did you learn…?

• To identify and work up metastatic bone disease?

• The importance of sending any and all tissue obtained at the time of surgical procedure for biopsy?

CASE 43

A 45-year-old male is taken to the emergency room after sustaining a motor vehicle accident. An Orthopaedic consult is placed after a unexpected finding is seen on the X-ray of his left hip. The X-rays is shown is Figure 8-40A and an MRI is shown is Figure 8–40B.

What is the most likely diagnosis?

A. Osteosarcoma

B. Chronic osteomyelitis

C. Aneurysmal bone cyst

D. Fibrous dysplasia

Discussion

The correct answer is (D). Fibrous dysplasia is characterized by a fibro-osseous tissue within the bone and is often asymptomatic and found incidentally. Lesions can be expansile with cortical thinning and a sclerotic rim, around central lucent lesions within the medullary canal. When it occurs in the proximal femur, a coxa vara deformity can result, termed the "shepherd's crook" deformity.

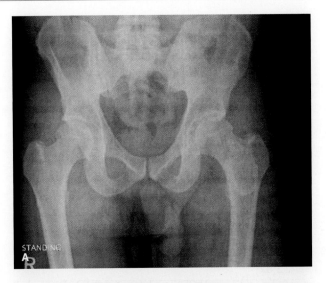

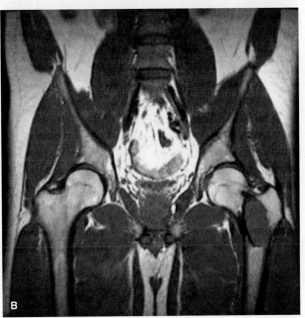

Figure 8–40 **A–B**

The biopsy of this lesion is shown in Figure 8–41. What of the following histologic features is characteristic of this lesion?

A. "Alphabet soup" pattern of bony trabeculae

B. Chondroid, myxoid, and fibrous areas

C. Bland cartilage

D. Areas of aneurysmal degeneration

Discussion

The correct answer is (A). Histologically, fibrous dysplasia appears as poorly mineralized immature fibrous tissue surrounding islands of irregular trabeculae of

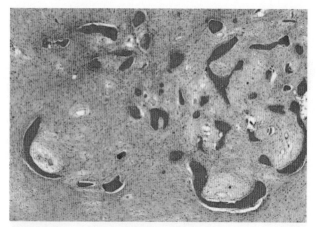

Figure 8–41

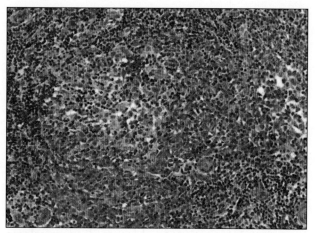

Figure 8–42

woven bone, termed "Chinese letters" or "alphabet soup." These lesions can be associated with secondary aneurysmal bone cysts, so sometimes cavernous blood-filled spaces are seen on histology, but this is not a characteristic feature and cannot be used alone to make the diagnosis.

He has no symptoms in his left hip. What is the most appropriate management at this time?

A. Observation

B. Curettage and bone graft using cortical allograft

C. Curettage and bone graft using cancellous allograft

D. Arthroplasty

Discussion

The correct answer is (A). Asymptomatic patients may be observed. Surgical indications include painful lesions, impending/actual pathologic fracture, severe deformity, and neurologic compromise. When curettage and bone grafting is performed, cortical allograft should be used. Internal fixation is usually recommended to achieve adequate stabilization and pain control.

Objectives: Did you learn...?

• To recognize fibrous dysplasia?

• To understand the treatment options for impending fracture?

CASE 44

An 8-year-old female complains of pain in her lower back. She is an active, otherwise healthy child, and the pain started indolently about 4 weeks ago, without history of trauma. Her parents report that it keeps her up at night, and her performance in sports has begun to suffer as result of the pain. She denies fever, chills, or constitutional symptoms. She denies pain, weakness, or sensory changes in the legs, and denies bladder/bowel dysfunction. X-rays of the spine shows vertebra plana of one of the lumbar vertebrae. A biopsy is performed and the histology is shown in Figure 8–42.

What is the most likely diagnosis?

A. Osteomyelitis

B. Congenital vertebral anomaly

C. Langerhans cell histiocytosis

D. Acute fracture

Discussion

The correct answer is (C). Wafer-shaped collapsed vertebra (termed "vertebra plana") in a child is typical of histiocytosis. The disk height above and below the involved level is increased. This can cause back pain but in the absence of acute trauma should not be confused with an acute compression fracture. Vertebral osteomyelitis is less likely to cause such a compression, unless it is chronic and destructive over years. This patient has no signs of osteomyelitis (fever, chills, etc.). A congenital vertebral anomaly would usually have caused symptoms prior to age 8, as well as a coronal plane deformity which the patient does not have.

Langerhans cell histiocytosis/eosinophilic granuloma is the most common tumor of the:

A. Clavicle

B. Scapula

C. Fibula

D. Distal radius

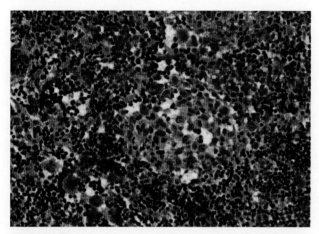

Figure 8–43

Discussion

The correct answer is (A). This benign but painful lytic bone lesion is commonly in children and is the most common tumor of the clavicle.

A high power biopsy slide is shown in Figure 8–43. Which of the following characteristic findings is not usually seen with Langerhans cell histiocytosis?

A. Hemosiderin laden tissues
B. Indented and lobular nuclei
C. Bilobed or coffee bean shaped nuclei
D. High proportion of eosinophils

Discussion

The correct answer is (A). Histopathologic examination of this lesion reveals eosinophils with typical eosinophilic cytoplasm and bilobed nucleus and the diagnostic Langerhans cells, which have an indented and lobular nucleus.

What is the most appropriate recommendation for treatment in this patient?

A. In situ posterior spinal fusion
B. Cortisone injection
C. Observation
D. Bisphosphonates

Discussion

The correct answer is (C). In the absence of cord compression, no treatment is necessary for vertebra plana. Eighty percent of patients will at least partially spontaneously reconstitute vertebral height at the affected level.

Objectives: Did you learn...?

• To recognize vertebra plana?
• To recognize Langerhans cell histiocytosis?
• Treatment of LCH?

CASE 45

A 46-year-old male presents to you for a second opinion. He recently underwent surgery to remove a mass from his forearm. His surgeon told him he had a benign tumor of his nerve sheath, but he is extremely anxious about the potential for malignancy. He brings with him the histology slides from his excisional biopsy and asks you to review them. Histology slides are shown in Figure 8–44A and B.

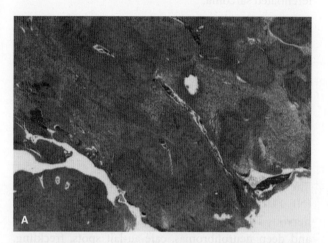

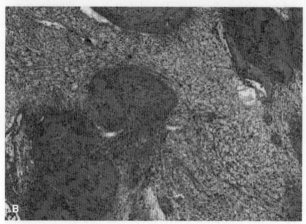

Figure 8–44 **A–B**

What is the most likely diagnosis?

A. Schwannoma
B. MPNST
C. Neurofibroma
D. Undifferentiated sarcoma

Discussion

The correct answer is (A). Schwannomas demonstrate two types of histologic features. On the left is a region of palisading spindle cells (Antoni A areas) and on the right is an area with myxoid background (Antoni B area). The presence of these two distinctively characteristic areas is suggestive of schwannoma. Histologic examination of MPNST reveals spindle cells that resemble fibrosarcoma with patterns of sweeping fascicles and Schwann cells arranged asymmetrically. Neurofibromas demonstrate a more disorganized pattern in comparison to the palisading spindle cells of schwannoma. There is nothing atypical about these cells that would suggest undifferentiated sarcoma.

He explains that he was concerned because his mother had neurofibromatosis. What is the inheritance pattern of this condition?

A. Autosomal recessive
B. Autosomal dominant
C. X-linked recessive
D. X-linked dominant

Discussion

The correct answer is (B). Type 1 neurofibromatosis (NF-1) is the most common single-gene disorder of the nervous system. It presents with numerous cutaneous and deep neurofibromas, café-au-lait spots, freckling, and cognitive disorder. The defect is on chromosome 17a11.2 in a gene encoding for neurofibromin, a tumor suppressor gene. Its inheritance pattern is autosomal dominant, although 50% of cases are new mutations.

Objectives: Did you learn...?

• To recognize a schwannoma by histology?

CASE 46

A 71-year-old male is brought to the ER after sustaining a motor vehicle crash. During routine trauma workup, a CT of the thorax is performed, and you are consulted regarding a lesion on the posterior chest wall. An MRI is also available for you to review, which demonstrates a soft-tissue mass on the posterior chest wall deep to the scapula with no particularly defining characteristic features. On interview, he denies recent pain in this area. He denies weakness or sensory changes in the upper extremity.

Which of the following lesions is found almost exclusively between the scapula and chest wall?

A. Desmoid tumor
B. Chordoma
C. Atypical lipoma
D. Elastofibroma

Discussion

The correct answer is (D). Elastofibroma is a slow-growing, reactive lesion found almost exclusively between the scapula and chest wall. It can present as a slowly enlarging mass that sometimes causes pain with shoulder movement but is often an incidental finding on imaging performed for another reason.

A needle biopsy is performed, which confirms the diagnosis. What is the best recommended treatment at this time?

A. Marginal resection
B. Wide resection and radiation
C. Observation
D. Neoadjuvant chemotherapy followed by resection

Discussion

The correct answer is (C). Elastofibroma is a slow-growing, benign lesion that can be observed if asymptomatic. There is no malignancy potential. Excision is reserved for symptomatic lesions, which usually cause pain in the area with shoulder motion.

Objectives: Did you learn...?

• Understand the clinical features of Elastofibroma?
• Potential treatment options for Elastofibroma?

CASE 47

A 38-year-old female presents to the emergency room with knee pain and swelling that began this morning when she woke up. She denies recent trauma. Over the past 6 months, this has occurred several times, and she has had frank blood aspirated from her knee at an urgent care center. She denies fever, chills, or pain in other joints. An MRI is conducted in the emergency room, which is displayed below in Figure 8–45A and B.

What is the most likely diagnosis?

A. Medial meniscus tear
B. Pigmented villonodular synovitis
C. Septic arthritis
D. ACL tear

Discussion

The correct answer is (B). Recurrent atraumatic hemarthroses in one joint is suggestive of PVNS. This benign tumor of synovium creates low signal on T1 and T2, illustrated in these images. Injuries to both the medial meniscus and ACL would be evident on the MRI, and neither of these findings is shown in the image. She has no signs or symptoms of septic arthritis, which usually

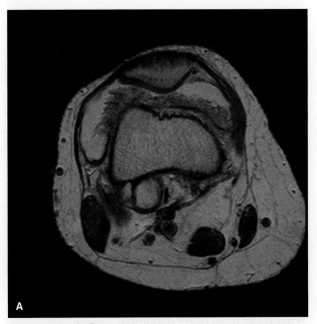

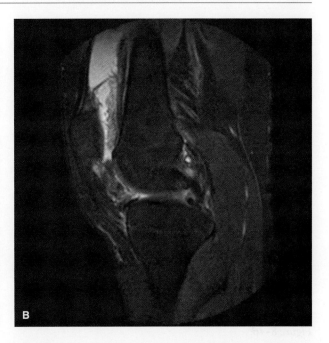

Figure 8–45 **A–B**

is associated with aspiration of purulent fluid, not bloody fluid.

What is the molecular mechanism that leads to the development of PVNS?

A. t(1;2) translocation leading to CSF1-COL6A3 fusion product
B. t(11:22) translocation leading to the EWS-FLI1 fusion product
C. 17q11.2 defect
D. EXT1 and EXT2 gene abnormality

Discussion

The correct answer is (A). The underlying pathologic molecular mechanism for PVNS has recently been elucidated. A specific t(1;2) translocation fuses the colony stimulating factor-1 (CSF1) gene to the collagen type Via3 (COL6A3) promoter, leading to the attraction of non-neoplastic inflammatory cells expressing the CSF1 receptor. The t(11;22) translocation leads to Ewing sarcoma; the 17q11.2 defect leads to neurofibromatosis type 1, and the EXT1 or EXT2 genetic defects leads to multiple hereditary exostoses.

The patient's MRI reveals diffuse PVNS. What is the recommended treatment?

A. Observation and symptomatic treatment with NSAIDs
B. Total knee arthroplasty
C. Total synovectomy
D. Chemotherapy and radiation

Discussion

The correct answer is (C). The standard of care for the diffuse form of PVNS is total synovectomy, often via an anterior and posterior approach. Eventually, these patients may require total knee replacement due to chondral erosion from recurrent tumor. This patient does not have any arthritis at this point, therefore arthroplasty would be premature. There is no role for NSAIDs or radiation in treating this condition. Medical therapies are on the horizon, currently in clinical trials since the underlying molecular mechanism of this disease has been defined.

Objectives: Did you learn...?

• Mechanism of development of PVNS?
• Treatment of PVNS?

CASE 48

A 14-year-old female presents to your office complaining of pain in her lower leg. She reports progression of pain over the past 3 months, especially at night. She has good temporary relief with ibuprofen but limits her intake due to GI upset. CT scan is shown in Figure 8–46.

All of the following statements are true of this lesion except:

A. The lesion is always painful and in the epiphysis of a child

B. They are most commonly diaphyseal and intracortical

C. Spinal lesions can cause a painful scoliosis; lesion is on concave side of curve

D. Bone scan often shows the "double density" sign

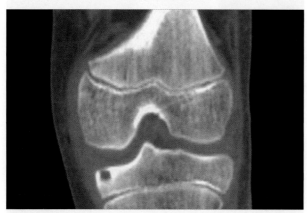

Figure 8–46

Discussion

The correct answer is (A). Osteoid osteomas are small, painful bone lesions that are usually intracortical. They are hot on bone scan, showing "double density sign" caused by diffuse uptake in the surrounding reactive region and higher uptake by the central nidus. When they develop in the spine, they can cause a painful scoliosis with the lesion on the concave side of the curvature; the scoliosis usually resolves without further treatment once the osteoid osteoma is treated. Chondroblastoma is the most common painful lesion found in the epiphysis of a child, not osteoid osteoma.

The patient is resistant to conservative management, as she cannot tolerate NSAIDs and is considerably bothered by the pain. What treatment would you recommend?

A. Curettage and bone graft

B. Wide resection and intercalary graft reconstruction

C. Marginal excision and prophylactic plating

D. Radiofrequency ablation

Discussion

The correct answer is (D). The preferred treatment is percutaneous radiofrequency ablation, typically performed by an interventional or musculoskeletal radiologist. Open curettage is recommended for lesions that present a high risk of complication with radiofrequency ablation, recurrent lesions, or in situations where the diagnosis is uncertain.

Objectives: Did you learn…?

• To recognize clinical and radiographic features of osteoid osteoma?

• Treatment of osteoid osteoma?

CASE 49

An 8-year-old male is brought in by his parents for "growing pains." He has been limping and has difficulty keeping up with other children on the playground secondary to pain in his legs. This has been progressive over the past 6 to 8 months. He is an otherwise healthy child without recent fever, chills, or significant past medical history. X-rays demonstrate a lesion in the anterior tibial cortex associated with some mild bowing of the bone. The lesion has a "soap-bubble" appearance and there are no other lesions seen.

What is the most likely diagnosis?

A. Osteosarcoma

B. Osteofibrous dysplasia

C. Enchondroma

D. Nonossifying fibroma

Discussion

The correct answer is (B). Osteofibrous dysplasia is a distinctive intracortical lesion almost always seen in the anterior tibial cortex, most commonly in children <10 years old. These x-rays reveal classic findings of an elongated, diaphyseal, intracortical, bubbly lytic lesion. Expansile remodeling can be seen, but there is no soft-tissue mass.

On histopathologic examination, what differentiates osteofibrous dysplasia from fibrous dysplasia?

A. Presence of osteoblastic rimming

B. Presence of eosinophils

C. Presence of epithelial nests

D. Presence of cigar-shaped nuclei

Discussion

The correct answer is (A). At low power, the features of osteofibrous dysplasia are very similar to those of fibrous dysplasia, including spicules of normal appearing bony trabeculae that are sometimes called "alphabet soup." However, osteofibrous dysplasia has osteoblastic rimming of these immature trabeculae, while fibrous dysplasia lacks this finding. Eosinophils are not predominant in either case. Epithelial nests are seen in adamantinoma, which differentiates osteofibrous dysplasia from this lesion. Cigar-shaped nuclei are associated with certain sarcomas.

If he remains symptomatic, what treatment is indicated?

A. Below-knee amputation

B. Wide resection with intercalary graft reconstruction and internal fixation

C. Curettage and bone grafting

D. Radiation therapy

Discussion

The correct answer is (C). Small, asymptomatic lesions may be observed, however, curettage and bone grafting is indicated for symptomatic lesions. A high recurrence rate has been reported with bone grafting, especially in younger children.

Objectives: Did you learn...?

• Clinical and radiographic figures of adamantinoma and osteofibrous dysplasia?

CASE 50

A 16-year-old female sprains her ankle playing lacrosse and is brought to the emergency room. X-rays are negative for fracture, but an orthopaedic consult is placed to evaluate a suspicious lesion in the distal tibia. Prior to her acute ankle injury, she denies any pain in her lower leg. Her father died at a young age of colon cancer, and she is anxious about this finding being suggestive of malignancy. X-ray is shown in Figure 8–47.

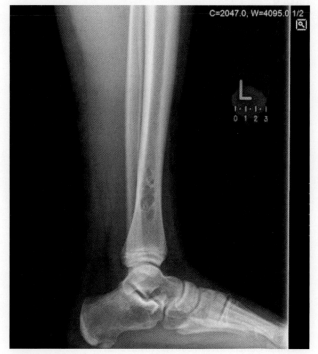

Figure 8–47

What is the most likely diagnosis?

A. Nonossifying fibroma

B. Metastatic carcinoma

C. Eosinophilic granuloma

D. Fibrous dysplasia

Discussion

The correct answer is (A). Nonossifying fibromas are most commonly discovered incidentally near the ends of long bones in the pediatric population. They are usually located in the metaphyseal portion of the bone, eccentrically located, with geographic lucency and a sclerotic border. Smaller lesions appear cortically based, but larger lesions can appear to involve the medullary cavity. They may expand and thin the cortex but are not associated with soft-tissue mass. Most will spontaneously ossify by skeletal maturity, starting in the periphery.

All of the following are true statements about fracture through a nonossifying fibroma <u>except</u>:

A. Fracture risk increases with age at time of diagnosis

B. Lesions greater than 3 cm in size are associated with higher fracture rate

C. Lesions affecting more than 50% bone width are associated with higher fracture rate

D. Fractures through nonossifying fibromas are particularly uncommon in the femur

Discussion

The correct answer is (C). The risk of pathologic fracture through a nonossifying fibroma is associated with the lesion's size (the percentage of cortical diameter consumed by the lesion, as well as its overall size), as well as where it is located: femoral fractures are particularly rare, while tibial fractures are more common. The age at time of diagnosis has not been shown to be associated with fracture rate, as these are often incidental findings on imaging studies performed for another reason.

What is the recommended management of this lesion?

A. Wide resection and reconstruction

B. Observation

C. Curettage and bone graft

D. Steroid injection into the lesion

Discussion

The correct answer is (B). Since she reports no symptoms prior to her ankle sprain, the risk of developing a pathologic fracture is low. Most patients require only observation, as the natural history for these lesions is to heal spontaneously. Repeat surveillance x-rays should be obtained to confirm the expected mineralization, starting peripherally, as the patient exits puberty. For large or painful lesions, intralesional excision (curettage) and bone grafting can be considered.

Objectives: Did you learn...?

• The clinical and radiographic feature of the NOF?

BIBLIOGRAPHY

Case 1

Ahn JI, Park JS. Pathological fractures secondary to unicameral bone cysts. *Int Orthop.* 1994;18(1):20–22.

Chang CH, Stanton RP, Glutting J. Unicameral bone cysts treated by injection of bone marrow or methylprednisolone. *J Bone Joint Surg Br.* 2002;84(3):407–412.

Leithner A, Windhager R, Lang S, Haas OA, Kainberger F, Kotz R. Aneurysmal bone cyst: a population based epidemiologic study and literature review. *Clin Orthop Relat Res.* 1999;(363):176–179.

Roposch A, Saraph V, Linhart WE. Flexible intramedullary nailing for the treatment of unicameral bone cysts in long bones. *J Bone Joint Surg Am.* 2000;82-A(10):1447–1453.

Case 2

Campanacci M, Capanna R, Picci P. Unicameral and aneurysmal bone cysts. *Clin Orthop Relat Res.* 1986;(204):25–36.

Cottalorda J, Bourelle S. Modern concepts of primary aneurysmal bone cyst. *Arch Orthop Trauma Surg.* 2007;127(2):105–114.

Kaufman RA, Towbin RB. Telangiectatic osteosarcoma simulating the appearance of an aneurysmal bone cyst. *Pediatr Radiol.* 1981;11(2):102–104.

Marcove RC, Sheth DS, Takemoto S, Healey JH. The treatment of aneurysmal bone cyst. *Clin Orthop Relat Res.* 1995;(311):157–163.

Case 3

Campanacci M. Osteoid osteoma. *Bone and Soft Tissue Tumors.* Vienna: Springer; 1999:391–414.

Cantwell CP, Obyrne J, Eustace S. Current trends in treatment of osteoid osteoma with an emphasis on radiofrequency ablation. *Eur Radiol.* 2004;14(4):607–617.

Lee EH, Shafi M, Hui JH. Osteoid osteoma: a current review. *J Pediatr Orthop.* 2006;26(5):695–700.

Saifuddin A, White J, Sherazi Z, Shaikh MI, Natali C, Ransford AO. Osteoid osteoma and osteoblastoma of the spine: factors associated with the presence of scoliosis. *Spine.* 1998;23(1):47–53.

Case 4

Mirra JM, Gold R, Downs J, Eckardt JJ. A new histologic approach to the differentiation of enchondroma and chondrosarcoma of the bones: a clinicopathologic analysis of 51 cases. *Clin Orthop Relat Res.* 1985;(201):214–237.

Murphey MD, Flemming DJ, Boyea SR, Bojescul JA, Sweet DE, Temple HT. Enchondroma versus chondrosarcoma in the appendicular skeleton: differentiating features. *Radiographics.* 1998;18(5):1213–1237.

Silve C, Jüppner H. Ollier disease. *Orphanet J Rare Dis.* 2006;1:37.

Case 5

Campanacci M. Multiple Hhereditary Eexostoses. *Bone and Soft Tissue Tumors.* Vienna: Springer;1999:197–205.

Kitsoulis P, Galani V, Stefanaki K, et al. Osteochondromas: review of the clinical, radiological and pathological features. *In Vivo.* 2008;22(5):633–646.

Nojima T, Yamashiro K, Fujita M, Isu K, Ubayama Y, Yamawaki S. A case of osteosarcoma arising in a solitary osteochondroma. *Acta Orthop Scand.* 1991;62(3):290–292.

Case 6

Arndt CA, Crist WM. Common musculoskeletal tumors of childhood and adolescence. *N Engl J Med.* 1999;341(5):342–352.

Tan JZ, Schlicht SM, Powell GJ, et al. Multidisciplinary approach to diagnosis and management of osteosarcoma—a review of the St Vincent's Hospital experience. *Int Semin Surg Oncol.* 2006;3:38.

Case 7

Dürr HR, Lienemann A, Nerlich A, Stumpenhausen B, Refior HJ. Chondromyxoid fibroma of bone. *Arch Orthop Trauma Surg.* 2000;120(1-2):42–47.

Case 8

Eckardt JJ, Grogan TJ. Giant cell tumor of bone. *Clin Orthop Relat Res.* 1986;204:45–58.

Case 9

Picci P, Rougraff BT, Bacci G, et al. Prognostic significance of histopathologic response to chemotherapy in nonmetastatic Ewing's sarcoma of the extremities. *J Clin Oncol.* 1993;11(9):1763–1769.

Case 10

Erlemann R. Imaging and differential diagnosis of primary bone tumors and tumor-like lesions of the spine. *Eur J Radiol.* 2006;58(1):48–67.

Saglik Y, Atalar H, Yildiz Y, Basarir K, Gunay C. Surgical treatment of osteoblastoma: a report of 20 cases. *Acta Orthop Belg.* 2007;73(6):747–753.

Samdani A, Torre-Healy A, Chou D, Cahill AM, Storm PB. Treatment of osteoblastoma at C7: a multidisciplinary approach. A case report and review of the literature. *Eur Spine J.* 2009;18(Suppl 2):196–200.

Case 11

Chauveinc L, Mosseri V, Quintana E, et al. Osteosarcoma following retinoblastoma: age at onset and latency period. *Ophthalmic Genet.* 2001;22(2):77–88.

Ferguson WS, Goorin AM. Current treatment of osteosarcoma. *Cancer Invest.* 2001;19(3):292–315.

Torti FM, Bristow MR, Howes AE, et al. Reduced cardiotoxicity of doxorubicin delivered on a weekly schedule assessment by endomyocardial biopsy. *Ann Inter Med.* 1983;99(6):745–749.

Case 12

Jacofsky DJ, Haidukewych GJ. Management of pathologic fractures of the proximal femur: state of the art. *J Orthop Trauma.* 2004;18(7):459–469.

Sukpanichnant S, Cousar JB, Leelasiri A, Graber SE, Greer JP, Collins RD. Diagnostic criteria and histologic grading in multiple myeloma: histologic and immunohistologic analysis of 176 cases with clinical correlation. *Hum Pathol.* 1994;25(3):308–318.

Zhang XG, Gaillard JP, Robillard N, et al. Reproducible obtaining of human myeloma cell lines as a model for tumor stem cell study in human multiple myeloma. *Blood.* 1994;83(12): 3654–3663.

Case 13

Getty PJ, Peabody TD. Complications and functional outcomes of reconstruction with an osteoarticular allograft after intra-articular resection of the proximal aspect of the humerus. *J Bone Joint Surg Am.* 1999;81(8):1138–1146.

Riedel RF, Larrier N, Dodd L, Kirsch D, Martinez S, Brigman BE. The clinical management of chondrosarcoma. *Curr Treat Options Oncol.* 2009;10(1-2):94–106.

Skrzynski MC, Biermann JS, Montag A, Simon MA. Diagnostic accuracy and charge-savings of outpatient core needle biopsy compared with open biopsy of musculoskeletal tumors. *J Bone Joint Surg Am.* 1996;78(5):644–649.

Case 14

Ahmed AR, Tan TS, Unni KK, Collins MS, Wenger DE, Sim FH. Secondary chondrosarcoma in osteochondroma: report of 107 patients. *Clin Orthop Relat Res.* 2003;(411):193–206.

Fiorenza F, Abudu A, Grimer RJ, et al. Risk factors for survival and local control in chondrosarcoma of bone. *J Bone Joint Surg Br.* 2002;84(1):93–99.

Kaim AH, Hügli R, Bonél HM, Jundt G. Chondroblastoma and clear cell chondrosarcoma: radiological and MRI characteristics with histopathological correlation. *Skeletal Radiol.* 2002;31(2):88–95.

Case 15

Scotlandi K, Baldini N, Cerisano V, et al. CD99 engagement: an effective therapeutic strategy for Ewing tumors. *Cancer Res.* 2000;60(18):5134–5142.

Turc-Carel C, Aurias A, Mugneret F, et al. Chromosomes in Ewing's sarcoma. I. An evaluation of 85 cases and remarkable consistency of t (11; 22)(q24; q12). *Cancer Genet Cytogenet.* 1988;32(2):229–238.

Yamaguchi U, Hasegawa T, Morimoto Y, et al. A practical approach to the clinical diagnosis of Ewing's sarcoma/ primitive neuroectodermal tumour and other small round cell tumours sharing EWS rearrangement using new fluorescence in situ hybridisation probes for EWSR1 on formalin fixed, paraffin wax embedded tissue. *J Clin Pathol.* 2005;58(10):1051–1056.

Case 16

Eckardt JJ, Grogan TJ. Giant cell tumor of bone. *Clin Orthop Relat Res.* 1986;204:45–58.

Case 17

Boccadoro M, Pileri A. Diagnosis, prognosis, and standard treatment of multiple myeloma. *Hematol Oncol Clin North Am.* 1997;11(1):111–131.

Riedel DA, Pottern LM. The epidemiology of multiple myeloma. *Hematol Oncol Clin North Am.* 1992;6(2):225–247.

Silvestris F, Cafforio P, Tucci M, Dammacco F. Negative regulation of erythroblast maturation by Fas-L+/TRAIL +highly malignant plasma cells: a major pathogenetic mechanism of anemia in multiple myeloma. *Blood.* 2002;99(4):1305–1313.

Case 18

Bielack SS, Kempf-Bielack B, Delling G, et al. Prognostic factors in high-grade osteosarcoma of the extremities or trunk: an analysis of 1,702 patients treated on neoadjuvant cooperative osteosarcoma study group protocols. *J Clin Oncol.* 2002;20(3):776–790.

Mervak TR, Unni KK, Pritchard DJ, McLeod RA. Telangiectatic osteosarcoma. *Clin Orthop Relat Res.* 1991;(270): 135–139.

Tan JZ, Schlicht SM, Powell GJ, et al. Multidisciplinary approach to diagnosis and management of osteosarcoma— a review of the St Vincent's Hospital experience. *Int Semin Surg Oncol.* 2006;3:38.

Case 19

Björkstrand BB, Ljungman P, Svensson H, et al. Allogeneic bone marrow transplantation versus autologous stem cell transplantation in multiple myeloma: a retrospective case-matched study from the European Group for Blood and Marrow Transplantation. *Blood.* 1996;88(12):4711–4718.

Mirels H. Metastatic disease in long bones A proposed scoring system for diagnosing impending pathologic fractures. *Clin Orthop Relat Res.* 1989;(249):256–264.

Case 20

Leibel SA, Wara WM, Hill DR, et al. Desmoid tumors: local control and patterns of relapse following radiation therapy. *Int J Radiat Oncol Biol Phys.* 1983;9(8):1167–1171.

Case 21

Lin J, Martel W. Cross-sectional imaging of peripheral nerve sheath tumors: characteristic signs on CT, MR imaging, and sonography. *AJR Am J Roentgenol.* 2001;176(1):75–82.

Matsunou H, Shimoda T, Kakimoto S, Yamashita H, Ishikawa E, Mukai M. Histopathologic and immunohistochemical study of malignant tumors of peripheral nerve sheath (malignant schwannoma). *Cancer.* 1985;56(9):2269–2279.

Case 22

Kooby DA, Antonescu CR, Brennan MF, Singer S. Atypical lipomatous tumor/well-differentiated liposarcoma of the extremity and trunk wall: importance of histological subtype with treatment recommendations. *Ann Surg Oncol.* 2004;11(1):78–84.

Case 23

Boyer MI. *AAOS Comprehensive Orthopaedic Review 2.* Rosemont, IL: American Academy of Orthopaedic Surgeons, Copyright; 2014:558–559.

Case 24

Boyer MI. *AAOS Comprehensive Orthopaedic Review 2.* Rosemont, IL: American Academy of Orthopaedic Surgeons, Copyright; 2014:566–567.

Case 25

Fisher C. Synovial sarcoma. *Ann Diagn Pathol.* 1998;2(6):401–421.
Kawai A, Woodruff J, Healey JH, Brennan MF, Antonescu CR, Ladanyi M. SYT–SSX gene fusion as a determinant of morphology and prognosis in synovial sarcoma. *N Engl J Med.* 1998;338(3):153–160.

Case 26

Dei Tos AP. Classification of pleomorphic sarcomas: where are we now?. *Histopathology.* 2006;48(1):51–62.
Strander H, Turesson I, Cavallin-Ståhl E. A systematic overview of radiation therapy effects in soft tissue sarcomas. *Acta Oncol.* 2003;42(5–6):516–531.

Case 27

Shives TC. Biopsy of soft-tissue tumors. *Clin Orthop Relat Res.* 1993;(289):32–35.

Case 28

Boyer MI. *AAOS Comprehensive Orthopaedic Review 2.* Rosemont, IL: American Academy of Orthopaedic Surgeons, Copyright; 2014:557.

Case 29

Ikeda T, Tada H. Arthroscopic surgery for synovial chondromatosis of the hip. *J Bone Joint Surg [Br].* 1989;989(71-B):l98–199.

Case 30

Lisa C. *Orthopaedic Knowledge Update 11.* Rosemont, IL: American Academy of Orthopaedic Surgeons, Copyright; 2014:278.

Case 31

Lisa C. *Orthopaedic Knowledge Update 11.* Rosemont, IL: American Academy of Orthopaedic Surgeons, Copyright; 2014:278.

Case 32

Lisa C. *Orthopaedic Knowledge Update 11.* Rosemont, IL: American Academy of Orthopaedic Surgeons, Copyright; 2014:279.
Mirels H. Metastatic disease in long bones A proposed scoring system for diagnosing impending pathologic fractures. *Clin Orthop Relat Res.* 1989;(249):256–264.
Redmond BJ, Biermann JS, Blasier RB. Interlocking intramedullary nailing of pathological fractures of the shaft of the humerus. *J Bone Joint Surg Am.* 1996;78(6):891–896.

Case 33

Lisa C. *Orthopaedic Knowledge Update 11.* Rosemont, IL: American Academy of Orthopaedic Surgeons, Copyright; 2014:279.
Grill V, Martin TJ. Hypercalcemia of malignancy. *Rev Endocr Metab Disord.* 2000;1(4):253–263.

Case 34

Lisa C. *Orthopaedic Knowledge Update 11.* Rosemont, IL: American Academy of Orthopaedic Surgeons, Copyright; 2014:279.
Olerud C, Jónsson H Jr, Löfberg AM, Lörelius LE, Sjöström L. Embolization of spinal metastases reduces peroperative blood loss: 21 patients operated on for renal cell carcinoma. *Acta Orthop Scand.* 1993;64(1):9–12.

Case 35

Schneiderbauer MM, von Knoch M, Schleck CD, Harmsen WS, Sim FH, Scully SP. Patient survival after hip arthroplasty for metastatic disease of the hip. *J Bone Joint Surg Am.* 2004;86-A(8):1684–1689.

Case 36

Boyer MI. *AAOS Comprehensive Orthopaedic Review 2.* Rosemont, IL: American Academy of Orthopaedic Surgeons, Copyright; 2014:557.

Case 37

Miller MD, ed. *Review of Orthopaedics.* 6th ed. Philadelphia, PA: WB Saunders; 2012:665.
Lisa C. *Orthopaedic Knowledge Update 11.* Rosemont, IL: American Academy of Orthopaedic Surgeons, Copyright; 2014:199.

Case 38

Cho HY, Lee M, Takei H, Dancer J, Ro JY, Zhai QJ. Immunohistochemical comparison of chordoma with chondrosarcoma, myxopapillary ependymoma, and chordoid meningioma. *Appl Immunohistochem Mol Morphol.* 2009; 17(2):131–138.
Miller MD, ed. *Review of Orthopaedics.* 6th ed. Philadelphia, PA: WB Saunders; 2012:653–654.
Romeo S, Hogendoorn PC. Brachyury and chordoma: the chondroid–chordoid dilemma resolved? *J Pathol.* 2006; 209(2):143–146.

Case 39

Ramakrishnan M, Prasad SS, Parkinson RW, Kaye JC. Management of subtrochanteric femoral fractures and metastases using long proximal femoral nail. *Injury.* 2004;35(2):184–190.

Case 40

Abbas JS, Holyoke ED, Moore R, Karakousis CP. The surgical treatment and outcome of soft-tissue sarcoma. *Arch Surg.* 1981;116(6):765–769.
Henson, JS, et al. *AJCC cancer staging manual.* 5th ed. Philadelphia, PA: Lippincott-Raven; 1997.
Munk PL, Lee MJ, Janzen DL, et al. Lipoma and liposarcoma: evaluation using CT and MR imaging. *AJR Am J Roentgenol.* 1997;169(2):589–594.

Case 41

Gebhardt MC, Lord FC, Rosenberg AE, Mankin HJ. The treatment of adamantinoma of the tibia by wide resection and allograft bone transplantation. *J Bone Joint Surg Am.* 1987; 69(8):1177–1188.

Case 42

Lisa C. *Orthopaedic Knowledge Update 11.* Rosemont, IL: American Academy of Orthopaedic Surgeons, Copyright; 2014:265–268.

Miller MD, ed. *Review of Orthopaedics.* 6th ed. Philadelphia, PA: WB Saunders; 2012:663–664.

Case 43

Floman Y, Bar-On E, Mosheiff R, Mirovsky Y, Robin GC, Ramu N. Eosinophilic granuloma of the spine. *J Pediatr Orthop B.* 1997;6(4):260–265.

Case 44

Miller MD, ed. *Review of Orthopaedics.* 6th ed. Philadelphia, PA: WB Saunders; 2012:665.

Case 45

Boyer MI. *AAOS Comprehensive Orthopaedic Review 2.* Rosemont, IL: American Academy of Orthopaedic Surgeons, Copyright; 2014:548.

Friedman JM, Gutmann DH, Maccollin M, Riccardi VM. *Neurofibromatosis, Phenotype, Natural History Pathogenesis.* Baltimore, MD: Johns Hopkins University Press; 1999:1–296.

Case 46

Muramatsu K, Ihara K, Hashimoto T, Seto S, Taguchi T. Elastofibroma dorsi: diagnosis and treatment. *J Shoulder Elbow Surg.* 2007;16(5):591–595.

Case 47

Boyer MI. *AAOS Comprehensive Orthopaedic Review 2.* Rosemont, IL: American Academy of Orthopaedic Surgeons, Copyright; 2014:557.

Case 48

Campanacci M. Osteoid osteoma. *Bone and Soft Tissue Tumors.* Vienna: Springer; 1999:391–414.

Cantwell CP, Obyrne J, Eustace S. Current trends in treatment of osteoid osteoma with an emphasis on radiofrequency ablation. *Eur Radiol.* 2004;14(4):607–617.

Case 49

Park YK, Unni KK, McLeod RA, Pritchard DJ. Osteofibrous dysplasia: clinicopathologic study of 80 cases. *Hum Pathol.* 1993;24(12):1339–1347.

Case 50

Boyer MI. *AAOS Comprehensive Orthopaedic Review 2.* Rosemont, IL: American Academy of Orthopaedic Surgeons, Copyright; 2014:503–504.

Miller MD, ed. *Review of Orthopaedics.* 6th ed. Philadelphia, PA: WB Saunders; 2012:649.

9

Sports Medicine

Joseph DeAngelis

CASE 1

A 22-year-old, female jogger presents complaining of right knee pain. She describes an insidious onset of her symptoms during the last 3 months. She enjoys running most days and is training for a five-mile road race. Recently, she has been running more and has added hill training. Her pain is centered around the patella with little swelling. She has crepitus and pain when climbing stairs or getting out of a chair. X-rays are shown in Figure 9–1A–C.

The most likely diagnosis for the condition described is:

A. Patellofemoral syndrome (runner's knee)
B. Osgood–Schlatter disease
C. Femoral stress fracture
D. Meniscal tear
E. ACL rupture

Discussion

The correct answer is (A). Patellofemoral syndrome (runner's knee) is very common, resulting from overuse. It

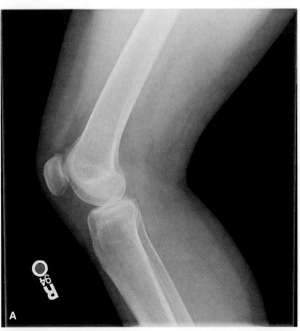

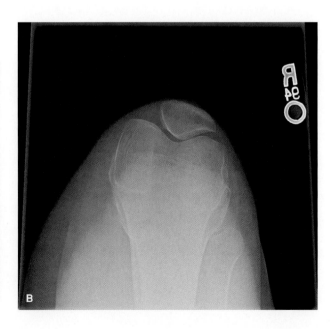

Figure 9–1 **A–B**

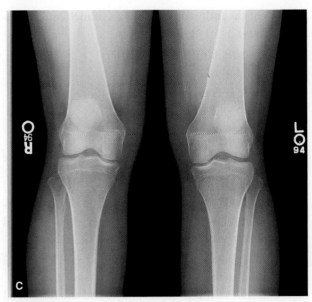

Figure 9–1 **C**

is seen frequently in runners and active women. Many believe that it results from maltracking of the patella within the femoral groove due to vastus medialis weakness.

Osgood–Schlatter's disease also results from overuse. It is more common in men and jumping athletes who have not reached skeletal maturity. Stress fractures can result from a sudden increase in activity and cause pain with all weight-bearing activities. Meniscal tears cause mechanical symptoms and are associated with knee swelling. Athletes with ACL tears complain of knee instability following an injury.

What is the preferred treatment for this female runner?

A. Corticosteroid injection
B. Knee arthroscopy
C. Activity modification and physical therapy
D. Endocrine evaluation
E. Strict immobilization

Discussion

The correct answer is (C). Increasing vastus medialis strength is believed to balance the pull on the patella. Lower extremity mechanics and function are thought to improve with combining increased quadriceps flexibility, balance, and proprioceptive training. Oral anti-inflammatories and cross-training will provide symptomatic improvement while maintaining fitness.

Three months later, she presents with recurrent right knee pain, medial to the patella. As before, her pain is exacerbated by knee flexion. On examination, there is tenderness and an area of fullness about 1 cm medial to the patella. The most likely diagnosis is:

A. Meniscal tear
B. Pigmented villonodular synovitis
C. Medial collateral ligament (MCL) strain
D. Plica syndrome
E. Patellofemoral pain syndrome

Discussion

The correct answer is (D). Her symptoms and examination are typical of plica syndrome. The synovial fold on the medial knee becomes irritated in sports that require repeated flexion of the knee (running, biking, rowing, etc.). Treatment should address the local inflammation with rest, ice, and oral anti-inflammatories. In recalcitrant cases, local corticosteroid injections may be helpful. If conservative management fails, arthroscopic resection is an option.

Objectives: Did you learn...?

• Identify runner's knee?
• Understand conservative treatment of anterior knee pain?
• Recognize plica syndrome?

CASE 2

An 18-year-old soccer player injures her knee during competition. She reports her knee buckled when stepping to kick the ball. She fell to the ground after hearing a pop and was unable to stand on her right leg. Since then, she has been able to bear some weight, but she does not trust her leg.

On examination, she has a large swollen knee.

The MOST likely isolated injury experienced by this athlete is:

A. Anterior cruciate ligament (ACL) rupture
B. Medial meniscus tear
C. Medial collateral ligament (MCL) sprain
D. Quadriceps tendon rupture

Discussion

The correct answer is (A). Following this noncontact soccer injury, the athlete has a sense of instability and a large swollen knee which is most consistent with an ACL rupture. Although acute meniscal tears can result in large effusions, typically they present as mechanical symptoms such as catching and locking. Collateral ligament injuries do not typically present with swelling. Commonly, these injuries feel stable when moving straight ahead but are painful with side-to-side movements.

A quadriceps rupture is uncommon in a young, healthy athlete and would result in an inability to stand or extend the knee.

In the acutely injured knee, the best test to confirm the diagnosis would be:

A. X-rays
B. McMurray test
C. Lachman test
D. Pivot shift test
E. Grind test

Discussion

The correct answer is (C). The most useful diagnostic test for an acute ACL rupture is the Lachman test. It is the most sensitive test for ACL insufficiency (80–95%). Radiographs can be helpful in affirming that there is no bony injury. The McMurray test is an assessment of meniscal pathology. The pivot shift test is pathognomonic for ACL tears but is best suited for a chronic injury. The grind test is a measure of patellofemoral pain.

The primary blood supply to the ACL is the:

A. Lateral superior geniculate artery
B. Descending geniculate artery
C. Middle geniculate artery
D. Recurrent anterior tibial artery

Discussion

The correct answer is (C). The middle geniculate artery provides the primary blood to the ACL.

Which of the following vessels is a branch of the femoral artery?

A. The descending geniculate artery
B. The superior geniculate arteries
C. The inferior geniculate arteries
D. The middle geniculate artery

Discussion

The correct answer is (A). The descending geniculate artery is a branch of the femoral artery.

An MRI of the injured knee shows a characteristic pattern of bony edema following this injury. Where would you typically see the bone bruising in this athlete?

A. Anterior lateral femoral condyle and anterior medial tibial plateau
B. Posterior lateral femoral condyle and anterior lateral tibial plateau
C. Anterior medial femoral condyle and posterior lateral tibial plateau
D. Anterior medial femoral condyle and posterior medial tibial plateau
E. Anterior lateral femoral condyle and posterior lateral tibial plateau

Discussion

The correct answer is (E). MRI of an ACL tear is shown in Figure 9–2A. The ACL rupture results in a sudden translation of the tibia anterior relative to the femur, resulting in a transchondral fracture (bone bruise) of

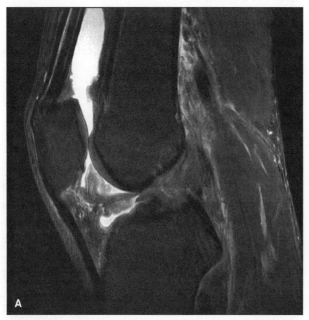

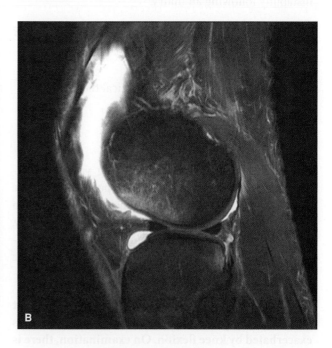

Figure 9–2 **A–B**

the anterior lateral femoral condyle and the posterior lateral tibial plateau (Fig. 9–2B).

Initial treatment of this athlete should include all of the following EXCEPT:

A. Quadriceps strengthening
B. Hamstring strengthening
C. Proprioceptive training
D. Lateral movement drills
E. Effusion control

Discussion

The correct answer is (D). Lateral movements, like planting, cutting, and pivoting are contraindicated in patients with ACL ruptures and can result in recurrent instability and/or additional injury.

If she elects to treat her injury without surgery, which activities are appropriate?

A. Running
B. Biking
C. Rowing
D. Swimming
E. All of the above

Discussion

The correct answer is (E). Individuals with ACL-deficient knees have very good outcomes with nonsurgical treatment if they can avoid cutting and pivoting movements. Activity modification should include any sport that does not put them at risk.

Objectives: Did you learn...?

• The diagnosis of an acute knee injury?
• To understand the presentation of an ACL rupture?
• To anticipate the relevant findings on MRI?
• The role of nonoperative treatment in ACL injuries?

CASE 3

A 44-year-old man slips while dancing at a wedding. With the help of his spouse, he is able to get home safely, but the next morning he has difficulty standing on his left leg. His knee is swollen, with little pain. If he gets on his feet, he is able to get around the house, but he is unable to go up or down stairs and feels unsteady on his feet.

His examination reveals a large swollen knee, held at 30 degrees of knee flexion. He has little pain with passive flexion or extension and no tenderness to

palpation. He is unable to actively extend his leg when supine. When lying on his right side, however, he can make his left leg straight.

What is the most likely diagnosis?

A. Quadriceps tendon rupture
B. Meniscal tear
C. ACL rupture
D. Patella fracture
E. Patella dislocation

Discussion

The correct answer is (A). An MRI of a quadriceps tendon rupture is demonstrated in Figure 9–3. The inability to extend the leg against gravity is most consistent with an injury to the extensor mechanism. The absence of tenderness on palpation and pain with passive motion makes a patella fracture unlikely. A transient patella dislocation can result in swelling but does not prevent a straight-leg raise. Placing the patient in the lateral decubitus position eliminates gravity as a resisting force.

In an active young man, the best outcomes will result from what treatment?

A. Early range of motion
B. Cast immobilization
C. Bracing
D. Surgical repair

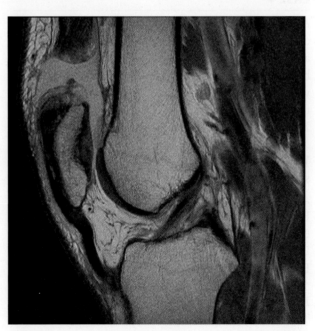

Figure 9–3

Discussion

The correct answer is (D). Extensor mechanism repairs are recommended in all patients in whom surgery is not contraindicated in order to restore normal function to the leg. Nonoperative treatment is reserved for incomplete (partial) injuries (<50%) and people unable to tolerate surgery.

Immediately following surgery, which of the following activities is appropriate?

A. Range of motion as tolerated
B. Closed chain strengthening
C. Open chain strengthening
D. Prone active knee flexion
E. Assisted passive knee flexion

Discussion

The correct answer is (D). Following surgical repair of the extensor mechanism, range of motion and strengthening should be limited to allow for tendon to bone healing. Assisted passive knee flexion can negatively affect the healing process. Prone, active knee flexion promotes motion without stressing the repair site.

Objectives: Did you learn...?

• Recognize extensor mechanism injury?
• Describe treatment options?
• Understand rehabilitation of tendon to bone healing?

CASE 4

A 54-year-old skier injures his right knee on the last run of the day. He describes getting his ski stuck in the snow and having an immediate onset of pain on the inside of his knee. He did not hear a pop and was able to make his way down the slope under his own power. Over the last few days, the pain has been worse when bearing weight. X-rays are shown in Figure 9–4A–C.

Which of the following structures provides dynamic stability to the medial knee?

A. The semimembranosus complex
B. The sartorius
C. The gracilis
D. The semitendinosus
E. The biceps femoris

Discussion

The correct answer is (A). On examination, there is swelling and bruising on the medial knee. He has increased laxity in response to valgus stress at 30 degrees of knee flexion when compared to the contralateral leg. At terminal extension, the valgus stress response is symmetric. His Lachman and anterior drawer tests are symmetric with the left knee.

What is his diagnosis?

A. ACL rupture with grade 1 MCL sprain
B. ACL rupture

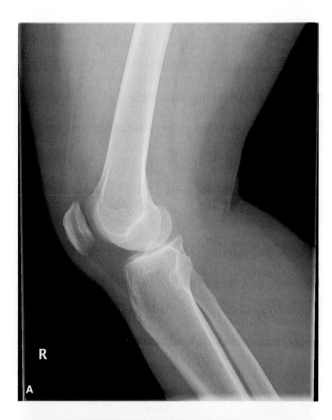

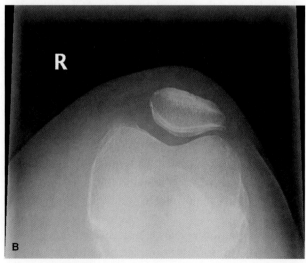

Figure 9–4 **A–B**

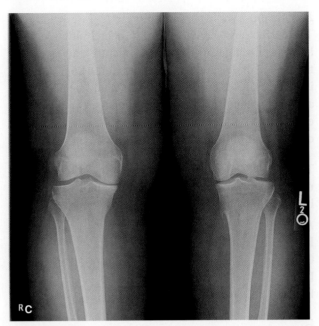

Figure 9–4 **C**

C. Grade 2 MCL sprain
D. Grade 3 MCL sprain
E. ACL rupture with grade 2 MCL sprain

Discussion

The correct answer is (C). Increased laxity at 30 degrees of knee flexion suggests an MCL sprain (grade 1 or 2). The lack of laxity to valgus stress at terminal extension (0 degrees) is only seen in grade 3 MCL sprains. The symmetric Lachman and anterior drawer tests make an ACL rupture less likely.

Treatment of this injury should include all of the following EXCEPT:

A. Immediate return to sports
B. Crutches
C. Knee immobilizer
D. Hinged knee brace
E. Quad strengthening

Discussion

The correct answer is (A). The timing for return to sports is related to the severity of the injury. Grade 1 injuries may return in 5 to 7 days. Grade 2 sprains generally require 2 to 4 weeks. Grade 3 injuries can take 4 to 8 weeks to recover. Protected weight bearing with crutches, immobilization, assistive devices, and strengthening can be of assistance.

Objectives: Did you learn…?
• The dynamic stabilizers of the knee?
• The physical examination of MCL injury?
• The treatment of MCL sprain?

CASE 5

A 24-year-old graduate student twists her knee while walking in high heels on a cobble stone street. She has an acute onset of pain and deformity. On presentation to the emergency department, she is uncomfortable and maintains her knee in a flexed position. As her leg is gradually extended, an audible "clunk" is heard, and her knee can rest flat on the stretcher. Moments later, she is able to complete a straight-leg raise.

What structure was most likely injured in her accident?

A. Medial meniscus
B. Medial patellofemoral ligament
C. Anterior cruciate ligament
D. Patellar tendon
E. Medial collateral ligament

Discussion

The correct answer is (B). The student sustained a patellar dislocation. With passive extension of the knee, the patella reduced causing an audible clunk. Lateral dislocations are the most common, and the medial patellofemoral ligament is injured as a result. While other intra-articular structures can be injured in twisting injuries, the restoration of function following passive leg extension makes a patella dislocation the most likely.

Radiographs of her knee reveal no fracture. If an MRI were ordered, which of the following is the least likely finding?

A. MPFL rupture
B. Bone edema on the lateral femoral condyle
C. Osteochondral injury to the medial patellar facet
D. Loose body in the medial gutter
E. Lipohemarthrosis

Discussion

Correct answer is "E." In the absence of fracture, a lipohemarthrosis is unlikely. Injury to the medial patellofemoral ligament results from a lateral dislocation. As the medial facet of the patella strikes the lateral femoral condyle, a bone bruise may result along with an injury to the patellar articular cartilage. If injured, a loose piece may be found on the MRI.

After the first event, she undergoes conservative treatment. Unfortunately, she has several recurrent episodes. A CT scan reveals excessive lateralization of the tibial tuberosity. If she undergoes a reconstruction of the medial patellofemoral ligaments, what other procedure should be performed simultaneously?

A. Distal tibial tuberosity transfer
B. Trochleoplasty
C. Femoral/tibial derotational osteotomy
D. Medial tibial transfer

Discussion

The correct answer is (D). Distal tibial tuberosity transfers are indicated with patella alta. Trochleoplasty should be used to address severe trochlear dysplasia. Excessive limb rotation can be corrected with combined femoral and tibial derotational osteotomies, while lateralization of the tibial tubercle benefits from a medial tibial transfer.

Objectives: Did you learn...?

• The signs and symptoms of MPFL injury?
• The imaging findings of MPFL injury?
• The treatment of MPFL injury?

CASE 6

During a recreational game of basketball, a 47-year-old man twists his right knee while defending an opponent. Initially, he had some swelling and walked with a limp. Over the next 2 weeks, he had continued pain with occasional symptoms of catching in his knee.

On examination, he cannot fully extend his knee and has tenderness on the medial joint line with a positive McMurray test.

What is the most appropriate next step in his evaluation?

A. Weight-bearing radiographs
B. MRI
C. MR arthrogram
D. Examination under anesthesia
E. Diagnostic arthroscopy

Discussion

The correct answer is (A). In an acutely injured athlete, it is essential to rule out a fracture and to assess the degree of degenerative changes in the knee. If there is no fracture or arthritis, an MRI would be appropriate. Meniscal injuries do not require an arthrogram. An examination under anesthesia and diagnostic arthroscopy are not indicated.

The patient is found to have a displaced tear of the medial meniscus. Which pattern of meniscal tearing is most amenable to repair?

A. Radial
B. Bucket-handle
C. Oblique
D. Horizontal cleavage
E. Vertical

Discussion

The correct answer is (B). Tear types that are most appropriate for repair include vertical tears in the vascular zone of the meniscus and bucket-handle tears that are in good condition when reduced. The other patterns have a lower propensity to heal and are treated with excision.

Which of the following factors does NOT coincide with better, long-term function following a partial meniscectomy?

A. Age older than 40 years
B. Normal limb alignment
C. Single tear
D. Minimal arthritis

Discussion

The correct answer is (A). Better, long-term function has been reported in patients who underwent partial meniscectomy, that were less than 40 years old, had normal limb alignment, a single tear, and little arthritis at the time of arthroscopy.

Which of the following statement is true regarding the function of the meniscus?

A. The meniscus absorbs more load in flexion than extension
B. The meniscus is primarily composed of type 2 collagen
C. 90% of the meniscus is water
D. The medial meniscus provides more support than the lateral meniscus
E. A partial meniscectomy decreases contact pressure

Discussion

The correct answer is (A). The meniscus absorbs up to 50% of the load across the knee in extension and 90% when the knee is flexed to 90 degrees. Type 1 collagen is the predominate type in the meniscus. Water makes up 70% of the meniscus. The lateral meniscus provides more support than the medial. Following a partial meniscectomy, the contact pressure on the articular cartilage increases.

Objectives: Did you learn...?

- The diagnostic algorithm of suspected meniscal injury?
- The anatomy and physiology of the meniscus?

CASE 7

An otherwise healthy 30-year-old carpenter presents with left knee pain and swelling. He has had intermittent symptoms that are worse with activity. Occasionally, his knee will get stuck such that he is unable to bend or straighten it. His knee is warm and full on examination, but his ligamentous examination is symmetric with the right.

Which of the following is the likely diagnosis?

A. Gout
B. Lyme disease
C. Gonococcal arthritis
D. Synovial chondromatosis

Discussion

The correct answer is (D). Infectious and crystalline causes of knee swelling do not present with mechanical symptoms. Proliferation of hyaline cartilage nodules in the synovial membrane can limit motion.

An MRI is obtained which demonstrates numerous cartilage nodules throughout the knee. What is the next best step in treatment?

A. Physical therapy
B. Immobilization
C. Corticosteroid injection
D. Radiation treatment
E. Synovectomy

Discussion

The correct answer is (E). Arthroscopic and/or open synovectomy can be effective at removing the cartilage nodules to address the mechanical symptoms and limiting recurrence. However, incomplete resection increases the chance of recurrence. Physical therapy, immobilization, corticosteroid injections, and radiation treatment have not been shown to address the mechanical symptoms or to facilitate recovery.

Objectives: Did you learn...?

- The signs of synovial chondromatosis?
- The treatment of synovial chondromatosis?

CASE 8

A 35-year-old triathlete has mechanical symptoms in her left knee and is diagnosed with a medial meniscal tear via MRI. At the time of her arthroscopic partial meniscectomy, a full-thickness cartilage defect (outerbridge IV) is found on the medial femoral condyle that measures 2 cm × 1.5 cm.

What is the best treatment for this lesion?

A. Nonoperative care
B. Microfracture
C. Autologous chondrocyte implantation
D. Osteochondral transplantation

Discussion

The correct answer is (B). A full-thickness defect is found in 4% of knee arthroscopies. Microfracture as a reparative technique has been shown to offer better results with lower morbidity in comparison to other restorative techniques currently available.

Which of the following are NOT considered a reparative marrow stimulation technique?

A. Microfracture
B. Drilling
C. Mosaicplasty
D. Abrasion chondroplasty

Discussion

The correct answer is (C). The use of osteochondral plugs is a restorative method like autogenous chondrocyte implantation. Microfracture, drilling, and abrasion chondroplasty are reparative techniques that promote a fibrocartilage repair of the exposed bone by stimulating bleeding in the area of concern.

Objectives: Did you learn...?

- The treatment of full-thickness chondral defects?
- The different treatments for reparative marrow stimulation?

CASE 9

A running back is struck on the outside of his right knee as he crosses the goal line. His cleats hold onto the turf and his knee hyperextends before giving way. The medical staff transports him to the locker room for a prompt examination. With his leg straight on the examination table, he has increased laxity to both a varus and valgus stress. With the knee bent to 30 degrees, the tibia translates more than one centimeter anterior to the femur and one centimeter posterior to the femur. His initial vascular examination on the field revealed a threaded, asymmetric pulse. Upon repeat examination, his distal pulses are symmetric. Radiographs at the stadium reveal no fracture or dislocation.

Initial management of this injury should include:

A. Immobilization

B. Immobilization and serial examinations

C. Immediate surgical reconstruction

D. Serial examinations

Discussion

The correct answer is (B). The athlete sustained a multiligamentous knee injury and experienced a transient dislocation of his right knee. The severity of this injury places him at increased risk for a vascular injury. Immobilization provides stability to the injured knee, while serial examinations should monitor the arterial flow and compartment pressures. Immediate reconstruction is not indicated in a complex knee injury in an athlete of any level.

Which ligaments are likely to be injured?

A. ACL

B. ACL, PCL

C. ACL, PCL, MCL

D. ACL, PCL, MCL, LCL

Discussion

The correct answer is (D). The examination reveals increased anterior and posterior translation consistent with a combined ACL and PCL injury. The varus and valgus laxity suggest an injury to the MCL and LCL.

What physical examination finding should be carefully assessed as a common sequelae of this injury?

A. Great toe extension

B. Great toe flexion

C. Hindfoot inversion

D. Hindfoot eversion

E. Heel pad two-point discrimination

Discussion

The correct answer is (A). Peroneal nerve palsy occurs in almost one-third of knee dislocations. Evaluation of the nerve's motor and sensory function is an essential part of a comprehensive examination.

Objectives: Did you learn...?

- The initial management of multiligamentous knee injury?
- The sequelae of MLI?

CASE 10

A 24-year-old, ultimate frisbee player reinjures his previously reconstructed left knee. He explains that 4 years ago he ruptured his ACL playing basketball. He had an allograft repair followed by an uneventful recovery. He returned to sports 8 months after surgery. X-rays are shown in Figure 9–5A and B.

Which element made the greatest contribution to his graft failure?

A. Graft fixation

B. Femoral tunnel position

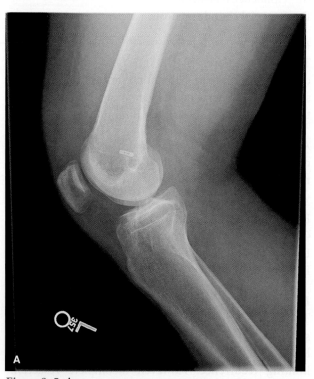

Figure 9–5 **A**

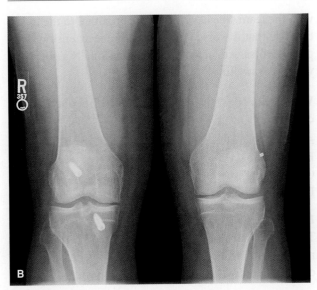

Figure 9–5 **B**

C. Graft type
D. Meniscal pathology
E. Tibial tunnel position

Discussion

The correct answer is (C). In younger people, allograft ACL reconstructions have been found to have a significantly higher failure rate than autograft reconstructions. Inadequate fixation can result in residual laxity following surgery. Tunnel position is important to restoring normal function of the knee. Meniscal pathology carries a worse prognosis over time but has not been associated with re-tears.

After careful consideration, he elects to proceed with a revision ACL reconstruction. In choosing between a single-stage ACL revision and a two-step, staged ACL revision (removal of hardware with bone grafting, followed by later revision ACL reconstruction), which finding most strongly favors a staged revision?

A. Tunnel widening
B. Vertical femoral tunnel
C. Retained hardware
D. Prior autograft reconstruction
E. Meniscal tear

Discussion

The correct answer is (A). A staged revision is necessary when the existing tunnels are too wide to achieve reliable fixation or if their position compromises the accurate reconstruction of the ACL. Vertical femoral tunnel placement is usually easily avoided during a revision

ACL. Retained hardware can be removed in one sitting. Prior autograft reconstruction and the presence of a meniscal tear should not affect the decision.

During the revision ACL reconstruction, the graft impinges in the notch as the knee is extended, making terminal extension 5 degrees short of straight. Which factor is responsible for the limitation in range of motion?

A. Femoral tunnel too anterior
B. Femoral tunnel too posterior
C. Tibial tunnel too anterior
D. Tibial tunnel too posterior
E. Use of autograft

Discussion

The correct answer is (C). The tibial tunnel is too anterior and the graft is impinging as the knee extends. The femoral tunnel position will not affect knee extension. A tibial tunnel that is posterior will not impede extension. The graft type should not affect knee motion.

Objectives: Did you learn...?

- The most common cause of graft failure?
- The indications of staged revision?
- The causes of graft impingement?

CASE 11

A 44-year-old waiter slips on a wet floor in the kitchen, hyperextending his right knee. He has an acute onset of swelling and pain with weight bearing. Three days later, radiographs reveal a minimally displaced fracture of the tibial spine.

What would you expect to find on his physical examination?

A. Laxity on valgus stress at 30 degrees of knee flexion
B. Increased external rotation of the tibia at 30 degrees of knee flexion
C. Positive patellar apprehension sign
D. Increase anterior translation of the tibia

Discussion

The correct answer is (D). Tibial spine avulsion injuries occur more frequently in children than adults. However, this injury can result in ACL laxity. Tibial spine fractures are not associated with valgus laxity (MCL sprain), a posterior lateral corner injury, or patellar instability.

The initial conservative treatment of this fracture may include all of the following EXCEPT:

A. Activity modification
B. Open chain strengthening
C. Immobilization
D. Aspiration

Discussion

The correct answer is (B). Activity modification and immobilization are essential steps to limit motion and prevent fracture displacement. Aspiration of the associated effusion may help to minimize pain due to capsular distention and help the patient achieve terminal extension. Open chain exercises will stress the knee with resistance and should not be performed early in the plan of care.

Six months following the injury, the patient reports his knee giving way when changing directions suddenly at work. His examination reveals increased anterior translation of the tibia, and the x-rays show a healed tibial spine without evidence of displacement.

What study will provide the best insight into his condition?

A. EMG
B. 3-ft standing films
C. MRI right knee
D. MRI lumbar spine
E. CT arthrogram right knee

Discussion

The correct answer is (C). An MRI will illustrate the integrity of the ACL and meniscal cartilage as a possible source of his instability and laxity. EMG will assess his nerve function, while 3-ft standing films can offer a perspective on the limb alignment. There is no evidence of lumbar disease contributing to his right knee disability. A CT arthrogram can be used to assess the ACL and menisci, but it does not offer the resolution or fidelity of an MRI.

Objectives: Did you learn...?

• The physical examination findings of tibial spine avulsion in adult?
• The initial management of tibial spine avulsion in adults?

CASE 12

A 19-year-old, college freshman has increased left anterior knee pain two weeks into her pre-season training with the team. She has tenderness proximal to the tibial tubercle that is worse with resisted knee extension. The pain is worse with activity and is occasionally associated with local swelling.

What sports is she most likely to be playing in college?

A. Ice hockey
B. Field hockey
C. Archery
D. Track & field

Discussion

The correct answer is (D). Patellar tendinitis occurs most commonly in athletes who engage in forceful, eccentric contractions of the knee as in jumping sports.

Her treatment may include all of the following except:

A. Activity modification
B. Immobilization
C. Progressive flexibility
D. Eccentric strengthening
E. Corticosteroid injection

Discussion

The correct answer is (E). Corticosteroid injections are contraindicated because of the increased risk of tendon rupture. Activity modification and immobilization can help encourage symptoms to subside. Flexibility and eccentric strengthening are essential to the resolution of the condition.

Objectives: Did you learn...?

• The causes and treatment of patellar tendinitis?

CASE 13

A 56-year-old mason presents with acute swelling of his left knee. He explains that he has been laying a tile floor in a large bathroom and has continued to work 10-hour days since misplacing his knee pads at the end of last week. The left knee became large and swollen in the absence of any acute trauma. It is firm but not tender. There is no surrounding erythema, and the overlying skin is intact.

What is the best next step in management of this problem?

A. Aspiration
B. Get new knee pads
C. One week of oral antibiotics

D. Immobilization

E. Corticosteroid injection

Discussion

The correct answer is (B). The mason's prepatellar bursa is swollen after the prolonged period of kneeling without his usual protection. Aspiration may provide temporary relief, but the fluid usually quickly re-accumulates. Because there is a significant risk of infection, aspiration is discouraged as a first step in treatment. In the absence of erythema or pain, antibiotics are not necessary. Immobilization can help reduce swelling if initial treatments are unsuccessful. Similarly, injecting the bursa with a corticosteroid can offer some benefit for recalcitrant bursitis.

In this case, which bursa is LEAST likely to be involved?

A. Pes bursa

B. Infrapatellar bursa

C. Prepatellar bursa

D. Deep patellar bursa

Discussion

The correct answer is (A). The bursa deep to the pes anserinus is rarely affected in housemaid's knee. The prepatellar bursa is most commonly involved, followed by the infrapatellar and deep patellar bursa.

Which physical finding is LEAST suggestive of septic bursitis?

A. Fever >37.8°C

B. Pre-bursal temperature difference greater 2.2°C

C. Pain with passive range of motion

D. Skin lesions

Discussion

The correct answer is (C). A recent literature review found that fever >37.8°C, pre-bursal temperature difference >2.2°C, and skin lesions were suggestive of septic bursitis. Pain with passive range of motion did not help differentiate septic from nonseptic bursae.

Objectives: Did you learn...?

- The causes of prepatellar bursitis?
- The physical examination findings of septic bursitis?

CASE 14

A 27-year-old soccer player injures himself in a fall onto a flexed knee, after colliding with an opponent. He describes a sense of his knee giving way when planting and pushing off to run. On examination, the knee demonstrates a slight sag, but the posterior translation of the tibia is less than one centimeter.

If the remainder of the knee examination is normal, which statement is most likely to be true?

A. His foot was dorsiflexed when he hit the ground

B. His foot was plantar flexed when he hit the ground

C. His posterior translation will increase when the tibia is internally rotated

D. He will be unable to complete a straight-leg raise

E. His anterior drawer test will be positive

Discussion

The correct answer is (B). The plantar-flexed ankle decreases the tension on the gastrocnemius, allowing the PCL to absorb the full force applied to the tibia. Internal rotation will decrease the posterior translation. There is no evidence of an injury to the extensor mechanism or the ACL.

The initial management of this injury should emphasize:

A. Quadriceps strengthening

B. Hamstring strengthening

C. Open chain rehabilitation

D. Strict immobilization

Discussion

The correct answer is (A). Quadriceps strengthening provides a dynamic stabilizing force for the knee to counteract the PCL laxity. Hamstring strengthening will not address the injury, and open chain exercises can increase patellar pain. Initial immobilization should only be relative. Patients should perform range of motion exercises daily to prevent arthrofibrosis and quadriceps atrophy.

Despite aggressive physical therapy, the patient has continued instability. With which movement would you expect the greatest disability?

A. Side stepping

B. Cross over drills

C. Single-leg stance

D. Descending stairs

Discussion

The correct answer is (D). Lateral movements like side-stepping and crossover drills are not typically a source of instability for patients with PCL injuries. Similarly, balance training on one-leg is often beneficial to knee function. Descending stairs and inclines often are problematic.

Objectives: Did you learn...?

- The management of PCL laxity?
- The disability associated with PCL laxity?

CASE 15

A 39-year-old, catcher has an acutely locked knee. She was standing up quickly to throw to second base on an attempted steal when her right knee became stuck, and she was unable to straighten it. She has been unable to move the knee since the injury. On examination, the right knee has a limited range of motion, moving from 30 to 45 degrees of knee flexion. Beyond this arc, the endpoint is firm and painful. Anterior–posterior and lateral x-rays reveal an aligned knee without fracture or dislocation.

Your next step in her care is to:

A. Administer a corticosteroid injection
B. Obtain an MRI
C. Provide her with oral anti-inflammatories and an appointment in 5 to 7 days
D. Apply a long-leg splint

Discussion

The correct answer is (B). MRI has been shown to offer considerable guidance when evaluating patients with a traumatic knee extension deficit (locked knee). The normal radiographs offer assurance that there is no fracture or dislocation preventing knee motion. Injection with a corticosteroid alone will not offer a prompt analgesic benefit. Similarly, oral anti-inflammatories with prompt follow-up do not address the acuity of the patient's problem. Immobilization in a long-leg splint may provide the patient with some comfort but does not advance her care.

She is found to have a loose body and a full-thickness cartilage defect on the medial femoral condyle. Which of the following reasons is the LEAST relevant indication for knee arthroscopy?

A. Recurrent mechanical symptoms
B. Risk of additional injury to articular cartilage
C. Prevention of arthritis
D. Treatment of cartilage defect
E. Harvesting chondrocytes for autologous chondrocyte implantation (ACI)

Discussion

The correct answer is (C). Removal of the loose body will decrease the risk of repeat catching, locking, or giving way as well as lowering the risk of additional injury. If appropriate, the defect could be treated at the initial arthroscopy, or cells could be collected for subsequent treatment. Removal of the loose body with or without a cartilage procedure has not been shown to prevent arthritis.

Objectives: Did you learn...?

- The imaging for a traumatic knee extension deficit (locked knee)?
- The indications for knee arthroscopy?

CASE 16

A 17-year-old runner has increased leg pain in the last week of her pre-season training for cross-country. The pain began without trauma and is present every time she tries to run.

What is the most common site of a stress fracture?

A. Calcaneus
B. Distal femur
C. Femoral neck
D. Pubic ramus
E. Tibia

Discussion

The correct answer is (E). In general, stress fractures occur more frequently in the lower extremities, with the tibia and metatarsals being the most common sites. They occur in the upper extremities although less frequently.

Which of the following is NOT part of the female athlete triad?

A. Amenorrhea
B. Disordered eating
C. Osteoporosis
D. Abulia

Discussion

The correct answer is (D). The female athlete triad consists of amenorrhea, disordered eating, and osteoporosis, and should be considered in all female athletes with a stress fracture. Evaluation of this condition and its underlying causes are essential to the athlete's long-term health.

The benefits of an MRI in the diagnosis of a stress fracture is best described as:

A. Very sensitive in identifying the presence and location of a stress fracture without visualization of a macroscopic fracture line
B. Able to identify bony edema associated with an early stress fracture as well as the presence of a fracture
C. Ideal for evaluating the location and extent of a fracture line
D. Effective overview of anatomic alignment, but limited in early stress fractures

Discussion

The correct answer is (B). Bone scans are very sensitive in identifying the presence and location of a stress fracture without visualization of a macroscopic fracture line. MRI is able to identify bony edema in an early stress fractures. CT scans are ideal for evaluating the location and extent of a fracture line. Plain radiographs provide an effective overview of anatomic alignment but are limited in early stress fractures and may not show the fracture.

When imaging is complete, her radiographs do not show a clear fracture line. However, there is edema on the MRI. Her pain is present with weight bearing. Which of the following locations presents the highest risk of fracture?

A. Calcaneus
B. Medial malleolus
C. First metatarsal
D. Anterior tibial diaphysis
E. Inferior femoral neck

Discussion

The correct answer is (D). The lateral malleolus, calcaneus, and first through fourth metatarsals are at low risk for fracture propagation. The medial malleolus and inferior femoral neck represent an intermediate risk. High-risk locations include the superior femoral neck, the anterior tibial diaphysis, the navicular, the base of the fifth metatarsal, and the neck of the talus.

Objectives: Did you learn...?

• The epidemiology of stress fractures?
• The three parts to the female athlete triad?

CASE 17

During a football game, a 21-year-old, right-hand-dominant male experiences a numb and tingling sensation in his right arm after making a tackle. With his elbow at his side, his arm is weak in external rotation when compared to his left.

Which finding is LEAST likely to accompany this injury?

A. Pain with lateral head turning toward the affected side
B. Transient symptoms
C. Positive Spurling test
D. History of prior symptoms
E. Bilateral symptoms

Discussion

The correct answer is (E). Stingers are transient and unilateral. Turning the head toward the affected side may compress the nerve roots causing symptoms as would the Spurling maneuver. Patients who have a stinger are three times more likely to have another.

All of the following findings are concerning for a more serious injury EXCEPT:

A. Circumferential distribution
B. Neck pain
C. Symptoms lasting more than 3 weeks
D. Abnormal EMG

Discussion

The correct answer is (A). Burners often cause transient pain, burning or tingling in a circumferential, not dermatomal, distribution. Limited neck motion or pain requires additional evaluation. Players with persistent symptoms or EMG changes should not return to sports participation.

Objectives: Did you learn...?

• The history and physical examination findings of stingers?
• The red flags associated with this injury?

CASE 18

A 17-year-old, right-hand-dominant, volleyball player presents for worsening right shoulder pain. Over the summer, she played more than usual having joined a travel team. Her pain is worse after playing, and she has noticed that her power has decreased when she strikes the ball. There has been no numbness or tingling in her arm, and she denies any trauma. Strength testing reveals no weakness when her arm is at her side. When outstretched, her right arm is weaker than the left. When completing wall push-up, her back is asymmetric.

The prominence in her back is best described as:

A. Postural kyphosis
B. Scapular winging
C. Congenital scoliosis
D. Hemihypertrophy

Discussion

The correct answer is (B). Long-thoracic nerve palsy can present in overhead athletes in the absence of trauma. The repetitive motion may result in nerve traction and resulting dysfunction in the serratus anterior leading to medial scapular winging. Postural kyphosis will result in a symmetric prominence of the upper back. Congenital scoliosis presents early in life. Hemihypertrophy is a congenital syndrome resulting in one side of the body or one limb larger than the other.

Which nerve root is LEAST likely involved in her injury?

A. C5
B. C6
C. C7
D. C8
E. T1

Discussion

The correct answer is (D). The long thoracic nerve arises predominantly from C5 to C7. In 8% of people, C8 contributes.

The best test to confirm the diagnosis and grade the severity is:

A. MRI
B. Metabolic panel
C. Muscle biopsy
D. EMG
E. Serial examinations

Discussion

The correct answer is (D). EMG with nerve conduction velocity will evaluate the function of the long-thoracic nerve and can offer an assessment of the severity of the injury. In long-thoracic nerve palsy, blood work and muscle function are normal. Repeat examination can be used to monitor recovery over 12 to 24 months but offer little confirmation or assessment of severity.

Objectives: Did you learn...?

• The pathophysiology of medial scapular winging?
• The diagnostic findings of medial scapular winging?

CASE 19

The mother of twin, 12-year-old girls contacts your office because her daughters are interested in playing soccer in the fall. The league requires a preparticipation physical examination.

All of the following are addressed by a preparticipation physical EXCEPT:

A. Assessment of life-threatening conditions that may be revealed by sports participation
B. Evaluation of current injuries to be treated before returning to play
C. Impartial documentation of skill and fitness
D. Create an opportunity to address injury prevention
E. Address legal and insurance requirements for the sponsoring organization/institution

Discussion

The correct answer is (C). The goal of preparticipation physical examinations is to diagnosis medical conditions that place an athlete at risk during sports participation. It also provides an opportunity to ensure the appropriate treatment of existing problems while also planning for prevention and safety. Legal concerns and insurance policies often require certification of the athlete's health prior to competition. In amateur athletes, the preparticipation physical is not a resource for player assessment.

When taking a history for the preparticipation examination, which of the following is LEAST worrisome?

A. Long QT syndrome
B. Healed long-bone fracture
C. Shortness of breath
D. Missed or absent menses
E. Prior heat stroke

Discussion

The correct answer is (B). The history should be examined for cardiac disease (hypertrophic cardiomyopathy, sudden death, long QT, or Marfan syndromes), exertional symptoms (shortness of breath, heart palpitations, chest pain, orthopnea), neurologic disorders (seizures, concussions, stingers), prior heat-related illnesses, as well as signs of female athlete triad (amenorrhea, disordered eating, and osteoporosis). Prior fracture history is important and should be carefully reviewed.

Cardiac auscultation is recommended with the patient standing, sitting and supine. Which of the following murmurs does NOT require further evaluation before participation?

A. Systolic murmur, squatting, 2/6 intensity
B. Murmur that worsens with Valsalva
C. Diastolic murmur
D. Systolic murmur, supine, 4/6 intensity
E. Murmur that worsens with standing

Discussion

The correct answer is (A). Mild systolic murmurs that do not worsen with Valsalva or change in position do not require additional workup. All diastolic murmurs, any systolic murmur that changes with provocation, and any systolic murmur with 3/6 intensity or higher needs to be evaluated.

Objectives: Did you learn...?

• The purpose of a preparticipation physical?
• The murmurs that require further workup?

CASE 20

Which of the following is NOT a cause of sudden cardiac death in athletes?

A. Hypertrophic cardiomyopathy
B. Coronary artery abnormalities
C. Situs inversus
D. Long QT syndrome
E. Commotio cordis

Discussion

The correct answer is (C). Situs inversus is not a cause of sudden cardiac death in athletes. While it is associated with a number of anatomic variations, it is not a contraindication for participation.

The most common cause of sudden cardiac death in athletes is:

A. Hypertrophic cardiomyopathy
B. Coronary artery abnormalities
C. Long QT syndrome
D. Commotio cordis

Discussion

The correct answer is (A). Hypertrophic cardiomyopathy is characterized by left ventricular hypertrophy that causes an obstruction to ventricular outflow. It is best diagnosed by echocardiography.

Objectives: Did you learn...?

• The causes of cardiac sudden death?
• The most common cause of cardiac sudden death?

CASE 21

A 15-year-old wrestler presents with a scaly rash on his chest halfway through the season. Several of his teammates have the same round, scaly patches, and applying skin lotion has not made any improvement. Because of the cold winter, he has not been outdoors.

What is the most likely diagnosis?

A. Tinea corporis
B. Tinea capitis
C. Lyme disease
D. Eczema
E. Psoriasis

Discussion

The correct answer is (A). Ring worm is common in wrestlers because of their many close contacts. All participants should be screened prior to the season. Tinea capitis is localized to the head. Lyme disease is unlikely without prior tick exposure. Eczema can have scaly plaques, but is not contagious.

Upon microscopic examination, the scaly edges of the wound should be scraped and examined after treatment with what compound?

A. Prussian blue
B. Silver nitrate
C. Potassium hydroxide
D. Methylene blue
E. Ziehl–Neelsen stain

Discussion

The correct answer is (C). Potassium hydroxide. This treatment will reveal the characteristic hyphae found in fungal infections. In tinea corporis, dermatophytes can be recognized under the microscope by their long branch-like tubular structures called hyphae. Fungi causing ringworm have a distinct appearance.

Objectives: Did you learn...?

• The clinical and microscopic findings of tinea corporis?

CASE 22

A 14-year-old, soccer player presents for his preseason physical. He describes having difficulty breathing during sport participation and occasionally after he exerts himself.

Which of the following symptoms is NOT consistent with exercise-induced bronchospasm?

A. Dry cough
B. Dizziness
C. Wheezing
D. Shortness of breath
E. Chest tightness

Discussion

The correct answer is (B). Dizziness following exertion is not a common symptom of exercise-induced bronchospasm (EIB), nor is a productive cough or persistent chest pressure. A dry, unproductive cough is commonly present along with wheezing, shortness of breath and chest tightness.

Which environmental factor is LEAST likely to exacerbate exercise-induced bronchospasm (EIB)?

A. Intense exercise
B. Cold weather
C. Air pollution
D. Endurance sports
E. Viral respiratory illness

Discussion

The correct answer is (D). Endurance sports have not been associated with increase rates of exercise-induced bronchospasm. Conversely, intense exercise, cold weather, air pollution, viral respiratory illnesses, and seasonal allergens frequently result in bronchospasm.

When appropriate, in-office spirometry testing can help diagnose underlying asthma in patients with EIB. What value of forced expiratory volume (FEV$_1$) would confirm the diagnosis?

A. 100%
B. 99%
C. <95%
D. <90%
E. <50%

Discussion

The correct answer is (D). FEV$_1$ <90% of predicted value can confirm the diagnosis of asthma, even when patients are believed to have EIB.

Which of the following options is NOT beneficial in the treatment of EIB?

A. Activity modification
B. Warm-up programs
C. Inhaled albuterol
D. Leukotriene modifiers
E. Allergen desensitization

Discussion

The correct answer is (E). Avoidance of environmental allergens or strenuous exercise and implementing warm-up exercises may reduce a patient's symptoms. Pharmacologic treatment with inhaled albuterol, leukotriene modifiers, or inhaled corticosteroids can be beneficial. Allergen desensitization has not been helpful.

Objectives: Did you learn...?

• The symptoms of EIB?
• The exacerbating factors of EIB?
• The treatment of EIB?

CASE 23

At a 10-km fun run, a 42-year-old woman collapses near the finish line. She is responsive but confused. Her blood pressure is 80/40. Which of the following findings are most concerning?

A. Core temperature >40.5°C
B. Headache
C. Tachycardia
D. Profuse sweating
E. Nausea/vomiting

Discussion

The correct answer is (A). Heat stroke is the most severe form of heat-induced illness. A core temperature >40.5°C combined with mental status changes and/or the lack of sweating are sign of a medical emergency.

Which of the following treatments is essential for patients with heat stroke?

A. Rest
B. Intravenous fluids
C. Whole-body immersion
D. Oral salt replacement

Discussion

The correct answer is (C). Whole-body immersion in an ice bath is the most efficient method for achieving rapid cooling in patients with heat stroke. Rest, IV fluids and salt replacement are helpful, but less urgent when trying to prevent end-organ failure and death.

Objectives: Did you learn...?
* The alarming signs and symptoms of heat stroke?
* The treatment of heat stroke?

CASE 24

A 32-year-old, competitive cross-country skier presents to the ski clinic with a painful right hand one hour after completing a 20-km race. The conditions were colder than he had expected, but he is pleased with his decision to wear less because he set a personal record for the distance. His right thumb and ring finger are numb despite his efforts to warm them up in the shower.

Which of the following is the LEAST likely diagnosis?

A. Superficial frostbite
B. Deep frostbite
C. Acute carpal tunnel syndrome
D. Acute rhabdomyolysis
E. Hypothermia

Discussion

The correct answer is (D). Prolonged exposure to cold temperatures can lead to temperature-related illnesses like hypothermia, superficial frostbite, and deep frostbite. Periods of intense exertion in sports requiring prolonged use of the hands for gripping have been associated with carpal tunnel syndrome. Rhabdomyolysis can be seen in athletes following periods of intense or prolonged exertion. Localized numbness and pain in the hand are an unlikely presentation.

All of the following treatments are helpful in the management of hypothermia EXCEPT:

A. Transition to a warmer environment
B. Removal of wet clothing
C. Consuming warm liquids
D. Warming bath immersion

Discussion

The correct answer is (D). Changing to a warmer environment (removal from the cold), removing wet clothing, and consumption of warm liquids are helpful in treating mild hypothermia. Warm water immersion may be dangerous in more severe cases if the process is too rapid.

Objectives: Did you learn...?
* The causes of acute rhabdomyolysis?
* The treatment of cold exposure?

CASE 25

A 15-year-old football player is interested in gaining weight in order to be more competitive next season. He has been eating more, lifting weights, and taking supplements. His mother has concerns about his decision.

Which of the following substances are banned in competition?

A. Methionine
B. Creatine phosphate
C. Caffeine
D. Arginine
E. Testosterone

Discussion

The correct answer is (E). Anabolic steroids are illegal at all levels of competition. Amino acids, like methionine and arginine are not regulated nor is the use of creatine. Caffeine intake is regulated, but its use is permitted below a designated blood plasma concentration.

Use of exogenous testosterone has a number of effects when consumed. Which of the following is NOT true?

A. Can be used orally or via intramuscular injection
B. Side effects are believed to be reversible following cessation
C. Resistance may occur following prolonged use
D. Aggression and mood disturbances occur commonly
E. A ratio of testosterone to epitestosterone greater than 6 to 1 is abnormal

Discussion

The correct answer is (C). Repeated use of human growth hormone (HGH) has been shown to result in the development of resistance. This finding has not been seen with the repeated use of testosterone or other anabolic steroids. These compounds can be administered orally, transcutaneously or via intramuscular injection. While their side effects include aggression and mood disturbances, these changes are believed to be reversible following cessation. Drug tests focus on the ratio of testosterone to its precursor, epitestosterone.

Objectives: Did you learn...?

• The exogenous effects of testosterone?

CASE 26

A 14-year-old wrestler has been experiencing left leg pain during practice and competition. He explains that the pain comes on quickly and is proportional to how hard he is pushing himself. There have been occasions when his leg felt clumsy and weak late in a match. He has no pain when riding a stationary bicycle.

Which test offers the best insight into his diagnosis?

A. MRI
B. MRI spectroscopy
C. Nuclear medicine blood flow studies
D. Compartment pressure measurements
E. EMG

Discussion

The correct answer is (D). The relationship of his symptoms to activity suggests exertional compartment syndrome. To assess any potential changes, compartment pressures should be measured.

When the symptoms are present, he has difficulty landing on his left foot and lifting it off of the ground due to pain. What other finding is most likely present on his examination during an episode?

A. Weak ankle plantar flexion
B. Diminished Achilles reflex
C. Decreased posterior tibial pulse
D. Down going Babinski reflex
E. Weak great toe extension

Discussion

The correct answer is (E). The increased pressure affects the anterior compartment of the lower leg resulting in diminished strength in the anterior tibialis and extensor hallucis longus. The posterior compartment does not appear to be involved, and there is no suggestion of upper motor neuron dysfunction.

A positive test for exertional compartment syndrome will reveal:

A. Resting pressure greater than 15 mm Hg
B. Exertional pressure greater than 30 mm Hg
C. Failure of pressure to return to baseline after 15 minutes

D. Pressure greater than 15 mm Hg at 15 minutes after exercise
E. All of the above

Discussion

The correct answer is (E). All of the above answers are consistent with acute exertional compartment syndrome.

Objectives: Did you learn...?

• Diagnosis exertional compartment syndrome?

CASE 27

In comparing the medial and lateral femoral condyles, the lateral femoral condyle:

A. Is larger than the medial
B. Projects farther posteriorly
C. Is more distal than the medial
D. Has greater width than the medial

Discussion

The correct answer is (D). The medial femoral condyle is larger than the lateral. It projects farther posteriorly and is more distal. The lateral femoral condyle projects more anteriorly and is wider medial to lateral than the medial femoral condyle.

Which of the following provides the greatest innervation to the intra-articular knee?

A. Posterior tibial nerve
B. Femoral nerve
C. Obturator nerve
D. Sciatic nerve

Discussion

The correct answer is (A). The posterior articular branch of the posterior tibial nerve is the largest nerve that innervates the intra-articular knee.

Objectives: Did you learn...?

• The anatomy of the knee?

CASE 28

The best clinical test(s) for determining the presence of a meniscal injury is (are):

A. Posterior sag test
B. Apley test
C. McMurray test
D. Pivot shift test
E. B and C

Discussion

The correct answer is (C). The McMurray test is the best test for determining meniscal injury. This is done by flexing the knee and then extending the knee while performing internal and external rotation of the tibia/fibula.

Objectives: Did you learn...?

• The test for diagnosing meniscal injury?

BIBLIOGRAPHY

Case 1

Arroll B, Ellis-Pegler E, Edwards A, Sutcliffe G. Patellofemoral pain syndrome a critical review of the clinical trials on nonoperative therapy. *Am J Sports Med.* 1997;25(2):207–212.

Fulkerson JP. Diagnosis and treatment of patients with patellofemoral pain. *Am J Sports Med.* 2002;30(3):447–456.

Hardaker WT, Whipple TL, Bassett FH 3rd. Diagnosis and treatment of the plica syndrome of the knee. *Bone Joint Surg Am.* 1980;62(2):221–225.

Case 2

Arnoczky SP. Anatomy of the anterior cruciate ligament. *Clin Orthop Relat Res.* 1983;(172):19–25.

Katz JW, Fingeroth RJ. The diagnostic accuracy of ruptures of the anterior cruciate ligament comparing the Lachman test, the anterior drawer sign, and the pivot shift test in acute and chronic knee injuries. *Am J Sports Med.* 1986;14(1):88–91.

Liu SH, Osti L, Henry M, Bocchi L. The diagnosis of acute complete tears of the anterior cruciate ligament. Comparison of MRI, arthrometry and clinical examination. *J Bone Joint Surg Br.* 1995;77(4):586–588.

Sanders TG, Medynski MA, Feller OF, Lawhorn KW. Bone contusion patterns of the knee at MR imaging: footprint of the mechanism of injury. *Radiographics.* 2000;20(suppl 1):S135–S151.

Case 3

Ilan DI, Tejwani N, Keschner M, Leibman M. Quadriceps tendon rupture. *J Am Acad Orthop Surg.* 2003;11(3):192–200.

Case 4

Ballmer PM, Ballmer FT, Jakob RP. Reconstruction of the anterior cruciate ligament alone in the treatment of a combined instability with complete rupture of the medial collateral ligament. *Arch Orthop Trauma Surg.* 1991;110(3):139–141.

Hughston JC, Andrews JR, Cross MJ, Moschi A. Classification of knee ligament instabilities. Part I. The medial compartment and cruciate ligaments. *J Bone Joint Surg Am.* 1976;58(2):159–172.

Case 5

Lee JH, Weissman BN, Nikpoor N, Aliabadi P, Sosman JL. Lipohemarthrosis of the knee: a review of recent experiences. *Radiology.* 1989;173(1):189–191.

Nomura E, Horiuchi Y, Inoue M. Correlation of MR imaging findings and open exploration of medial patellofemoral ligament injuries in acute patellar dislocations. *Knee.* 2002;9(2):139–143.

Case 6

Fanelli GC, Orcutt DR, Edson CJ. The multiple-ligament injured knee: evaluation, treatment, and results. *Arthroscopy.* 2005;21(4):471–486.

Sauren AA, Huson A, Schouten RY. An axisymmetric finite element analysis of the mechanical function of the meniscus. *Int J Sports Med.* 1984;5(1):S93–S95.

Shakespeare DT, Rigby HS. The bucket-handle tear of the meniscus. A clinical and arthrographic study. *J Bone Joint Surg Br.* 1983;65(4):383–387.

Case 7

Dorfmann H, De Bie B, Bonvarlet JP, Boyer T. Arthroscopic treatment of synovial chondromatosis of the knee. *Arthroscopy.* 1989;5(1):48–51.

Ogilvie-Harris DJ, Saleh K. Generalized synovial chondromatosis of the knee: a comparison of removal of the loose bodies alone with arthroscopic synovectomy. *Arthroscopy.* 1994;10(2):166–170.

Case 8

Hangody L, Feczkó P, Bartha L, Bodó G, Kish G. Mosaicplasty for the treatment of articular defects of the knee and ankle. *Clin Orthop Relat Res.* 2001;(391 Suppl):S328–S336.

Williams RJ 3rd, Harnly HW. Microfracture: indications, technique, and results. *Instructional Course Lectures.* 2006;56:419–428.

Case 9

Giuseffi SA, Bishop AT, Shin AY, Dahm DL, Stuart MJ, Levy BA. Surgical treatment of peroneal nerve palsy after knee dislocation. *Knee Surg Sports Traumatol Arthrosc.* 2010;18(11):1583–1586.

Levy BA, Dajani KA, Whelan DB, et al. Decision making in the multiligament-injured knee: an evidence-based systematic review. *Arthroscopy.* 2009;25(4):430–438.

Case 10

Fink C, Hoser C. ACL graft failure. *The ACL-Deficient Knee.* London: Springer; 2013:329–341.

Maak TG, Voos JE, Wickiewicz TL, Warren RF. Tunnel widening in revision anterior cruciate ligament reconstruction. *J Am Acad Orthop Surg.* 2010;18(11):695–706.

Romano VM, Graf BK, Keene JS, Lange RH. Anterior cruciate ligament reconstruction The effect of tibial tunnel placement on range of motion. *Am J Sports Med.* 1993;21(3):415–418.

Case 11

Kendall NS, Hsu SY, Chan KM. Fracture of the tibial spine in adults and children. A review of 31 cases. *J Bone Joint Surg Br.* 1992;74(6):848–852.

Lubowitz JH, Grauer JD. Arthroscopic treatment of anterior cruciate ligament avulsion. *Clin Orthop Relat Res.* 1993;(294):242–246.

Case 12

Cook JL, Khan KM, Purdam CR. Conservative treatment of patellar tendinopathy. *Phys Ther Sport.* 2001;2(2):54–65.

Peers KH, Lysens RJ. Patellar tendinopathy in athletes. *Sports Med.* 2005;35(1):71–87.

Case 13

Ho G, Tice AD, Kaplan S. Septic bursitis in the prepatellar and olecranon bursae: an analysis of 25 cases. *Ann Interl Med.* 1978;89(1):21–27.

Mysnyk MC, Wroble RR, Foster DT, Albright JP. Prepatellar bursitis in wrestlers. *Am J Sports Med.* 1986;14(1):46–54.

Case 14

Keller PM, Shelbourne KD, McCarroll JR, Rettig AC. Nonoperatively treated isolated posterior cruciate ligament injuries. *Am J Sports Med.* 1993;21(1):132–136.

Rubinstein RA Jr, Shelbourne KD, McCarroll JR, VanMeter CD, Rettig AC. The accuracy of the clinical examination in the setting of posterior cruciate ligament injuries. *Am J Sports Med.* 1994;22(4):550–557.

Case 15

Helmark IC, Neergaard K, Krogsgaard MR. Traumatic knee extension deficit (the locked knee): can MRI reduce the need for arthroscopy? *Knee Surg Sports Traumatol Arthrosc.* 2007;15(7):863–868.

Case 16

Brunet II. Female athlete triad. *Clin Sports Med.* 2005;24(3):623–636.

Matheson GO, Clement DB, McKenzie DC, Taunton JE, Lloyd-Smith DR, MacIntyre JG. Stress fractures in athletes A study of 320 cases. *Am J Sports Med.* 1987;15(1):46–58.

Stafford SA, Rosenthal DI, Gebhardt MC, Brady TJ, Scott JA. MRI in stress fracture. *AJR Am J Roentgenol.* 1986;147(3):553–556.

Case 17

Cantu RC. Stingers, transient quadriplegia, and cervical spinal stenosis: return to play criteria. *Med Sci Sports Exerc.* 1997;29(7 Suppl):S233–S235.

Safran MR. Nerve injury about the shoulder in athletes, part 2 long thoracic nerve, spinal accessory nerve, burners/stingers, thoracic outlet syndrome. *Am J Sports Med.* 2004;32(4):1063–1076.

Case 18

Kuhn JE, Plancher KD, Hawkins RJ. Scapular winging. *J Am Acad Orthop Surg.* 1995;3(6):319–325.

Martin RM, Fish DE. Scapular winging: anatomical review, diagnosis, and treatments. *Curr Rev Musculoskelet Med.* 2008;1(1):1–11.

Case 19

Runyan DK. The pre-participation examination of the young athlete defining the essentials. *Clin Pediatr (Phila).* 1983;22(10):674–679.

Seto CK. Preparticipation cardiovascular screening. *Clin Sports Med.* 2003;22(1):23–35.

Case 20

Wyman RA, Chiu RY, Rahko PS. The 5-minute screening echocardiogram for athletes. *J Am Soc Echocardiogr.* 2008;21(7):786–788.

Case 21

Adams BB. Transmission of cutaneous infections in athletes. *Br J Sport Med.* 2000;34(6):413–414.

Adams BB. Tinea corporis gladiatorum. *J Am Acad Dermatol.* 2002;47(2):286–290.

Adams BB. Skin infections in athletes. *Dermatol Nurs.* 2008;20(1):39–44.

Case 22

Meltzer SS, Hasday JD, Cohn J, Bleecker ER. Inhibition of exercise-induced bronchospasm by zileuton: a 5-lipoxygenase inhibitor. *Am J Respir Crit Care Med.* 1996;153(3):931–935.

Rundell KW, Jenkinson DM. Exercise-induced bronchospasm in the elite athlete. *Sports Med.* 2002;32(9):583–600.

Storms WW. Exercise-induced bronchospasm. *Curr Sport Med Rep.* 2009;8(2):45–46.

Wilber RL, Rundell KW, Szmedra L, Jenkinson DM, Im J, Drake SD. Incidence of exercise-induced bronchospasm in Olympic winter sport athletes. *Med Sci Sports Exerc.* 2000;32(4):732–737.

Case 23

Armstrong LE, Crago AE, Adams R, Roberts WO, Maresh CM. Whole-body cooling of hyperthermic runners: comparison of two field therapies. *Am J Emerg Med.* 1996;14(4):355–358.

Bouchama A, Knochel JP. Heat stroke. *N Engl J Med.* 2002;346(25):1978–1988.

Case 24

Gentilello LM. Advances in the management of hypothermia. *Surg Clin North Am.* 1995;75(2):243–256.

Case 25

Haupt HA., Rovere GD. Anabolic steroids: a review of the literature. *Am J Sports med.* 1983;12(6):469–484.

Case 26

Wilder RP, Magrum E. Exertional compartment syndrome. *Clin Sports Med*. 2010;29(3):429–435.

van den Brand JG, Nelson T, Verleisdonk EJ, van der Werken C. The diagnostic value of intracompartmental pressure measurement, magnetic resonance imaging, and near-infrared spectroscopy in chronic exertional compartment syndrome a prospective study in 50 patients. *Am J Sports Med*. 2005;33(5):699–704.

Case 27

Goldblatt JP, Richmond JC. Anatomy and biomechanics of the knee. *Oper Techn Sport Med*. 2003;11(3):172–186.

Case 28

O'Shea KJ, Murphy KP, Heekin RD, Herzwurm PJ. The diagnostic accuracy of history, physical examination, and radiographs in the evaluation of traumatic knee disorders. *Am J Sports Med*. 1996;24(2):164–167.

10

Pediatrics

Coleen S. Sabatini

CASE 1

Dr. Coleen S. Sabatini

An 8-year-old girl is brought to the ER by her mother after she fell from the monkey bars during recess at school. She had immediate pain, deformity, and swelling of the elbow after the fall. Upon arrival to the ER, the following radiographs were obtained (Figs. 10–1 and 10–2).

On examination, the patient is cooperative, but not able to move her fingers in all the ways that you ask her to do. The most likely nerve injury with this fracture is:

A. Radial nerve
B. Axillary nerve
C. Median nerve
D. Ulnar nerve
E. Anterior interosseus nerve

Discussion

The correct answer is (A). With supracondylar humerus fractures, the humeral shaft is what causes the nerve

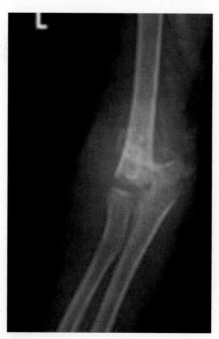

Figure 10–1

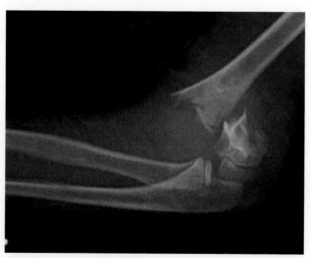

Figure 10–2

injury. The direction that the humeral shaft displaces tells you which nerve is injured. For this patient, the distal fragment is posterior and medial, which means the shaft is anterior and lateral. The nerve most likely injured by a shaft that goes anterior and lateral is the radial nerve. If the shaft had gone anteromedially and the distal fragment posterolateral, the anterior interosseus branch of the median nerve would have been the correct answer. A preoperative ulnar nerve neurapraxia occurs in the setting of a flexion-type supracondylar humerus fracture. The axillary nerve is not usually injured in a supracondylar humerus fracture.

The patient is taken to the operating room and a reduction is successfully obtained via closed means. Three lateral pins are placed to hold the reduction. Following surgery, the nerve is still not functioning. The most appropriate next step would be:

A. Immediately return to OR for nerve exploration.
B. Observe overnight and take back to OR the following day if the fingers are not moving normally.
C. Observe for a week.
D. Observe for 6 weeks and then obtain EMG/nerve conduction studies if nerve function has not recovered.
E. Observe for 3 to 6 months and then obtain EMG/nerve conduction studies if nerve has not recovered.

Discussion

The correct answer is (E). Most nerve injuries that occur with supracondylar humerus fractures are neuropraxias, and resolve without any further intervention. Three to six months is given to allow for spontaneous resolution before considering further testing. If the nerve was out preoperatively, then persistent nerve dysfunction is expected in the first several days/weeks postoperatively. The other answers are incorrect because they do not allow for sufficient time for self-recovery of the nerve and expose the patient to potentially unnecessary surgical intervention.

This patient was treated with three lateral pins. Which nerve is at risk with this technique? Had a medial wire been used for a crossed-pin technique, which nerve would have been at risk?

A. Radial and ulnar
B. Median and ulnar
C. Ulnar with both
D. Median for both
E. Radial and median

Discussion

The correct answer is (B). Meta-analysis data has shown us that the lateral wires can put the median nerve at risk. Multiple studies have shown that medial wire placements put the ulnar nerve at increased risk.

Objectives: Did you learn...?

- Neurapraxias about the elbow associated with different fracture displacement patterns in supracondylar humerus fractures?
- The appropriate management of neurapraxias that occurs at the time of injury in fractures of the distal humerus?
- The nerves at risk with pin fixation for supracondylar humerus fractures?

CASE 2

Dr. Coleen S. Sabatini

A 6-year-old boy fell from the monkey bars a few hours ago and had immediate pain and deformity of his elbow. He was seen at his local ER which transferred him to your Level 1 pediatric trauma center for further evaluation and treatment. On arrival at midnight, he complains of pain at the elbow but not anywhere else. He reports normal sensation in the hand. His hand is warm and well-perfused, but you cannot feel a radial pulse. His motor examination is intact. X-rays reveal a type III supracondylar humerus fracture. Your next step in management is:

A. Apply a splint and discharge to home, have patient return in the morning for surgery.
B. Apply a splint and admit to the floor for surgery as an add-on to the end of the OR day tomorrow, ask nurses to do neurovascular checks every shift.
C. Apply a splint and admit to the floor for serial neurovascular checks every couple of hours with an early first case start in the morning.
D. Call the OR and demand to bump the urgent appendectomy that is going into the OR in a few minutes.

Discussion

The correct answer is (C). The child has a pulseless, but perfused supracondylar humerus fracture. Given the potential vascular status change that could occur, close monitoring is imperative. Since the hand is perfused, it is not an emergency (thus choice D is incorrect). The child does need to be monitored closely with vascular status checks every few hours, so sending the child home or having a nurse do checks only once every shift is not sufficient monitoring, since you then may have a delay in recognizing decreasing perfusion to the hand. Thus, answer C is correct—the patient should be splinted, admitted, and closely monitored. Should there be a decline in vascular status, the patient should be taken emergently to the OR. Some surgeons would prefer to take the child to the OR as soon as possible rather than waiting until the morning, but that is surgeon preference.

You get an early start time, and the child is in the OR by 7 AM. The child was monitored by nursing and the on-call resident every 1 to 2 hours overnight, and the hand remained warm and well-perfused. There is still no pulse preoperatively. In the OR, the child is placed under general anesthesia. After positioning, prep/drape, and time-out, you proceed with fracture reduction. You perform the milking maneuver and then traction to bring the fracture out to length. You then perform the reduction maneuver to reduce the distal fragment to the shaft. You obtain AP, lateral, and column views with the fluoroscan, and the fracture is anatomically reduced. You stabilize the fracture with three lateral k-wires with at least 2 mm of pin spread at the fracture site and bicortical purchase. You then obtain additional images to ensure the fracture fixation is stable, and you note that there is not a gap anteriorly at the fracture site. The hand remains warm and well-perfused with brisk cap refill once you extend the arm out of the flexed position that it was in for pinning. You still do not feel a radial pulse.

Your next step in management is:

A. Explore the brachial artery.
B. Perform an angiogram.
C. Monitor the patient in the OR for an hour, and if the pulse does not return, explore the artery.
D. Splint the arm and monitor the child in the PACU for an hour—if the examination is stable postoperatively, compared to preoperatively, child can be discharged to home.
E. Splint the arm and monitor the child in the hospital for at least 24 hours with frequent, regular vascular checks to ensure no decline in perfusion.

Discussion

The correct answer is (E). Immediate exploration of the brachial artery is not indicated if the child's hand has remained warm and well-perfused. An angiogram also is not indicated. Studies have shown that a perfused hand immediately post-op can change, and the limb can become dysvascular postoperatively. Children with a pulseless, but perfused supracondylar fracture are therefore monitored for 24 to 72 hours postoperatively in the hospital before discharge to ensure that if there is vascular change or issues with swelling, this is caught and acted upon as soon as possible.

About 12 hours after the patient was taken to the recovery room, you are paged by the floor nurse. He report that the child has been requiring increasing frequency of pain medication since the postoperative check and has maxed out on what you ordered. On examination, the child appears anxious. You find that the splint is not too tight. Hand is warm and well-perfused with brisk cap refill; there is still no radial pulse. Sensory examination is stable compared to preoperative examination. There is increased pain when the fingers are passively extended. You look back over the medication record and see that initially no pain medication was required, but since about 3 hours post-op, the patient has been requesting it with increasing frequency.

What do you do next for management?

A. Apply ice to the forearm and elbow regions.
B. Elevate the arm so hand is as high above the heart as possible.
C. Obtain an MRI to assess the soft tissues and the fracture reduction.
D. Return to OR to measure compartments and fasciotomy.
E. Increase pain medication dose and check on patient every 2 hours to ensure that sensory and motor examination remain stable.

Discussion

The correct answer is (D). The clinical scenario presented is consistent with compartment syndrome. Bae showed that in children, pain, pallor, paresthesia, paralysis, and pulselessness were relatively unreliable signs and symptoms of compartment syndrome. An increasing analgesia requirement was a more sensitive indicator of compartment syndrome—particularly when combined with clinical findings such as pain with passive range of motion, anxiety and agitation, as seen in this patient. Compartment syndrome is an emergency and therefore ice, elevation, and more pain medication will only serve to mask/worsen the problem. An MRI is not indicated nor helpful in this scenario. For this child, you would return to the OR for compartment pressure checks and releases to prevent further damage from compartment syndrome.

Objectives: Did you learn...?

- Evaluation and initial treatment of a pulseless supracondylar humerus fracture?
- Differences in management between pulseless and perfused versus pulseless and nonperfused scenarios?
- Management of the persistent pulseless, but perfused limb after fracture reduction?
- Signs of compartment syndrome in children?

CASE 3

Dr. Coleen S. Sabatini

It is a busy night in the emergency room—you have just been consulted on two patients with "elbow fractures." The first one is a 5-year-old girl who was climbing on a playground structure and fell off. She has pain in her left elbow and is refusing to move the arm normally. She is neurovascularly intact on examination.

What is the next imaging study you should order if the AP and lateral films show the following (Fig. 10–3A and B)?

A. Comparison views of the other elbow
B. Internal oblique view of the elbow
C. External oblique view of the elbow
D. CT scan of the elbow
E. MRI of the elbow

Discussion

The correct answer is (B). This is a lateral condyle fracture. The internal oblique view is imperative because the fracture fragment often lies posterolateral, and the amount of displacement can be missed on just an AP and lateral x-ray. The internal oblique view is obtained to better evaluate the fracture pattern and the amount of displacement. Comparison views of the other elbow are rarely indicated if you know your pediatric elbow anatomy and would not be helpful in this case—you already know what the fracture is, but you need to know how much displacement there is. The external oblique view is helpful for evaluation of the medial epicondyle and condyle, not the lateral condyle. A CT scan of the elbow would have certainly given you a lot of data, but the single internal oblique view would likely give you sufficient information and avoid a larger radiation dose to the child that would come with the CT scan. An MRI would also provide a lot of data but not the necessary next step—an MRI at this age would likely require general anesthesia.

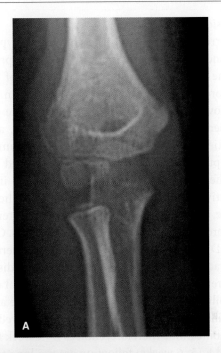

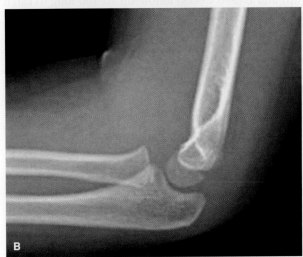

Figure 10–3 **A–B**

An internal oblique view is obtained for the patient above. It shows less than 2 mm of displacement. What is your recommended treatment?

A. Application of long-arm splint or cast with follow-up in 5 to 7 days
B. Application of long-arm cast with follow-up in 3 weeks
C. Application of a Munster cast with follow-up in 3 to 5 days
D. Application of a Munster cast with follow-up in 3 weeks
E. Application of a long-arm cast with follow-up in 5 to 6 weeks

Discussion

The correct answer is (A). The child has a type I lateral condyle fracture. A long-arm splint is preferred by some to allow for easy removal at time of follow-up in order to get clearer x-rays rather than having to remove a whole cast. The internal oblique view is most sensitive for evaluating displacement, and for this patient, the displacement is less than 2 mm which is acceptable. Since surgery is not indicated at this time, the appropriate treatment is in a cast—in order to effectively immobilize the arm to stabilize the lateral condyle, a long-arm cast is necessary; a Munster cast is not appropriate for a fracture of the humerus. Choices C and D are therefore incorrect. Because lateral condyle fractures, even non- and minimally displaced ones, are known to displace in the first several days of immobilization, close follow-up is imperative as up to 10% will displace enough to need surgical reduction and stabilization. Therefore, choices B (3-week follow-up) and E (5–6 weeks) follow-up are too long to catch those that displace.

In the room next door, there is a 6-year-old girl who also fell from a playground structure and has the following injury (Fig. 10–4A and B):

What is the appropriate treatment for this fracture?

A. Application of long-arm cast, immobilization for 4 weeks
B. Closed reduction in the ER and immobilization in long-arm cast for 6 weeks
C. Open reduction and percutaneous pinning
D. Open reduction and internal fixation with a screw and washer
E. Open reduction and internal fixation with plate and screws

Discussion

The correct answer is (C). This is a displaced lateral condyle fracture and needs surgical reduction and stabilization—therefore A and B are incorrect. Lateral condyle fractures can be closed reduced and pinned in the OR. An arthrogram is then performed, and if the intra-articular fracture is anatomically reduced and there is no articular step-off, then an open procedure does not need to be performed. Many surgeons will by-pass attempted closed reduction for notably displaced fractures and go straight to open reduction (note that the attempted closed reduction was not an option in this question due to this being a sur-

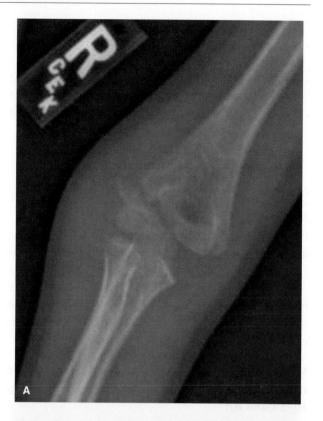

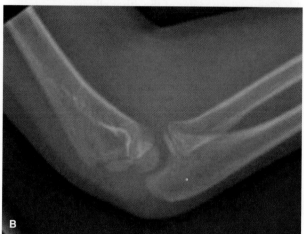

Figure 10–4 **A–B**

geon preference issue). If you are going to do an open reduction, then use stabilization with smooth k-wires as your first choice. If the patient is older or the fracture cannot be stabilized with pins, then some surgeons would use a screw. This is not usually the first choice however. For a 6-year old with a straightforward lateral condyle fracture, plates and screws are not necessary. When making the surgical approach to the lateral condyle, you want to avoid dissecting posteriorly to help mobilize the fragment.

What is the most concerning potential risk of posterior dissection?

A. Damage to cartilage due to rotation of the fragment
B. Osteonecrosis due to loss of blood supply
C. No increased risk with posterior dissection
D. Delayed healing

Discussion

The correct answer is (B). A Kocher approach is used to perform an open reduction of a lateral condyle fracture. During the approach and reduction of the fracture, the surgeon should avoid posterior dissection in order to avoid disrupting the blood supply of the lateral condyle fragment—the blood supply comes in posteriorly. If you were to dissect posteriorly, you could injure the blood supply and cause osteonecrosis. AVN of the lateral condyle is the main reason to avoid posterior dissection.

Objectives: Did you learn...?

- Correct radiographic evaluation of a lateral condyle fracture?
- Treatment of nondisplaced and displaced lateral humeral condyle fractures?
- Risk of displacement in type 1 fractures?
- Safe approach to the lateral condyle, importance of avoiding posterior dissection?

CASE 4

Dr. Coleen S. Sabatini

An 11-year-old girl was transferred from an outside hospital for further evaluation and treatment. Earlier that day, she had been at a gymnastics meet when, upon dismount, she over-rotated and landed on her arm rather than sticking the landing. She had immediate pain and gross deformity of her elbow. She was transported to her local emergency room. An orthopaedic surgeon was called in after x-rays confirmed elbow dislocation. The surgeon performed a reduction in the ER and then splinted the elbow. Postreduction x-rays were obtained (Fig. 10–5A and B) and revealed the following.

What is the appropriate treatment at this point?

A. Long-arm cast for 2 weeks, followed by hinged elbow brace for additional 2 weeks
B. Long-arm cast for 2 weeks, followed by physical therapy
C. Hinged elbow brace with immediate initiation of range of motion

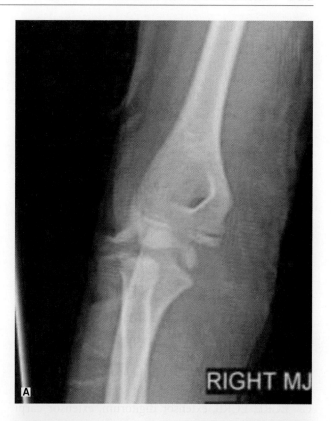

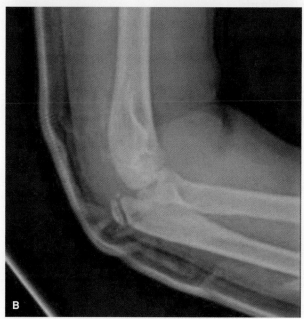

Figure 10–5 **A–B**

D. Closed reduction and percutaneous pin fixation
E. Open reduction and internal fixation

Discussion

The correct answer is (E). The radiographs of the elbow demonstrate an incarcerated medial epicondyle. Medial epicondyle fractures occur from a valgus stress across the elbow. About 50% are associated with an elbow dislocation. The flexor-pronator mass originates on the medial epicondyle and, with a valgus force across the elbow, can avulse the medial epicondyle off the humerus. If there is a dislocation, sometimes with reduction, the medial epicondyle is pulled into the joint and becomes incarcerated. An incarcerated medial epicondyle is the undisputed indication for surgical intervention for a medial epicondyle fracture. Open reduction with screw fixation (usually with a washer) is the preferred method of treatment as it allows for early motion. Percutaneous pinning is an option for young children. Casting is an option if the fracture is not incarcerated, the elbow is stable, and there is not significant displacement (amount of displacement that indicates operative intervention remains controversial).

What muscles attach to the avulsed structure?

A. Flexor carpi radialis, flexor digitorum superficialis, flexor carpi ulnaris

B. Extensor carpi radialis longus, extensor carpi radialis brevis, extensor digitorum

C. ECRL, ECRB, extensor digitorum, extensor carpi ulnaris

D. Pronator teres, flexor carpi radialis, palmaris longus, flexor digitorum superficialis, flexor carpi ulnaris

E. Pronator teres, flexor carpi radialis, palmaris longus, flexor digitorum superficialis

Discussion

The correct answer is (D). The flexor-pronator mass is what originates on the medial epicondyle. The flexor-pronator mass is comprised of pronator teres, flexor carpi radialis, palmaris longus, flexor digitorum superficialis, and flexor carpi ulnaris. The extensors originate on the lateral aspect of the humerus.

The medial epicondyle ossification center appears around what age in boys?

A. Before the age of 2

B. Between ages 2 and 5

C. Between ages 7 and 8

D. Between ages 10 and 12

E. After age 12

Discussion

The correct answer is (C). We are classically taught that the appearance of elbow ossification centers occurs in a predictable pattern—although it has also been shown that ossification can be quite varied among individuals.

The capitellum ossifies first—by around age 1. The radial head develops second. In boys, this occurs at age 5 to 6 (4–5 in girls). The third ossification center is the medial epicondyle—it appears around the age of 7 to 8 (5–6 in girls). The trochlea and olecranon ossification centers follow—around age 10. The lateral epicondyle develops after age 10. It is important to know what structures ossify when in order to evaluate the radiographs of pediatric patients and assess for injury/alterations in normal anatomy. Not knowing that the medial epicondyle ossifies before the trochlea, olecranon and lateral epicondyle can lead to a missed medial epicondyle incarceration after elbow trauma.

Objectives: Did you learn…?

- The anatomy of the medial epicondyle and mechanism of avulsion?
- Absolute indication for surgical fixation of medial epicondyle fracture?
- Ossification pattern of the pediatric elbow?

CASE 5

Dr. Coleen S. Sabatini

A 4-year-old girl fell from a playground structure, suffering the injury shown in the x-ray (Fig. 10–6A and B).

On examination, she is complaining of pain in her right arm. Her motor examination and sensation are intact. The forearm has some swelling with deformity, but there is no concern for compartment syndrome at this time.

What is your approach to treatment of this fracture?

A. Closed reduction and casting with the forearm pronated, elbow to 110 degrees flexion

B. Closed reduction and casting with the forearm in supination, elbow to 110 degrees flexion

C. Closed reduction and casting with the forearm neutral and elbow at 90 degrees

D. Open reduction and internal fixation of the ulna and pinning of the radiocapitellar joint

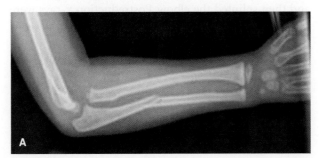

Figure 10–6 **A**

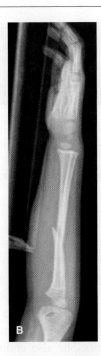

Figure 10–6 **B**

Discussion

The correct answer is (B). Closed reduction and casting with the forearm in supination and elbow flexed above 90 degrees. This is a Bado 1 Monteggia fracture. Fracture reduction is achieved by longitudinal traction of the forearm to reduce the ulna along with flexion, supination, and direct pressure over the radial head to reduce the radiocapitellar joint. The fracture is then casted in flexion of about 110 degrees, supinated to tighten the interosseous membrane, and then relaxation of the biceps to help hold the reduction. Close follow-up is imperative given the high risk of displacement. Many would advocate for treatment of this fracture with closed reduction and fixation of the ulnar fracture with an intramedullary wire. This method is often preferred due to the low risk of complications and the increase in stability of the reduction. This however was not an option here. "A" is incorrect because supination helps stabilize the reduction, not pronation. The forearm and elbow in neutral, choice C, also does not optimize stability of the reduction so would not be the preferred option. "D" is incorrect because pinning of the radiocapitellar joint is not needed nor recommended.

The patient is discharged home with strict instructions to follow-up within the week for x-rays to ensure that the ulna and radiocapitellar joint remain reduced. They end up not coming back in for 4 weeks because "some things came up," and they didn't show for their appointments. On follow-up x-rays, the ulna fracture has healed with an apex radial malunion of about 10 degrees, and the radiocapitellar joint is again dislocated.

What is your recommendation?

A. Observation
B. Open reduction of the radiocapitellar joint and reconstruction of the annular ligament
C. Ulnar osteotomy, reduction of the radiocapitellar joint, and reconstruction of the annular ligament
D. Radial head resection

Discussion

The correct answer is (C). The child has a chronic Monteggia fracture and the recommendation would be to try to restore normal anatomic alignment of the limb. Because the ulna has a malunion in the position where it would encourage the radial head to dislocate, the ulna needs to be cut, lengthened, and the angulation corrected. This change in the ulnar anatomy will then allow for the radial head to be reduced back into alignment with the capitellum, and the joint can be stabilized with annular ligament reconstruction. Because of the deformity of the ulna, trying to reduce the radiocapitellar joint would be quite difficult, and even if you were able to obtain a reduction intraoperatively, angulation of the ulna may push the radial head back out over time. Therefore "B" is not correct because it does not do enough to restore anatomy of the elbow and forearm. "D" is incorrect because we do not resect the radial head in children.

After seeing the above patient in follow-up in your clinic, you move to the next room and meet a 7-year-old who had a fall about 5 days ago. She has pain in the elbow when her splint is removed, and there is tenderness over the radial head and swelling of the soft tissues. Her distal motor, sensory, and vascular examinations are normal. You order new x-rays of the elbow and see the following (Fig. 10–7A and B).

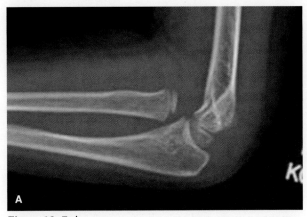

Figure 10–7 **A**

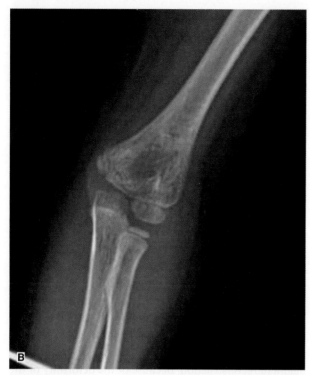

Figure 10–7 **B**

What is your next step in management of this patient?

A. Obtain x-rays of the contralateral elbow

B. Obtain x-rays of the ipsilateral forearm

C. Perform a closed reduction in the ER followed by an arthrogram

D. Obtain a CT scan of the elbow

E. Obtain an MRI of the elbow

Discussion

The correct answer is (B). Obtaining x-rays of the ipsilateral forearm would be the next step for evaluation of this child. She has an obvious radial head dislocation. Isolated radial head dislocations are thought to not happen in children—they are usually associated with an injury to the ulna which can be a very subtle ulnar bow. Failure to recognize the ulna deformity can compromise the success of any attempt at radiocapitellar joint reduction—the ulna often has to be corrected via an osteotomy to allow for the radiocapitellar joint reduction. A full forearm x-ray on this patient confirmed that there was a subtle ulnar bow relative to a straight line drawn down the x-ray (Fig. 10–8).

Objectives: Did you learn...?

• The importance of checking the radiocapitellar alignment on every pediatric elbow x-ray?

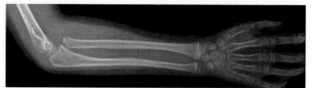

Figure 10–8

• The classification of Monteggia fractures and treatment options for acute injuries?

CASE 6

Dr. Jennifer Tangtiphaiboontana

A 12-year-old girl presents to clinic with complaints of right hip pain over the last 2 weeks. She reports that her pain has progressively worsened and has had difficulty bearing weight. She denies any trauma to her hip, fevers, chills, or night sweats. She also endorses a 2-year history of intermittent left hip pain. Physical examination is notable for a well-appearing adolescent girl, weight of 85 kg, and bilateral hip pain (right > left) with range of motion, pain with logroll, and limited internal rotation. X-rays of the pelvis/hip were obtained (Fig. 10–9A–C).

Which of the following are risk factors associated with the condition shown in Figure 10–9A–C?

A. Age

B. Weight

C. Femoral anteversion

D. Endocrinopathies

E. A, B, and D

F. All of the above

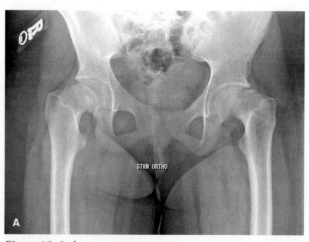

Figure 10–9 **A**

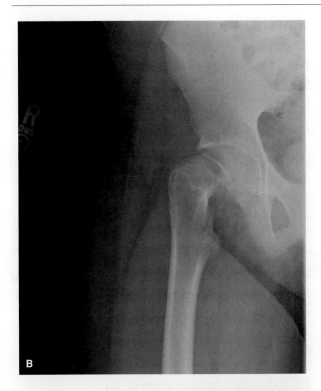

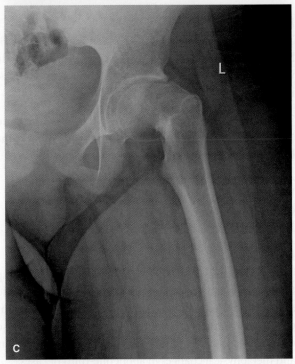

Figure 10–9 **B–C**

Discussion

The correct answer is (E). Obesity has been found to be the greatest risk factor for developing slipped capital femoral epiphysis (SCFE). The etiology of this condition is thought to be a combination of biomechanical and biochemical factors that weaken the physis. Femoral retroversion is thought to increase the load across the physis, particularly when in an obese patient. It is femoral retroversion, not femoral anteversion, that is a risk factor for SCFE. SCFE has also been shown to be associated with endocrine disorders such as hypothyroidism, osteodystrophy of chronic renal failure, and hypogonadism. SCFE is most common in children ages 10 to 16 (12–16 for boys and 10–14 for girls).

You discuss the risk and benefits of surgical management with the patient's parents, and they elect to proceed with surgery. You recommend single-screw fixation.

What is the ideal position of the screw in single-screw fixation?

A. Anteroinferior to the epiphysis, perpendicular to the physis, and <5 threads engaged in the epiphysis

B. Center of the epiphysis, perpendicular to the physis, and ≥5 threads engaged in the epiphysis

C. Center of the epiphysis, perpendicular to the physis, and <5 threads engaged in the epiphysis

D. Posterosuperior to the epiphysis, oblique to the physis, and ≥5 threads engaged in the epiphysis

E. Posterosuperior to the epiphysis, perpendicular to the physis, and <5 threads engaged in the epiphysis

Discussion

The correct answer is (B). The ideal position for single-screw fixation is in the center of the epiphysis, perpendicular to the physis (best achieved with a start point on the anterior surface of the femoral neck), and at least 5 threads engaged in the epiphysis. Carney et al. reported progression of greater than 10 degrees in 9 out of 22 patients with <5 threads across the physis versus none in patients with ≥5 threads engaged in the epiphysis. Placement of the screw into the posterosuperior femoral neck can disrupt the vascular supply and result in osteonecrosis.

Which of the following statements is true with regards to the development of osteonecrosis of the affected hip?

A. Complete or partial reduction of an unstable SCFE increases the risk of osteonecrosis

B. Screw position has not been shown to affect the rate of osteonecrosis

C. Higher rates of osteonecrosis are associated with grade 1 (mild) SCFE

D. Multiple screw fixation has been shown to decrease the rate of osteonecrosis

Discussion

The correct answer is (A). A study by Tokmakova found that complete or partial reduction of an unstable SCFE, greater severity of slip at time of presentation, multiple pin fixation, pin penetration, and pin position are associated with increased risk of osteonecrosis.

If this patient had presented to your clinic prior to the acute slip of her right hip, what would be the indications for prophylactic screw fixation?

A. Age at presentation <10 years
B. Family history of SCFE
C. History of endocrinopathies (hypothyroidism or growth hormone deficiency)
D. A and B
E. A and C

Discussion

The correct answer is (E). Although there is controversy with recommendations for prophylactic fixation of an asymptomatic contralateral hip, there are studies to support prophylactic fixation in patients with risk factors for bilateral hip involvement. The overall reported rate of bilateral hip involvement ranges from 17% to 50% in all-comers and higher in those with endocrine disorders. Loder et al. reported a prevalence of bilateral hip involvement in 61% of patients with hypothyroidism or growth hormone deficiency. A decision analysis model developed by Schultz et al. also supported prophylactic pining in patients at high risk for contralateral slip, including those with endocrinopathies, obese children, age <10 years, or open triradiate cartilage.

Objectives: Did you learn...?

- The risk factors associated with slipped capital femoral epiphysis?
- Ideal positioning for single-screw fixation?
- Risks associated with osteonecrosis?
- Indications for prophylactic fixation of an asymptomatic contralateral hip?

CASE 7

Dr. Amanda T. Whitaker

A 6-year-old boy presents to your office with a limp. It is difficult for you to examine him because he will not stay still. He is thin, 3′10″ tall with a Trendelenburg gait. He has normal, painless range of motion of his feet, ankles, and knees with limited abduction of his right hip. Radiographs are normal. Laboratory values demonstrate an erythrocyte sedimentation rate of 36.

What is the next step?

A. Aspirate hip
B. Ultrasound hip
C. Irrigation and debridement of hip
D. Technetium 99m radionucleotide scan

Discussion

The correct answer is (D). This is a picture of Legg–Calvé–Perthes, a condition often affecting boys between the ages of 4 and 8 and often they are of short stature and hyperactive. They present with a painless limp, limited abduction of the hip, and normal radiographs. The ESR may be elevated and the Technetium 99m radionucleotide scan is positive in the early stages of the disease.

Bone scan demonstrates activity and a diagnosis of Legg–Calvé–Perthes is made. What is the best treatment option?

A. Bedrest, adductor stretching
B. Proximal varus femoral osteotomy
C. Shelf osteotomy
D. Valgus-flexion femoral osteotomy

Discussion

The correct answer is (A). Children <6 with <50% head necrosis and those <8 with lateral pillar A or B do well regardless of the treatment. Answer A is the least invasive.

The next boy is 9 years old with a painless limp and >50% fragmentation of the femoral head. What is the best treatment option?

A. Bedrest, adductor stretching
B. Proximal femoral osteotomy
C. Shelf osteotomy
D. Valgus-flexion femoral osteotomy

Discussion

The correct answer is (B). The Norwegian Study Group found that a femoral osteotomy in a child >6 years old and >50% of femoral head necrosis did better than without surgery. Surgery during the fragmentation phase also decreases the length of the disease, femoral head extrusion, and metaphysical changes in about one-third of cases.

He elects not to have surgery. Twelve years later he presents with an incongruent joint, coxa magna, lateral hinging, and no evidence of arthritis. What is the most important predictor of outcome on examination?

A. Incongruent joint
B. Coxa magna

C. Lateral hinging

D. No evidence of arthritis

Discussion

The correct answer is (A). Patients with aspherical, incongruent joints develop osteoarthritis in their 40s. Coxa magna or lateral hinging has not been shown to increase the development of arthritis. At the age of 21, the cartilage space should still be present on x-ray.

At this time, what is the best salvage option for his hip?

A. Observation

B. Proximal varus femoral osteotomy

C. Shelf osteotomy

D. Valgus-flexion femoral osteotomy

Discussion

The correct answer is (D). The valgus-flexion femoral osteotomy with or without an acetabular procedure to correct the dysplasia or retroversion has been shown to decrease pain in symptomatic hips after skeletal maturity with impingement, instability, and poor range of motion without signs of arthritis.

Objectives: Did you learn...?

• Clinical presentation of a child with Legg–Calvé–Perthes disease?

• Treatment for LCP at different stages of severity?

• Risk of future arthritis at younger age?

CASE 8

Dr. Coleen S. Sabatini

A 7-year-old girl is transferred to the ER after suffering an injury playing tackle football with her older brothers. She has notable deformity of the right thigh and was in significant pain. She was placed in a traction splint at the outside hospital and sent with the following x-ray (Fig. 10–10).

You call for a portable x-ray (Fig. 10–11) to assess her alignment in traction while you obtain a full history from the family. They report that she is otherwise healthy and a very active "tomboy." The nursing staff attempts to weigh her in the bed as part of her assessment and the weight is 35 kg. You find her to be hemodynamically stable on examination. She has no abdominal tenderness and the other extremities have full, painless ROM of every joint and no tenderness or swelling. Her distal motor and sensory examination is intact in the injured leg.

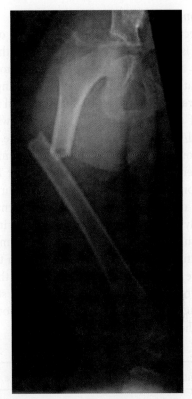

Figure 10–10

What is the treatment of choice for this patient?

A. Reduction and immediate spica cast

B. Lateral trochanteric intramedullary nail fixation

C. Traction followed by delayed spica casting

D. Flexible intramedullary nails

E. External fixation

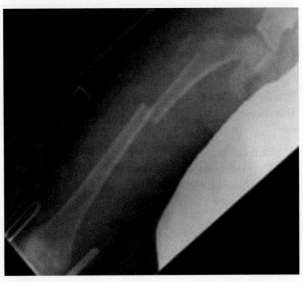

Figure 10–11

Discussion

The correct answer is (D). Spica cast is an option, but the child is large enough and old enough that flexible nailing is an option and has been found to be better for the patient and family than spica casting (with or without traction). A lateral trochanteric nail is used for a child of at least 9 years of age or older who is over 49 kg and/or has a length unstable fracture. There are risks to consider of the trochanteric entry nail including greater trochanteric apophyseal arrest leading to growth abnormalities of the proximal femur and osteonecrosis of the femoral head (rare). External fixation is certainly an option for fracture treatment in children, but is usually reserved for severely comminuted or open fractures, or treatment of fractures in the setting of damage control orthopaedics. Thus, for this 7-year-old girl who weighs 35 kg and has a length stable fracture, reduction and flexible nail fixation would be the optimal choice.

Treatment Options of Femur Fractures by Age	
Less than 6 months	Splint or Pavlik harness
6 months–2 years	Spica cast
2–5 years	Spica cast or flexible nails
6–8 years	Flexible nails, submuscular plate, spica cast
>8 years to adolescent	Flexible nails (if under 50 kg), lateral trochanteric entry nail, submuscular plate
Skeletally mature patient	Adult implant

*An external fixator would be an option throughout these age groups if necessary.
**The fracture pattern and surgeon preference will significantly impact the type of fixation chosen.

You measure the preoperative x-ray at the isthmus. The measurement is 7.5 mm. You therefore decide to use _____ mm nails to obtain __% canal fill.

A. Two 2.5-mm nails, 67% canal fill
B. Two 3-mm nails, 80% canal fill
C. One 3.0-mm nail and one 3.5-mm nail, 87% canal fill

Discussion

The correct answer is (B). The patient's isthmus is 7.5 mm and the goal for flexible intramedullary nail fixation of a femur fracture is 80% canal fill. Available flexible nails come in increasing sizes with 0.5 mm difference. Since the goal is 80% fill, "B" is the correct answer because it uses two nails of the same size that together will fill 80% of the canal. "A" is not correct because that is less than ideal canal fill and could put the child at risk of failure of fixation. "C" is incorrect because using two nails of different sizes can contribute to loss of reduction and malalignment of the femur. Also, trying to obtain canal fill greater than 80% can lead to increased risk of complications.

The most common complication that you should inform parents about when recommending this form of treatment is:

A. Infection
B. Bleeding
C. Pain at the knee (insertion sites)
D. Loss of reduction

Discussion

The correct answer is (C). Pain/irritation at insertion sites. Available studies have shown low rates of infection, bleeding, and loss of reduction (with length stable fractures). The most common complication is irritation of the soft tissues at the end of the nails. It has been suggested that nails be left no more than 25 mm out of the bone to decrease this risk.

When discussing complications of femur fractures in general with the family preoperatively, what do you tell them about the amount of overgrowth that may occur?

A. There is no risk of overgrowth at this age, overgrowth only happens in children under 2.
B. Ipsilateral overgrowth does occur, average is less than 5 mm.
C. Ipsilateral overgrowth does occur, usually around 9 mm in 2 to 10 year olds.
D. Ipsilateral overgrowth does occur, usually between 15 and 20 mm in the 2 to 10 year olds.
E. Overgrowth is a risk in children over 10, not in those younger than 10.

Discussion

The correct answer is (C). Children ages 2 to 10 are at risk for ipsilateral overgrowth after femur fracture. Although the range is around 4 to 25 mm, the average is around 9 mm. Children under 2 and those over 10 are not as likely to have overgrowth, so choices A and E are incorrect. Choices B and D are incorrect because they under- and overestimate the amount of likely overgrowth, respectively.

Objectives: Did you learn...?

- Treatment options for diaphyseal femur fractures in children of various ages?
- Indications for flexible nail fixation in children and proper nail selection?
- Risk of overgrowth in children who sustain diaphyseal femur fractures?

CASE 9

Dr. Coleen S. Sabatini

A 14-year-old boy is brought to the ER with complaints of right knee pain after he was injured playing basketball. X-rays and a CT scan (CT Shown in Fig. 10–12) were done at an outside hospital and he was transferred to you for care.

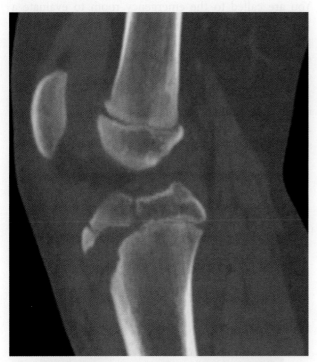

Figure 10–12

What condition is thought to be a risk factor for this fracture?

A. Patellofemoral syndrome

B. Osgood–Schlatter disease

C. Sinding-Larsen–Johansson syndrome

D. Patellar tendonitis

Discussion

The correct answer is (B). Tibial tubercle fractures occur more commonly in adolescents with a history of

Osgood–Schlatter disease, but a causal relationship has yet to be demonstrated. Osgood–Schlatter disease is an overuse injury caused by repetitive strain across the tibial tubercle apophysis. Tibial tubercle avulsion fractures are not known to occur more commonly in young people who have patellofemoral syndrome (anterior knee pain associated with overuse), Sinding-Larsen–Johansson syndrome (a condition similar to Osgood–Schlatter, affects the lower pole of the patella, not the tibial tubercle and therefore not associated with tibial tubercle fractures), nor in people who have inflammation of the patella tendon. Therefore, choices A, C and D are not correct.

You perform a thorough evaluation of the patient in the ER. He is neurovascularly intact—no weakness, no parasthesias. The soft tissues over the tibial tubercle are swollen, but there is no tenting of the skin. The OR is not available, so you splint the patient and admit to the floor in anticipation of the OR in the morning. You monitor him closely for compartment syndrome because you know that there is a risk of developing compartment syndrome with this injury.

What compartment are you most concerned about and what vessel is at risk with this fracture?

A. Anterior compartment—medial inferior geniculate

B. Anterior compartment—recurrent anterior tibial artery

C. Anterior compartment—anterior tibial artery

D. Lateral compartment—recurrent anterior tibial artery

E. Lateral compartment—fibular artery

Discussion

The correct answer is (B), Anterior compartment from injury to the recurrent anterior tibial artery. Knowledge of anatomy will allow you to come to the correct answer. Studies of this fracture have shown risk of isolated anterior compartment syndrome. It is very important in the perioperative period to monitor the neurovascular examination of patients with this injury—particularly of the anterior compartment. Most surgeons will release the anterior compartment fascia at the time of surgery to help reduce risk of anterior compartment syndrome postoperatively.

What treatment would you utilize to care for this patient?

A. Closed reduction and application of cast

B. Closed reduction and pinning

C. Open reduction and pinning

D. Open reduction and fixation with cannulated screws, arthrotomy

E. Open reduction and suture fixation, arthrotomy

Discussion

The correct answer is (D). This patient has a type III fracture, and given the amount of displacement, an open reduction is necessary. Choices A and B can be excluded because a closed reduction with casting or pinning are not sufficient treatment methods for this fracture. Given the association of type III fractures with intra-articular pathology, it is recommended to perform an arthrotomy at the time of surgery to ensure that there is no meniscal injury or soft tissue incarceration and to ensure that the joint surface is anatomically reduced. Some advocate using arthroscopy for this purpose rather than doing a full arthrotomy—this would depend on surgeon's preference, but regardless of technique, it is important to evaluate. Screw fixation is preferred over pins or sutures, particularly in larger adolescents because of the significant pulling force that the quadricep exerts on the tibial tubercle. In children/very young adolescents (who very rarely get this injury) you may consider suture fixation with cast augmentation if there is concern regarding the growth plates, but the injury occurs far more commonly in adolescents in whom the growth plate is already closing, so screw fixation is preferred to give more stable fixation and allow an earlier return to range of motion (Fig. 10–13).

Objectives: Did you learn...?

- What a tibial tubercle fracture is and potential risk factors?
- Risk of compartment syndrome with tibial tuberosity fractures?
- Treatment considerations for these fractures?
- Potential for other intra-articular pathology with tibial tubercle fractures?

CASE 10

Dr. Cordelia W. Carter

You are called to the emergency room to evaluate a 13-year-old male complaining of acute right ankle pain. He reports that he injured his ankle earlier in the day when another player "took him out" during a soccer match. He was unable to bear weight through the right lower extremity and was brought promptly to the hospital for evaluation and management of his injury. An anteroposterior radiograph of the patient's ankle is shown in Figure 10–14.

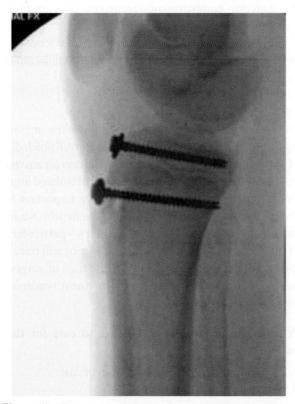

Figure 10–13

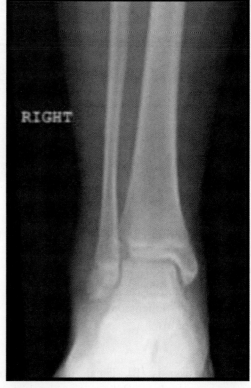

Figure 10–14

Which of the following answers correctly pairs the eponym commonly used to describe this injury with the affected anatomic structure?

A. Tillaux fracture; ATFL (anterior talofibular ligament)

B. Tillaux fracture; AITFL (anterior inferior tibiofibular ligament)

C. Chopart fracture; ATFL (anterior talofibular ligament)

D. Chopart fracture; AITFL (anterior inferior tibiofibular ligament)

E. Chaput fracture; ATFL (anterior talofibular ligament)

Discussion

The correct answer is (B). The radiograph shown demonstrates a Tillaux fracture, the eponym used to describe transitional ankle fractures in adolescents characterized by two main fragments: one fragment being the anterolateral distal tibial epiphysis and the second including the tibial metadiaphysis, the physis, and the posteromedial epiphysis. On an anteroposterior radiograph, the fracture line appears to run through the physis and exit through the epiphysis. The anatomic structure attached to this piece is the anterior inferior tibiofibular ligament (AITFL), one of the primary syndesmotic ligaments of the ankle. Chopart injuries involve the midtarsal joint. The Chaput fragment is another eponym (used more commonly in adult ankle fractures) to describe the fracture piece that remains attached to the AITFL. The anterior talofibular ligament (ATFL) is the most commonly injured structure in lateral ankle sprains.

After reviewing the patient's radiographic imaging, you diagnose an injury involving the growth plate of the distal tibia. Which of the following answers correctly pairs the description of this injury with its associated Salter–Harris fracture classification?

A. The fracture involves the physis only; Salter–Harris I or V

B. The fracture exits from the physis into the metaphysis; Salter–Harris III

C. The fracture exits from the physis into the metaphysis; Salter–Harris IV

D. The fracture exits from the physis into the epiphysis; Salter–Harris III

E. The fracture exits from the physis into the epiphysis; Salter–Harris IV

Discussion

The correct answer is (D). The Salter–Harris classification system for describing fractures in skeletally immature individuals is as follows: Salter–Harris I fractures involve the growth plate only and are not usually evident on plain radiographs. This is usually a clinical diagnosis. Salter–Harris II injuries involve the physis (growth plate) and then the fracture line "exits" into the metaphysis (away from the joint). This metaphyseal fragment is often called a "Thurston–Holland" fragment. Salter–Harris III injuries involve the physis and then the fracture exits into the epiphysis (towards the joint). The injury depicted in Figure 10–14 is a Salter–Harris III. Salter–Harris IV injuries involve the growth plate, with extension of the fracture into both the epiphysis and metaphysis. Salter–Harris V injuries are crush injuries through the growth plate that are often radiographically indistinguishable from Salter–Harris I injuries initially, but have higher rates of physeal arrest due to the increased force that produces this injury.

The typical pattern of closure of the distal tibial physis is best described by which of the following?

A. Medial → Central → Lateral

B. Medial → Lateral → Central

C. Central → Medial → Lateral

D. Central → Lateral → Medial

E. Lateral → Central → Medial

Discussion

The correct answer is (C). The pattern of physeal closure for the distal tibia is central-medial-lateral. This fact, coupled with the fact that the cartilaginous physis is the "weak link" in the chain (e.g., more likely to sustain injury than bone or ligament) helps explain the predictable patterns of ankle injury seen in adolescent "transitional" ankle fractures during the period of physeal closure.

The primary mechanism for this injury is _____ _____ (choose the best answer).

A. Internal rotation of the foot

B. External rotation of the foot

C. Adduction of the foot

D. Supination of the foot

E. Dorsiflexion of the ankle

Discussion

The correct answer is (B). The classic cadaveric studies performed by Paul Jules Tillaux (a French surgeon), demonstrated that external rotation of the foot is the primary force that reliably reproduces an avulsion fracture of the distal anterolateral tibia at the insertion of the AITFL, now eponymously termed the Tillaux fragment.

Coincidentally, a 13-year-old male (a player for the opposing team) is in the next bed in the emergency room, awaiting evaluation of a left ankle injury that was sustained in a similar fashion later in the game. Upon your evaluation, his skin is closed, his foot and ankle are swollen, and he is able to actively flex and extend his toes with minimal discomfort. His initial radiographs are shown (Fig. 10–15A–C). Based on the available imaging you diagnose this patient with a _____ (choose the correct group of answers).

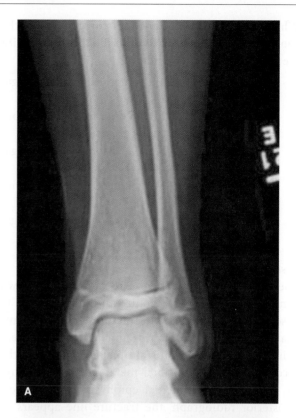

A. Triplane fracture; Salter–Harris III on sagittal view; Salter–Harris II on anteroposterior (AP) view

B. Triplane fracture; Salter–Harris II on sagittal view; Salter–Harris III on AP view

C. Triplane fracture; Salter–Harris III on sagittal view; Salter–Harris III on AP view

D. Tillaux fracture; Salter–Harris III on sagittal view; Salter–Harris II on AP view

E. Tillaux fracture; Salter–Harris II on sagittal view; Salter–Harris III on AP view

Discussion
The correct answer is (B). Classically, triplane fractures have the radiographic appearance of a Salter–Harris II fracture on lateral radiographs and of a Salter–Harris III fracture (this is the Tillaux fragment) on coronal imaging.

You discuss this patient with the on-call attending and decide to perform closed reduction and long-leg splint application. The reduction maneuver should consist primarily of _____ (choose the best answer).

A. Traction, internal rotation of the foot, and dorsiflexion of the ankle

B. Traction, internal rotation of the foot, and plantarflexion of the ankle

C. Traction, external rotation of the foot, and dorsiflexion of the ankle

D. Traction, external rotation of the foot, and plantarflexion of the ankle

E. Traction, abduction of the foot, and plantarflexion of the ankle

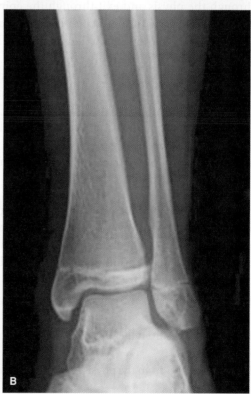

Figure 10–15 **A–B**

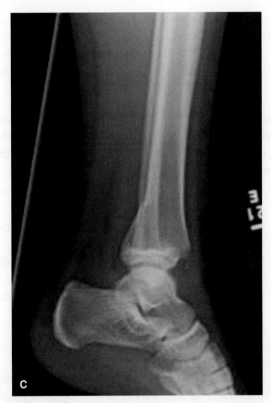

Figure 10–15 **C**

Discussion

The correct answer is (A). Sustained axial traction followed by maximal internal rotation and supination of the foot with dorsiflexion of the ankle is the maneuver employed to affect reduction of triplane ankle fractures in adolescents.

You recognize the importance of re-evaluating the fracture alignment following your reduction attempt. Therefore, the next step in evaluation of this patient's injury might include (choose the best answer):

A. Magnetic resonance imaging (MRI) without contrast of the left ankle

B. Magnetic resonance imaging (MRI) with contrast of the left ankle

C. Delayed gadolinium-enhanced MRI of cartilage (dGEMRIC) of the left ankle

D. Computed tomography scan (CT) without contrast of the left ankle

E. Computed tomography scan (CT) with contrast of the left ankle

Discussion

The correct answer is (D). In general, MRI is considered the "gold standard" for evaluation of soft tissue injuries, such as ligaments and tendons. dGEMRIC imaging (as

its name implies) is used primarily to evaluate injury to the articular cartilage. CT scanning is generally considered the "gold standard" for evaluation of bony injury and alignment. Because your goal in evaluation post-reduction is assessment of the fracture alignment at the articular surface, a noncontrast CT scan is the best choice. Contrast enhancement in this setting would not add additional useful information.

Post-reduction CT images are shown (Fig. 10–16A and B). Based on the images and measurement shown, you recommend (choose the best answer):

A. Continued immobilization, protected weightbearing with crutches, and serial radiographs to ensure maintenance of reduction

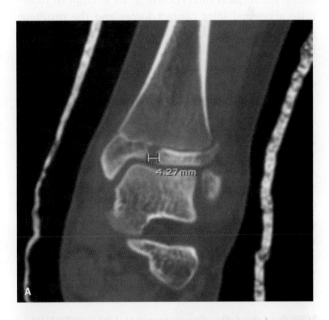

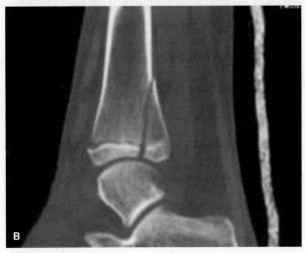

Figure 10–16 **A–B**

B. Continued immobilization, protected weightbearing with crutches, and serial three-dimensional imaging to ensure maintenance of reduction

C. Surgical reduction and internal fixation using a metaphyseal lag screw(s) construct

D. Surgical reduction and internal fixation using an all-epiphyseal lag screw(s) construct

E. Surgical reduction and internal fixation using a construct involving placement of lag screws in both the epiphyseal and metaphyseal fracture fragments

F. Surgical reduction and internal fixation using a physeal-spanning compression plate construct

Discussion

The correct answer is (E). In general, >2 mm of residual articular diastasis on radiographs is considered an indication for surgical intervention in an attempt to minimize abnormal joint contact forces and the resultant joint degeneration that occurs over time. This patient has >4 mm of residual articular gap measured on CT scan and is therefore a candidate for surgery. While surgical approaches to treatment of triplane fractures vary, one traditional approach is to reduce the articular surface (either open or percutaneously) and fix it in place using all-epiphyseal lag screws (with or without washers) placed perpendicular to the fracture line in an extraphyseal and extra-articular fashion. Depending on the size of the metaphyseal fragment, additional fixation with lag screws placed across the metaphyseal spike may optimize fracture fixation. This patient has a large metaphyseal fragment and would likely benefit from lag screw fixation in both the epiphyseal and metaphyseal fragments. Compression plating across a growth plate is not typically indicated.

Which of the following statement(s) is(are) TRUE?

A. Fractures with greater residual physeal diastasis following reduction are thought to be more likely to go on to physeal arrest

B. Fractures with greater residual articular diastasis following reduction are thought to be more likely to go on to physeal arrest

C. Fractures with greater residual articular diastasis following reduction are thought to more likely to result in degenerative changes in the tibiotalar joint

D. A and C

E. B and C

Discussion

The correct answer is (D). One generally accepted goal for treatment of triplane fractures is to achieve and maintain <2 mm of fracture diastasis at the articular surface, in an attempt to minimize arthritic degeneration. Additionally, >3 mm residual physeal diastasis is significantly more likely to result in physeal closure following injuries involving the distal tibial physis.

Nine months after his initial presentation, the patient returns to your office for follow-up. You tell him that the most likely sequela of his injury to occur at this point is:

A. Posttraumatic physeal closure of the distal tibia that does not require additional treatment

B. Posttraumatic physeal closure of the distal tibia that requires corrective valgus osteotomy

C. Posttraumatic physeal closure of the distal tibia that requires corrective varus osteotomy

D. Posttraumatic physeal closure of the distal tibia that requires corrective extension osteotomy

E. Nonunion of the Thurston–Holland fragment

Discussion

The correct answer is (A). Because transitional ankle fractures such as the Tillaux and triplane fractures occur at the time of physiologic physeal closure, clinically significant physeal arrest is unlikely to result. Nonunion of the Thurston–Holland fragment has not been reported.

Objectives: Did you learn...?

- Relevant anatomy for transitional ankle fractures?
- Proper application of the Salter–Harris classification system for fractures involving the growth plate?
- Proper steps for initial work-up and treatment of transitional ankle fractures?
- Indications and approaches for surgical treatment of transitional ankle fractures?

CASE 11

Dr. Coleen S. Sabatini

A 3-month-old boy is sent in to the ER by the pediatrician. Grandmother, who is babysitting today, brought the child in because she noticed that the child's thigh was swollen, and the baby cried whenever she would move the leg for diaper changes. She also noticed that the baby was kicking one leg normally, but the baby was not voluntarily moving the leg that was swollen. The ER ordered an x-ray of the leg and called an Orthopaedic consult for evaluation. You see the x-ray prior to examining the child (Fig. 10–17):

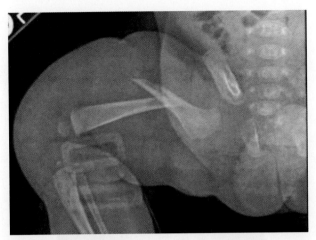

Figure 10–17

What are you immediately concerned about, even before meeting the patient and family?

A. Compartment syndrome
B. Birth trauma
C. Nonaccidental trauma
D. Osteogenesis imperfecta

Discussion

The correct answer is (C). This is a femur fracture in a nonambulatory child less than 1 year of age. It is estimated that approximately 80% of femur fractures in nonambulatory children are due to nonaccidental trauma (NAT). Compartment syndrome of the thigh after femur fracture is quite rare and is something that should be checked for on examination, but not the most likely issue in this clinical scenario. Birth trauma (B) is not correct because this child is 3 months old, and if the child had suffered a fracture at birth, it would be healed with a robust callus at this point. Osteogenesis imperfecta is certainly something to consider, to discuss with the family and to assess for on examination, but nonaccidental trauma is more common and must not be missed. If there is concern for OI based on history and examination, work-up can be included as part of the overall evaluation of potential nonaccidental trauma.

What is your next step in evaluation?

A. Perform only a physical examination of the child's leg to assess neurovascular status in the setting of fracture.
B. Perform a thorough physical examination including removal of all the child's clothing to evaluate the skin.
C. Ensure that baby is moving the arms and other leg normally, then focus in on the injured leg.

D. Order an x-ray of the whole baby ("babygram") to screen for other injuries.

Discussion

The correct answer is (B). Fractures are the second most common physical manifestation of child abuse—skin lesions (bruises, burns) are the most common, therefore a thorough examination of the skin is important. Option A is incorrect because you must examine the entire child, not just the leg known to be injured. This is the same for option C. D is incorrect because the child needs a full physical examination first before determining what imaging studies should be done. Further, a "babygram" is not the study of choice because it does not show enough detail and injuries can be easily missed.

You complete your history and physical examination. Grandmother is not the primary caregiver and does not know how the injury occurred. She contacts the child's parents and neither of them can offer up any explanation—one parent is rather defensive when you try to speak with them and the other simply cannot think of anything that happened that could have led to the femur fracture. Your examination is concerning because there is tenderness over one of the forearms and there is some bruising on the chest. You therefore talk to the ER and a skeletal survey is ordered.

The skeletal survey confirms that there is a both-bone forearm fracture that has callus formation present, the distal tibia of the contralateral leg has corner fractures, and there are posteromedial rib fractures—some that are healed and some that look fresh.

In general on a skeletal survey, which fractures are most specific for child abuse?

A. The femur fracture since the child is nonambulatory
B. Multiple fractures
C. The femur, the tibia, and the both-bone forearm fracture in different stages of healing.
D. The rib fracture and corner fractures

Discussion

The correct answer is (D). Although all of the above are concerning for child abuse, some are more specific for abuse than others. The fractures with the highest specificity for nonaccidental trauma are corner fractures, rib fractures (particularly posteromedial rib fractures), scapular fractures, sternal fractures, and spinous process fractures. Fractures with moderate specificity for abuse include fractures in different stages of healing, multiple fractures, finger fractures, vertebral body fractures, transphyseal separations, and complex skull fractures. Long-bone shaft fractures have low specificity for abuse.

Given the high suspicion for nonaccidental trauma in this patient, the child is admitted to the hospital and child protective services is called.

Objectives: Did you learn...?

- Orthopaedic surgeons must consider the possibility of nonaccidental trauma when evaluating injured children?
- The history and injury red flags that should raise suspicion for nonaccidental trauma?
- The differences in specificity for NAT of different fractures?
- Importance of involving your hospital's Child Protection Team/local Child Protective Services with any child for whom there is a concern for NAT?

CASE 12

Dr. Coleen S. Sabatini

You are in your scoliosis clinic today and your patients are already in the room.

In room 1, you meet a girl who turned 10 years old 5 days ago. She has not yet started her menses. She is here with the chief complaint of "scoliosis." She was recently seen by her pediatrician for a "well-child" visit, and as part of evaluation, a forward-bend test was performed that raised concern for a spine curvature. A PA full spine x-ray was performed (Fig. 10–18) and she was referred to you for evaluation.

After performing a physical examination in which there are no neurologic abnormalities detected, you measure her x-ray, and the curve measures 48 degrees. She is hyperkyphotic on the lateral x-ray. There is no spondylolysis or spondylolisthesis.

What is your next step in her evaluation/treatment?

A. Order laboratory tests including a CBC, ANA, and HLA-B27.
B. Order a bone density scan.
C. Prescribe a brace.
D. Order an MRI of the thoracic and lumbar spine.
E. Order an MRI of the cervical, thoracic, and lumbar spine.

Discussion

The correct answer is (E). This is a patient who just turned 10 years old this week and has a large scoliotic

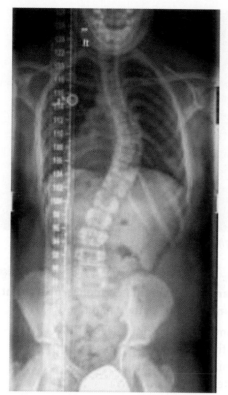

Figure 10–18

curve. This is clearly onset before the age of 10 in this premenarchal girl, therefore this is classified as juvenile scoliosis. It has been estimated that approximately 20% of children who have juvenile scoliosis (age of onset 3–10 years old) have an intraspinal anomaly; obtaining an MRI of the spine is important in their evaluation. You want to look for a Chiari malformation, syringomyelia (syrinx) and tethered cord, as well as less common findings such as a spinal cord tumor. In order to evaluate for those potential underlying diagnosis, the entire spine must be imaged and therefore choice E is the correct answer. "A" is not correct because, although a CBC may be desired before any potential surgical intervention, it is not needed now. The ANA and HLA-B27 are not needed in this case scenario. A bone density scan is also not a necessary part of the work-up of juvenile scoliosis. It can be obtained in selected patients for whom there is concern about underlying bone density. Bracing for a curve of this magnitude is not likely to be effective. Even if the curve were smaller and bracing was a consideration, you would still get an MRI for this child. "D" is not correct because in order to thoroughly evaluate for potential problems with the neural axis, you need base of brain/cervical spine imaging to evaluate for Chiari malformation, as this patient has.

After ordering the MRI for the above patient and concluding discussion with her family, you move to the next room.

In room 2 you met a 3-year-old boy who is here with both of his parents. They report that over the last year, they have noticed that his spine "looks crooked" and they think that it is getting worse. On examination, you agree that his spine appears to have a curvature, and you order x-rays (Fig. 10–19).

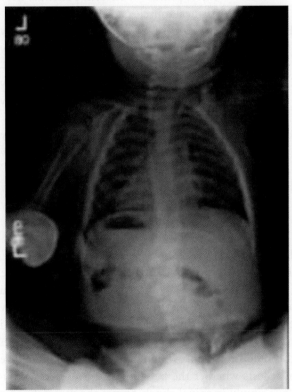

Figure 10–19

The x-ray is as above and you explain to the parents that their child has:

A. Infantile scoliosis
B. Juvenile scoliosis
C. Congenital scoliosis
D. Idiopathic scoliosis
E. A positional curve

Discussion

The correct answer is (C). This child has a hemivertebrae in the lumbar spine. The other options are not correct because A, B, and D assume that there is not an underlying structural issue with the osseus structures of the spine other than the curve itself. Given the obvious structural abnormality in the lumbar spine, this is not just a curve related to position at time of x-ray, so "E" is incorrect.

With congenital scoliosis, there are multiple anomalies of the vertebrae that can occur. What is the correct order of anomaly type from that which is most likely to result in progressive scoliosis to least likely to progress?

A. Hemivertebra, unilateral bar, wedge vertebra, unilateral bar with contralateral hemivertebra, block vertebra
B. Unilateral bar, wedge vertebra, unilateral bar with contralateral hemivertebra, block vertebra, hemivertebra
C. Wedge vertebra, unilateral bar with contralateral hemivertebra, block vertebra, hemivertebra, unilateral bar
D. Block vertebra, wedge vertebra, hemivertebra, unilateral bar, unilateral bar with contralateral hemivertebra
E. Unilateral bar with contralateral hemivertebra, unilateral bar, hemivertebra, wedge vertebra, block vertebra

Discussion

The correct answer is (E). This requires knowledge of the basic vertebral anomalies that occur with congenital scoliosis. The anomaly most likely to cause the most severe scoliosis is the unilateral bar with contralateral hemivertebra. This is followed by a unilateral bar, a hemivertebra, and then the wedge vertebra. Block vertebrae are unlikely to cause scoliosis. For the patient in this scenario, he has a hemivertebra. You can explain to the family that there is on average a 2- to 5-degree progression per year associated with the hemivertebra. For children with congenital scoliosis, curve progression occurs more rapidly during periods of rapid spine growth—this is during the first 5 years of life and then during the adolescent growth spurt.

Objectives: Did you learn...?

• The importance of evaluating for intraspinal anomalies in children with juvenile and congenital scoliosis?
• Recognize the differences in scoliosis diagnosed at different ages?
• Know the different types of vertebral anomalies and how they contribute to the development of scoliosis during growth?

CASE 13

Dr. Jaysson Brooks

A 15-year-old male is unable to move his bilateral lower extremities after being involved in an ATV accident where the vehicle rolled over multiple times during a jump. There was positive loss of consciousness at the scene. Upon arrival to your tertiary pediatric trauma center he has a Glasgow Coma Score of 15, a left wrist deformity, and reports that he is unable to move or feel his legs. His blood pressure is 105/68, heart rate is 102, respiratory rate is 26, and SpO$_2$ is 98% on room air. He is in a hard cervical collar, lying comfortably in no acute distress.

Your next action is:

A. Immediate CT scan of cervical, thoracic, and lumbar spine
B. Exchange of hard cervical collar for a Miami-J collar
C. Neurosurgical consultation
D. Evaluation of lungs with stethoscope
E. Obtain radiographs of left wrist to evaluate for fracture

Discussion

The correct answer is (D). Never forget the ABCDEs of Advanced Trauma Life Support (ATLS) when evaluating pediatric trauma patients. Regardless of the various coinciding injuries, all pediatric trauma patients should first be evaluated for (a) maintenance of their airway, (b) breathing and ventilation, (c) circulation and hemorrhage control, (d) evaluation of disability which includes an assessment of neurological status, and (e) environment and exposure of all body surfaces to look for hypothermia, burns, lacerations, ballistic wounds, etc. All of these items should be part of the primary trauma survey and should be evaluated before further work-up into musculoskeletal injuries. The other options are all reasonable choices once evaluation of his air, breathing, and circulation have been evaluated and stabilized.

You undertake a detailed physical examination, which reveals that his skin is closed, and his sensation is not intact distal to the level of his umbilicus. He had no sensation around his rectum and no voluntary rectal tone. He has 5/5 strength in his bilateral upper extremities. He has 0/5 strength in his iliopsoas, quadriceps, hamstrings, tibialis anterior, gastrocnemius, extensor hallucis longus, and flexor hallucis

longus bilaterally. He had a negative Babinski test and no signs of clonus bilaterally. He has palpable pulses in his bilateral lower extremities. When his glans penis is squeezed during a simultaneous digital rectal examination, the muscles surrounding his rectum contract around your finger.

What is the neurophysiological pathway by which the bulbocavernosus reflex works?

A. Genitofemoral nerve → afferent pudendal nerve fibers → sacral plexus → efferent pudendal nerve fibers → perineal muscle
B. Genitofemoral nerve → afferent obturator nerve fibers → sacral plexus → efferent obturator nerve fibers → perineal muscle
C. Dorsal penile nerve → afferent ilioinguinal nerve fibers → sacral plexus → efferent ilioinguinal nerve fibers → perineal muscle
D. Dorsal penile nerve → efferent pudendal nerve fibers → sacral plexus → afferent pudendal nerve fibers → perineal muscle
E. Dorsal penile nerve → afferent pudendal nerve fibers → sacral plexus → efferent pudendal nerve fibers → perineal muscle

Discussion

The correct answer is (E). The bulbocavernosus reflex (BCR) is clinically elicited by squeezing the glans penis and digitally palpating the contraction of the bulbocavernosus (BC) muscle. This test was first used for examination of the neurogenic bladder. It is important to test this reflex in patients with potential spinal cord injuries as it tests whether the patient has a true spinal injury or is simply in spinal shock. Spinal shock is defined as temporary loss of spinal cord function and reflex activity below the level of a spinal cord injury. It is characterized by flaccid areflexic paralysis, bradycardia, hypotension, and as previously mentioned, an absent BCR. If the BCR is intact, then there is a significant chance of their neurological deficit being final. The other pathways listed are not involved in the BCR.

Based on his physical examination, what would the patient's classification according to the American Spinal Injury Association (ASIA) impairment scale?

A. A
B. B
C. C
D. D
E. E

Discussion

The correct answer is (A). The ASIA classification is still widely used today to classify various types of traumatic spinal cord injuries that can occur. The classification is as follows:

A = **Complete.** No sensory or motor function is preserved in the sacral segments S4–5.

B = **Sensory incomplete.** Sensory but not motor function is preserved below the neurological level and includes the sacral segments S4–5 (light touch or pin prick at S4–5 or deep anal pressure) AND no motor function is preserved more than three levels below the motor level on either side of the body.

C = **Motor incomplete.** Motor function is preserved below the neurological level,** and more than half of key muscle functions below the neurological level of injury (NLI) have a muscle grade less than 3 (Grades 0–2).

D = **Motor incomplete.** Motor function is preserved below the neurological level,** and at least half (half or more) of key muscle functions below the NLI have a muscle grade >3.

E = **Normal.** If sensation and motor function as tested with the ISNCSCI are graded as normal in all segments, and the patient had prior deficits, then the AIS grade is E. Someone without an initial SCI does not receive an AIS grade.

Plain radiographs were taken of the patient's spine and displayed in Figure 10–20A and B.

Given the clinical and radiographic findings, what is the next step in management to definitively diagnose the patient?

A. Obtain a CT scan of the thoracic and lumbar spine.

B. Obtain an MRI without contrast of the thoracic and lumbar spine.

C. Obtain bending radiographs to observe for instability of the thoracolumbar spine.

D. Obtain electromyogram and nerve conduction studies of the patient's bilateral lower extremities.

Discussion

The correct answer is (B). The patient's clinical picture points toward a spinal cord injury, however the plain radiographs seen above show no evidence of any fractures or displacements. Detailed evaluation of the spinal cord and its surrounding paraspinal ligaments is needed in this case, of which only an MRI can reveal. A standard CT scan provides excellent bony detail but does not give much information about the spinal cord unless a CT myelogram is obtained. Given the patient's clinical findings, obtaining bending radiographs in a potentially unstable spine is not recommended. EMG and nerve conduction studies are not indicated in this patient.

An MRI is obtained and a sagittal view is displayed in Figure 10–21.

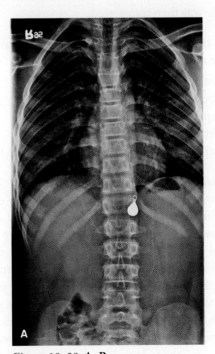
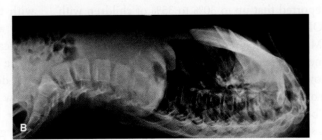

Figure 10–20 **A–B**

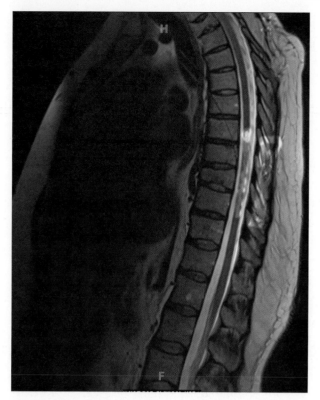

Figure 10–21

Given the findings on MRI, what is the best predictor of long-term neurologic outcome in this condition?

A. Age at the time of injury
B. Sex
C. Mechanism of injury
D. Neurologic status at time of presentation
E. Socioeconomic status

Discussion

The correct answer is (D). This patient has a spinal cord injury without radiographic abnormality (SCIWORA), and it was defined by Pang and Wilberger in 1982 as the presence of myelopathy as a result of trauma with no evidence of fracture or ligamentous instability on plain radiographs or tomography. MRI is the gold standard currently to diagnose this condition, however it has been reported that up to 30% to 35% of children with SCIWORA have no evidence of spinal cord abnormality on MRI. The main predictor of long-term neurologic outcome is the neurologic status at the time of presentation; however, in the subset of patients with only minor edema or hemorrhage on MRI, an MRI has been shown to be a better predictor of long-term outcome than neurologic status at presentation. This patient does not have minor edema on MRI. Children with complete lesions

very rarely improve, and those with incomplete but severe spinal cord lesions may improve but not to pre-injury levels. None of the other listed items have been shown to affect long-term outcomes in patients with SCIWORA.

Objectives: Did you learn...?

• The importance of adhering to the basics of ATLS when evaluating all trauma patients regardless of other reported injuries?
• The mechanism of action behind the bulbocavernosus reflex and the important ramifications if it is not present?
• How to use imaging and the process of deduction to diagnosis SCIWORA?
• The best predictor of outcome for patients presenting with SCIWORA?

CASE 14

Dr. Coleen S. Sabatini

A 5-year-old boy has been transferred from an outside hospital to your hospital's ER for further evaluation. Last evening, he developed pain in his left groin/testicle/hip. By this morning, he was limping and his mother took him to the ER. There, he had a temperature of 102.5°F (39.2°C) and his WBC was 15. They did an ultrasound which showed no testicular torsion, but there was some fluid in the left hip. They did not ultrasound the other side. He was then transferred.

Other than performing a physical examination, what is your next step in evaluation?

A. Obtain an MRI.
B. Obtain a CT scan.
C. Repeat the CBC, but add a differential.
D. Obtain an ESR and CRP.
E. Start antibiotics and observe response to treatment.

Discussion

The correct answer is (D). The evaluation of a child with this presentation includes a physical examination and laboratory evaluation. There are multiple clinical findings and laboratory studies that help make the diagnosis of septic arthritis. From a study first done by Kocher and then repeated by others, we know that if all four of the following are present— fever higher than 38.5°C, inability to bear weight, ESR greater than 40 mm/h and WBC greater than 12,000/µL—there is a 59% to 99.6% probability of septic arthritis. A CRP level greater than 2.0 mg/dL is an independent risk factor for septic arthritis. The CRP is also more helpful early on because it elevates within about 6 hours of infection, whereas the ESR becomes elevated within 24 to 48 hours of infection. An MRI and a CT scan are not needed when diagnosing septic arthritis and can delay treatment. MRIs are sometimes obtained if there is low clinical suspicion for septic joint. You have already been told that the WBC was 15 and a differential is helpful (there will be a left shift in the setting of infection), but having the differential will not be as helpful as knowing the patient's CRP. You would not start antibiotics in a nonseptic child until the work-up is complete and hopefully not until after a specimen has been obtained so that the organism causing the infection can be identified and subsequent antibiotics tailored appropriately.

For your physical examination you note the following—the patient is laying with leg extended and externally rotated on the bed. The patient appears somewhat toxic and is refusing to move the leg. He is now unable to bear weight and his temperature is now 38.6°C.

What part of this presentation is less consistent with septic arthritis of the hip?

A. Position of the leg
B. Refusal to move leg
C. Temperature
D. Refusal to bear weight

Discussion

The correct answer is (A). Patients with a septic joint will hold the joint in the position that maximizes the volume of the joint, thereby helping to reduce the pain. For the hip, in the setting of septic arthritis, the patient usually holds the hip in flexion, abduction and external rotation to maximize the hip capsule volume. Perhaps this patient may not have a large effusion yet, so does not need to maximize capsular volume, but the other factors in the presentation are suggestive of septic hip.

His labs come back as WBC 12.8, ESR of 20, and CRP of 3. In the short time that he has been in your ER, his hip examination has worsened. Given the elevated temperature >38.5, the CRP >2, refusal to bear weight, and the elevated WBC, you determine that he likely has a septic hip (ESR may not yet be elevated above 40 because his symptoms onset less than 24 hours ago). You take him to the OR and perform a needle aspiration of the hip and aspirate purulent material. You send that material

to the laboratory for cell count, Gram stain and culture, but given the clinical picture and frank pus in the joint, you proceed with a formal arthrotomy before waiting for the cell count results.

Other than a septic joint, what other conditions may give you similar WBC and PMN results on the cell count?

A. Toxic synovitis
B. Acute rheumatic fever
C. Juvenile inflammatory arthritis
D. Lyme arthritis
E. B and D
F. C and D

Discussion

The correct answer is (F). Septic arthritis has a leukocyte count greater than 50,000 cells/mL and there are greater than 75% PMs. Toxic synovitis—the condition that we are most often trying to distinguish septic arthritis from—has a leukocyte count of about 5,000 to 15,000 cells/mL with less than 25% PMNs. Joint effusions associated with acute rheumatic fever have WBC in the range of 10,000 to 15,000 cells/mL and there are around 50% PMNs. Juvenile inflammatory arthritis effusions have a wider range of leukocytes, ranging from 15,000 to 80,000 with around 75% PMNs—this overlaps with septic arthritis as septic arthritis can have a left shift around 75%. Lyme disease can cause a joint effusion that on cell count has leukocytes of 40,000 to 140,000 cells/mL with over 75% PMNs—same as septic arthritis.

In children with septic joints, the infection can come from a hematogenous source during a period of bacteremia, from direct inoculation, or from spread from an adjacent osteomyelitis.

Which joints are at risk of septic arthritis from direct spread from an adjacent osteomyelitis?

A. Shoulder, wrist, hip, knee
B. Shoulder, elbow, wrist, hip, ankle
C. Shoulder, elbow, hip, ankle
D. Shoulder, elbow, hip, knee
E. Elbow, hip, knee, ankle

Discussion

The correct answer is (C). Bones that have an intracapsular metaphysis are a potential source of septic arthritis due to direct spread of the infection from the bone directly into the joint. The proximal humerus, proximal radius, proximal femur, and distal tibia/fibula have intracapsular metaphyses in children, and these four joints are at risk of direct spread of infection from the bone into the joint.

Objectives: Did you learn...?

- The clinical presentation of a child with a septic hip?
- The evaluation of a child with a possible septic hip?
- The differential for hip effusion in children based on cell count?
- The joints most at risk of developing septic arthritis in the setting of osteomyelitis?

CASE 15

Dr. Nirav K. Pandya

A 12-year-old male presents to the orthopaedic clinic with several months of right knee pain which limits his ability to participate in sports. The patient cannot recollect a history of trauma but notes pain over the medial aspect of his knee. He is able to participate in most sporting activities but occasionally notes minor swelling. On physical examination, he has a trace effusion with tenderness to palpation over the medial aspect of the knee; particularly over the medial femoral condyle. He has full knee range of motion without any ligamentous instability. Pain is exacerbated when the patient's leg is flexed 90 degrees, the tibia is internally rotated, and the knee is extended. Pain is relieved when the tibia is externally rotated.

Your next action is:

A. Reassure the patient and have them take anti-inflammatory medications.
B. Prescribe a course of physical therapy.
C. Order an MRI of the patient's knee.
D. Obtain plain films including a tunnel (notch view) of the knee.

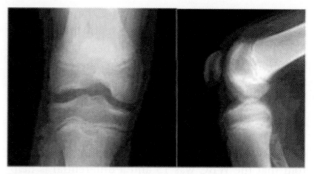

Figure 10–22

Discussion

The correct answer is (D). The patient has several months of localized knee pain which is limiting his ability to engage in age-appropriate activities (i.e., sports). The physical examination maneuver described (Wilson's test) is utilized to diagnose an osteochondritis dissecans (OCD) lesion of the knee. In a pediatric patient with localized pain which is limiting his/her activities, the next step in management should include a radiographic work-up prior to prescribing treatment (i.e., reassurance or physical therapy). Plain films should precede advanced imaging such as an MRI. The tunnel/notch view profiles the posterosuperior articular surface of the medial and lateral condyles where many OCD lesions of the knee are located which can be missed on a standard AP and lateral series of the knee.

The patient then obtains the following radiograph (Fig. 10–22) which confirms the diagnosis of an OCD lesion of the medial femoral condyle. An MRI is then ordered to examine the lesion further. A T2 image is shown in Figure 10–23.

Your next action is:

A. Arthroscopically drill the lesion in an antegrade manner

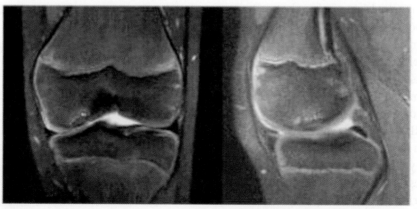

Figure 10–23

B. Arthroscopically drill the lesion in a retrograde manner

C. A period of protected weight bearing and bracing

D. Open reduction and internal fixation of the lesion

Discussion

The correct answer is (C). The patient has an OCD lesion of the posterolateral aspect of the medial femoral condyle which is the most common location for these lesions. Pediatric patients have a much better prognosis for OCD lesions as open distal femoral physes are the best predictor of a successful outcome with nonoperative management. Lesions which have synovial fluid behind the lesion on MRI are potentially unstable and require much more aggressive surgical management to prevent detachment and separation. As this patient is young, has open distal femoral physes, and has no instability on MRI, a trial of conservative treatment is appropriate. Arthroscopic drilling (either antegrade or retrograde) can be performed for stable lesions which have not responded to a trial of conservative management (Fig. 10–24). Open reduction and internal fixation should be reserved for unstable lesions.

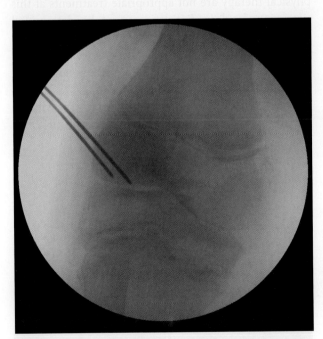

Figure 10–24

The patient responds well to a period of nonoperative management and returns to sporting activity. He is playing basketball when he has acute onset of pain, swelling, and decreased range of motion after an awkward landing. Plain radiographs are unremarkable, and a repeat MRI (Fig. 10–25) is obtained.

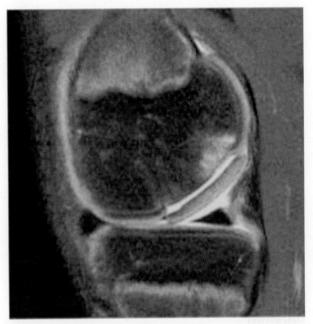

Figure 10–25

Which of the following is NOT recommended?

A. Fixation of the unstable lesion

B. Drilling of the unstable lesion

C. Microfracture

D. Fragment removal and chondroplasty

Discussion

The correct answer is (D). The patient has an unstable lesion on MRI which is acute; therefore every attempt should be made to salvage the lesion. The ideal treatment would be fixation of the lesion although the determination for treatment cannot be made until it is examined arthroscopically. If the lesion is not deemed stable during arthroscopy, then drilling would be a reasonable option (and can be combined with fixation). If the fragment is nonviable, microfracture would be a reasonable option to stimulate fibrocartilage formation as long as the donor site is not too large. Fragment removal and chondroplasty is not ideal for a young patient; particularly one who is engaged in sporting activities. Every attempt should be made to salvage the lesion and/or stimulate new cartilage formation if the fragment is unsalvageable.

The lesion is shown arthroscopically (Fig. 10–26). The appropriate treatment option is:

A. Fixation of the unstable lesion

B. Drilling of the unstable lesion

C. Microfracture

D. Mosaicplasty

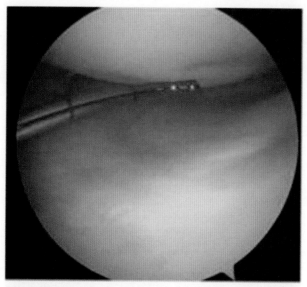

Figure 10–26

Discussion

The correct answer is (A). The patient has an unstable lesion on MRI and is demonstrating instability on arthroscopic examination. The fragment is viable therefore fixation of the lesion is optimal. Drilling would be appropriate for a stable lesion but both imaging and clinical findings suggest instability. As the lesion is viable, it should not be removed. Therefore, microfracture and mosaicplasty in the absence of exposed subchondral bone should not be utilized.

Objectives: Did you learn...?

- The clinical presentation and physical examination findings of OCD lesions of the knee?
- The appropriate initial radiographic work-up including tunnel/notch views of the knee?
- The radiographic criteria for determining stability versus instability of the lesion on MRI?
- The criteria for nonoperative treatment of OCD lesions of the knee as well as favorable prognostic factors?
- The various surgical treatment options for OCD lesions?

CASE 16

Dr. Drew Lansdown

A 12-year-old boy presents to your office 2 days after sustaining a noncontact injury to his left knee. He was playing soccer when he injured the knee, though he does not recall any other details about the injury. He could not continue playing due to pain and swelling. He is otherwise healthy and has no prior knee injuries. On physical examination, his left knee range of motion is 10 to 70 degrees, and he has a large effusion. Your

ligamentous examination and meniscal tests are equivocal and limited due to guarding. Radiographs show an effusion, but no obvious fracture.

The next best step in treatment is:

A. Place the patient in a hinged knee brace and follow-up in 3 to 4 weeks.
B. Order a CT scan of the knee to evaluate for an occult fracture.
C. Prescribe physical therapy with a focus on regaining range of motion.
D. Order an MRI of the knee to evaluate for ligamentous or meniscal injuries.

Discussion

The correct answer is (D). An acute knee effusion in an adolescent patient is often associated with an ACL rupture or patellar dislocation. Physical examination in this setting may be challenging due to patient guarding and pain with physical examination. Abbasi et al. reported that the two most common injuries in 10- to 14-year-old patients with an acute knee effusion were patellar dislocations (36%) and ACL tears (22%). Bracing and physical therapy are not appropriate treatments at this time since a clear diagnosis cannot be determined from the history and physical examination. An occult fracture is not likely given this patient's age and presentation. CT will not offer the same ability to visualize soft tissue injuries as does the MRI scan.

The MRI is obtained, and the patient returns with his parents to review the images (Figs. 10–27 and 10–28).

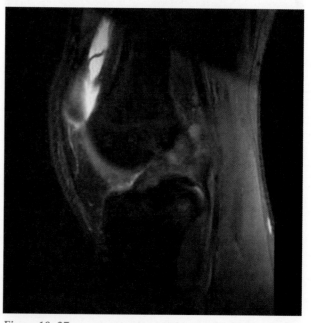

Figure 10–27

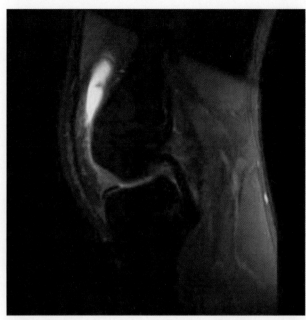

Figure 10–28

The diagnosis most consistent with the images shown in Figures 10–27 and 10–28 is:

A. Mid-substance ACL rupture
B. Tibial eminence avulsion fracture
C. Lateral patellar dislocation
D. Bucket-handle medial meniscus tear

Discussion

The correct answer is (A). The patient has sustained an ACL tear. Once thought to be uncommon amongst pediatric populations, recent studies have shown these injuries are frequently encountered. A tibial eminence avulsion fracture is of concern in adolescent patients, though there is no evidence of injury at this location. The axial view of the patella shows no injury to the medial patellofemoral ligament or bone marrow edema at the patella or femoral trochlea which are signs of a possible patellar dislocation. The medial meniscus is intact.

Follow-up physical examination reveals a 2A Lachman and a positive pivot shift. The remainder of the MRI is negative for meniscal or cartilage lesions. The patient and his parents elect to undergo surgical treatment for his ACL tear. They are interested in reviewing different potential surgical options and are concerned about the possible impacts of this surgery on the patient's remaining growth.

Which of the following treatment options carries the highest risk of growth disturbance?

A. Transphyseal ACL reconstruction with anteromedial portal drilling for the femoral tunnel and hamstring autograft
B. All-epiphyseal ACL reconstruction with outside-in drilling for the femoral tunnel and hamstring autograft
C. Transphyseal ACL reconstruction with anteromedial portal drilling for the femoral tunnel and patellar tendon autograft
D. All-epiphyseal ACL reconstruction with outside-in drilling for the femoral tunnel and posterior tibialis allograft

Discussion

The correct answer is (C). Options for ACL reconstruction in patients with open growth plates include transphyseal and all-epiphyseal reconstruction. For transphyseal reconstructions, multiple studies have demonstrated that the greatest risk for growth disturbance is with a bony block across the physis, such as with patellar tendon autograft. Soft tissue placed across the physis carries little risk for growth disturbance.

You are counseling the patient and his family about graft choices. They inquire about the possibility of using allograft tissue and ask about the risks associated with this selection.

The greatest risk associated with using allograft tissue is:

A. Graft failure
B. HIV transmission
C. Superficial surgical site infection
D. Postoperative septic arthritis

Discussion

The correct answer is (A). Allograft ACL reconstruction in the adolescent population is associated with an increased risk of graft failure relative to an autograft reconstruction. This risk has been estimated to be greater than 20% over 2 years in pediatric and adolescent patients. Viral transmission from musculoskeletal allograft tissue is a rare complication and estimated to be approximately 1 in 1 million. Infections following ACL reconstruction, regardless of graft choice, occur infrequently. Deep infection occurs in less than 1% of cases, while the rate for superficial infection is reported at 2.3%.

Objectives: Did you learn…?

• The importance of obtaining advanced imaging for a pediatric patient with an acute knee effusion?

- The MRI appearance of an acute ACL rupture and that these injuries are frequently encountered in pediatric patients?
- Understanding different options for femoral tunnel drilling in the pediatric patient and the importance of avoiding a bony block across the physis to limit the potential for growth disturbance?
- The risk of graft failure observed in pediatric patients with allograft reconstruction?

CASE 17

Dr. Nirav K. Pandya

A 10-year-old female soccer player presents to the sports clinic with a several month history of knee pain and swelling along the lateral joint line. The patient notes pain and a snapping sensation laterally. She also describes occasional mechanical symptoms as well. On physical exam she is unable to fully extend the knee. The patient otherwise has a stable ligamentous examination of the knee. Radiographs are obtained and shown in Figure 10–29.

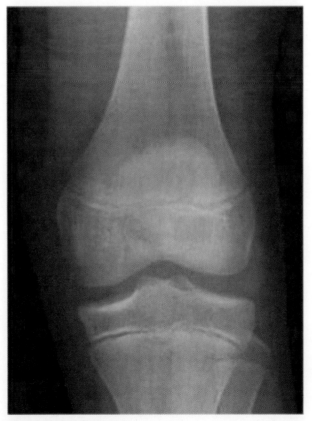

Figure 10–29

The next course of action is:

A. Physical therapy for iliotibial band tendonitis
B. MRI of the knee
C. Corticosteroid injection
D. Reassurance

Discussion

The correct answer is (B). The patient's clinical examination is concerning for meniscal injury (lateral joint line pain) with the snapping sensation concerning for an unstable meniscus. The radiographs demonstrate lateral joint space widening, cupping of the lateral tibial plateau, and a hypoplastic lateral tibial spine—all suggestive of a discoid meniscus. Discoid menisci are classified using the Watanabe classification as complete, incomplete, or Wrisberg (lack of posterior meniscotibial attachment to the tibia). Unstable variants create the classic "snapping" sensation. The diagnosis of a discoid meniscus can be made with three or more 5-mm sagittal images with meniscal continuity. As the patient has had several months of pain with mechanical symptoms and swelling, reassurance is not appropriate. Although IT band tendonitis can cause "snapping" it is not accompanied by loss of extension and swelling. Corticosteroid injections should be utilized sparingly in the pediatric population; particularly when a diagnosis has not been made.

The patient then obtains an MRI which is shown in Figure 10–30. The next appropriate step in management is:

A. Lateral compartment unloader bracing and physical therapy
B. Arthroscopy
C. Long-leg casting × 6 weeks
D. Return to unrestricted sporting activity

Discussion

The correct answer is (B). If the patient were asymptomatic, then the discoid meniscus could simply be observed with a return to unrestricted sporting activity. For a younger patient who is intermittently symptomatic and/or elects to not undergo operative intervention, lateral compartment unloader bracing may be appropriate until the patient and/or family agree to intervention. Long-leg casting is not appropriate and will do nothing more than cause stiffness, loss of strength, and range of motion. As the patient is symptomatic, has mechanical symptoms, and has potential tearing seen on MRI, arthroscopic intervention is indicated to examine the meniscus and intervene.

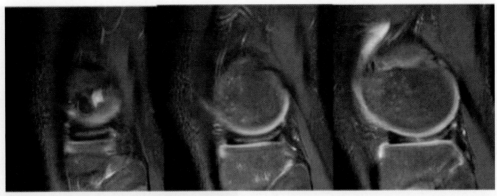

Figure 10–30

The patient is taken to surgery, and intraoperative images (Figs. 10–31 and 10–32) are shown. The next step in management is:

A. Complete meniscectomy
B. No intervention; the knee looks normal
C. Saucerization
D. Chondroplasty

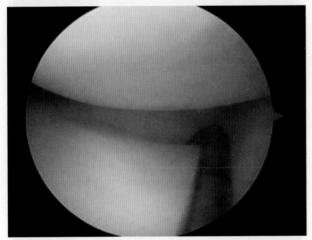

Figure 10–31

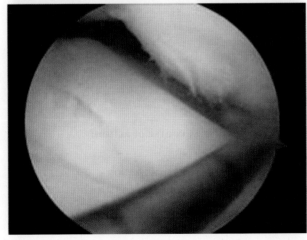

Figure 10–32

Discussion
The correct answer is (C). The arthroscopic images demonstrate a complete discoid meniscus which is covering the entire lateral tibial plateau. As the patient is symptomatic from the meniscus, saucerization is the first step in management. The meniscus is trimmed back using a combination of shavers and biters to a stable peripheral rim, which replicates the width of the native meniscus. Complete meniscectomy would not be indicated in a patient of this age due to the high risk of early onset degenerative arthritis. In fact, even prior to intervention, many discoid menisci have been associated with the development of lateral hemijoint osteochondral lesions. Although chondroplasty may be necessary, the meniscus is the underlying problem causing chondral wear and must be dealt with first.

After saucerization is performed, the meniscus is probed and the following arthroscopic image is seen (Fig. 10–33). The next step in management is:

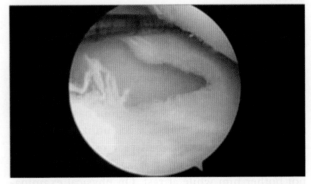

Figure 10–33

A. No further work is necessary; the meniscus has been returned to a stable rim
B. Continuation of the saucerization; too much meniscus remains

C. Microfracture of the lateral femoral condyle

D. Repair of the unstable peripheral rim of the meniscus

Discussion

The correct answer is (D). The arthroscopic image demonstrates an unstable peripheral rim of the meniscus which an attempt should be made to repair. The meniscus has been trimmed adequately but instability remains. Further saucerization without repair may lead to very little to no meniscus remaining which can lead to early degeneration. Although chondral damage may be present in association with the meniscus, there is no exposed subchondral bone to suggest the need for microfracture. Various repair techniques (inside-out, outside-in, all-inside) are available to the surgeon and should be utilized based on surgeon preference and experience.

Objectives: Did you learn...?

- The clinical presentation and physical examination findings of discoid meniscus?
- The MRI criteria for diagnosis of discoid menisci?
- The Watanabe classification of discoid menisci?
- The indications for operative intervention and the surgical approach to discoid menisci?
- The importance of saucerization and assessment of peripheral rim instability?
- The increased risk of OCD lesions and arthritis with this pathology, particularly after total meniscectomy?

CASE 18

Dr. Nirav K. Pandya

You are performing preparticipation physicals for the local youth sports team. An 11-year-old male presents with 6 weeks of medial elbow pain that is aggravated by throwing. He notes a vague history of a "pop" while playing 6 weeks ago in baseball game. He pitches multiple times a week utilizing a variety of pitches. He plays baseball year round and chose to specialize in this sport at age 9. The pain does not bother him while at rest. On physical examination, he is tender to palpation over the medial side of the elbow with slightly decreased range of motion. Radiographs of the affected and normal elbow are obtained (Figs. 10–34 and 10–35).

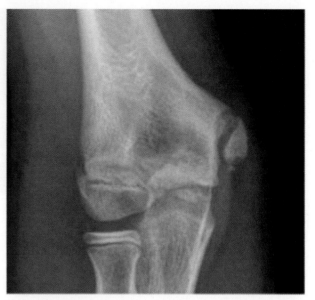

Figure 10–34

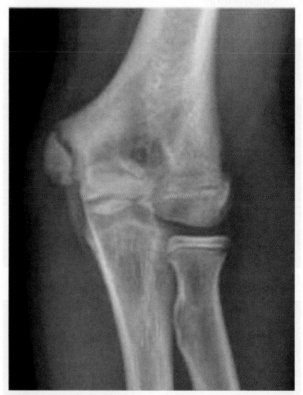

Figure 10–35

What is the next best course of action?

A. MRI of the right elbow

B. Open reduction internal fixation

C. Ulnar collateral ligament reconstruction

D. Cessation of all throwing activity and physical therapy

Discussion

The correct answer is (D). The patient has "Little league elbow" due to repetitive throwing which causes valgus stress on the medial elbow structures. On radiographs, there is widening of the medial epicondyle apophysis compared to the contralateral side. Poor throwing mechanics, overuse, and single sport specialization are risk factors for the development of this condition. As this is an overuse/mechanical problem, cessation of throwing activity and an examination of mechanics/physical therapy are key in treatment. The patient does not require an MRI given his history, physical examination, and radiographic findings; failure of conservative treatment should warrant an MRI. The patient is too young to have suffered a UCL injury. Furthermore, the patient's widening of the medial epicondylar apophysis is due to overuse not an acute fracture; therefore fixation is not necessary.

The next patient arrives in clinic complaining of increasing knee pain and a "bump" over his proximal tibia. This 10-year-old patient plays basketball and notes this "bump" has been increasing in size over the past several months. He has pain with repetitive running and jumping activities. On physical examination, he has exquisite tenderness over the proximal tibia and pain with resisted knee extension. He has very tight popliteal angles. There is no ligamentous instability about the knee. Radiographs of the affected knee are obtained (Fig. 10–36).

What is the next best course of action?

A. MRI of the knee to evaluate for malignancy
B. Open reduction internal fixation
C. Reassurance
D. Arthroscopy

Discussion

The correct answer is (C). The patient has Osgood–Schlatter's disease. This is a condition which occurs in children who are engaged in repetitive explosive activities, which can cause a painful bump over the proximal tibia. This bump is due to the patellar tendon pulling on the tibial tubercle apophysis during explosive activities; particularly during periods of rapid growth. Symptoms typically abate once growth ceases, although the bump may persist into adulthood. The vast majority of cases can be treated with rest, ice, activity modification, and stretching. An MRI is not necessary as the "bump" is due

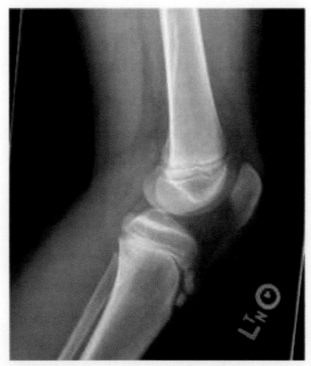

Figure 10–36

to traction apophysitis; not a malignancy. The patient's presentation is not consistent with a fracture, and fixation of the fragment in a child of this age could lead to a recurvatum deformity. Finally, as the patient's pain is due to an extra-articular process, arthroscopy is not indicated.

The younger brother of the patient above is the next patient that you see in clinic. He is complaining of "heel pain." He enjoys playing soccer. This pain has waxed and waned over the past several months and is worse with running and kicking. On physical examination, he is tender over the calcaneus with weakness in plantarflexion and limited dorsiflexion. There is some localized swelling over the calcaneus.

The patient is at greatest risk for the following if he continues to play:

A. Achilles tendon rupture
B. Calcaneal fracture
C. Growth arrest
D. Increased pain and duration of symptoms

Discussion

The correct answer is (D). The patient's clinical presentation is consistent with Sever's disease which is a traction apophysitis of the calcaneus. This occurs during periods of growth causing pain and swelling. There is no association of this condition with Achilles tendon rupture (which would be rare in this age group regardless), calcaneal fracture, or growth arrest. Continuing activity will increase the intensity and duration of symptoms. Patients can be treated for this condition with rest, ice, anti-inflammatory medications, gastroc-soleus stretching, and limited wear of unsupportive shoes such as cleats.

At the end of clinic, the parents of the previous three patients ask you advice as to how to best manage their children's athletic career in regards to injury prevention; particularly overuse.

Which of the following is an appropriate recommendation?

A. Single sport specialization before age 13 to prevent stress from playing multiple sports
B. 6 months of complete rest during the year in which no active sporting activity takes place
C. A well-designed weight lifting and plyometric program to build muscle bulk and explosive strength
D. Periods of active rest in which athletes are playing multiple different sports

Discussion

The correct answer is (D). The concept of active rest (taking a break from one sport by playing another sport) is essential in preventing overuse injuries in young athletes. Active rest not only provides physiologic benefits through the utilization of different movement patterns and muscle groups, but it also provides emotional and social benefits through different teammates and coaches. Although periods of complete rest should be incorporated, 6 months of complete rest is extreme. Although weight lifting and plyometrics are an important component of a well-designed athletic program, it is not indicated for prepubertal patients. Finally, the detrimental physical, social, and emotional effects of early single sport specialization have been well documented. Burnout, both emotional and physical, can be avoided by encouraging a breadth of activities.

Objectives: Did you learn...?

• The history, physical examination, and radiographic findings of Little league elbow?
• The initial treatment for throwing injuries in the young athlete (i.e., cessation)?

• The clinical presentation of Osgood–Schaltter's disease?
• The treatment modalities for Sever's disease?
• The risk factors for overuse injuries and the modalities to combat its occurrence?

CASE 19

Dr. Nirav K. Pandya

A 14-year-old female soccer player presents with a 1 year history of anterior knee pain. The pain presents when the patient is warming up, abates in the heat of competition, and re-presents again after sporting activity. She uses her entire hand to describe the location of the pain in her knee. She has discomfort going up and down stairs and when she sits for long periods of time. She feels as if "sandpaper" is under her knee. She denies any effusion, fevers, chills, night sweats, or sick contacts. Besides generalized tenderness over the patellar facets, her knee examination is unremarkable.

What is the next best course of action?

A. AP and frog pelvis radiographs
B. MRI of the knee to rule out an osteochondral lesion
C. AP, lateral, notch, and merchant views of the affected knee
D. Assessment of flexibility and strength

Discussion

The correct answer is (D). The vast majority of patients with anterior knee pain possess deficits in core strength, single leg balance, and flexibility. This should be assessed prior to further imaging. The patient is not of the typical age for a slipped capital femoral epiphysis nor does she present as such; therefore imaging of the pelvis is not necessary. Physical examination should always proceed a radiographic work-up (and may not be necessary if there is no concerning physical examination findings); as a result both plain films and an MRI are not necessary at this time.

After a thorough physical examination, it is noted that the patient does lack flexibility and strength contributing to her anterior knee pain. Beyond the principles of rest, ice, and anti-inflammatory medications, you decide that a course of physical therapy would be appropriate.

What area should the physical therapists concentrate on?

A. Core and hip muscle stretching/strengthening
B. Quadriceps and hamstring strengthening

C. Massage of the peripatellar region

D. Upper body weight lifting

Discussion

The correct answer is (A). Proximal stretching and strengthening has been shown to be extremely effective in the management of anterior knee pain in the literature. Traditionally, quadriceps and hamstring strengthening was utilized in the treatment of anterior knee pain. This ignored the fact that the body's inability to stabilize itself and absorb load appropriately proximally was a much larger risk factor when compared to developing muscles which were likely already developed in athletic individuals. Upper body weight lifting has no role in the management of anterior knee pain. Although peripatellar massage may help, it should not be the central aspect of rehabilitation.

Which of the following modalities has NOT been shown to be effective in reducing anterior knee pain arising from patellofemoral syndrome?

A. McConnell taping

B. Bracing

C. Physical therapy

D. Rest from activity

Discussion

The correct answer is (B). Bracing has not been shown to be effective for pain reduction in patients with patellofemoral syndrome. Although the mechanism is not clear, McConnell taping has been shown to reduce pain. Not surprisingly, rest from activity and physical therapy is beneficial as well.

After a course of appropriate physical therapy, the patient's pain is isolated to the medial aspect of the knee in the distribution shown in Figure 10–37. Pain is particularly present between 30 and 70 degrees of flexion and is accompanied by a snapping sensation.

What is the most likely structure causing the pain?

A. Medial plica

B. Medial meniscus

C. Medial collateral ligament

D. OCD lesion

Discussion

The correct answer is (A). The patient's pain is in the location of the medial patellar plica which can cause a snapping sensation between 30 and 70 degrees of flexion as the synovial fold is caught between the patella and femur. The medial meniscus would present with pain

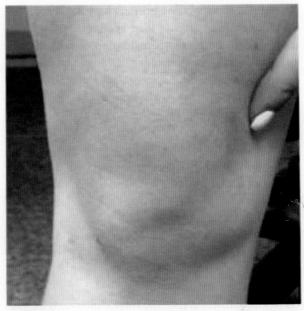

Figure 10–37

located more posteriorly over the joint line. The medial collateral ligament would give the patient instability rather than localized pain in a certain arc of movement. Although pain from an OCD could potentially give pain in the region described, the snapping sensation as well as the isolated arc over which the pain is occurring is atypical for an OCD.

Objectives: Did you learn...?

• The clinical presentation of anterior knee pain?

• Key assessment principles of the young patient with anterior knee pain?

• The emphasis on proximal rehabilitation in anterior knee pain?

• The efficacy of various treatment modalities for pain in patellafemoral syndrome?

• The presence of medial plica syndrome in the diagnosis of anterior knee pain?

CASE 20

Dr. Cordelia W. Carter

A 16-year-old, right-handed female presents to your office with complaint of bilateral shoulder pain, worse on the right than the left, that has been present for "as long as she can remember." She cannot recall a specific injury. She tells you the pain is achy in nature and is worse when she does overhead activities, including volleyball. She feels like her shoulders "pop in and out." On physical examination, she exhibits scapular dyskinesis, 2+ anterior and posterior load-and-shift testing bilaterally, and 10 degrees hyperextension of both elbows. Her active and passive shoulder ROM is equal, with 180 degrees of forward flexion and 180 of abduction.

What physical examination finding would suggest incompetence of her rotator interval?

A. A positive "hornblower's" sign
B. A positive "bear-hug" test
C. A sulcus sign with the arm held in neutral rotation
D. A sulcus sign with the arm held in 30 degrees of external rotation
E. A sulcus sign with the arm held in 30 degrees of internal rotation

Discussion

The correct answer is (D). The rotator interval is an anatomic structure whose boundaries include the superior edge of the subscapularis tendon and the anterior edge of the supraspinatus tendon. The contents of the rotator interval include the coracohumeral ligament, the glenohumeral capsule, the superior glenohumeral ligament, and the biceps tendon. The rotator interval has been shown to play an important role in glenohumeral stability; laxity of the rotator interval is associated with increased glenohumeral motion and increased humeral head translation. Competence of the rotator interval is commonly evaluated by looking for the disappearance of the sulcus sign with the arm held in an externally rotated position. (A positive sulcus sign is the appearance of a gap greater than 1 to 2 cm inferior to the acromion when a downward-directed pressure is applied to the adducted arm held in a neutral position, and is considered indicative of ligamentous laxity and/or inferior humeral instability.) Repeating this maneuver with the arm held in external rotation normally results in the disappearance of the sulcus sign. For patients with pathologic laxity of the rotator interval, however, the sulcus sign persists in this position.

Additional examination findings include a positive anterior apprehension test on the right, and you become concerned for an injury to the anterior-inferior glenoid labrum. Her radiographs do not reveal a frank bony lesion. What is the best study to further evaluate her shoulder for this injury?

A. A three-dimensional computed tomography (3D-CT) scan of the shoulder
B. Magnetic resonance imaging (MRI) of the shoulder performed with and without IV contrast
C. An MRI arthrogram of the shoulder
D. A delayed gadolinium-enhanced MRI of cartilage (dGEMRIC) of the shoulder
E. A three-phase bone scan

Discussion

The correct answer is (C). 3D-CT is a powerful test to evaluate osseous anatomy and injury. However, it is not the best test to evaluate injuries that primarily involve soft tissue, such as labral or cartilage lesions. Additionally, CT imaging carries with it an inherent risk of exposure to radiation, which ideally is avoided in young patients. While an MRI of the shoulder with and without IV contrast may be useful in this setting, it is unlikely to be as useful for evaluating labral pathology as an MRI arthrogram. An MRI arthrogram of the shoulder, in which radiopaque dye is injected into the shoulder prior to image acquisition, is the "gold standard" test for evaluating labral pathology. The MRI arthrogram for patients with labral tears will exhibit a characteristic appearance in which the dye "turns the corner," tracking underneath the labrum and around the glenoid (see Figure 10–38). dGEMRIC MRI is most helpful for assessing cartilage injury. Three-phase bone scans may be used to identify areas of high metabolic activity (such as tumor, injury, or infection) but would not be useful in this setting.

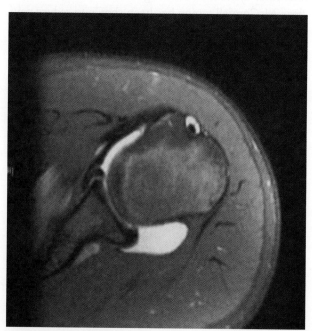

Figure 10–38 T2 axial image of an MRI arthrogram of the shoulder, exhibiting an anterior labral tear.

Review of your patient's diagnostic imaging does not reveal a discrete injury in the shoulder, although the axillary pouch appears "patulous" and the rotator interval is widened. You decide to recommend physical therapy and oral nonsteroidal anti-inflammatory medicine as a first line of treatment.

In addition to core strengthening, physical therapy should focus on achieving what goal(s)?

A. Strengthening the static stabilizers of the shoulder
B. Strengthening the dynamic stabilizers of the shoulder
C. Restoration of normal muscle coordination through proprioceptive and neuromuscular retraining
D. A and B
E. A and C
F. B and C
G. A, B, and C

Discussion

The correct answer is (F). You have diagnosed this patient with atraumatic multidirectional shoulder instability, and physical therapy remains a first line of treatment for this clinical entity. Physical therapy should include strengthening of the core musculature and the entire kinetic chain. Strengthening the dynamic stabilizers of the shoulder, including the rotator cuff musculature, the periscapular musculature, the biceps and the deltoid, is a critical component of therapy. Additionally, patients with MDI frequently exhibit uncoordinated muscle activity patterns, abnormal scapulothoracic motion, and overall poor shoulder kinematics; neuromuscular/proprioceptive retraining to improve these parameters is also a cornerstone of non-operative treatment. The static stabilizers of the shoulder include the glenohumeral ligaments, the glenoid labrum, and the bony congruity of the glenoid/humerus articulation. These cannot be changed with physical therapy.

Your patient returns for follow-up after completing 12 months of your prescribed physical therapy regimen and reports little symptomatic improvement. Her examination continues to reveal unrestricted shoulder motion, 2+ load-and-shift testing, inferior laxity, and mild anterior apprehension. Based on her failure to respond to what you consider appropriate nonoperative therapy, you initiate a discussion about possible surgical treatments, including both open and arthroscopic capsular plication/shift procedures.

You counsel her that:

A. She is more likely to have recurrent instability with an arthroscopic procedure.

B. She is more likely to return to sports with an arthroscopic procedure.
C. There is a higher rate of postoperative complications with an open procedure.
D. She may lose roughly 10 degrees of external rotation with either an open or an arthroscopic procedure.
E. Thermal capsulorrhaphy is a safe and effective adjunctive arthroscopic tool.

Discussion

The correct answer is (D). While an open capsular shift procedure has been the standard of treatment for decades, arthroscopic capsular plication using either suture-only or suture anchor constructs has been shown to have similar rates of failure (<10% re-dislocation rate); similar return-to-sport rates (~85%) and similar complication rates. Both procedures are associated with minor losses in shoulder motion, specifically external rotation, although there is no significant difference in loss of external rotation between patients treated with open inferior capsular shift and arthroscopic capsular plication. The use of thermal capsulorrhaphy for treatment of MDI has been associated with catastrophic complications, including glenohumeral chondrolysis, capsular necrosis, and injury to the axillary nerve.

During the course of the follow-up office visit, your patient's mother asks if you would evaluate her younger daughter, who is 14. This patient also has achy bilateral shoulder pain and reports discomfort when doing activities of daily life, such as brushing her hair or pulling on a shirt. Additionally, she reports that she has dislocated both of her kneecaps and has had recurrent ankle sprains. You notice that she is 5′10″, quite thin, and towers over her mother and older sister.

In addition to performing a thorough musculoskeletal examination, what other referrals might you consider making?

A. Genetics, cardiology, ophthalmology
B. Genetics, rheumatology, ophthalmology
C. Nephrology, cardiology, ophthalmology
D. Nephrology, cardiology, rheumatology
E. Nephrology, genetics, rheumatology

Discussion

The correct answer is (A). This patient has symptoms of generalized ligamentous laxity in addition to clinical findings (tall stature, thin habitus) that are suggestive of a connective tissue disorder, such as Marfan's syndrome. Marfan's syndrome is a genetic disease affecting the protein Fibrillin-1 that is inherited in an autosomal dominant pattern. The most common extraskeletal manifestations of Marfan's syndrome are cardiovascular (mitral valve prolapse, aortic aneurysm) and ophthalmologic (ectopia lentis—lens subluxation; astigmatism, nearsightedness, detachment of the retina). Common musculoskeletal manifestations include scoliosis, pectus excavatum, hypermobility of the joints, and arachnodactyly. Shoulder instability in the setting of Marfan's syndrome is a different clinical entity from multidirectional shoulder instability, with poorer outcomes resulting from both surgical and nonoperative treatment.

Objectives: Did you learn...?

- Key components of history and physical examination for MDI?
- Appropriate selection of diagnostic tests for MDI?
- Basic treatment algorithm for MDI?
- Underlying genetic disorders that may be associated with MDI?

CASE 21

Dr. Jaysson Brooks

A 4-year-old male presents to your office as a self-referral by his mother. She is concerned that something is wrong with her little boy, as he does not seem to be reaching his motor milestones. She reports that he started walking at the age of 3, and currently has difficulty running and jumping along with his friends. On physical examination he is normocephalic, with normal appearing facies, and proportional arm and leg length. He has enlarged calf muscles and prominent lumbar lordosis. While the child is supine on the examination table, you ask him to stand up; he rolls to the prone position and uses his arms to progressively stand from a crawling position to standing.

The disorder that this child has is caused by a defect in the gene coding for what protein?

A. Cartilage oligomeric matrix protein (COMP)
B. Dystrophin
C. Fibrillin
D. Vitronectin
E. Core-binding factor subunit alpha-1 (CBFA-1)

Discussion

The correct answer is (B). This patient has Duchenne's muscular dystrophy (DMD) which most commonly presents in boys that are between 3 and 5 years old. They

tend to gain motor milestones from 6 to 7 years old but often transition to a wheel chair secondary to proximal muscle weakness by age 12. Dystrophin helps to form a complex that mechanically links the sarcomere to the extracellular matrix. Remember to check creatinine kinase (CK) levels, which are often elevated between 10 and 200 times the normal reference levels. COMP is a protein that when mutated can result in pseudo-achondroplasia or multiple epiphyseal dysplasia. Mutations in the gene encoding for fibrillin result in Marfan's syndrome. Vitronectin is a protein involved in tumor metastasis due to its function in cell adhesion. CBFA-1 is encoded by the RUNX2 gene and its dysfunction results in cleidocranial dysplasia.

What is the inheritance pattern of patients with this disorder?

A. Autosomal dominant
B. Autosomal recessive
C. X-linked dominant
D. X-linked recessive
E. Mitochondrial inheritance

Discussion

The correct answer is (D). Examples of autosomal dominant disorders include syndactyly, Marfan's syndrome, achondroplasia, and Ehlers–Danlos syndrome. Examples of autosomal recessive disorders include diastrophic dysplasia, Friedreich's ataxia, spinal muscle atrophy, and Gaucher's disease. An example of an X-linked dominant disorder includes hypophosphatemic rickets. Myoclonic epilepsy and ragged-red fibers (MERRF) are examples of a disease with a mitochondrial inheritance pattern.

As part of your general work-up for patients with DMD you tell the mother that you plan to get a standing scoliosis radiograph in clinic which is displayed in Figure 10–39. You relay to the mother that his radiograph shows no sign of scoliosis, however his mother is deeply concerned about the possible development of scoliosis in the future.

If left untreated and once the patient is weak enough to need a wheelchair, you tell the mother that the chance of progression of scoliosis is:

A. 10%
B. 30%
C. 50%
D. 70%
E. 90%

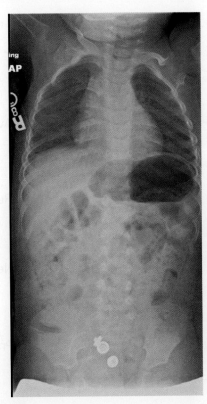

Figure 10–39

Discussion

The correct answer is (E). Patients with DMD become wheelchair bound secondary to progressive muscle weakness. This muscle weakness also involves the paraspinal muscles which leads to a lack of trunk control. If left untreated, this results in progressive scoliosis in almost all patients.

Relieved that she finally has a diagnosis, his mother asks about the best treatment options available to improve her son's overall prognosis in regards to muscle weakness and progression of his scoliosis.

What is the best treatment that can be offered to patients with DMD which improves overall prognosis?

A. Early posterior spinal fusion for Cobb angles >20 degrees
B. Corticosteroid treatment starting before the age of 5
C. Physical therapy focused on gait training and strengthening
D. Methotrexate treatment
E. Recombinant dystrophin injections before the age of 5

Discussion

The correct answer is (B) Glucocorticoid treatment starting before the age of 5. Corticosteroids should be offered

to all patients with DMD. Treatment helps to prolong walking, transiently increases muscle strength, reduces falls, improves pulmonary function and cardiac function, and slows the progression of scoliosis. Its effect on scoliosis is quite profound; a recent study by Lebel et al. compared boys with DMD who were treated with glucocorticoids to boys with DMD who were not treated with steroids; both were walking prior to treatment. They found that 20% of boys in the treatment group developed scoliosis while 92% in the untreated group developed scoliosis. The general rule before steroid use became prevalent was to perform a posterior spinal fusion on patients with DMD who had 20-degree curves because of the rapid progression. The literature does not show that physical therapy, methotrexate, or recombinant dystrophin affect overall prognosis of DMD.

Objectives: Did you learn...?

- The inheritance pattern of DMD and other common musculoskeletal disorders?
- The importance of obtaining scoliosis films of patients with DMD?
- The rate of progression of scoliosis in patients with DMD who go untreated?
- The importance of corticosteroids in slowing the progression of pulmonary, cardiac, and spine dysfunction in patients with DMD?

CASE 22

Dr. Andrea S. Bauer

You are called to the newborn nursery to evaluate a 1-day-old girl who has not moved her right arm since birth. She was the product of spontaneous vaginal delivery at 41 weeks' gestation. The mother's pregnancy was complicated by gestational diabetes mellitus. Birth weight was 10 lb 2 oz (4,590 g). The delivery was complicated by shoulder dystocia lasting 1 minute, and the vacuum suction was used to facilitate delivery. The newborn girl now holds her arm in an extended and internally rotated position, with no active movement of the right upper extremity. She does not seem to respond to touch on that arm. She moves her left arm and both legs normally. There is no ecchymosis or swelling to suggest a fracture.

Your diagnosis is:

A. Cerebral palsy
B. Brachial plexus birth palsy
C. Congenital muscular torticollis
D. Arthrogryposis multiplex congenita

Discussion

The correct answer is (B). Prenatal risk factors for brachial plexus birth palsy include preeclampsia and gestational diabetes. Perinatal risk factors include macrosomia, shoulder dystocia, and the use of devices such as forceps and vacuum suction for delivery.

The differential diagnosis includes pseudoparalysis due to a fracture of the clavicle or humerus sustained during the birth practice. If local swelling or bruising suggests a fracture, x-rays should be obtained.

Upper extremity monoplegic type cerebral palsy can be mistaken for a brachial plexus birth palsy. Risk factors for cerebral palsy include prematurity and low birth weight.

Congenital muscular torticollis is due to a shortening or overactivity of the sternocleidomastoid muscle. The head is laterally tilted towards the affected muscle and rotated away from it.

Arthrogryposis multiplex congenital, or amyoplasia, is a condition of multiple congenital joint contractures. Hypoplasia of muscles leads to decreased joint movement in utero. Usually both arms and both legs are involved, with the arms generally positioned in shoulder internal rotation, elbow extension, wrist flexion, and a thumb-in-palm deformity.

You notice that the newborn has ptosis of the eyelid on the same side as the paralyzed arm. On closer inspection, you also notice that the pupil is smaller than the contralateral side (miosis). You recognize that these signs, along with anhydrosis and enopthalmos, are known together as Horner's syndrome.

Horner's syndrome is a concomitant injury to the ____, and denotes a ____ prognosis for this infant's brachial plexus recovery:

A. Facial nerve, favorable
B. Facial nerve, unfavorable
C. Cervical sympathetic chain, favorable
D. Cervical sympathetic chain, unfavorable

Discussion

The correct answer is (D). Horner's syndrome arises from injury to the cervical sympathetic chain. Because the cervical sympathetic chain is in very close proximity to the spinal cord, Horner's syndrome is pathognomonic for a brachial plexus injury that consists of a nerve root avulsion from the spinal cord. Birth injuries to the brachial plexus can occur along a continuum of severity (Fig. 10–40), of which nerve root avulsion is the most severe type.

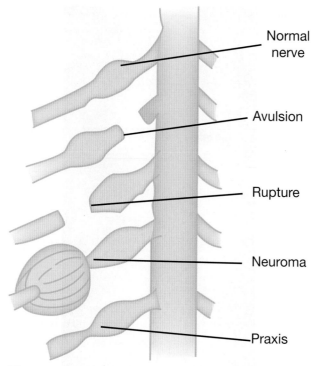

Figure 10–40

Injury to the facial nerve is also possible during a difficult delivery. This would cause paralysis of the voluntary facial muscles, with facial drooping, on the affected side. There is no known prognostic value of a concomitant facial nerve injury.

You follow the patient's recovery as an outpatient over the next few months. At the age of 6 months, you notice that her Horner's syndrome has resolved. She can now move her fingers and wrist spontaneously, and she is able to internally rotate her shoulder. However, she still does not bend her elbow actively against gravity (AMS score of 3) and cannot elevate her shoulder in either forward flexion or abduction beyond 30 degrees even with gravity eliminated (AMS score of 2 for each).

Based on these physical examination findings, your next course of action is:

A. Schedule for exploration of the brachial plexus with microsurgical reconstruction
B. Schedule for Botox injections into her triceps and pectoralis major
C. Begin functional electrical stimulation therapy
D. Continue regular observation

Discussion

The correct answer is (A). Exact indications for microsurgical exploration and reconstruction of the brachial plexus are controversial in brachial plexus birth palsy. However, it is commonly agreed that for infants who do not recover the ability to flex the elbow against gravity by the age of 6 months, the course of their recovery will be improved by microsurgical treatment. The AMS or Active Movement Scale measures the active motion of 15 different movements of the upper extremity on a 0–7 scale, based on how much movement the child can produce with gravity eliminated (scores 0–4) or against gravity (scores 5–7).

Botox injections can be used as an adjunctive treatment in brachial plexus birth palsy, generally to assist in the treatment of secondary joint contractures.

On her preoperative examination, you notice that the passive range of motion of her shoulder has decreased from your prior examination. Specifically, it is difficult to passively externally rotate her shoulder while her arm is adducted to her side. You obtain an ultrasound of the shoulder, shown in Figure 10–41.

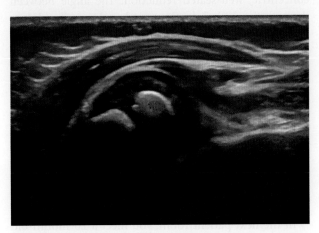

Figure 10–41 (Courtesy of Dr. Andrea Bauer)

The * in Figure 10–41 demonstrates:

A. The ossific nucleus of the humeral head, which is well-reduced in the glenoid
B. The ossific nucleus of the humeral head, which is posteriorly dislocated to the glenoid
C. The ossific nucleus of the humeral head, which is anteriorly dislocated to the glenoid
D. The ossific nucleus of the humeral head, which is superiorly dislocated to the glenoid

Discussion

The correct answer is (B). Ultrasound is a safe and reliable method of detecting glenohumeral dysplasia in infants with brachial plexus birth palsy. Through mechanisms that are still not completely understood, infants

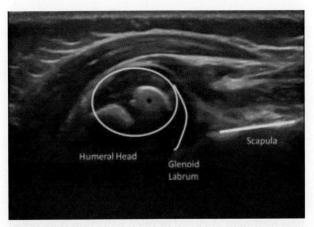

Figure 10–42

with brachial plexus birth palsy are at risk for developing glenohumeral dysplasia. The characteristic positioning is that of glenoid flattening and retroversion along with a flattened and posteriorly dislocated humeral head. Figure 10–42 demonstrates this positioning on ultrasound, this time with labels.

Objectives: Did you learn...?

- The differential diagnosis of neonatal brachial plexus birth palsy?
- The definition of a Horner's syndrome and its prognostic value in brachial plexus birth palsy?
- Indications for microsurgical repair for infants with brachial plexus birth palsy?
- How to use ultrasound to evaluate for glenohumeral dysplasia in an infant with brachial plexus birth palsy?

CASE 23

Dr. Amanda T. Whitaker

A 2-week-old girl, born to a G1P1 mother, is brought to you for evaluation due to concern for "hip click." On examination, she has full range of motion of the hips. She is Ortolani negative on examination bilaterally, but you do note a positive Barlow on one side. The rest of her examination is unremarkable.

What is the next step in treatment?

A. Pavlik harness
B. Closed reduction
C. Observation
D. Open reduction
E. Double diaper

Discussion

The correct answer is (C). Hip clicks are nonspecific physical findings and can be seen in children with normal hips. This child is only 2 weeks old. The hips are reduced on examination (Ortolani negative). Eighty percent of hips with evidence of dysplasia or that can subluxate/dislocate with a Barlow maneuver resolve in the first 6 weeks. Therefore, for this patient you would observe and reassess at age 6 weeks with a physical examination and ultrasound if there are risk factors or positive findings on examination. If the hips are dysplastic at that time, then you would initiate Pavlik harness treatment. A closed or open reduction is incorrect because the hips are not dislocated. Double diapering is not effective for treatment of hip dysplasia.

If the mother had a history of DDH and another daughter with DDH, what is the likelihood the second daughter will have DDH?

A. Not related
B. 6%
C. 12%
D. 36%

Discussion

The correct answer is (D). DDH etiology is multifactorial with a genetic component. Family history is important to obtain. With a parent and a sibling with DDH, the likelihood that the child will have DDH is 36%. With just a parent the likelihood is 12% and if just a sibling it is 6%.

At 6 weeks, the ultrasound demonstrates an alpha angle of 40 degrees with <50% of the femoral head covered on one side, the other hip is normal. She is treated in a Pavlik harness.

What are the risks associated with Pavlik harness?

A. Inferior head dislocation
B. Femoral nerve palsy
C. Osteonecrosis
D. All of the above

Discussion

The correct answer is (D). Inferior head dislocation is associated with flexing the hips >90 degrees. Femoral nerve palsy is usually in older infants with increased hip flexion. The harness is stopped until the nerve palsy recovers. Osteonecrosis is from forced abduction and traction on the hip for reduction. All are potential risks that the family needs to be educated about, and the harness position needs to be monitored and adjusted to minimize these risks.

Another patient returns to your clinic for follow-up. She is a 3 month old you met a few weeks ago, and she was found to have an Ortolani positive hip on examination for which you started Pavlik harness treatment to try to reduce and hold the hip. On examination today, you note that the hip is dislocated and no longer reducible.

What is your next step in treatment?

A. 2 more weeks of Pavlik harness
B. Closed reduction in clinic
C. Closed reduction in OR
D. Open reduction

Discussion

The correct answer is (C). The baby is placed under anesthesia to allow the muscles to relax, and the hip can often then be reduced. An adductor tenotomy is usually performed to help prevent dislocation as it widens the safe zone. An arthrogram is performed to ensure a concentric, well-seated reduction. The angle between the maximum abduction and minimum abduction in which the hip remains reduced, is determined and referred to as the safe zone. A spica cast is placed with the hip maintained between about 90 and 100 degrees of flexion and less than 60 degrees of abduction to reduce the risk of osteonecrosis. An MRI or CT is done after spica cast placement to determine if the hip remains reduced once the spica cast is on. If the hip is reduced in the cast, casting is continued for 3 to 4 months (with a spica cast change at the mid-point) and then the child is continued in an abduction brace until the dysplasia has fully resolved.

In the next patient room, you meet a 20-month-old girl who, since she started walking at age 14 months, has had "an odd-gait" per her parents. They recently took her to their new pediatrician for this concern. The pediatrician agreed with them and also noticed that one hip did not abduct as much as the other. The pediatrician ordered an AP pelvis x-ray and referred them to you for evaluation. On the x-ray, you note that one hip is dislocated, and there is a pseudoacetabulum forming. You speak to the family about the need for an open hip reduction.

Which of the following is not included as a part of an open hip reduction (at any age)?

A. Traction
B. Femoral shortening osteotomy
C. Lengthening of adductors
D. Abductor release

Discussion

The correct answer is (D). Gentle traction is used to assess reduction. Femoral shortening osteotomy is performed when the hip is really high-riding and too much force is required to reduce the hip—this is frequently necessary in children older than 2 years of age. The adductors are often lengthened or released. The iliopsoas, pulvinar, labrum, inferomedial capsule, ligamentum teres, and transverse acetabular ligament are often barriers to reduction that are addressed at the time of an open reduction. The abductors are not included in open hip reductions as they do not contribute to the dislocation or prevent reduction.

Your final patient of the morning is a 5-year old with a fixed dislocation of the left hip that was just adopted, and her new family has been trying to establish medical care for her. She was seen by a pediatrician recently and referred. She has a notable limp on examination and is Galeazzi positive on the right. She has limited hip abduction on the left compared to the right. You confirm the diagnosis of unilateral hip dislocation on her x-rays.

What is the next step?

A. Traction
B. Closed reduction
C. Open reduction
D. Pelvic osteotomy

Discussion

The correct answer is (D). With a fixed unilateral dislocation under age 8, you would do an open reduction with a pelvic osteotomy to improve anterior and lateral coverage of the femoral head. A femoral shortening osteotomy may be needed in addition to the pelvic osteotomy. The other answers are not sufficient to reduce and stabilize a hip dislocation in a 5-year old.

CASE 24

Dr. Melinda Sharkey

A healthy, 1-month-old baby is brought to see you because the right lower extremity is shorter than the left. This was noticeable at birth. The baby is otherwise healthy and growing normally. Examination shows a healthy infant with a shortened and bulbous right thigh with palpable flexion deformity at the proximal thigh. The right lower extremity is externally rotated and abducted compared to the left. An x-ray taken at the visit is shown (Fig. 10–43).

Based on the clinical examination and radiograph the correct diagnosis is:

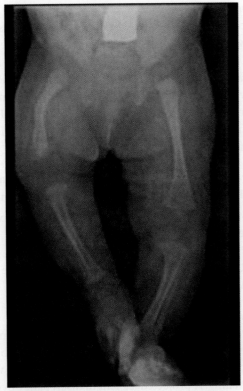

Figure 10–43

A. Healing femoral shaft fracture
B. Proximal femoral focal deficiency (congenital femoral deficiency)
C. Congenital coxa vara
D. Osteogenesis imperfect

Discussion

The correct answer is (B). The described clinical examination and radiograph are consistent with proximal femoral focal deficiency (PFFD), also known as congenital femoral deficiency. This is a condition involving abnormal development of the acetabulum and proximal femur. The condition demonstrates variable degrees of severity. In its most severe form the acetabulum, femoral head and most of the femur is absent. A subtrochanteric deformity including flexion, abduction, and external rotation is present and distinguishes this from congenital coxa vara.

PFFD is commonly associated with all the following congenital anomalies EXCEPT:

A. Fibular deficiency
B. Other limb anomalies
C. Absent cruciate ligaments
D. Congenital vertical talus

Discussion

The correct answer is (D). PFFD is commonly associated with all of the above except for congenital vertical talus. Some degree of fibular deficiency (fibular hemimelia) is seen in the majority of patients with PFFD. Many are also found to have other limb anomalies. Absence of cruciate ligaments is the rule in both PFFD and fibular deficiency. Congenital vertical talus is not specifically associated with PFFD.

Prior to undertaking a femoral lengthening in a patient with PFFD, the following requirement must be met:

A. Stability of the hip joint via pelvic and/or proximal femur osteotomies when necessary
B. Projected leg length discrepancy over 30 cm
C. Reconstruction of the cruciate ligaments of the knee
D. Age 8 or greater

Discussion

The correct answer is (A). Prior to a planned femoral lengthening in PFFD, the hip joint must be stable or surgically stabilized to prevent hip dislocation while lengthening. A projected leg length discrepancy over 30 cm would be a contraindication for lengthening. Reconstruction of the deficient cruciate ligaments is not routinely carried out, but the knee joint must be stabilized externally during lengthening so as not to dislocate. Lengthening is often carried out at ages much younger than 8, especially if multiple lengthenings are planned due to large leg length discrepancies.

Objectives: Did you learn...?

- Proximal femoral focal deficiency is an uncommon congenital anomaly resulting in varying degrees of under-development or even absence of the acetabulum and proximal femur?
- PFFD is often associated with other extremity anomalies?
- In the majority of cases, PFFD is associated with some degree of fibular deficiency?
- Amputation as well as hip reconstruction and femoral lengthening are treatment options depending on the degree of shortening of the affected extremity?

CASE 25

Dr. Amanda T. Whitaker

A 6-year-old boy with leg length difference presents to your clinic. He has a history of right distal femoral osteomyelitis at the age of 3. Full length radiographs demonstrate the left femur is 1.5 cm longer than the right.

What is the most predictable growth pattern disruption?

A. Postinfectious
B. Hemihypertrophy
C. Proximal femoral focal deficiency
D. Fibular hemimelia
E. Posttraumatic

The correct answer is (E). The most predictable growth disturbance is a post traumatic growth arrest at the physis (E). Postinfectious (A) and hemihypertrophy (B) have unpredictable growth disturbance patterns. Proximal femoral focal deficiency (C) and fibular hemimelia (D) have deformities and deficiencies that can add to the leg length difference at maturity.

What is the appropriate treatment at this time?

A. Epiphysiodesis of the left distal femur
B. Hemiepiphysiodesis
C. Shortening osteotomy left femur
D. Lengthening right femur
E. Right shoe lift and observation

Discussion

The correct answer is (E). A 2- to 2.5-cm leg length discrepancy is treated with observation and a shoe lift. Epiphysiodesis (A) or shortening left femoral osteotomy (C) is reserved for predicted final discrepancies between 2 and 5 cm. Lengthening of the right femur (D) is reserved for predicted final discrepancies >5 cm. Hemiepiphysiodesis (B) is indicated with angular deformities of the leg.

What is the predicted leg length difference at maturity?

A. 6.5 cm
B. 7.8 cm
C. 8.8 cm
D. 9.0 cm
E. 10.5 cm

Discussion

The correct answer is (E). The physis of the lower extremity grow at these approximate rates per year: 3 mm for the proximal femoral physis, 9 mm for the distal femoral physis, 6 mm for the proximal tibial physis, and 5 mm for the distal tibial physis. The distal femoral physis consists of approximately 37% of the total limb growth. For a 6-year old with a distal femoral disruption, current 1.5-cm leg length difference, and estimated end of growth at the age of 16, he will have a 10.5-cm leg length difference ([10 years growth remaining × 9 mm/year] + 1.5 cm) at maturity. He should be followed closely because a large difference in leg lengths such as predicted here may require multiple procedures during growth to maintain a <2-cm discrepancy.

The child returns at age 11 for follow-up. He has a predicted leg length discrepancy of 4.5 cm at maturity. His bone age is equal to his chronologic age as demonstrated by hand radiographs. What should his treatment consist of?

A. Epiphysiodesis of left femur
B. Lengthen right femur
C. Epiphysiodesis of left distal femur and lengthen right femur
D. Shorten left femur
E. Shoe lift and observe

Discussion

The correct answer is (A). For a 4.5-cm leg length discrepancy, epiphysiodesis of the long side (the left femur) is the recommended treatment. Lengthening of the femur (B) is recommended for deformities >5 cm due to the complications associated with lengthening (pin tract infections, neurovascular stretch injuries) but these risks and alternatives should be discussed with the family. Dual procedures such as epiphysiodesis of the left distal femoral physis and lengthening of the right femur (C) are reserved for large deformities predicted >15 cm. Shortening of the left femur (D) greater than 4 cm leads to quadriceps weakness and difficulty with gait. Shoe lifts and observation are for discrepancies less than 2 to 2.5 cm. Hand radiographs using a Greulich and Pyle atlas is a method of confirming skeletal age for accurate timing of epiphysiodesis.

When should the epiphysiodesis be done?

A. Now
B. 11.5 years
C. 12 years
D. 12.5 years
E. 13 years

Discussion

The correct answer is (A). To obtain 4.5 cm of length from the contralateral femur at a rate of 9 mm per year, 5 years from the time of skeletal maturity must be used to correct the difference. Therefore, he should

have the epiphysiodesis now in order to make up the 4.5-cm leg length inequality. The following differences can be accounted for by the other answers: 11.5 years (B) 4 cm, 12 years (C) 3.6 cm, 12.5 years (D) 3.1 cm, and 13 years (E) 2.7 cm. All options, however, will allow him to wear a shoe lift without anticipated complications.

Objectives: Did you learn...?

• Common causes of leg length discrepancies in children?
• How to estimate final leg length discrepancies in children?
• Treatment algorithm of treating leg length discrepancies in children?

CASE 26

Dr. Amanda T. Whitaker

A 2-year-old African-American girl presents with progressive bowing of her legs. On physical examination, she has asymmetric genu vara with a lateral thrust. Radiographs demonstrate bilateral Langenskiöld stage II proximal tibial changes.

What treatment should this child undergo?

A. Gradual corrective proximal osteotomies with multiplanar frame
B. Hemiepiphysiodesis of the lateral proximal tibae
C. Valgus osteotomies of the proximal tibiae
D. Knee–ankle–foot orthoses (KAFO)
E. Observation

Discussion

The correct answer is (D). For Langenskiöld stage II changes in the proximal tibia for infantile Blount disease, which is the most common form of the disease, KAFO wear has been shown to improve the lower extremity deformity in children less than 3 years old with stage I and II changes. Valgus osteotomies of the proximal tibias are reserved for Langenskiöld stages II to VI changes in ages <3 years old, stages I to II changes in children >3 years old, or failure of KAFO treatment. Hemiepiphysiodesis has been attempted in younger children with uncertain results and is reserved for adolescent (>10 years old) Blount disease treatment. Gradual corrective osteotomies are reserved for the skeletally mature patient to limit neurovascular stretch injury. Observation is not recommended for Langenskiöld stage II infantile Blount disease.

She returns at age 3 for follow-up. What metaphyseal–diaphyseal angle (Drennan's angle) is consistent with a 95% chance of progression?

A. Less than 5 degrees
B. 5 to 10 degrees
C. 12 degrees
D. 16 degrees

Discussion

The correct answer is (D). The angle between the metaphyseal beak, proximal tibial metaphysis, and perpendicular to the tibia at the physis is the metaphyseal–diaphyseal angle (Drennan's angle). An angle of >16 degrees (answer D) is considered abnormal and has a 95% chance of progression. A Drennan's angle of <10 degrees has a 95% chance of resolving over time.

For a 3-year old who has progressive tibia vara despite KAFO treatment and a Drennan's angle of >16 degrees, what is the treatment?

A. Gradual corrective proximal osteotomies with multiplanar frame
B. Hemiepiphysiodesis of the lateral proximal tibia
C. Valgus osteotomies of the proximal tibia to neutral alignment
D. Valgus osteotomies of the proximal tibia with overcorrection
E. Continue knee–ankle–foot orthoses (KAFO)

Discussion

The correct answer is (D). As discussed, treatment for children with failure of KAFO treatment (progression of deformity), valgus osteotomies are the treatment of choice in this age group with approximately 10 degrees of overcorrection to decrease recurrence and decrease the load on the medial tibia (answer D). Anterior compartment releases are often performed to decrease the risk of compartment syndrome. Recurrence of the deformity decreases if the osteotomies are performed before age 4.

At her post-op visit, the family presents her 10-year-old sister with unilateral tibia vara. You would like to get a radiograph and the technician is having difficulty achieving a true AP.

What other rotational deformities are present in adolescent Blount disease?

A. Distal tibial varus
B. Internal tibial torsion
C. Recurvatum of the proximal tibia
D. Femoral valgus

Discussion

The correct answer is (B). Secondary deformities are present in Blount disease that often interfere with gait and obtaining a true AP radiograph. These include distal tibial valgus (not varus as in A), procurvatum of the proximal tibia (not recurvatum as in C), femoral varus (not valgus as in D), and internal tibia torsion (the correct answer B). With internal tibial torsion, the knee will be externally rotated on an AP radiograph with the foot pointed forward. The patella must be faced forward to obtain a true AP. Adolescent Blount disease is unilateral and presents in children older than 10 years of age. It is less common than the infantile form.

The family returns, and the 10-year-old sister has a metaphyseal–diaphyseal angle of 17 degrees and 8 degrees of varus at the femur.

What is her treatment?

A. KAFO
B. Hemiepiphysiodesis of the lateral proximal tibia
C. Hemiepiphysiodesis of the lateral proximal tibia and lateral distal femur
D. Osteotomy of the proximal tibia
E. Osteotomy of the proximal tibia and distal femur

Discussion

The correct answer is (C). At this stage, KAFO treatment (A) is not indicated, as indications are for children <3 years old with Langenskiöld stage I to II changes. Hemiepiphysiodesis of the lateral proximal tibia (B) would only correct the tibia and not the femoral varus. Osteotomies (choices D and E) are reserved for younger children or with gradual correction and multiplanar frame for the complex form of adolescent Blount disease. This is performed to decrease neurovascular stretch injury. Hemiepiphysiodesis of the lateral proximal tibia and lateral distal femur (C) is the appropriate surgical treatment, but 25% of these children may require corrective osteotomies in the future.

Objectives: Did you learn...?

- Treatment for infantile Blount disease?
- Indications for surgical correction of Blount disease?
- Secondary deformity in Blount disease?
- Differences in infantile and adolescent Blount disease?

CASE 27

Dr. Melinda Sharkey

A healthy, 9-month-old baby is brought in by her parents. At birth, it was noted that she only had three toes

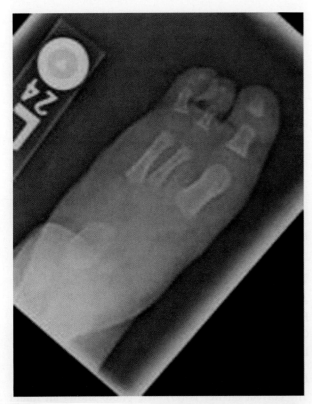

Figure 10–44

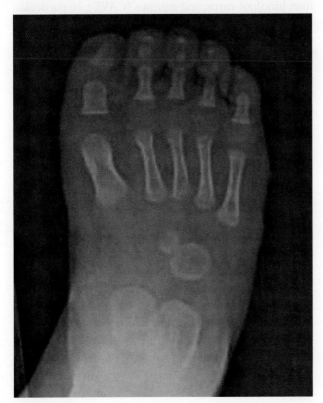

Figure 10–45

on the left foot. It appears the lateral two rays are absent. Radiographs of both feet are shown (Figs. 10–44 and 10–45). The left leg appears well formed but the entire lower extremity is slightly shorter compared to the other side.

How do you counsel the parents? (Figs. 10–44 and 10–45)

A. Absence of the lateral rays will unlikely affect her function
B. Absence of lateral ray(s) is associated with fibular deficiency
C. She will require an amputation in the future
D. She should be evaluated for cervical spine anomalies

Discussion

The correct answer is (B). Absence of lateral ray/rays of the foot is typical of fibular deficiency. Fibular deficiency is a spectrum of congenital malformations affecting postaxial limb development. Findings include absence of lateral rays of the foot, coalitions of the foot, ball and socket ankle, varying degrees of shortening or even absence of the fibula, as well as tibial shortening and genu valgum. Fibular deficiency is often associated with some degree of shortening of the femur as well.

The full-length lower extremity radiograph of the child is shown (Fig. 10–46). The difference in tibial lengths is approximately 2 cm. All of the following are true EXCEPT:

A. This small length difference will remain the same or even improve with growth
B. This difference in tibial lengths will increase with growth
C. The calculated leg length difference at skeletal maturity is most important
D. Amputation is indicated for projected leg length discrepancies greater than 30%

Discussion

The correct answer is (B). Congenital leg length discrepancies will increase with growth. Projected length discrepancy is most important in determining the best treatment option. Patients with large projected length discrepancies, especially those greater than 30% of the contralateral limb, are best served with a Syme or Boyd amputation and prosthetic fitting. Patients with a nonfunctional foot may also be better served with an amputation.

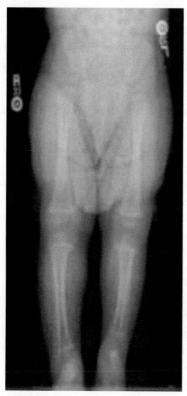

Figure 10–46

Objectives: Did you learn...?

• Fibular deficiency is a congenital longitudinal deficiency involving abnormalities of the fibula, tibia, ankle, foot, and often the femur as well?

• Projected leg length discrepancy at skeletal maturity is very important in determining treatment options?

• Mild to moderate leg length differences associated with a functional foot and ankle may be treated with contralateral epiphysiodesis or limb lengthening?

• Very large projected length discrepancies (over 30% of the contralateral side) are treated with amputation and prosthetic fitting?

CASE 28

Dr. Melinda Sharkey

A 10-day-old male is brought into your office for evaluation of foot deformities. The parents say the foot deformity was noted on prenatal ultrasound but they did not come in for prenatal counseling. The mother's pregnancy and delivery were uncomplicated. There is no family history of foot deformity. The parents are healthy. The infant is healthy. The babies' feet appear as follows (Fig. 10–47):

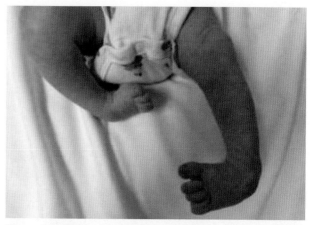

Figure 10–47 Pictures courtesy of Melinda Sharkey, MD.

The deformities are consistent with:

A. Metatarsus adductus
B. Calcaneovalgus
C. Congenital vertical talus
D. Clubfoot

Discussion

The correct answer is (D). The photo shows an infant with bilateral clubfoot deformities. Clubfoot deformity can be conceptualized as four separate components including **c**avus, **a**dductus of the midfoot on the hindfoot, hindfoot **v**arus, and **e**quinus (CAVE). In particular, the adductus and cavus can be appreciated in the photo. Calcaneovalgus is a transient, positional deformity due to in-utero positioning and presents as extreme dorsiflexion and eversion of the foot (opposite of clubfoot). Congenital vertical talus deformity, like clubfoot, is a structural abnormality and presents as a stiff rocker-bottom deformity with abduction and dorsal dislocation of the forefoot on the hindfoot (again opposite of clubfoot, but stiff unlike calcaneovalgus). Metatarsus adductus strictly involves the forefoot and is not associated with cavus or hindfoot abnormalities and is often very flexible.

The Ponseti method of clubfoot treatment is described to the parents. Figure 10–48 is a photograph of the first cast placed on the left foot. The goal of the first cast is to correct:

A. Cavus
B. Equinus
C. Adductus
D. Supination

Discussion

The correct answer is (A). The Ponseti method requires correction of the midfoot cavus prior to correction of

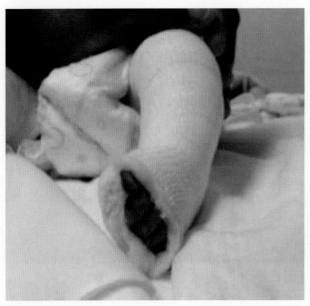

Figure 10–48

the other parts of the foot deformity. The first ray, which is pronated relative to the hindfoot, is supinated, as shown in the cast, in order to bring the forefoot/first ray in line with the hindfoot and stretch the tight plantar structures of the foot (cavus).

The feet correct with serial casting and heelcord tenotomies. The parents are compliant with long-term bracing. At about 2.5 years of age it is noted that the deformity is starting to recur. This is especially obvious when the patient is walking and the forefoot supinates. The patient is tending to walk on the lateral border of the foot. The table examination shows the foot is totally flexible with adequate dorsiflexion at the ankle and good subtalar joint motion including the ability to position the heel in valgus.

Appropriate treatment at this time includes:

A. Repeat serial casting
B. Physical therapy
C. Anterior tibialis tendon transfer
D. Watchful waiting

Discussion

The correct answer is (C). The patient demonstrates dynamic supination with walking in the presence of a foot that remains supple including the subtalar joint evidenced by the observation of heel valgus. Appropriate treatment at this time is anterior tibialis tendon transfer (split transfer or complete transfer) to one of the dorsolateral foot bones (cuneiform or cuboid).

Objectives: Did you learn...?

• Clubfoot deformity can be conceptualized as four component deformities: cavus, adductus, varus, and equinus?
• Serial casting followed by heelcord tenotomy, as described by Ponseti, is the standard of care for infant clubfoot deformity?
• Long-term bracing (up to 4 years) is important to prevent recurrence of clubfoot deformities?
• Roughly ¼ of patients with clubfoot will benefit from an anterior tibialis tendon transfer for dynamic supination with walking?

CASE 29

Dr. Coleen S. Sabatini

A 6-month-old baby is referred to your clinic for evaluation of her feet. Her parents and pediatrician are concerned because her feet do not look "normal." Clinically, both feet have the appearance of the photo shown in Figure 10–49. The Achilles is palpably tight, there is an empty heelpad, the arch does not reconstitute with hyperextension of the great toe, and the talar head is prominent in the plantar surface of the foot.

You want to order imaging studies to evaluate the foot to help you confirm the diagnosis. Which images do you order?

A. AP and lateral x-rays of the foot
B. AP, lateral, and maximum dorsiflexion view x-rays of the foot

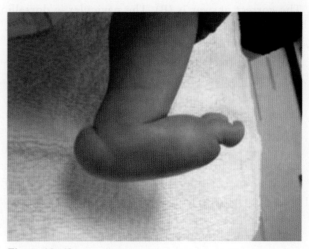

Figure 10–49

C. AP, lateral, and maximum plantarflexion view x-rays of the foot
D. AP and lateral x-rays of the tibia
E. MRI of the foot

Discussion

The correct answer is (C). This patient has a rocker bottom foot deformity and a clinical description (prominent talar head, no arch reconstitution, Achilles contracture) consistent with a congenital vertical talus. When evaluating the foot radiographically for this condition, the lateral view with the foot in forced plantarflexion is diagnostic. Choice A is not correct because it does not provide you with sufficient information to make the diagnosis. Choice B, which includes an x-ray of the foot in maximum dorsiflexion, is what you order for evaluation of clubfoot, not CVT. X-rays of the tibia (choice D) are not necessary here and do not help confirm the diagnosis. An MRI of the foot is unnecessary at this time and would require a general anesthetic at this age.

Assuming this is congenital vertical talus, what would you expect to see on the lateral maximum plantarflexion x-ray?

A. Irreducible plantar dislocation of the navicular on the talus
B. Irreducible dorsal dislocation of the navicular on the talus
C. Apparent dislocation of the navicular relative to the talus on the lateral view and then reduction of the navicular on the maximum plantarflexion lateral view
D. Normal alignment of the talus and the navicular

Discussion

The correct answer is (B). The navicular is dorsally dislocated on the talus. The x-ray is shown (Fig. 10–50):

"A" is incorrect because the navicular is dorsal to the talus, not plantar. "C" is what happens in the setting of an oblique talus—the navicular reduces on the plantarflexion view. "D" is incorrect because by definition in CVT, the anatomy is not normal.

You have confirmed the diagnosis of CVT and explained this to the family. You have educated them that this is a rare condition that occurs in about 1:150,000 births. You have explained that in approximately 50% of patients with CVT, there is an associated neuromuscular disease or chromosomal abnormality, and you therefore are going to refer them to genetics.

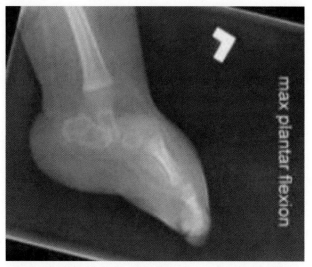

Figure 10–50

For orthopaedic treatment of the feet, you recommend the following:

A. Observation, the condition will eventually resolve on its own
B. Surgical intervention at age 3
C. Serial manipulation and casting only
D. Serial manipulation and casting, followed by surgery
E. Pantalar release and fusion now

Discussion

The correct answer is (D). CVT will not correct on its own and observation is not appropriate for children with this condition, thus choice A is incorrect. Current treatment involves serial manipulation and casting of the foot to stretch the dorsal soft tissues. In some cases, reduction of the talar head can be obtained. After casting, surgery is needed to reduce the talonavicular joint, lengthen the Achilles, and possibly additional soft tissue releases and transfers depending on the correction obtained with casting and the age of the child. The traditional pantalar release is not usually performed until the patient is over 12 months old, and a fusion is not a first-line treatment for this condition.

Objectives: Did you learn...?

- The clinical findings in congenital vertical talus?
- The radiographic findings in CVT?
- Importance of evaluation for other conditions since there is a high rate of associated neuromuscular or chromosomal abnormalities in patients with CVT?
- Treatment for patients with CVT?

CASE 30

Dr. Coleen S. Sabatini

A 1-year-old male is brought to your clinic by his parents for evaluation. He has shortened limbs with the proximal aspects more involved than the distal aspect, frontal bossing, and midface hypoplasia. He cannot bring his middle and ring fingers together, and he has genu varum. His feet are not clubbed.

The mutation responsible for his skeletal dysplasia causes a defect in what gene?

A. CBFA-1
B. Sulfate transporter
C. COMP
D. EXT1
E. FGFR-3

Discussion

The correct answer is (E). The patient has achondroplasia— the features described above are consistent with this diagnosis (rhizomelic shortening of the limbs, frontal bossing with midface hypoplasia, trident hands, and genu varum). FGFR-3 is the gene affected in achondroplasia. The mutation inhibits chondrocyte proliferation in the zone of proliferation of the growth plate. CBFA-1 is the gene affected in cleidocranial dysplasia. Although there is frontal bossing with cleidocranial dysplasia, the other features of that condition are not present with this patient. The sulfate transporter gene is affected in diastrophic dysplasia. This condition also has short stature with rhizomelic shortening of the limbs, the hand deformity is a hitchhiker thumb rather than a trident hand, the ears are described as "cauliflower" ears, and the feet are clubbed. Mutations in COMP result in pseudoachondroplasia. Given the face abnormalities, this patient does not have pseudoachondroplasia as it is associated with normal facies. EXT1 is involved in multiple hereditary exostosis.

On examination, you notice that when he is sat up, he has kyphosis of his thoracolumbar spine. What is your recommendation for treatment of this?

A. Observation
B. Traction
C. Casting
D. Surgical decompression with stabilization via a growing rod construct

Discussion

The correct answer is (A). Thoracolumbar kyphosis is seen in many children with achondroplasia. It is thought to be related to hypotonia of the core muscles combined with a relatively large head. It usually resolves when the child begins walking. The other options are incorrect because they are unnecessary in the setting of a condition that usually self-resolves. The spine condition to be aware of in the growing child and adult with achondroplasia is the decreased interpedicular distance in the lumbar vertebrae and lumbar stenosis with short pedicles.

There has been some concern of sleep apnea for this child. What should the orthopaedic surgeon order (if not already ordered by others previously) in children with achondroplasia, particularly when there are apnea issues?

A. Pulmonary function tests
B. Chest x-ray
C. MRI of the chest
D. MRI of the base of brain and cervical spine
E. ENT consult

Discussion

The correct answer is (D). In a child with achondroplasia there is a need to screen for foramen magnum and upper cervical spine stenosis. Should these be present, they can cause central sleep apnea and lead to sudden death.

Objectives: Did you learn...?

- The clinical findings associated with achondroplasia?
- The gene affected in patients with achondroplasia?
- The appropriate management of thoracolumbar kyphosis in this population?
- Importance of screening for foramen magnum stenosis?

CASE 31

Dr. Coleen S. Sabatini

A 13-year-old girl presents to your office, having just moved to your area in recent months. Her parent reports that she and other family members were followed by an Orthopaedic surgeon where they lived previously. She has never had any surgery. She reports some medial-sided knee pain with activity—both proximal and distal to the joint. No pain at rest. No constitutional symptoms. Her x-ray is shown (Fig. 10–51).

Mutations in which gene are associated with this disorder?

A. RUNX2
B. EXT2

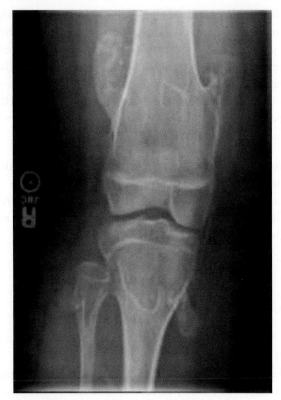

Figure 10–51

C. COMP
D. FGFR3
E. FMR1

Discussion

The correct answer is (B). The RUNX2 gene encodes runt-related transcription factor 2 (also known as core-binding factor subunit alpha-1 [cbfa-1]). This is associated with osteoblast differentiation. Mutations in RUNX2 are associated with cleidocranial dysplasia. Disorders of the COMP gene ("cartilage oligomeric matrix protein") are associated with pseudoachondroplasia. FGFR3 is the gene associated with achondroplasia. FMR1 is the gene mutation associated with Fragile X syndrome. Mutations in EXT 1 and EXT2 are associated with multiple hereditary exostosis, the condition depicted above (Fig. 10–51).

Which of the following has the same inheritance pattern as this condition?

A. Rett syndrome
B. Limb-girdle muscular dystrophy
C. Charcot–Marie–Tooth
D. Sickle cell disease
E. Friedreich's ataxia

Discussion

The correct answer is (C). Rett syndrome is a sex-linked dominant condition. Limb-girdle muscular dystrophy is autosomal recessive. Charcot–Marie–Tooth is autosomal dominant, the same as multiple hereditary exostosis. Sickle cell and Friedreich's ataxia are autosomal recessive.

What should you tell the family about the overall risk of malignant transformation?

A. There is no risk of malignant transformation
B. 1% to 25%
C. 26% to 50%
D. 51% to 75%
E. Over 75%

Discussion

The correct answer is (B). Patients with MHE do have a risk of malignant transformation. The percent of those that go on to have malignant transformation is not clear but is thought to be in the range of 1% to 25%. Patients without MHE who have just a solitary osteochondromas have a less than 1% risk of malignant transformation.

Should any of the patient's lesions undergo malignant transformation, which location is most likely, and to what lesion type will it most likely transform?

A. Distal femur, osteosarcoma
B. Distal femur, chondrosarcoma
C. Proximal humerus, osteosarcoma
D. Pelvis, chondrosarcoma
E. Pelvis, osteosarcoma

Discussion

The correct answer is (D). When there is malignant transformation of osteochondromas, they transform most commonly to chondrosarcoma. Lesions in the pelvis are more likely than peripheral lesions to have malignant degeneration.

What is the most common ankle deformity that you need to monitor for in patients with MHE?

A. Varus
B. Valgus
C. Equinus
D. Recurvatum

Discussion

The correct answer is (B). About half of patients with MHE develop ankle valgus. Depending on the severity of the deformity and growth remaining, sometimes excision of exostosis is all that is needed, but other times the addition of a medial hemiepiphysiodesis is needed to correct the deformity. The other deformities listed are not the most common deformity seen in patients with MHE.

Objectives: Did you learn...?

- Multiple hereditary exostosis is an autosomal dominant disorder?
- Mutations in the EXT family of tumor suppressor genes are found in the majority of patients with MHE?
- Risk of malignant transformation for both solitary osteochondromas and in patients with MHE?
- Important of monitoring for ankle valgus in patients with MHE?

CASE 32

Dr. Coleen S. Sabatini and Dr. Amanda T. Whitaker

You are called to the emergency room to evaluate an 11-month-old, nonambulatory girl with a femur fracture. On examination, she is in the bottom 5% for height and weight. She has a triangular face, white sclerae, normal dentition, and reacts to your words with turning of the head to follow you. There is an obvious deformity of the right femur with tenderness to palpation and deformity of the left tibia without any tenderness to palpation. There is no bruising or skin lesions. On skeletal survey she has irregular intrasutural bones in addition to the normal cranial bones. There are multiple vertebral compression fractures, a right midshaft femur fracture, and deformity of the left tibia with evidence of healing.

What is causing these fractures?

A. Child abuse
B. Nutritional deficiency
C. Abnormal collagen type I
D. Normal

Discussion

The correct answer is (C). This case describes a classical presentation of osteogenesis imperfecta (OI). Osteogenesis imperfecta is a condition of abnormal collagen type I, either quantitative or qualitative. The most popular described mutation is a glycine substitution that decreases cross-linking and prevents the formation of the triple helix. Child abuse (A) should always be considered in a child who presents with multiple fractures, but other features (triangular face, wormian bones, vertebral compression fractures) suggest osteo-

genesis imperfecta. Long bone fracture in a nonambulatory child is never a normal presentation (D), and child abuse or bone disease should always be considered.

What type of OI is this?

A. I
B. II
C. III
D. V
E. VIII

Discussion

The correct answer is (A). Type I OI is mild and presents with blue sclerae, 50% have hearing deficits, may have dental involvement, and is autosomal dominant (A). Type II OI is lethal at birth with blue sclerae and is autosomal recessive (B). Type III OI is described in the above scenario with normal sclerae, triangular face, wormian bones, multiple fractures, vertebral compression fractures, or "codfish" vertebrae, can have basilar invagination, and is autosomal recessive (C). This is the most severe of the survivable types. Type V OI is autosomal recessive and presents with hypertrophic callus formation and ossification of the interosseus membranes between the radius and ulna and tibia and fibula (D). Type VIII OI has white sclera, bulbous metaphyses, involves a mutation in the LEPRE 1 gene, is often lethal at birth, and is autosomal recessive (E).

This child has another tibia and femur fracture over the past year. What is treatment?

A. Vitamin D
B. Vitamin D and calcium
C. Vitamin C
D. Bisphosphonates

Discussion

The correct answer is (D). While vitamin D (A) and vitamin D with calcium (B) may improve the mineral availability to build stronger bones, they have not been shown to decrease fracture rates in children with osteogenesis imperfecta. Vitamin C (C) deficiency results in abnormal cross-linking of collagen, but this is not the underlying cause of OI and has not been demonstrated to change bone health in children with OI. Bisphosphonate treatment (D) is the correct answer and has been shown to decrease fracture frequency and increase cortical thickness in children with OI. Bisphosphonate therapy is recommended for children with OI who sustain two or more fractures within a year.

The radiographs at age 5 have multiple horizontal densities at the metaphyses, most notably at the distal femoral metaphyses.

What is the most likely cause?

A. A change in the child's nutritional status
B. The child has had multiple significant illnesses
C. Multiple fractures at physis with growth arrest
D. Increased densities corresponding to bisphosphonates
E. This is a common finding due to OI collagen disruption

Discussion

The correct answer is (D). Nutritional status (A) and illnesses (B) can often cause changes in bone density with recovery described above and referred to as Harris growth lines (or growth arrest lines), these also are a key finding with cyclical bisphosphonate treatment in children with OI (D). A fracture at the physis can cause a growth line, growth arrest with shortening, or angular deformity (C), but is not the most likely cause in this case with multiple horizontal densities). Growth arrest lines are common in OI due to bisphosphonate treatment, but are not common in untreated OI (E).

At age 6, despite bisphosphonate treatment she fractured her right femur again. What is the appropriate treatment?

A. Cast
B. Flexible nails
C. Expandable rod
D. Traction

Discussion

The correct answer is (C). While in children with normal bones cast treatment (A) or flexible nail (B) would be appropriate, children with osteogenesis imperfecta should be treated with an expandable rod (C). Traction may be used for older children in developing nations, but this is not the most appropriate treatment.

At age 11 the child develops scoliosis with a curve of 37 degrees. What is the treatment for her scoliosis?

A. Observe
B. Brace
C. Tethering
D. Fusion

Discussion

The correct answer is (D). In children with OI and scoliosis, bracing is ineffective (B) and should be treated with a fusion (D). Fusion is recommended in curves greater than 45 degrees for mild types of OI and 35 degrees for severe OI, such as in this case. Fusion is often difficult and accompanied by halo traction and multiple rods due to the poor bone quality and high pullout rate. Tethering is not an indicated procedure for OI scoliosis (C). Observation is not recommended for curves in severe scoliosis greater than 35 degrees (A).

Objectives: Did you learn...?

- Common findings in osteogenesis imperfecta?
- Fracture treatment for children with OI?
- Radiographic findings in children with OI?
- Scoliosis treatment for children with OI?

CASE 33

Dr. Jasmin McGinty

A 3-year-old girl presents to your clinic with her mother. The patient's mother states that she has noted over the past few months that her daughter's right leg has begun to bow slightly, and she has begun to limp. She does not report any recent trauma. She has been well and does not report any fevers or recent illness. She walked at 16 months old and all other developmental milestones were met on time. You notice that indeed she has a bowed right shin and order an x-ray of her right tibia and fibula. X-ray results are shown in Figure 10–52A and B.

On closer examination you notice that the patient has multiple light brown spots with smooth borders in her axilla bilaterally and in her groin. What is the diagnosis?

A. Adamantinoma
B. McCune–Albright syndrome
C. Fibrous dysplasia
D. Neurofibromatosis type 1
E. Fibular hemimelia

Discussion

The correct answer is (D). Diagnostic criteria for a conclusive diagnosis of neurofibromatosis type I are put forth in the consensus statement from the National Institutes of Health. A patient with two or more of the following criterion is diagnosed with neurofibromatosis. The following criteria include:

- 6 or more café-au-lait spots
- Neurofibromas or plexiform neurofibromas
- Axillary freckling
- Optic glioma
- Lisch nodules (iris hamartomas)
- Distinctive osseus lesion
- First-degree relative with neurofibromatosis type 1

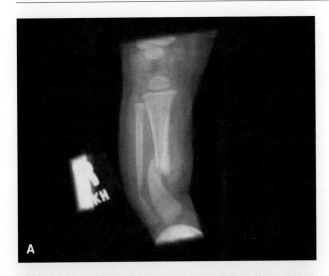

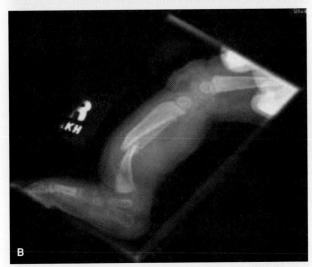

Figure 10-52 **A–B.** All images in this case are courtesy of Jasmin McGinty, MD.

The patient described in this case has pseudoarthrosis of the tibia (distinctive osseus lesion) and axillary freckling and therefore meets the criteria for the diagnosis of neurofibromatosis type 1.

What risk does this patient have of passing her diagnosis to her future children?

A. 50%
B. 25%
C. 0%
D. 100%
E. 20%

Discussion

The correct answer is (A). Neurofibromatosis has an autosomal dominant inheritance pattern. The disease manifestations occur due to a defect in the gene encoding for neurofibromin. Neurofibromin assists in cell growth regulation via the *RAS* signaling pathway. Because one of the pathways for cell growth regulation is defective, patients with neurofibromatosis are at risk of developing tumors. These tumors can be benign or malignant. Common benign tumors seen in NF1 are plexiform neurofibromas and neurofibromas. Patients with NF1 have a 10% lifetime risk of developing a malignancy. Common malignant tumors seen in patients with NF1 are astrocytomas, malignant nerve sheath tumors, pheochromocytomas, and brainstem gliomas.

What treatment is indicated at this time?

A. Long-leg cast
B. Total contact brace
C. Reassurance and physical therapy
D. Referral to orthopaedic oncologist
E. Amputation

Discussion

The correct answer is (B). Initial treatment for pseudoarthrosis of the tibia is bracing.

The patient does well with your selected treatment for 2 years. She now returns to your clinic with moderate to severe pain while walking. Her current radiographs are shown in Figure 10–53A and B. Mother would like to pursue surgery at this time.

What is your best indicated surgical option at this time?

A. Amputation
B. Open reduction and internal fixation with locking plate
C. Intramedullary nail with bone stimulator
D. Intramedullary nail with excision of pseudoarthrosis, allograft
E. Intramedullary nail with excision of pseudoarthrosis, autograft

Discussion

The correct answer is (E). This treatment can also be augmented with a spatial frame. Even with surgical treatment, there is a high rate of nonunion. After approximately three unsuccessful attempts at fusion, amputation should be considered.

Objectives: Did you learn...?

• Clinic features of NF1?
• Inheritance pattern of NF1?
• Orthopaedic manifestations of NF1?

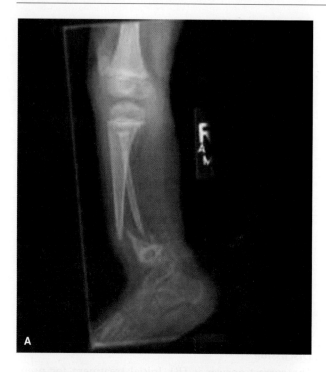

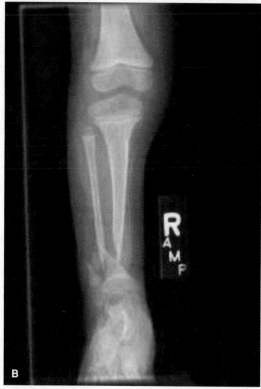

Figure 10–53 **A–B**

CASE 34

Dr. Alexander A. Theologis

You see a 14-year-old girl in your clinic for the first time who has a chief complaint of right medial ankle pain. While doing physical therapy for a contralateral ankle injury, her right ankle was noted to have decreased inversion. Upon further questioning you find that the patient has also noted pain on the medial aspect of the ankle that is described as vague and deep in the ankle joint. The pain has caused her to adjust her gait during activities. There is no history of antecedent trauma or sprains. She denies constitutional symptoms. There is no family history of foot abnormalities.

On examination, there is decreased subtalar motion on the right side when compared to the left. She is tender to palpation on the medial aspect of her hindfoot slightly distal to the tip of the medial malleolus. There is a negative anterior drawer test. There is no tenderness to palpation over the sinus tarsi, midfoot, and forefoot. There is no ankle effusion. Her hindfoot rests in slight valgus, which corrects when the foot is plantarflexed, although subtly less on the right side than the left side.

What is the most likely cause of her medial ankle pain?

A. Accessory navicular
B. Talocalcaneal coalition
C. Calcaneonavicular coalition
D. Talar dome osteochondral defect (OCD)
E. Osteomyelitis
F. Tumor

Discussion

The correct answer is (B). The patient presents with vague symptoms, which makes pinpointing a definitive diagnosis challenging. However, there are important features of her history and physical examination that are most consistent with a **talocalcaneal coalition**.

A talocalcaneal coalition is a fibrous, cartilaginous, or bony connection between the talus and calcaneus. It forms as a result of failure of segmentation of primitive mesenchymal tissue and has an incidence of 1%. Patients with talocalcaneal coalitions commonly describe a vague, deep discomfort on the medial aspect of the ankle. Symptoms are most prevalent between 12 and 16 years of age, which coincides with increasing ossification of a cartilaginous or fibrous coalition. Clinical symptoms also frequently follow ankle sprains. On physical examination, there may be a lump under the tip of the medial malleolus. This is in contrast to patients with calcaneonavicular coalitions who present with lateral sided ankle pain and tenderness to palpation over the sinus tarsi between the ages of 8 and 12 years. While your patient does not have a rigid flatfoot, she does have limited subtalar motion, which is common with talocalcaneal coalitions and can lead to a severe valgus hindfoot with time.

The other diagnosis options are unlikely but should be considered. An accessory navicular commonly presents with tenderness over the medial midfoot, and a medial sided talar dome OCD often manifests with recurrent ankle effusions, both of which were not discovered on physical examination. Osteomyelitis and tumor should be included in the differential diagnosis; however, they are less likely than a tarsal coalition given the lack of constitutional symptoms. Additional imaging should be obtained to pinpoint a definitive diagnosis.

You discuss the aforementioned diagnosis with the patient and her family. They ask you how you will definitively diagnose the condition.

Your next step is:

A. No further work-up is needed
B. Obtain radiographs (3-views) of the foot and ankle
C. Order a bone scan of the foot and ankle
D. Obtain radiographs (3-views) AND a CT scan and MRI of the foot and ankle

Discussion

The correct answer is (B). Diagnosis of a tarsal coalition starts with obtaining plain radiographs of the foot and ankle. The most helpful radiographs are the internal oblique and weight-bearing lateral views. On the internal oblique view, a calcaneonavicular coalition is best visualized (Fig. 10–54). On the lateral radiograph there are numerous secondary signs that are associated with talar coalitions. A few notable ones include the "anteater nose," the "C" sign, and talar beaking. The "anteater nose" is formed by the extension of the anterior process of the calcaneus past the calcaneocuboid joint in calcaneonavicular coalitions. It has been reported to be present in 100% of patients with this type of coalition. The "C" sign is formed by a posterior continuity of the talus and sustentaculum tali as a result of coalition of the middle and posterior facets of the subtalar joint. As the most common talocalcaneal coalition involves the middle facets of the subtalar joint, the "C" sign may be posteriorly disrupted if the posterior facet is not involved, and therefore, the sign has low specificity. Another sign of a talocalcaneal coalition is talar beaking, which forms as a result of increased stress at the talonavicular joint and traction from the talonavicular ligament. Talar beaking does not represent degenerative changes and does not predict degenerative changes of the joint. It can also be associated with other conditions that cause decreased subtalar motion, such as trauma, rheumatoid arthritis, acromegaly, and hypermobile flatfeet.

Calcaneonavicular coalitions are nearly all diagnosed reliably with plain radiographs. However, talocalcaneal coalitions can be easily missed on conventional radiographs, as the subtalar joint is incompletely visualized. The most definitive method to diagnose a talocalcaneal coalition is with advanced imaging, including CT and MRI scans. The CT scan allows for assessment of bony bridging while the MRI is more accurate for diagnosing, partial osseous coalitions, and fibrous or cartilaginous coalitions. Advanced imaging may also detect other asymptomatic coalitions, such as the uncommon talonavicular and calcaneocuboid coalitions. Radionuclide scanning of the foot with 99m-technetium can also be used to assess for talar coalitions if radiographs are unremarkable;

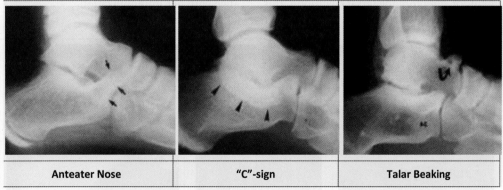

| **Anteater Nose** | **"C"-sign** | **Talar Beaking** |

Figure 10–54 Primary and secondary radiographic findings of tarsal coalitions on the lateral projection (Reproduced with permission from Newman JS, Newberg AH. Congenital Tarsal Coalition: Mutimodal Evaluation with Emphasis on CT and MR Imaging. *Radio Graphics* 2000;20:321–332.).

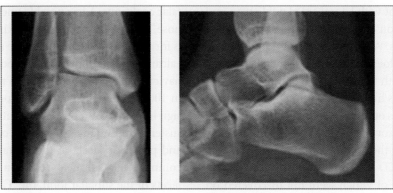

Figure 10–55 Anteroposterior and lateral radiographs of your patient.

however, bone scans lack anatomic detail and are non-specific. Therefore, the next best step in management of your patient is to obtain radiographs (3-views) and a CT scan and MRI of the foot and ankle (D).

You order and review the foot radiographs with the patient and her parents in clinic (Fig. 10–55).

As the radiographs demonstrate an equivocal C-sign and subchondral sclerosis of the subtalar joint, you suggest that the patient has a subtalar coalition and explain the importance of also obtaining CT and MRI scans.

Before her next follow-up appointment, you also recommend:

A. Nothing additional
B. Manipulation
C. Physical therapy
D. Nonsteroidal inflammatory medications, immobilization, and physical therapy
E. Subtalar corticosteroid injection

Discussion

The correct answer is (D). Nonoperative care is the first line of treatment for symptomatic tarsal coalitions. This involves the use of nonsteroidal anti-inflammatory medications, immobilization, and physical therapy of the ankle with a CAM boot or short leg cast. Anti-inflammatory medications are used to decrease pain acutely, while immobilization prevents subtalar motion and progressive deterioration of the subtalar cartilage. Other nonoperative options for the supple foot include orthotics, heel wedges, and arch supports. Despite a myriad of nonoperative options, success of conservative treatment for patients with talocalcaneal coalitions is guarded with a reported range between 0% and 46%. Calcaneonavicular coalitions are less likely to respond to conservative treatment. Patients and families should be made aware of the unpredictable success with non-operative treatment for talocalcaneal coalitions.

You see the patient and her family back for follow-up 6 weeks later. Both the CT (Fig. 10–56) and MRI (Fig. 10–57) scans were completed and they confirm an incomplete talocalcaneal coalition that involves <50% of the subtalar joint surface There are no degenerative changes of the subtalar or talonavicular joints noted on MRI. The patient reports persistent pain despite compliance with her immobilization.

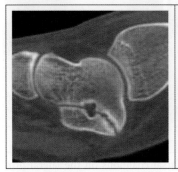
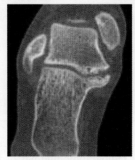
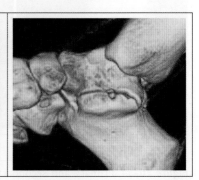

Figure 10–56 Lateral (**left**) and coronal (**middle**) CT scan images and a 3D-reconstruction (**right**) of the ankle of your patient.

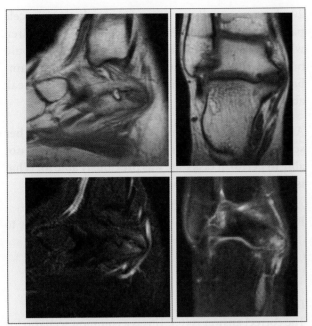

Figure 10–57 Sagittal (**left**) and coronal (**right**) MR images (T1: upper row; T2: bottom row) of the ankle of your patient.

What is the next step in management?

A. Continued immobilization

B. Subtalar corticosteroid injection

C. Talocalcaneal resection

D. Subtalar arthrodesis

Discussion

The correct answer is (A). The patient has persistent pain despite a course of NSAIDs and immobilization. Surgical intervention is a consideration; however, a **second course of immobilization** is often recommended before proceeding with surgical care. If the patient's pain persists despite a second round of immobilization, she would be a good candidate for a talocalcaneal resection, as she would have failed nonoperative management, the coalition involves <50% of the subtalar joint surface, the foot has good overall alignment (heel valgus angle <16 degrees), and she has no subtalar or talonavicular arthritis. The success rates of operative treatment for calcaneonavicular and talocalcaneal coalitions vary. The success rate after calcaneonavicular coalition resection via a lateral approach and placement of interposing extensor digitorum brevis muscle ranges from 73% to 90%. For talocalcaneal coalitions, surgical resection from a medial approach and placement of interposing fat has a reported success of 33% to 80%. Best outcomes are seen in younger patients (i.e., <16 years), when the coalition involves <50% of the subtalar joint sur-

face, and if degenerative changes are absent. A subtalar arthrodesis is indicated if a coalition and/or pain recurs after resection if the talocalcaneal coalition involves >50% of the subtalar joint, and if there are degenerative changes of the talonavicular and/or subtalar joints.

Objectives: Did you learn...?

- The common distinguishing clinical features between the two most common tarsal coalitions (calcaneonavicular and talocalcaneal)?
- The appropriate imaging evaluation of a patient with a suspected tarsal coalition?
- The necessary nonoperative management of tarsal coalitions?
- The unique surgical indications for tarsal coalitions?

CASE 35

Dr. Amanda T. Whitaker

A couple comes to you for counseling regarding their unborn child. They have been told that the child has spina bifida.

What should the family be told?

A. Your child will unlikely walk

B. Your child will not be of normal intelligence

C. You should have a natural birth

D. You should have a cesarean section

Discussion

The correct answer is (D). Myelomeningocele is a failure of closure of the spinal elements at 26 to 28 days of development or a re-opening of the spinal elements. Children with exposed neural elements should be born via cesarean section to avoid injury to the sac. Children with lumbar lesions usually can walk and those without hydrocephalus have normal intelligence. Also, outcomes are better if the defect is closed early within 24 hours of life.

Supplementation with what has decreased the incidence of myelomeningocele in the United States?

A. Vitamin A

B. Vitamin D

C. Folic acid

D. Vitamin B12

Discussion

The correct answer is (C). Myelomeningocele is associated with folate deficiency. There has been a 23%

decrease in spina bifida since the supplementation of grains in the United States in 1998. There is also an increased incidence in first-degree relatives.

The child is born with a thoracic myelomeningocele and clubfoot deformity. What is the recurrence rate after Ponseti casting?

A. 10%
B. 26%
C. 44%
D. 68%

Discussion

The correct answer is (D). Children with high-level lesions often have clubfoot. Sixty-eight percent of patients recur with approximately one-third of those requiring a posteromedial release. Other foot conditions associated with myelomeningocele are calcaneovarus, calcaneovalgus, and vertical talus. The goal of treatment is a braceable foot that is plantigrade. This is critical due to their decreased sensation on their feet and tendency to ulcerate.

At the age of 4, she is not walking. Both hips are dislocated. What should be done?

A. Observation
B. Closed reduction in the OR with spica cast
C. Open reduction in the OR with spica cast
D. Dega osteotomy, proximal femoral osteotomy, and spica cast

Discussion

The correct answer is (A). In this case, the child has a high-level myelomeningocele, does not walk, and has bilateral hip dislocations. The best treatment is observation because the hips will not stay in due to the abnormal muscle forces across the joint.

At age 10 the child has had a rapidly progressing scoliosis of over 15 degrees in 6 months to a curve magnitude of 30 degrees. What should be done?

A. Observation to 50 degrees
B. MRI
C. Posterior spinal fusion
D. Anterior spinal fusion

Discussion

The correct answer is (B). In myelomeningocele, a rapidly progressing curve should be concerning for a tethered cord and should undergo neurosurgical evaluation for detethering. Curves greater than

20 degrees usually progress in myelomeningocele patients and warrant surgical evaluation. In children who are ambulatory, however, spinal fusion should be approached with caution as many use their lumbar spine to assist with ambulation due to weak abductors.

At the age of 12 the child is unable to complete her schoolwork, her grades are suffering and she is not able to perform tasks she was previously able to. What is the most likely etiology?

A. Natural history of the condition
B. Too many surgeries at a young age and exposure to anesthesia
C. Shunt malfunction
D. Depression

Discussion

The correct answer is (C). This is a common scenario for patients with myelomeningocele, especially after spinal fusion. A deterioration in cognitive status is most commonly associated with shunt malfunction. During their lifetime, 86% require a shunt with 95% needing a revision due to increasing hydrocephalus.

Objectives: Did you learn...?

• Early treatment of myelomeningocele?
• Prevention of myelomeningocele?
• Associated conditions with myelomeningocele?
• Treatment and outcomes of thoracic level myelomeningocele orthopaedic conditions?

CASE 36

Dr. Coleen S. Sabatini

A 12-year-old boy is brought to your clinic for evaluation after being seen in the ER yesterday due to a twisting injury to his left leg from a bike fall. He had intense pain in the knee which started to swell almost immediately. On examination, you note that he has an effusion and is holding the leg in about 10 degrees of flexion. He is very guarded on examination, making ligamentous testing unreliable. You order knee x-rays to further assess (Figs. 10–58 and 10–59).

Based on the x-rays, you explain to the family that the patient has the following:

A. ACL tear
B. Tibial tubercle fracture
C. Tibial eminence fracture

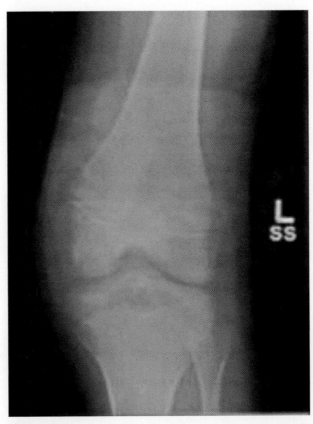

Figure 10–58

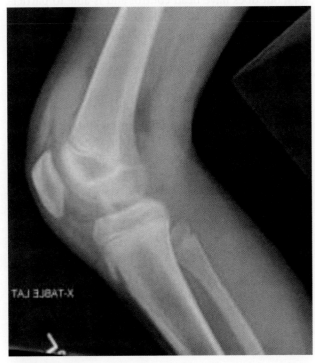

Figure 10–59

D. Osteochondral defect

E. A transient patella dislocation

Discussion

The correct answer is (C). The patient has a tibial eminence fracture. On the AP view, there is an irregularity of the tibial spine that can be seen, but the lateral view is the view that best shows this injury. You can clearly see that the tibial spine is displaced on this view. The Meyers and McKeever classification is what is used to describe tibial eminence fractures—type 1 injury is a minimally displaced fracture of the tibial eminence. A type 2 tibial eminence fracture is lifted anteriorly, but has an intact posterior hinge. In a type 3 fracture, the fracture fragment is completely displaced.

You explain to the family that the fracture is displaced and you would like to get additional information before making a recommendation as to how to proceed. You order the following:

A. Ultrasound of the knee

B. Bone scan and MRI

C. Ultrasound and MRI

D. CT and MRI

E. CT and ultrasound

Discussion

The correct answer is (D). A CT scan is useful in visualizing the details of the fracture pattern, the shape, size, and position of the tibial spine. The MRI is very important because in nearly 40% of patients there are associated injuries such as meniscus, capsule, collateral ligament injuries, or an osteochondral fracture. Ultrasounds and bone scans are not utilized in the evaluation of tibial spine fractures. Some surgeons who have access to high-resolution MRI are no longer obtaining CT scans (or doing so much more selectively) because the high-resolution MRI is providing sufficient information about the bony anatomy as well as the soft tissue involvement and the radiation associated with a CT scan can be avoided.

The advanced imaging studies show a completely displaced tibial eminence fracture, and you recommend surgery. You explain that your preferred surgical technique is an arthroscopic approach, but an open arthrotomy would also be acceptable (no studies yet show one to be superior to the other you explain, but your personal preference is arthroscopic repair). At the time of surgery, you find that there is soft tissue

blocking the reduction. What anatomic structure is most likely to be blocking the reduction?

A. Anterior horn of lateral meniscus
B. Posterior horn of medial meniscus
C. Anterior horn of medial meniscus
D. Intermeniscal ligament
E. Plica

Discussion

The correct answer is (A). Kocher found that there was soft tissue entrapment in 26% of type 2 fractures and 65% of type 3 fractures. In cases where there was soft tissue entrapment, the anterior horn of the medial meniscus was the most likely culprit, followed by inter-meniscal ligament and rarely the anterior horn of the lateral meniscus. The posterior horn of medial menis-cus and plicas are not in an anatomic location to affect the tibial spine reduction.

Surgery goes well and you are confident with your surgical fixation of the tibial eminence fracture. You explain to the family that after an initial brief period of rest and limited ROM, you would like to start range of motion exercises. If ROM is started more than 4 weeks after surgery, the child is at risk of what?

A. Arthrofibrosis
B. Nonunion
C. ACL laxity
D. No risk—waiting more than 4 weeks to begin ROM is your plan

Discussion

The correct answer is (A). Patel et al. showed, in a retro-spective review of 40 patients, that patients who didn't start range of motion exercises until more than 4 weeks after surgery were 12 times more likely to develop arthrofibro-sis. Nonunion is very rare—especially in patients who had surgery. ACL laxity is a known finding after tibial emi-nence fractures. A study by Willis showed that as many as 74% of patients had ACL laxity on KT-1,000 testing when compared to the uninjured side, but this was not clini-cally relevant in the majority of patients. Laxity is more common in those treated nonsurgically than in surgical patients. D is not correct since there has been increased risk of arthrofibrosis shown in patients who do not begin ROM until more than 4 weeks after surgery.

Objectives: Did you learn…?

- The classification of tibial eminence fractures?
- The diagnostic imaging evaluation of tibial eminence fractures?

- Nonsurgical and surgical options for tibial eminence fractures?
- Blocks to reduction?
- Outcomes and anticipated complications?

CASE 37

Dr. Coleen S. Sabatini

A 4-year-old male with cerebral palsy is brought to your clinic for evaluation. He is nonambulatory but is able to hold his head up against gravity. He can sit on the floor with assistance. He can help stand for transfers but does not take any steps.

As part of his assessment, you document his GMFCS level as:

A. GMFCS I
B. GMFCS II
C. GMFCS III
D. GMFCS IV
E. GMFCS V
F. Not enough information provided to classify

Discussion

The correct answer is (D). The Gross Motor Function Classification System (GMFCS) is an ordinal grading system used to describe the gross motor function of children with cerebral palsy. This child is nonambula-tory, but does have head control and is able to partici-pate with transfers which classifies him at a level 4. A thorough description of GMFCS classification can be found at http://motorgrowth.canchild.ca/en/GMFCS/resources/GMFCS-ER.pdf. A brief summary of Palis-ano et al.'s work is as follows:

LEVEL I—Walks without limitations. They can run and jump, but speed and coordination are limited.
LEVEL II—Have some limitations in walking long dis-tances and with balance. Need a railing for going up and down stairs. May use wheeled mobility devices when traveling longer distances. Have more difficulty with running and jumping than level 1 children. After age 4 can often walk without a handheld mobil-ity device.
LEVEL III—Walk using a handheld mobility device to walk indoors. Often will use a wheelchair when outside. Are able to sit on their own either with no, or very little, support. They can be independent for standing transfers.
LEVEL IV—Need a manual or powered wheelchair, can sit upright with assistance.

LEVEL V—Have severe limitations in head and trunk control, they are transported in a manual wheelchair and require extensive assistance.

The parents report that they recently moved to the area and are hoping to establish care with you for the orthopaedic care of their child. They note that he has a history of botox injections that were "helpful," but they have noticed that his hips are "more tight" now than they were previously.

What is the mechanism by which botox works?

A. Inhibits the release of calcium into the sarcoplasmic reticulum

B. Inhibits the release of acetylcholine at the neuromuscular junction

C. Promotes binding of GABA to GABA type A receptors

D. Binds to a synaptic vesicle glycoprotein and inhibits presynaptic calcium channels

E. Functions as a gamma-aminobutyric acid (GABA) analog that inhibits calcium influx into presynaptic terminals and suppresses the release of excitatory neurotransmitters

Discussion

The correct answer is (B). A is the mechanism of dantrolene. C is the mechanism of benzodiazepenes. D is the mechanism of levetiracetam (Keppra). E is the mechanism of action for baclofen.

On examination, his hip abduction is less than 30 degrees and his migration index is 35%. What do you recommend?

A. Continued observation

B. Nighttime hip abduction bracing

C. Physical therapy

D. Surgery—soft tissue releases

E. Surgery—soft tissue releases and pelvic osteotomy

Discussion

The best answer is "D." Soft tissue lengthenings are indicated for children who are less than 8 years of age, who have hip abduction less than 30 degrees, and have a migration index greater than 25% but less than 60%. For patients with a migration index greater than 60%, bony reconstruction is indicated. This 4-year-old child's MI is only 35% therefore bony work is not pursued at this time. High success rates have been seen with soft tissue lengthenings alone for children with migration index less than 40%. Choice B is incorrect because hip

abduction bracing has not been found to prevent hip dislocation. A and C would be correct if the child's abduction was greater than 45 degrees and the MI was less than 25%—if the abduction is less and the MI is higher, the hip is at risk. Once abduction is less than 30 degrees and the MI is over 25%, surgical intervention is considered.

The patient does well after surgery with no immediate postoperative complications. He continues in a physical therapy program and his parents are very attentive to a home exercise program. They move away for a few years but return to your care at age 8. On examination you note limited ROM of the right hip and the parents report that he now seems more uncomfortable with transfers and sitting. You order an AP pelvis x-ray (Fig. 10–60).

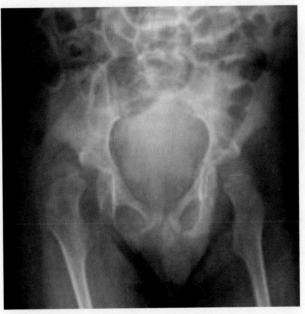

Figure 10–60

What is your current recommendation of treatment for this new presentation?

A. Observation

B. Botox and bracing

C. Soft tissue lengthenings (revision)

D. Pelvic osteotomy

E. Varus derotation osteotomy of the femur with possible shortening, soft tissue lengthenings, acetabuloplasty

Discussion

The correct answer is (E). Since the patient is older than 4 years of age, has a migration index greater than 40%, and does not have evidence of advanced degenerative changes of the femoral head, hip reconstruction is recommended. Choices A, B, and C will not help a child with a dislocation/severe subluxation. A pelvic osteotomy alone would likely not be enough to reduce and stabilize this hip given the significant coxa valga. There is increasing support for combined procedures that address both the proximal femoral deformity as well as the insufficiency of the acetabular coverage.

Objectives: Did you learn...?

- The GMFCS classification of children with cerebral palsy?
- The mechanism of action of Botox—an agent frequently used in the soft tissue management of children with cerebral palsy?
- Considerations and indications for surgery in children with cerebral palsy depending on both clinical and radiographic measures?

CASE 38

Dr. Coleen S. Sabatini

You are on-call in the emergency room and are paged to see three different patients who came in around the same time with trauma to their wrists.

Your first patient is a 6-year old who fell off a swing and complained of pain in the wrist. Her family iced it overnight, and she was able to use the arm some, so they decided to monitor for a day. When she continued to have pain into the next day (today), they brought her in for evaluation. On examination, she is tender over the distal radius. There is no tenderness over the ulna. She has full elbow flexion and extension with no pain. You order an x-ray and it shows (Figs. 10–61 and 10–62):

What do you offer the family in terms of treatment options?

A. Long-arm cast
B. Nothing
C. Short-arm cast
D. Velcro wrist brace
E. C or D

Discussion

The correct answer is (E). The patient has a distal radius buckle fracture, and this fracture is at low risk of displacement due to the stability conferred by the intact volar cortex. Long-arm cast is more immobilization than is needed for this fracture and would be unnecessarily

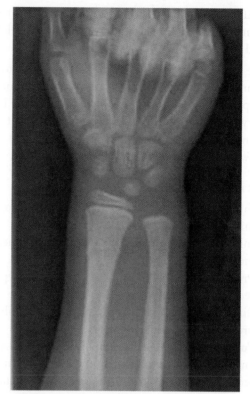

Figure 10–61

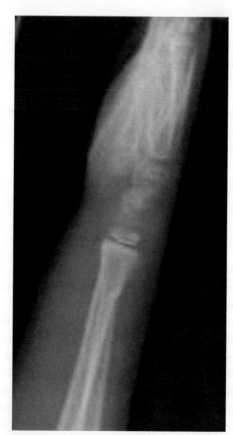

Figure 10–62

difficult for the patient and family. B is not a good option because the child has a broken bone and to give them no support is not appropriate since a nonimmobilized fracture is a source of pain. Either a prefabricated velcro wrist brace or a short-arm cast can be used effectively for this fracture. Williams et al. conducted a randomized trial for treatment of buckle fractures with wrist splints (Velcro wrist brace) versus cast finding that those in the splint group reported higher levels of satisfaction, preference, and convenience overall, but did have more pain than the casted group initially. You can therefore inform the family of this and give them the option of either.

After ordering a splint for your first patient, you move on to say hello to your next patient—a 6-year-old boy who fell while riding a scooter about 2 hours ago. The ER had already obtained x-rays, and you are able to review them before meeting the family. He has a distal radius fracture that is in bayonet apposition, there is no angulation and there is about 3 mm of shortening.

In discussing options with the family, what do you tell them about the current position of his radius?

A. It is unacceptable and a closed reduction under conscious sedation should be performed.
B. It is unacceptable and a closed reduction under general anesthesia should be performed.
C. It is acceptable and a cast is needed for immobilization.
D. It is acceptable and a wrist brace is all that is needed for immobilization.

Discussion
The correct answer is (C). This patient has a distal radius fracture with bayonet apposition and shortening of only 3 mm. Patients who undergo closed reduction to bring these fractures out to length often have redisplacement. Recent work by Crawford, Lee, and Izuka demonstrated that an overriding distal radius fracture (bayonet apposition) is acceptable and will sufficiently remodel under the age of 10. There is significant cost savings and good patient satisfaction associated with this treatment. A and B are not correct because the alignment as described is acceptable. A wrist brace, although acceptable for a buckle fracture, would not be acceptable for a complete fracture and one that needs to be held in a stable position.

You place a cast on the patient with gentle molding to prevent angulation. After instructing the family on cast care, you move on to the next patient.

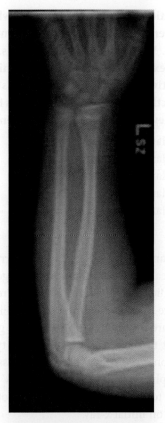

Figure 10–63

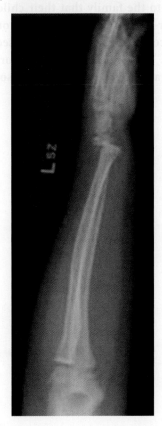

Figure 10–64

The third patient is an 11-year-old male who fell while playing soccer and had immediate pain and deformity of the wrist. You review the x-rays (Figs. 10–63 and 10–64) and explain the injury to the family. They are very inquisitive and ask a lot of questions—they want to know exactly what type of distal radius fracture this is. After reviewing the x-rays, you tell them:

A. Salter–Harris I fracture
B. Salter–Harris II fracture
C. Salter–Harris III fracture
D. Salter–Harris IV fracture
E. Salter–Harris V fracture

Discussion

The correct answer is (B). The Salter–Harris classification of physeal fractures is basic knowledge for anyone in orthopaedics. A Salter–Harris I fracture is a transverse fracture through the growth plate (Fig. 10–65). A type II fracture is through a portion of the growth plate, but goes out through the metaphysis. A type III goes into the epiphysis. Type IV fractures cross all three—metaphysis, physis, and epiphysis. A type V fracture is a crush injury to the physis and there are not necessarily any findings on initial x-ray.

You explain to the family that their child has a displaced Salter–Harris II fracture and you have recommended conscious sedation and closed reduction with casting. They agree, and you perform a reduction. You are able to reduce the fracture some, but not

completely—there is about 25% displacement and no significant angulation. What do you tell the family?

A. Alignment is unacceptable and you need to perform the reduction again.
B. Alignment is unacceptable and the child needs an operation to reduce and stabilize the fracture.
C. Alignment is acceptable because of remodeling potential of the distal radius, but there is no harm in trying again to "get it perfect," so you attempt another reduction.
D. Alignment is acceptable because of remodeling potential of the distal radius, and there is potential for harm if you do another reduction, so you will accept it as is. Follow-up in 1 week.

Discussion

The correct answer is (D). The alignment is acceptable in this patient because there is less than 50% displacement through the physis. There is not true consensus on the amount of angulation that is acceptable, but in general, angulation up to 20 degrees would be accepted in this patient over age 9 with open growth plates. Angulation as high as 25 to 30 degrees would be accepted in a child less than 9 years of age. Given that 75% of the growth happens from the distal growth plate in the radius, there is a fair amount of remodeling potential with distal radius fractures. A study by Lee demonstrated that premature arrest of the physis was related to multiple reduction attempts, not to degree of angulation. If you were to re-reduce this patient's fracture, you would be exposing him to the risk of premature physeal arrest unnecessarily.

Objectives: Did you learn...?

- Different types of distal radius fractures have different treatment options?
- Management of buckle fractures of the distal radius?
- Management of displaced distal radius fractures in children under age 10—nonprocedural options?
- Salter–Harris classification of physeal fractures?
- Treatment of distal radius physeal fractures in children given remodeling potential?
- Importance of knowing what is acceptable and what is not in terms of alignment so as to avoid performing unnecessary procedures on children?

CASE 39

Dr. Coleen S. Sabatini

A 12-year-old, premenarchal girl has been referred to you by her pediatrician after school screening for scoliosis

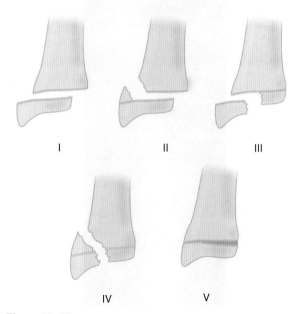

Figure 10–65

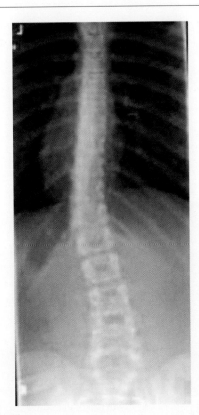

Figure 10-66

raised concern. On examination, she has a left thora-columbar prominence on Adam's forward bend test. She has normal, symmetrical reflexes. Her motor and sensory examinations are normal as well. She has no pain and no complaints at this time. Her standing spine film is as follows (Fig. 10–66):

You measure the Cobb Angle and obtain a value of 18 degrees. She is Risser 0. Her lateral x-ray shows hypokyphosis of the thoracic spine and no spondy-lolysis/spondylolisthesis. What do you recommend for treatment at this time?

A. Observation
B. X-ray of the left hand for bone age
C. MRI of the spine
D. Boston brace
E. Posterior spine instrumentation and fusion

Discussion

The correct answer is (A). This is a healthy, 12-year old who is premenarchal, neurologically normal, with a curve of only 18 degrees. For this patient, you would follow her examination and radiographs over time to see if there is progression. B—hand film for bone age—is not needed at this time because her curve magnitude

is not large enough to consider interventions for which knowing more about her skeletal maturity is necessary. C is not correct because she has a classic presentation for adolescent idiopathic scoliosis, and there is not anything in her history nor examination that would suggest the need for MRI. If she had an abnormal neurologic examination or red flags on history, then an MRI would be warranted. D is incorrect because a curve of 18 degrees does not warrant brace treatment. Curves greater than 25 degrees in patients who are still growing are candidates for bracing (Risser 0, 1, 2). E is incorrect because a curve of 18 degrees is not large enough to warrant surgical intervention—thoracic curves larger than 50 degrees or lumbar curves larger than 45 degrees are the curve magnitudes for which you would consider surgery (although smaller curves in the setting of significant decompensation or underlying conditions would also be considered, but that is not the case here).

A 13-year-old girl is next in your clinic. This patient is 2 months postmenarchal. She was recently seen by a pediatrician for the first time in about 4 years just last week, and her new pediatrician was very concerned given notable asymmetry on forward bend testing. She ordered an x-ray (Fig. 10–67) and referred her to you when she saw the following:

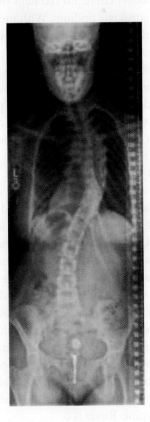

Figure 10-67

On examination, she has a notable right thoracic prominence on Adam's forward bend test. She has normal reflexes, normal strength, and normal sensation on examination. You measure her x-ray and note that she has a right thoracic curve that measures 56 degrees. She is Risser 1 on examination.

What do you recommend to the family?

A. Observation
B. MRI of the spine
C. Boston brace
D. Posterior spine instrumentation and fusion
E. Combined anterior and posterior fusion with posterior instrumentation

Discussion

The correct answer is (D). The curve magnitude is over 50 degrees and menarche was in the last few months, therefore she still has growth left—both of these put her at risk of curve progression over time. Spinal fusion is recommended for patients with curves larger than 50 degrees, as this patient has. A and C are incorrect. Her curve is past the point where a brace can be helpful—curves larger than 40 degrees do not respond well to bracing. An MRI is not needed because this is an adolescent onset curve, no red flags on history, and there are no neurologic findings. With modern surgical techniques and instrumentation, a combined anterior/posterior surgery is not needed in this patient as her curve is less than 75 degrees and she has no associated syndromes. For curves larger than 75 to 80 degrees, one may consider doing a combined anterior/posterior procedure or if the curve is particularly stiff as well. Excellent results can be obtained from a posterior fusion with instrumentation.

You go next to see a patient who is 13 years old and had spine asymmetry picked up on school screening. Her pediatrician saw her last year and obtained an x-ray that showed a curve of 17 degrees. At one year follow up with the pediatrician, it was found that the curve had progressed. Parents as well as the patient report occasional diffuse back pain without radiation, no weakness in the arms or legs. She functions well in PE and sports with no difficulties. She is premenarchal. Her examination is notable for an apex right thoracic prominence and an apex left lumbar prominence on Adam's forward bend test. Examination is otherwise normal. You review her x-ray (Fig. 10–68).

Upon measurement of the x-ray, you obtain a Cobb angle of 28 degrees in the thoracic spine and 17 degrees in the lumbar spine. Risser is 0.

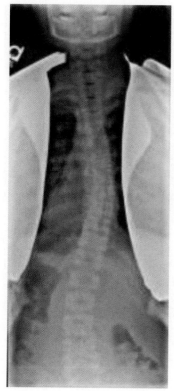

Figure 10–68

Given that she has a curve greater than 25 degrees and is still growing (premenarchal, Risser 0), you offer the patient a Boston brace for treatment of her scoliosis. What do you tell them about wearing the brace in order to help make it as effective as possible?

A. She should wear the brace just at night.
B. She should wear the brace for at least 8 hours a day during the daytime.
C. She should wear the brace for 18 to 20 hours a day with at least 12 hours in the daytime.
D. She should wear the brace at all times on weekends, but can wear on the weekdays just at night.
E. Wearing a brace probably won't help, but she can try it anyway.

Discussion

The correct answer is (C). Although it is true that earlier studies about bracing were not very conclusive as to whether or not bracing was helpful in the treatment of adolescent idiopathic scoliosis, earlier studies were flawed by having inaccurate data with regard to the amount of time patients were actually wearing the brace. Recent studies (Katz, Weinstein) have utilized temperature sensors in braces to get a true measurement of brace wear. These studies showed a dose-response relationship between amount of time in brace with prevention of progression of curve—within that, they found that brace wear for 12 or more hours during the daytime was most effective in preventing curve progression. Thus, of the options provided above, C is the best answer since it has the patient in the brace for at least 12 hours of daytime wear. A, B, and D are not enough time in the brace to benefit. E is incorrect based on these new studies—particularly given that this patient is Risser 0.

Objectives: Did you learn...?

- The evaluation of patients with scoliosis in adolescence?
- The curve magnitude indications for observation versus bracing versus surgery?
- The indications for brace treatment and the necessary time in brace to have potential benefit?

CASE 40

Dr. Coleen S. Sabatini

The ER requests your consultation on a 3-year-old boy who presented with 5 days of pain and refusal to bear weight in the right leg for the past day. He also had a fever of 39°C this morning. The ER ordered labs and are requesting your evaluation. The WBC is 8.9 cells/mm^3 and the C-reactive protein is 6.4 mg/dL (normal at your hospital is <1 mg/dL). They did not get an ESR. On examination, he looks unhappy but is not septic appearing. You see no evidence of rash. His right lower extremity examination reveals full and painless ROM of the hip, knee, and ankle. He is tender over the distal tibial metaphysis, not tender more distally, and no effusion appreciated in the knee or ankle on examination. You try to get him to walk, but he refuses to put weight on the leg. You confirm with mother that his symptoms began just yesterday—no pain, limp or other complaints prior to that.

You suspect osteomyelitis given the fever, tenderness over distal tibia, refusal to bear weight, and elevated CRP. The lack of elevation of the WBC doesn't change your thoughts on diagnosis because you know that in only around 25% of patients with osteomyelitis is the WBC elevated. For your next step in evaluation, you order x-rays.

What do you expect to see if your diagnosis is correct?

A. Lucency in the tibia
B. Periosteal reaction along the tibial cortex
C. Moth-eaten appearance throughout the distal tibia
D. Normal appearing bone

Discussion

The correct answer is (D). The patient's symptoms just began a few days ago, so this is a case of acute osteomyelitis. Changes in the bone aren't seen radiographically usually until 7 to 10 days after the onset of symptoms. Sometimes on early x-rays the soft tissue planes are obscured, but the bone is normal. By 7 to 10 days you can start to see periosteal bone along the cortex and then lucency in the metaphysis.

After reviewing the x-rays, you confirm that they appear normal. There is no evidence of fracture. He is admitted to the hospital for treatment of presumed osteomyelitis. He is started on antibiotics to cover the most common organism responsible for osteomyelitis in children over the age of 1 in the United States.

What organism is that?

A. *Streptococcus pyogenes*
B. Group B streptococci
C. *Kingella kingae*
D. Salmonella
E. *Staphylococcus aureus*

Discussion

The correct answer is (E). There are a number of pathogens that can cause osteomyelitis in kids (and all of those in the list do), *Staphylococcus aureus* accounts for 70% to 90% of pediatric acute hematogenous osteomyelitis. *Streptococcus pyogenes* does cause osteomyelitis in children, but is far less common than *S. aureus*. *Group B strep* is the most common in neonates, but this question specifically asked for children older than 1-year old. *Salmonella* is frequently associated with sickle cell because patients with sickle cell anemia are most at risk of having a *Salmonella* infection than the general population, but *S. aureus* is still more common in sickle cell than *Salmonella* is. *Kingella kingae* is increasingly the culprit in septic arthritis—in some places surpassing Staph as the primary cause of joint infection in young children. However, *Staph aureus* continues to be the most common etiologic agent in osteomyelitis and osteoarticular infections in children when all age groups are considered.

You work with the infectious disease service on this patient's care and he is put on the appropriate agent for the treatment of *S. aureus*. Over the next 36 hours he improves clinically and begins to weightbear normally. He is transitioned over to an oral antibiotic which he tolerates well and is ultimately discharged to home. The plan is for him to complete a 4- to 6-week course of antibiotics, per the ID service. They acknowledge that even their literature doesn't have great data on how long to treat for and even when they should have changed from IV to oral form, but they will monitor his continued response to treatment and respond as needed.

You reflect on the patient and think about how things could have been different if the child had community-acquired MRSA infection. You remember reading about kids that have the MRSA osteomyelitis. All of the following are true about children with multifocal MRSA osteomyelitis, EXCEPT:

A. They are less likely to need surgery.
B. They are more likely to need surgery.
C. They are more likely to need multiple surgeries.
D. They are at higher risk of developing DVT and septic pulmonary emboli.
E. They are more likely to be in the ICU and have a longer hospital course.

Discussion

The correct answer is (A), because it is NOT true that children with MRSA osteomyelitis are LESS likely to need surgery. Multiple studies have now shown that children with MRSA, when compared to kids with MSSA infections, are more likely to need surgery, they require more surgeries, they have longer hospital stays, they are more likely to require ICU support, and are more likely to develop DVT and septic pulmonary emboli.

Additional Questions

You are working in a remote clinic in an area with limited healthcare resources. A patient comes in, brought by their family, because they have had a problem with their leg for the past year. A year ago, she developed pain in the leg after a trauma. There was a skin wound that got infected, and she was on antibiotics for about a week which improved the infection briefly. They feel it never really went away though and over time, there was continued intermittent drainage, foul smell, and they could see the bone at times—this has worsened over the past 2 months. There is now continued drainage, and she is having difficulty walking. They were not able to access care until now. You are able to obtain an x-ray (Fig. 10–69).

What is the red arrow pointing at?

A. Cloaca
B. Sequestrum
C. Involucrum
D. Brodie's abscess
E. Fracture

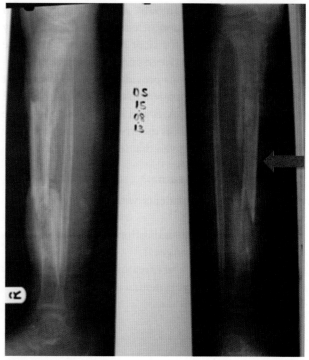

Figure 10–69

Discussion

The correct answer is (B). The patient has chronic osteomyelitis of their tibia. In chronic osteomyelitis, there can be increased pressure in the metaphysis where the infection first starts and the fluid can push out through the metaphyseal cortex and into the subperiosteal space. This communication is the cloaca (which ultimately communicates into the soft tissues and sometimes out of the skin). The fluid continues to build up in the subperiosteal space, further stripping the periosteum off the cortex. Both the stripping of the periosteum and the increased pressure from the fluid inside the bone leads to reduced vascular supply to the bone which can lead to necrosis. This necrotic bone is the sequestrum. The body then tries to heal along the periosteum that was lifted off, and this new bone is called the involucrum. On the x-ray shown in Figure 10–69, the arrow is pointed at the dysvascularized piece of bone which is the sequestrum. A Brodie's abscess is seen in subacute and chronic osteomyelitis and is a walled-off area of bone usually in the metaphysis—there is an inner lucency, surrounded by sclerotic bone. E is incorrect because this is simply not a fracture. Treatment of this chronic osteomyelitis will depend on what resources are available. Ultimately, a sequestrectomy will need to be performed to remove the sequestrum since it is a nidus for infection. The timing will depend on surgeon preference and if there is available equipment for stabilization of the involucrum. Because equipment often is not available, many surgeons will wait until the involucrum is in continuity and developed enough to minimize risk of fracture and segmental bone loss.

Objectives: Did you learn...?

- Differences in presentation and treatment between acute, subacute, and chronic osteomyelitis?
- The most common organisms that cause osteomyelitis in children?
- The increased risks associated with MRSA osteomyelitis?
- The presentation of chronic osteomyelitis?

BIBLIOGRAPHY

Case 1

Babal JC, Mehlman CT, Klein G. Nerve injuries associated with pediatric supracondylar humeral fractures: a meta-analysis. *J Pediatr Orthop.* 2010;30(3):253–263.

Otsuka NY, Kasser JR. Supracondylar fractures of the humerus in children. *J Am Acad Orthop Surg.* 1997;5:19–26.

Case 2

Bae DS, Kadiyala RK, Waters PM. Acute compartment syndrome in children: contemporary diagnosis, treatment, and outcome. *J Pediatr Orthop.* 2001;21(5):680–688.

Choi PD, Melikian R, Skaggs DL. Risk factors for vascular repair and compartment syndrome in the pulseless supracondylar humerus fracture in children. *J Pediatr Orthop.* 2010;30(1):50–56.

Scannell BP, Jackson JB 3rd, Bray C, Roush TS, Brighton BK, Frick SL. The perfused, pulseless supracondylar humeral fracture: intermediate-term follow-up of vascular status and function. *J Bone Joint Surg Am.* 2013;95(21):1913–1919.

Weller A, Garg S, Larson AN, et al. Management of the pediatric pulseless supracondylar humeral fracture: is vascular exploration necessary? *J Bone Joint Surg Am.* 2013;95(21):1906–1912.

Case 3

Pirker ME, Weinberg AM, Höllwarth ME, Haberlik A. Subsequent displacement of initially nondisplaced and minimally displaced fractures of the lateral humeral condyle in children. *J Trauma.* 2005;58(6):1202–1207.

Song KS, Kang CH, Min BW, Bae KC, Cho CH. Internal oblique radiographs for diagnosis of nondisplaced or minimally displaced lateral condylar fractures of the humerus in children. *J Bone Joint Surg Am.* 2007;89(1):58–63.

Tejwani N, Phillips D, Goldstein RY. Management of lateral humeral condylar fracture in children. *J Am Acad Orthop Surg.* 2011;19(6):350–358.

Weiss JM, Graves S, Yang S, Mendelsohn E, Kay RM, Skaggs DL. A new classification system predictive of complications in surgically treated pediatric humeral lateral condyle fractures. *J Pediatr Orthop.* 2009;29(6):602–605.

Case 4

Brodeur AE, Silberstein MJ, Graviss ER. *Radiology of the Pediatric Elbow.* Boston, MA: GK Hall Medical Publishers; 1981.

Gottschalk HP, Eisner E, Hosalkar HS. Medial epicondyle fractures in the pediatric population. *J Am Acad Orthop Surg.* 2012;20(4):223–232.

Mehlman CT, Howard AW. Medial epicondyle fractures in children: clinical decision making in the face of uncertainty. *J Pediatr Orthop.* 2012;32(Suppl 2):S135–S142.

Case 5

Lincoln TL, Mubarak SJ. "Isolated" traumatic radial-head dislocation. *J Pediatr Orthop.* 1994;14(4):454–457.

Ring D, Jupiter JB, Waters PM. Monteggia fractures in children and adults. *J Am Acad Orthop Surg.* 1998;6(4):215–224.

Speed JS, Boyd HB. Treatment of fractures of ulna with dislocation of head of radius (Monteggia fracture). *JAMA.* 1940; 115:1699–1705.

Case 6

Carney BT, Birnbaum P, Minter C. Slip progression after in situ single screw fixation for stable slipped capital femoral epiphysis. *J Pediatr Orthop.* 2003;23(5):584–589.

Loder RT, Wittenberg B, DeSilva G. Slipped capital femoral epiphysis associated with endocrine disorders. *J Pediatr Orthop.* 1995;15(3):349–356.

Schultz WR, Weinstein JN, Weinstein SL, Smith BG. Prophylactic pinning of the contralateral hip in slipped capital femoral epiphysis: evaluation of long-term outcome for the contralateral hip with use of decision analysis. *J Bone Joint Surg Am.* 2002;84-A(8):1305–1314.

Tokmakova KP, Stanton RP, Mason DE. Factors influencing the development of osteonecrosis in patients treated for slipped capital femoral epiphysis. *J Bone Joint Surg Am.* 2003;85-A(5):798–801.

Case 7

Joseph B, Rao N, Mulpuri K, Varghese G, Nair S. How does a femoral varus osteotomy alter the natural evolution of Perthes' disease? *J Pediatr Orthop B.* 2005;14(1):10–15.

Shah H. Perthes disease: evaluation and management. *Orthop Clin North Am.* 2014;45(1):87–97.

Wiig O, Terjesen T, Svenningsen S. Prognostic factors and outcome of treatment of Perthes disease: a prospective study of 368 patients with five-year follow-up. *J Bone Joint Surg Br.* 2008;90(10):1364–1371.

Case 8

Flynn JM, Schwend RM. Management of pedatric femoral shaft fractures. *J Am Acad Orthop Surg.* 2004;12(5):347–359.

Heffernan MJ, Gordon JE, Sabatini CS, et al. Treatment of femur fractures in young children: a multicenter comparison of flexible intramedullary nails to spica casting in young children aged 2 to 6 years. *J Pediatr Orthop.* 2014;35(2):126–129.

Holsaker HS, Pandya NK, Cho RH, Glaser DA, Moor MA, Herman MJ. Intramedullary nailing of pediatric femoral shaft fractures. *J Am Acad Orthop Surg.* 2011;19(8):472–481.

Kocher MS, Sink EL, Blasier RD, et al. AAOS clinical practice guideline summary: treatment of pediatric diaphyseal femur fractures. *J Am Acad Orthop Surg.* 2009;17(11):718–725.

Case 9

Mosier SM, Stanitski CL. Acute tibial tubercle avulsion fractures. *J Pediatr Orthop.* 2004;24(2):181–184.

Ogden JA, Tross RB, Murphy MJ. Fractures of the tibial tuberosity in adolescents. *J Bone Joint Surg Am.* 1980;62(2):205–215.

Pandya NK, Edmonds EW, Roocroft JH, Mubarak SJ. Tibial tubercle fractures: complications, classification, and the need for intra-articular assessment. *J Pediatr Orthop.* 2012; 32(8):749–759.

Pape JM, Goulet JA, Hensinger RN. Compartment syndrome complicating tibial tubercle avulsion. *Clin Orthop Relat Res.* 1993;(295):201–204.

Zionts LE. Fractures around the knee in children. *J Am Acad Orthop Surg.* 2002;10(5):345–355.

Case 10

Kay RM, Matthys GA. Pediatric ankle fractures: evaluation and treatment. *J Am Acad Orthop Surg.* 2001;9(4):268–278.

Koury SI, Stone CK, Harrell G, La Charité DD. Recognition and management of Tillaux fractures in adolescents. *Pediatr Emerg Care.* 1999;15(1):37–39.

Schnetzler KA, Hoernschemeyer D. The pediatric triplane ankle fracture. *J Am Acad Orthop Surg.* 2007;15(12):738–747.

Case 11

Baldwin KD, Scherl SA. Orthopaedic aspects of child abuse. *Instr Course Lect.* 2013;62:399–403.

Flaherty EG, Perez-Rossello JM, Levine MA, Hennrikus WL; American Academy of Pediatrics Committee on Child Abuse and Neglect; Section on Radiology, American Academy of Pediatrics; Section on Endocrinology, American Academy of Pediatrics; Section on Orthopaedics, American Academy of Pediatrics; Society for Pediatric Radiology. Evaluating children with fractures for child physical abuse. *Pediatrics.* 2014;133(2):e477–e489.

Kleinman P, ed. *Diagnostic Imaging of Child Abuse.* St Louis, MO: Mosby Inc; 1998.

Sink EL, Hyman JE, Matheny T, Georgopoulos G, Kleinman P. Child abuse: the role of the orthopaedic surgeon in nonaccidental trauma. *Clin Orthop Relat Res.* 2011;469(3):790–797.

Case 12

Diab M, Landman Z, Lubicky J, Dormans J, Erickson M, Richards BS; Members of the Spinal Deformity Study Group. Use and outcome of MRI in the surgical treatment of adolescent idiopathic scoliosis. *Spine (Phila Pa 1976).* 2011;36(8):667–671.

Gillingham BL, Fan RA, Akbarnia BA. Early onset scoliosis. *J Am Acad Orthop Surg.* 2006;14(2):101–112.

Hedequist D, Emans J. Congenital scoliosis: a review and update. *J Pediatr Orthop.* 2007;27(1):106–116.

McMaster MJ, Ohtsuka K. The natural history of congenital scoliosis. A study of two hundred and fifty-one patients. *J Bone Joint Surg Am.* 1982;64:1128–1147.

Case 13

Dickman CA, Zabramski JM, Hadley MN, Rekate HL, Sonntag VK. Pediatric spinal cord injury without radiographic abnormalities: report of 26 cases and review of the literature. *J Spinal Disord.* 1991;4(3):296–305.

Ditunno JF Jr, Young W, Donovan WH, Creasey G. The international standards booklet for neurological and functional classification of spinal cord injury. *Paraplegia* 1994;32(2): 70–80.

Kool DR, Blickman JG. Advanced Trauma Life Support®. ABCDE from a radiological point of view. *Emerg Radiol.* 2007;14(3):135–141.

Looby S, Flanders A. MRI of spinal cord injury. *Contem Diagnos Radiol.* 2012;35(1):1–5.

Yang CC, Bradley WE. Reflex innervation of the bulbocavernosus muscle. *BJU Int.* 2000;85(7):857–863.

Case 14

Boyer MI. *AAOS Comprehensive Orthopaedic Review 2.* Rosemont, IL: American Academy of Orthopaedic Surgeons, Copyright; 2014:659–661.

Miller MD, ed. *Review of Orthopaedics.* 6th ed. Philadelphia, PA: WB Saunders; 2012:99.

Case 15

Flynn JM, Kocher MS, Ganley TJ. Osteochondritis dissecans of the knee. *J Pediatr Orthop.* 2004;24(4):434–443.

Case 16

Abbasi D, May MM, Wall EJ, Chan G, Parikh SN. MRI findings in adolescent patients with acute traumatic knee hemarthrosis. *J Pediatr Orthop.* 2012;32(8):760–764.

Beck NA, Patel NM, Ganley TJ. The pediatric knee: current concepts in sports medicine. *J Pediatr Orthop B.* 2014;23(1): 59–66.

Finlayson CJ, Nasreddine A, Kocher MS. Current concepts of diagnosis and management of ACL injuries in skeletally immature athletes. *Phys Sportsmed.* 2010;38(2):90–101.

Frank SJ, Gambacorta PL. Anterior cruciate ligament injuries in the skeletally immature athlete: diagnosis and management. *J Am Acad Orthop Surg.* 2013;21:78–87.

Case 17

Aichroth PM, Patel DV, Marx CL. Congenital discoid lateral meniscus in children. A follow-up study and evolution of management. *J Bone Joint Surg Br.* 1991;73(6):932–936.

Klingele KE, Kocher MS, Hresko MT, Gerbino P, Micheli LJ. Discoid lateral meniscus: prevalence of peripheral rim instability. *J Pediatr Orthop.* 2004;24(1):79–82.

Silverman JM, Mink JH, Deutsch AL. Discoid menisci of the knee: MR imaging appearance. *Radiology.* 1989;173(2): 351–354.

Case 18

Crowther M. Elbow pain in pediatrics. *Curr Rev Musculoskelet Med.* 2009;2(2):83–87.

Wall EJ. Osgood-Schlatter disease. *Phys Sport Med.* 1998;26:3.

Williams B, Lindholm LH, Sever P. Systolic pressure is all that matters. *Lancet.* 2008;371(9631):2219–2221.

Case 19

Amatuzzi MM, Fazzi A, Varella MH. Pathologic synovial plica of the knee. Results of conservative treatment. *Am J Sports Med.* 1990;18(5):466–469.

Irha E, Vrdoljak J. Medial synovial plica syndrome of the knee: a diagnostic pitfall in adolescent athletes. *J Pediatr Orthop B.* 2003;12(1):44–48.

Shetty VD, Vowler SL, Krishnamurthy S, Halliday AE. Clinical diagnosis of medial plica syndrome of the knee: a prospective study. *J Knee Surg.* 2007;20(4):277–280.

Case 20

Burkhead WZ Jr, Rockwood CA Jr. Treatment of instability of the shoulder with an exercise program. *J Bone Joint Surg Am.* 1992;74(6):890–896.

Grahame R. Joint hypermobility and genetic collagen disorders: are they related? *Arch Dis Child.* 1999;80(2):188–191.

Iannotti JP, et al. Magnetic resonance imaging of the shoulder. Sensitivity, specificity, and predictive value. *J Bone Joint Surg.* 1991;73(1):17–29.

Morag Y, Bedi A, Jamadar DA. The rotator interval and long head biceps tendon: anatomy, function, pathology, and magnetic resonance imaging. *Magn Reson Imaging Clin N Am.* 2012;20(2):229–259.

Sugaya H, Kon Y, Tsuchiya A. Arthroscopic repair of glenoid fractures using suture anchors. *Arthroscopy.* 2005;21(5):635. e1–e635.e5.

Treacy SH, Savoie FH 3rd, Field LD. Arthroscopic treatment of multidirectional instability. *J Shoulder Elbow Surg.* 1999; 8(4):345–350.

Case 21

Lebel DE, Corston JA, McAdam LC, Biggar WD, Alman BA. Glucocorticoid treatment for the prevention of scoliosis in children with Duchenne muscular dystrophy: long-term follow-up. *J Bone Joint Surg Am.* 2013;95(12): 1057–1061.

Mah JK, Korngut L, Dykeman J, Day L, Pringsheim T, Jette N. A systematic review and meta-analysis on the epidemiology of Duchenne and Becker muscular dystrophy. *Neuromuscul Disord.* 2014;24(6):482–491.

Shapiro F, Zurakowski D, Bui T, Darras BT. Progression of spinal deformity in wheelchair-dependent patients with duchenne muscular dystrophy who are not treated with steroids: coronal plane (scoliosis) and sagittal plane (kyphosis, lordosis) deformity. *Bone Joint J.* 2014;96-B(1):100–105.

Wicklund MP. The muscular dystrophies. *Continuum (Minneap Minn).* 2013;19(6 Muscle Disease):1535–1570.

Case 22

Miller MD, ed. *Review of Orthopaedics.* 6th ed. Philadelphia, PA: WB Saunders; 2012:231.

Case 23

Guille JT, Pizzutillo PD, MacEwen GD. Developmental dysplasia of the hip from birth to six months. *J Am Acad Orthop Surg.* 2000;8(4):232–242.

Thomas SR, Wedge JH, Salter RB. Outcome at forty-five years after open reduction and innominant osteotomy for late-presenting developmental dislocation of the hip. *J Bone Joint Surg Am.* 2007;89(11):2341–2350.

Vitale MG, Skaggs DL. Developmental dysplasia of the hip from six months to four years of age. *J Am Acad Orthop Surg.* 2001; 9(6):401–411.

Case 24

Boyer MI. *AAOS Comprehensive Orthopaedic Review 2.* Rosemont, IL: American Academy of Orthopaedic Surgeons, Copyright; 2014:703.

Krajbich I. Proximal femoral focal deficiency. In "Congenital Lower Limb Deficiencies" A. Kalamchi (ed). New York, NY: Springer; 1989. 108–127.

Case 25

Gurney B. Leg length discrepancy. *Gait Posture.* 2002;15(2): 195–206.

Lisa C. *Orthopaedic Knowledge Update 11 .* Rosemont, IL: American Academy of Orthopaedic Surgeons, Copyright; 2014:886.

Miller MD, ed. *Review of Orthopaedics.* 6th ed. Philadelphia, PA: WB Saunders; 2012:265.

Case 26

Boyer MI. *AAOS Comprehensive Orthopaedic Review 2.* Rosemont, IL: American Academy of Orthopaedic Surgeons, Copyright; 2014:697–698.

Johnston CE 2nd.Infantile tibia vara. *Clin Orthop Relat Res.* 1990;(255):13–23.

Levine AM, Drennan JC. Physiological bowing and tibia vara. *J Bone Joint Surg Am.* 1982;64(8):1158–1163.

Richards BS, Katz DE, Sims JB. Effectiveness of brace treatment in early infantile Blount's disease. *J Pediatr Orthop.* 1998;18(3):374–380.

Case 27

Achterman C, Kalamchi A. Congenital deficiency of the fibula. *J Bone Joint Surg Br.* 1979;61-B(2):133–137.

Boyer MI. *AAOS Comprehensive Orthopaedic Review 2.* Rosemont, IL: American Academy of Orthopaedic Surgeons, Copyright; 2014:703.

Case 28

Diméglio A, Bensahel H, Souchet P, Mazeau P, Bonnet F. Classification of clubfoot. *J Pediatr Orthop B.* 1995;4(2):129–136.

Kuo KN, Hennigan SP, Hastings ME. Anterior tibial tendon transfer in residual dynamic clubfoot deformity. *J Pediatr Orthop.* 2001;21(1):35–41.

Morcuende JA, Dolan LA, Dietz FR, Ponseti IV. Radical reduction in the rate of extensive corrective surgery for clubfoot using the Ponseti method. *Pediatrics.* 2004;113(2):376–380.

Case 29

Alaee F, Boehm S, Dobbs MB. A new approach to the treatment of congenital vertical talus. *J Child Orthop.* 2007; 1(3): 165–174.

Merrill LJ, Gurnett CA, Connolly AM, Pestronk A, Dobbs MB. Skeletal muscle abnormalities and genetic factors related to vertical talus. *Clin Orthop Relat Res.* 2011;469(4):1167–1174.

Sullivan JA. Pediatric flatfoot: evaluation and management. *J Am Acad Orthop Surg.* 1999;7(1):44–53.

Case 30

Shirley ED, Ain MC. Achondroplasia: manifestations and treatment. *J Am Acad Orthop Surg.* 2009;17(4):231–241.

Wright MJ, Irving MD. Clinical management of achondroplasia. *Arch Dis Child.* 2012;97(2):129–134.

Case 31

Pierz KA, Stieber JR, Kusumi K, Dormans JP. Hereditary multiple exostoses: one center's experience and review of etiology. *Clin Orthop Relat Res.* 2002;(401):49–59.

Sonne-Holm E, Wong C, Sonne-Holm S. Multiple cartilaginous exostoses and development of chondrosarcomas—a systematic review. *Dan Med J.* 2014;61(9):A4895.

Stieber JR, Dormans JP. Manifestations of hereditary multiple exostoses. *J Am Acad Orthop Surg.* 2005;13(2):110–120.

Case 32

Barsh GS, David KE, Byers PH. Type I osteogenesis imperfecta: a nonfunctional allele for pro alpha 1 (I) chains of type I procollagen. *Proc Natl Acad Sci USA.* 1982;79(12):3838–3842.

Janus GJ, Finidori G, Engelbert RH, Pouliquen M, Pruijs JE. Operative treatment of severe scoliosis in osteogenesis imperfecta: results of 20 patients after halo traction and posterior spondylodesis with instrumentation. *Eur Spine J.* 2000;9(6):486–491.

Land C, Rauch F, Glorieux FH. Cyclical intravenous pamidronate treatment affects metaphyseal modeling in growing patients with osteogenesis imperfecta. *J Bone Miner Res.* 2006;21(3):374–379.

Luhmann SJ, Sheridan JJ, Capelli AM, Schoenecker PL. Management of lower-extremity deformities in osteogenesis imperfecta with extensible intramedullary rod technique: a 20-year experience. *J Pediatr Orthop.* 1998;18(1):88–94.

Phillipi CA, Remmington T, Steiner RD. Bisphosphonate therapy for osteogenesis imperfecta. *Cochrane Database Syst Rev.* 2008;(4):CD005088.

Rauch F, Glorieux FH. Osteogenesis imperfecta. *Lancet.* 2004; 363(9418):1377–1385.

Case 33

Boyer MI. *AAOS Comprehensive Orthopaedic Review 2.* Rosemont, IL: American Academy of Orthopaedic Surgeons, Copyright; 2014:550.

Boyer MI. *AAOS Comprehensive Orthopaedic Review 2.* Rosemont, IL: American Academy of Orthopaedic Surgeons, Copyright; 2014:617.

Case 34

Andreasen E. Calcaneo-navicular coalition. Late results of resection. *Acta Orthop Scand.* 1968;39(3):424–432.

Bohne WH. Tarsal coalition. *Curr Opin Pediatr.* 2001;13(1): 29–35.

Comfort TK, Johnson LO. Resection for symptomatic talocalcaneal coalition. *J Pediatr Orthop.* 1998;18(3):283–238.

Gonzalez P, Kumar SJ. Calcaneonavicular coalition treated by resection and interposition of the extensor digitorum brevis muscle. *J Bone Joint Surg Am.* 1990;72(1):71–77.

Kulik SA Jr, Clanton TO. Tarsal coalition. *Foot Ankle Int.* 1996;17(5):286–296.

Lateur LM, Van Hoe LR, Van Ghillewe KV, Gryspeerdt SS, Baert AL, Dereymaeker GE. Subtalar coalition: diagnosis with the C sign on lateral radiographs of the ankle. *Radiology.* 1994;193(3):847–851.

Morgan RC Jr, Crawford AH. Surgical management of tarsal coalition in adolescent athletes. *Foot Ankle.* 1986;7(3): 183–193.

Newman JS, Newberg AH. Congenital tarsal coalition: multimodality evaluation with emphasis on CT and MR imaging. *Radiographics.* 2000;20(2):321–332; quiz 526–527, 532.

Oestreich AE, Mize WA, Crawford AH, Morgan RC Jr. The "anteater nose": a direct sign of calcaneonavicular coalition on the lateral radiograph. *J Pediatr Orthop.* 1987;7(6):709–711.

Scranton PE Jr. Treatment of symptomatic talocalcaneal coalition. *J Bone Joint Surg Am.* 1987;69(4):533–539.

Swiontkowski MF, Scranton PE, Hansen S. Tarsal coalitions: long-term results of surgical treatment. *J Pediatr Orthop.* 1983;3(3):287–292.

Case 35

Gerlach DJ, Gurnett CA, Limpaphayom N, et al. Early results of the Ponseti method for the treatment of clubfoot associated with meylomeningocele. *J Bone Joint Surg Am.* 2009; 91(6):1350–1359.

Quinlivan EP, Gregory JF III. Effect of food fortification on folic acid intake in the United States. *Am J Clin Nutr.* 2003;77(1):221–225.

Talamonti G, D'Aliberti G, Collice M. Myelomeningocele: long-term neurosurgical treatment and follow-up in 202 patients. *J Neurosurg.* 2007;107(Suppl 5):368–386.

Case 36

Herman MJ, Martinek MA, Abzug JM. Complications of tibial eminence and diaphyseal fractures in children: prevention and treatmen. *J Am Acad Orthop Surg.* 2014;22:730–741.

Kocher MS, Mandiga R, Klingele K, Bley, L, Micheli LJ. Anterior cruciate ligament injury versus tibial spine fracture in the skeletally immature knee: a comparison of skeletal maturation and notch width index. *J Pediatr Orthop.* 2004;24(2):185–188.

Kocher MS, Micheli LJ, Gerbino P, Hrekso MT. Tibial eminence fractures in children: prevalence of meniscal entrapment. *Am J Sports Med.* 2003;31(3):404–407.

LaFrance RM, Giordano B, Goldblatt J, Voloshin I, Maloney M. Pediatric tibial eminence fractures: evaluation and management. *J Am Acad Orthop Surg.* 2010;18:395–405.

Patel NM, Park MJ, Sampson NR, Ganley TJ. Tibial eminence fractures in children: earlier posttreatment mobilization results in improved outcomes. *J Pediatr Orthop.* 2012; 32(2):139–144.

Case 37

Flynn JM, Miller F. Management of hip disorders in patients with cerebral palsy. *J Am Acad Orthop Surg.* 2002;10:198–209.

Koman LA, Paterson Smith B, Balkrishnan R. Spasticity associated with cerebral palsy in children: guidelines for the use of botulinum A toxin. *Paediatr Drugs.* 2003;5(1):11–23.

Palisano R, Rosenbaum P, Walter S, Russell D, Wood E, Galuppi B. Development and reliability of a system to classify gross motor function in children with cerebral palsy. *Dev Med Child Neurol.* 1997;39(4):214–223.

Palisano RJ, Hanna SE, Rosenbaum PL, et al. Validation of a model of gross motor function for children with cerebral palsy. *Phys Ther.* 2000;80(10):974–985.

Case 38

Crawford SN, Lee LSK, Izuka BH. Closed treatment of overriding distal radial fractures without reduction in children. *J Bone Joint Surg Am.* 2012;94(3):246–252.

Do TT, Strub WM, Foad SL, Mehlman CT, Crawford AH. Reduction versus remodeling in pediatric distal forearm fractures: a preliminary cost analysis. *J Pediatr Orthop B.* 2003;12:109–115.

Houshian S, Holst AK, Larsen MS, Torfing T. Remodeling of Salter-Harris type II epiphyseal plate injury of the distal radius. *J Pediatr Orthop.* 2004;24(5):472–476.

Lee BS, Esterhai JL Jr, Das M. Fracture of the distal radial epiphysis. Characteristics and surgical treatment of premature, post-traumatic epiphyseal closure. *Clin Orthop Relat Res.* 1984;(185):90–96.

Williams KG, Smith G, Luhmann SJ, Mao J, Gunn JD 3rd, Luhmann JD. A randomized controlled trial of cast versus splint for distal radial buckle fracture: an evaluation of satisfaction, convenience, and preference. *Pediatr Emerg Care.* 2013;29(5):555–559.

Case 39

Katz DE, Herring JA, Browne RH, Kelly DM, Birch JG. Brace wear control of curve progression in adolescent idiopathic scoliosis. *J Bone Joint Surg Am.* 2010;92(6):1343–1352.

Weinstein SL, Dolan LA, Wright JG, Dobbs MB. Effects of bracing in adolescents with idiopathic scoliosis. *N Engl J Med.* 2013;369(16):1512–1521.

Weinstein SL, Dolan LA, Spratt KF, Peterson KK, Spoonamore MJ, Ponseti IV. Health and function of patients with untreated idiopathic scoliosis: a 50-year natural history study. *JAMA.* 2003;289:559–567.

Weinstein SL, Ponseti IV. Curve progression in idiopathic scoliosis. *J Bone Joint Surg Am.* 1983;65(4):447–455.

Case 40

Gonzalez BE, Teruya J, Mahoney DH Jr, et al. Venous thrombosis associated with staphylococcal osteomyelitis in children. *Pediatrics.* 2006;117(5):1673–1679.

Mantadakis E, Plessa E, Vouloumanou EK, Michailidis L, Chatzimichael A, Falagas ME. Deep venous thrombosis in children with musculoskeletal infections: the clinical evidence. *Int J Infect Dis.* 2012;16(4):e236–e243.

Saavedra-Lozano J, Mejías A, Ahmad N, et al. Changing trends in acute osteomyelitis in children: impact of methicillin-resistant Staphylococcus aureus infections. *J Pediatr Orthop.* 2008;28(5):569–575.

Speigel DA, Penny JN. Chronic osteomyelitis in children. *Tech Orthop.* 2005;20(2):142–152.